Nutrition and Development
Short- and Long-Term Consequences for Health

Nutrition and Development
Short- and Long-Term Consequences for Health

The Report of a British Nutrition Foundation Task Force

Chaired by
Professor Thomas A. B. Sanders

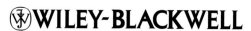

WILEY-BLACKWELL

A John Wiley & Sons, Ltd., Publication

Published by Wiley-Blackwell
for the British Nutrition Foundation

Library of Congress Cataloging-in-Publication Data

Nutrition and development : short- and long-term consequences for health / report of a British Nutrition Foundation Task Force chaired by Thomas A. B. Sanders ; edited by Laura Wyness, Sara Stanner, Judith Buttriss.
    p. ; cm.
  Includes bibliographical references and index.
  ISBN 978-1-4443-3678-8 (softback : alk. paper) – ISBN 978-1-118-54111-1 (ePub) – ISBN 978-1-118-54122-7 (eMobi) – ISBN 978-1-118-54123-4 (ePDF)
  I. Wyness, Laura. II. Stanner, Sara. III. Buttriss, Judith. IV. British Nutrition Foundation. [DNLM:
1. Nutritional Physiological Phenomena. 2. Human Development. 3. Nutrigenomics–methods. QU 145]
  613.2–dc23
                      2013001801

A catalogue record for this book is available from the British Library.

The British Nutrition Foundation would like to thank the copyright holders acknowledged in the text for permission to reproduce data and figures in this book. Every effort has been made to contact all copyright holders and to acknowledge the sources of copyright material. Any inadvertent omissions will be rectified in any future reprinting or edition of this work. We are also grateful to Hilary Bamforth for her help with proofreading.

Contents

This report is the collective work of all the members of the Task Force.
Authors of the final draft of each chapter are given below.

Foreword

The concept, that early growth and development determines health in animals, has been known to nutritional scientists for more than 70 years. However, the realisation that this concept has major implications for human health is much more recent. The importance of considering the effect of diet on the whole life-cycle, rather than focusing on middle-aged and older adults, is increasingly recognised, particularly when the seeds of adult disease may be sown *in utero* and in infancy.

There is now a considerable body of evidence to link risk of developing type 2 diabetes and raised blood pressure to patterns of fetal and infant growth, alongside emerging evidence that obesity, bone health, gut microbiota, immunity, lung function, mental health and risk of cancer may be influenced by events in early life. British researchers have played a leading role in these discoveries.

The pioneering work by Sir John Hammond at Cambridge showed how piglets fed different diets during early life could determine their relative size and proportions of fat to lean tissue. Professor RA McCance and Dame Elsie Widdowson took this work further and with Professor John Dobbing coined the term 'vulnerable phases of development'. The vulnerability of the human brain in early pregnancy explains why iodine deficiency in pregnancy, a major global problem, causes endemic deaf mutism and cretinism.

In the late 1950s the vulnerability of the fetus to 'toxic insults' in early pregnancy was highlighted, following the use of the drug thalidomide. More recent studies show that excessive intakes of a form of vitamin A (retinoic acid) also causes birth defects. Exposure to heavy metals, such as mercury and lead, in pregnancy may have long-term effects on intellectual capacity. On the positive side, Professor Richard Smithells was the first to show that high intakes of folic acid could prevent neural tube defects.

The ground-breaking work of Professor David Barker deserves special mention because it took research on the developmental origins of human disease onto another level. Professor Barker had been unable to find any relationship with current diet and risk of cardiovascular disease in his studies in the UK. However, he was able to show that low birthweight and the pattern of infant growth strongly predicted risk of type 2 diabetes and cardiovascular disease, in adult life. He introduced the concept of 'developmental programming' of adult disease. His work sparked off enormous interest and spawned many other studies, which we have attempted to summarise.

Recent advances in molecular biology have also provided insights into how cells in the body can be programmed. It would seem that this is to prepare us for the environment into which we are born and that problems arise if that environment is different to that expected.

This Task Force set out to summarise current knowledge on early life and later disease for a broader non-specialist audience and tried to identify gaps in knowledge where further research is needed. We have also attempted to try to translate the implications of these findings with regard to practical dietary advice for the population.

I am extremely grateful to the members of the Task Force for all their hard work and contributions and to Professor Judy Buttriss and her team at the British Nutrition Foundation for their patience and help putting the report together.

Professor Thomas A. B. Sanders
Chair of the Task Force

Terms of Reference

The Task Force was invited by the Council of the British Nutrition Foundation to:

1. Review the present state of knowledge of the importance of diet during early development.
2. Prepare a report and, should it see fit, draw conclusions, make recommendations and identify areas for future research.

British Nutrition Foundation
Nutrition and Development: Short- and Long-Term Consequences for Health Task Force Membership

Chair

Professor Thomas A. B. Sanders, Professor of Nutrition & Dietetics
Diabetes and Nutritional Sciences Division, School of Medicine, King's College London, Franklin-Wilkins Building, 150 Stamford Street, London SE1 9NH

Members

Professor Judith L. Buttriss
Director General
British Nutrition Foundation
Imperial House
15–19 Kingsway
London
WC2B 6UN

Professor Graham S. Devereux
Professor of Respiratory
   Medicine
Child Health
University of Aberdeen
Royal Aberdeen Children's
   Hospital
Aberdeen
AB25 2ZG

Professor Paul Haggarty
Head of Lifelong Health
University of Aberdeen
Rowett Institute of Nutrition and
   Health
Greenburn Road
Bucksburn
Aberdeen
AB21 9SB

Dr Nicholas C. Harvey
Senior Lecturer and Honorary
   Consultant Rheumatologist
MRC Lifecourse Epidemiology
   Unit
University of Southampton
Southampton General Hospital
Southampton
SO16 6YD

Dr Alison M. Lennox
Principal Investigator Scientist
MRC Human Nutrition
   Research
Elsie Widdowson Laboratory
120 Fulbourn Road
Cambridge
CB1 9NL

Professor Harry J. McArdle
Deputy Director of Science
University of Aberdeen
Rowett Institute of Nutrition and
   Health
Greenburn Road
Bucksburn
Aberdeen
AB21 9SB

Dr Anne L. McCartney
Senior Research Fellow
Microbial Ecology & Health
  Group
Department of Food and
  Nutritional Sciences
University of Reading
Reading
RG6 6AP

Professor Julian G. Mercer
Theme Leader, Obesity and
  Metabolic Health
University of Aberdeen
Rowett Institute of Nutrition and
  Health
Greenburn Road
Bucksburn
Aberdeen
AB21 9SB

Dr Susan E. Ozanne
Reader in Developmental
  Endocrinology
Institute of Metabolic Science
Metabolic Research Laboratories
University of Cambridge
Box 289, Level 4
Addenbrooke's Hospital
Cambridge
CB2 0QQ

Professor Lucilla Poston
Head of Division of Women's
  Health
Women's Health Academic
  Centre
King's College London
10th Floor, North Wing
St Thomas' Hospital
Westminster Bridge Road
London
SE1 7EH

Professor Marcus Richards
Programme Leader, Medical
  Research Council and
  Professor of Psychology in
  Epidemiology
Institute of Epidemiology and
  Health Care
University College London
MRC Unit for Lifelong Health
  and Ageing
33 Bedford Place
London
WC1B 5JU

Dr Siân Robinson
Principal Research Fellow
MRC Lifecourse Epidemiology
  Unit
University of Southampton
Southampton General Hospital
Southampton
SO16 6YD

Professor Richard M. Sharpe
Principal Investigator
MRC Centre for Reproductive
  Health
The Queen's Medical Research
  Institute
University of Edinburgh
47 Little France Crescent
Edinburgh
EH16 4TJ

Dr Paul D. Taylor
Senior Lecturer in
  Developmental Programming
Division of Women's Health
King's College London
Women's Health Academic
  Centre
10th Floor, North Wing
St Thomas' Hospital
1 Westminster Bridge
SE1 7EH

Observer

Rachel Marklew
Department of Health
133-155 Wellington House
Waterloo Road
London
SE1 8UG

Contributors

Professor Cyrus Cooper
Director and Professor of
  Rheumatology
MRC Lifecourse Epidemiology
  Unit
University of Southampton
Southampton General Hospital
Southampton
SO16 6YD

Dr Alan Dangour
Registered Public Health
  Nutritionist
London School of Hygiene and
  Tropical Medicine
Room 137
Keppel Street
London
WC1E 7HT

Professor Elaine Dennison
Professor of Musculoskeletal
  Epidemiology and Honorary
  Consultant in Rheumatology
MRC Lifecourse Epidemiology
  Unit
University of Southampton
Southampton General Hospital
Southampton
SO16 6YD

Dr Lorraine Gambling
Research Fellow
University of Aberdeen
Rowett Institute of Nutrition and
  Health
Greenburn Road
Bucksburn
Aberdeen
AB21 9SB

Professor Steven Darryll Heys
Head of Division of Applied
  Medicine and Co-Director of
  the Institute of Medical
  Sciences
Institute of Medical Sciences
Polwarth Building
Foresterhill
Aberdeen
AB25 2ZD

Dr Nanda Prabhu
Research Fellow
Child Health
University of Aberdeen
Royal Aberdeen Children's
  Hospital
Aberdeen
AB25 2ZG

Dr Vicki Quincey
Registrar in Rheumatology
MRC Lifecourse Epidemiology
  Unit
University of Southampton
Southampton General Hospital
Southampton
SO16 6YD

Professor Ricardo Uauy
Professor of Public Health
  Nutrition
London School of Hygiene &
  Tropical Medicine
Room 182
Keppel St
London
WC1E 7HT

Editors

Professor Judith L. Buttriss
Director General
British Nutrition Foundation
Imperial House
15–19 Kingsway
London
WC2B 6UN

Sara A. Stanner
Science Programme Manager
British Nutrition Foundation
Imperial House
15–19 Kingsway
London
WC2B 6UN

Dr Laura A. Wyness
Senior Nutrition Scientist
British Nutrition Foundation
Imperial House
15–19 Kingsway
London
WC2B 6UN

Secretariat

Helena J. Gibson-Moore
Research Assistant
British Nutrition Foundation
Imperial House
15–19 Kingsway
London
WC2B 6UN

Bethany C. Hooper
Research Assistant
British Nutrition Foundation
Imperial House
15–19 Kingsway
London
WC2B 6UN

1
Introduction to Early Life and Later Disease

1.1 Environmental influences on development

This report sets out our current understanding of the links between early life and later health, and examines the role played by variations in early diet and nutrition in the aetiology of adult disease. Every individual has a 'blueprint' for growth and development determined by their genome, but realisation of this growth potential is only possible if nutrient supplies in intrauterine life and in childhood are adequate (Jackson 1996). While it is widely recognised that low birthweight is common among babies born to chronically malnourished women, and that stunting in children is prevalent in communities where food supplies are insufficient, the importance of more moderate variations in diet and nutritional status and their influence on early growth and development are currently less well understood.

1.1.1 Nutrition and the early environment

The supply of nutrients to the growing fetus is influenced by the nature of the maternal diet and nutrient stores. Animal studies show clearly that the fetus is sensitive to variations in its nutrient supply (Harding 2001), and experimental manipulations of this supply can have a profound impact on growth and development (Luther *et al.* 2005; McArdle *et al.* 2006). Compared with many other species, human gestation is

long and the fetus is small in relation to maternal size (Widdowson 1976); thus synthetic demands and additional nutrient needs in pregnancy are relatively low. As most babies born to women in the Western world are above recognised cut-offs for low weight at birth, the human fetus has been regarded as being well protected from wide variations in maternal diet and nutritional status (Harding 2001; Jackson and Robinson 2001). However, although the intrauterine environment may be protective, there are well-known examples of adverse effects of variations in maternal nutrition – either from excessive exposure or due to insufficiency.

Damaging effects of alcohol have been recognised for many years, but a consistent pattern of malformations in children whose mothers consumed excessive alcohol in pregnancy was described around 40 years ago (Hoyme *et al.* 2005). The effects include a range of structural anomalies and behavioural and neurocognitive disabilities, and are now termed fetal alcohol spectrum disorders (FASD) (Hoyme *et al.* 2005). The specific effects on the fetus of variations in the level and frequency of maternal alcohol consumption, as well as its timing in pregnancy, are not fully understood and require further research. We currently do not have reliable estimates of the incidence of FASD in the UK (Morleo *et al.* 2011). Although FASD may not be common, as many women stop drinking alcohol in pregnancy (Crozier *et al.* 2009), it is considered to be an important cause of intellectual disability in the Western world (Abel and Sokol 1986). Another nutrient with recognised teratogenic effects when in excess in the diet is vitamin A (retinol). High intakes of retinol are associated with a specific pattern of craniofacial and other abnormalities in the fetus (Miller *et al.* 1998). The safe upper limit of intake is uncertain, but intakes from supplements above 10 000 IU have been associated with adverse outcomes (Rothman *et al.* 1995). Current UK guidance for pregnant women is that they should avoid eating liver, as it has a very high retinol content, and avoid dietary supplements that contain retinol (Department of Health 2009a).

In terms of effects of nutrient insufficiency, the clearest evidence we have is for the link between inadequate maternal folate status and the occurrence of neural tube defects (NTDs) in the fetus (De-Regil *et al.* 2010). A randomised controlled trial conducted in the 1980s provided conclusive evidence of the protective effects of folic acid supplementation (Medical Research Council 1991). It has since been shown that the inverse association between folate status and the risk of NTDs shows a dose–response relationship (Daly *et al.* 1995). A second nutrient for which there is good evidence of adverse developmental effects linked to insufficiency is iodine (Hetzel 2000). In areas of severe iodine deficiency, maternal and fetal hypothyroxinaemia can cause cretinism and have adverse effects on cognitive development in children (Zimmermann 2009). Whether mild or moderate maternal iodine deficiency causes more subtle changes in cognitive function in offspring is unclear as there are no controlled intervention studies in which long-term clinical outcomes have been assessed (Zimmermann 2009). For women living in iodine-deficient areas, maternal supplementation significantly reduces the incidence of these disorders. Ensuring adequate iodine status among women of reproductive age should thus be a high priority.

Developmental consequences of variation in nutrient intake are not restricted to fetal life. Growth faltering in infancy is widespread in many parts of the world and results in permanent height deficits. Stunting is linked to many indices of functional impairment, including intellectual development (Jackson 1996). The primary driver of infant growth is thought to be nutritional (Karlberg *et al.* 1994), and young children are vulnerable to the effects of chronic energy and nutrient restriction (SACN 2011a). The secular changes in height observed in most European populations since the nineteenth century are attributed to increased height gain in late infancy (Cole 2000), arising at least in part from improvements in diet and nutrition.

In each of these examples, there are adverse effects of inappropriate nutrition – with nutrients either acting as damaging teratogens, or being supplied in insufficient amounts to meet needs during intrauterine and early postnatal life. The key issue is that in all cases the effects are permanent – and they will have lifelong consequences. Exactly how they affect the individual will depend on the nature of the nutritional insult, its severity and timing. These examples describe the effects of extremes in nutrient intake that have measurable effects, allowing examination of the role of nutrition in their aetiology. What we need to understand more about are the developmental consequences of more modest variations in nutrition arising from existing differences in dietary habits and food choice.

1.1.2 Variations in growth and development

The measure that is widely used to judge the success of pregnancy is the weight of the baby at birth. This varies over a wide range: weights between 2.5 kg and 4 kg are considered normal for babies born at term. While babies of low birthweight (<2.5 kg) are recognised as being at increased risk of mortality in infancy (McCormick 1985), until recently, variations above 2.5 kg were seen as unremarkable and regarded as a result of differences in fetal growth due to genetic variation. A growing body of epidemiological data now shows that this may not be the case as these 'normal' variations in fetal growth and size at birth are predictive of differences in the incidence of specific disease conditions in adult life – and this is evident even in developed communities such as the UK (Barker 1998). If constraint of fetal growth is linked to changes in physiology that have long-term health consequences, we clearly need to reconsider whether we know enough about the current determinants of normal variations in fetal growth.

Variation in postnatal growth may also be important for long-term health. Growth monitoring is widely used to assess the nutritional status of infants and children and as an indicator of health and wellbeing. There are growth reference curves to enable judgement of adequacy of growth between birth and adulthood (see Chapter 2, Section 2.8). But what constitutes optimal growth in infancy and childhood is not clear. In the same way as for fetal growth, we need to reconsider what is an optimal pattern of infant growth. For example, although poor infant growth is clearly of concern as it may be an indicator of failure to thrive, systematic reviews of infant growth studies show that rapid infant growth (or 'catch-up' growth) is predictive of obesity in older children and adults (Baird *et al.* 2005; Ong and Loos 2006).

As we begin to take account of the long-term consequences of variations in early growth and development, we expose a lack of understanding of the importance of current variations in diet and nutrition, particularly in the developed world. As adequate nutrition is key to successful fetal and infant growth, to address differences in adult health and risk of disease, we need to define what is optimal in terms of maternal and infant diet and nutrition.

1.2 Links between early life and adult disease

1.2.1 Animal studies

The classic studies of McCance and Widdowson carried out five decades ago provided evidence that permanent changes can occur in response to manipulation of early nutrition. For example, in their studies of rats, they showed that by altering litter size at birth the pups were overfed or underfed during the period of lactation. The overfeeding of rats raised in small litters promoted early growth and, compared with rats raised in large litters, the achieved adult size was greater (Fig. 1.1) (McCance 1962). Altering the plane of nutrition between 9 and 12 weeks did not have this effect, suggesting that there is a critical period within which variations in postnatal nutrition determine growth and body composition. More recently, rats raised in small litters have been shown to develop hyperphagia and greater adiposity in adult life (Plagemann 2005). Other important early studies include the work of Stewart and colleagues who showed that, in rats maintained on a low-protein diet for 10–12 generations, refeeding for several generations was required in order to correct the physical and behavioural deficits in the offspring (Stewart *et al.* 1980). Thus the physiological changes resulting from dietary restriction were evident beyond the immediate offspring.

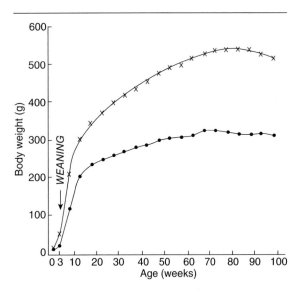

Figure 1.1 The growth of rats raised in small (x) or large (•) litters between birth and weaning. (Unlimited food was provided after weaning.) Reprinted from McCance RA (1962) Food, growth, and time. *Lancet*, **2**, 671–6, copyright 1962, with permission from Elsevier.

These studies clearly demonstrated the principle that permanent changes in physiology occur in early life as a result of variations in maternal and/or postnatal nutrition. Although at the time of these early studies the physiological mechanisms involved were not understood, recent experimental studies have made enormous progress in explaining these links (see Chapter 4).

1.2.2 Evidence from human populations

One of the earliest studies to propose a role for early experience in the aetiology of adult disease was carried out by Forsdahl (1977). In a comparison of the past infant mortality rates of Norwegian counties with their current mortality rates from arteriosclerotic heart disease, he showed that they were highly correlated (Fig. 1.2). Forsdahl proposed that the increased risk for adults living in some counties was a result of their experience of poverty earlier in life – and that poor living conditions in childhood and adolescence led to a lifelong vulnerability that remained, even if the environment improved in adult life.

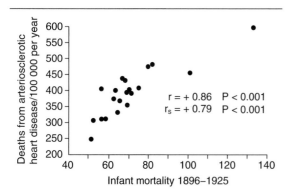

Figure 1.2 Correlation between mortality from arteriosclerotic heart disease (1964–7) in men aged 40–69 years (standardised rates/100 000 population) and infant mortality rates 1896–1925. Reproduced from Forsdahl A (1977) Are poor living conditions in childhood and adolescence an important risk factor for arteriosclerotic heart disease? *British Journal of Preventative and Social Medicine*, **31**, 91–5, copyright 1977, with permission from BMJ Publishing Group Ltd.

In the UK, Barker and colleagues showed that mortality rates for cardiovascular disease were also high in geographical areas that in the past had been areas with high infant mortality (Barker and Osmond 1986; Barker, Osmond *et al.* 1989). In these studies the authors were able to subdivide deaths occurring in the first year of life into those occurring in the first month (neonatal) and those occurring in the rest of the year (postneonatal). Stroke mortality was linked to neonatal mortality but not to postneonatal mortality (Table 1.1), while mortality from coronary heart disease (CHD) related to both neonatal and postneonatal mortality rates. In contrast, death rates from chronic bronchitis showed an association only with postneonatal mortality rates. These data suggested that the origins of cardiovascular disease might be even earlier in the life course than childhood and adolescence – and that events in fetal life were important in the aetiology of adult cardiovascular disease (see Chapter 10).

Table 1.1 Death rates (standardised mortality ratios) from stroke, coronary heart disease and chronic bronchitis (1968–78, men and women aged 35–74 years) in the 212 areas of England and Wales, grouped by neonatal and postneonatal mortality (1911–25)

		Postneonatal mortality					
		(low) 1	2	3	4	5	(high)
				Stroke			
Neonatal							
mortality	1 (low)	85	81	79	78	79	
	2	86	90	98	74	76	
	3	102	100	104	104	104	
	4	–	108	110	115	117	
	5 (high)	124	–	121	123	117	
				Coronary heart disease			
Neonatal							
mortality	1 (low)	84	89	91	88	98	
	2	85	93	95	88	91	
	3	86	94	99	106	113	
	4	–	98	109	111	115	
	5 (high)	83	–	114	119	116	
				Chronic bronchitis			
Neonatal							
mortality	1 (low)	67	78	106	115	161	
	2	64	84	85	104	126	
	3	69	65	89	88	151	
	4	–	91	99	120	142	
	5 (high)	41	–	108	123	144	

Reproduced from Barker DJ, Osmond C & Law CM (1989) The intrauterine and early postnatal origins of cardiovascular disease and chronic bronchitis. *Journal of Epidemiology and Community Health*, **43**, 237–40, copyright 1989, with permission from BMJ Publishing Group.

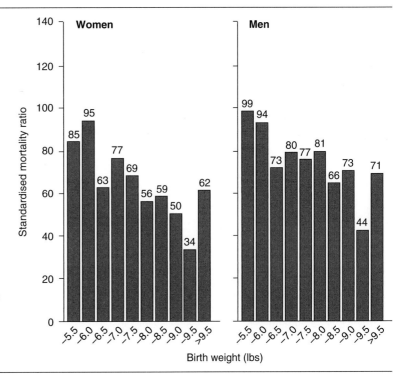

Figure 1.3 Mortality from cardiovascular disease before 65 years in 15 726 men and women who were born in Hertfordshire, UK. Reproduced from Osmond C, Barker DJ, Winter PD *et al.* (1993) Early growth and death from cardiovascular disease in women. *British Medical Journal*, **307**, 1519–24, with permission from BMJ Publishing Group.

Barker and colleagues went on to identify a number of cohorts of adult men and women whose early growth had been recorded, and whose records had survived to the present day. By tracing these men and women they were able to link measures of early growth to disease-specific mortality rates, as well as to risk factors for those conditions. Figure 1.3 shows the risk of dying prematurely from cardiovascular disease among 15 726 men and women who were followed up in this way (Osmond *et al.* 1993).

In both men and women there was a graded inverse association between weight at birth and risk of death from cardiovascular disease. Studies of other cohorts have shown that the associations are not explained by variations in gestational age at birth, or by differences in adult lifestyle. These associations have been replicated in a number of studies in a wide range of populations in Europe (Frankel *et al.* 1996; Leon *et al.* 1998; Lawlor, Ronalds *et al.* 2005), North America (Rich-Edwards *et al.* 1997) and India (Stein *et al.* 1996). We now know that there are similar associations between weight at birth and risk of hypertension and type 2 diabetes in adult life – two disorders closely linked to cardiovascular disease

(Hales *et al.* 1991; Curhan *et al.* 1996; Bergvall *et al.* 2005; Gamborg *et al.* 2007) (see Chapter 10).

It seems that people who were smaller at birth remain biologically different from people who were larger, consistent with Forsdahl's proposition that an adverse environment in early life results in a lifelong vulnerability to cardiovascular disease. The work of Barker and colleagues (Barker 1998) indicated that, for cardiovascular disease, the early environment included experience in fetal life as well as in later childhood.

1.2.3 The interaction of fetal and postnatal experience and adult disease

Many of the historical cohorts studied do not provide information about postnatal growth, and it is not possible to gain any insight into how postnatal experience impacts on the link between fetal growth and adult disease. Important information about the interaction of prenatal and postnatal experience on adult disease has therefore come from the study of men and women born in Helskinki, Finland, where birth records can be linked both to records of childhood

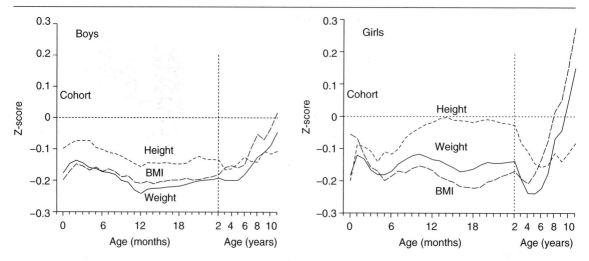

Figure 1.4   Growth of 357 men and 87 women born in Helsinki, Finland, who developed or died from coronary heart disease, relative to the rest of the cohort. Measurements at each age are expressed as Z-scores; the Z-score for the cohort is set at zero. Reproduced from Barker DJ, Osmond C, Forsen TJ *et al.* (2005) Trajectories of growth among children who have coronary events as adults. *New England Journal of Medicine*, **353**, 1802–9, copyright 2005, with permission from Massachussetts Medical Society.

growth and to hospital admission and mortality data (Eriksson *et al.* 1999). In a cohort of 8760 men and women who were born between 1934 and 1944, there were 357 men and 87 women who had developed or died from CHD (Barker *et al.* 2005). As in the Hertfordshire study (Osmond *et al.* 1993), the body size of children, who as adults had coronary events, was below average at birth. Between birth and 2 years their growth relative to other men and women in the cohort who did not develop the disease was poorer, and weight, height and body mass index (BMI) was low (Fig. 1.4). Beyond 2 years the men and women who went on to have CHD gained weight rapidly, such that they reached average or above average weight and BMI by the age of 11 years.

It has been shown that hypertension and type 2 diabetes are associated with the same general pattern of growth as CHD (Eriksson *et al.* 2000; Forsen *et al.* 2000). Similarly to CHD, the risk of disease is not determined only by the absolute value of BMI in childhood, but by the combination of body size at birth and during childhood (Eriksson *et al.* 2000; Forsen *et al.* 2000). The influence of different pathways of growth on later health has also been described in a study of young Indian adults (Bhargava *et al.* 2004). Thinness at the age of 2 years, but followed by rapid growth and a relatively high BMI at the

age of 12 years, was associated with the highest rates of impaired glucose tolerance or diabetes (see Chapter 9).

Singhal and Lucas (2004) have proposed that it is the effect of rapid postnatal growth that is particularly damaging in relation to cardiovascular disease. For example, in an intervention study they showed that feeding a high-nutrient diet to pre-term infants promoted weight gain, but that this was associated with later insulin resistance (Singhal, Fewtrell *et al.* 2003). Additionally, there is an increased risk of obesity in individuals who exhibited rapid infant growth (Baird *et al.* 2005; Ong and Loos 2006). These contrasting findings highlight our current lack of understanding about what is optimal in terms of pathways of postnatal growth.

1.2.4   Vulnerability to stressors acting in adult life

The American Nurses' Health Study found that in the men and women born in Helsinki, the significance of a single measure of their BMI at any age, in relation to cardiovascular risk and impaired glucose tolerance, differed according to earlier pathways of growth. The study also provided evidence that the effects of BMI are conditioned by early growth. Interactive effects were found, such that higher BMI in adulthood was an especially strong risk factor for CHD among women who were small at birth (Rich-Edwards *et al.* 2005). Such heterogeneity in response, originating in early life, could also apply to other influences. For example, variations in adult diet may have different metabolic effects among adults who differ in their early experience. There is some evidence that this is the case, as total and saturated fat intakes have been shown to differ in their associations with serum high-density lipoprotein (HDL) cholesterol concentrations, and with the ratio of HDL-cholesterol to low-density lipoprotein (LDL) cholesterol, in men of different birthweights (Robinson *et al.* 2006). In men in the Hertfordshire cohort, comparable interactive effects of early growth and adult lifestyle have also been described in relation to bone status (see Chapter 12), as smoking was associated with a lower bone mineral density, but only among men of lower birthweight (Moinuddin *et al.* 2008).

In addition there is evidence that adult responses to psychosocial stressors differ according to early experience. Among men studied in the Helsinki cohort, born between 1934 and 1944, low income was associated with increased rates of CHD (Barker *et al.* 2001). This effect has been described many times and is a major component of the social inequalities in health in Western countries (Marmot and McDowall 1986; Macintyre *et al.* 2001). In the Helsinki study,

however, the effect of low income was shown to be limited to men who were thin at birth, defined by a ponderal index less than 26kg/m^3 (Fig. 1.5). Men who were not thin at birth appeared to be resilient to the effects of low income on CHD.

One explanation of these findings is that perceptions of low social status and lack of success lead to changes in neuroendocrine pathways and hence to disease (Marmot and Wilkinson 2001), and that this may differ according to early experience. This possibility is consistent with the finding that there are persisting alterations in responses to stress, including raised serum cortisol concentrations in adults who were small at birth (Phillips *et al.* 2000).

The finding that there are interactive effects of early life and adult experience in determining disease risk is consistent with the ideas of Dubos (1987), who wrote: 'The effects of the physical and social environment cannot be understood without knowledge of individual history.'

1.3 Biological mechanisms

1.3.1 Fetal programming

The link between early experience and later disease was described by Lucas (1991) as 'programming'. This was defined as a process whereby a stimulus or insult, acting at a critical phase of development,

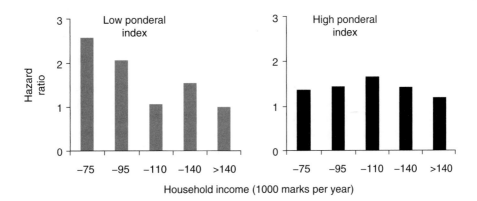

Figure 1.5 Hazard ratios for coronary heart disease in men according to ponderal index at birth and household income in adult life. Barker *et al.* (2005).

results in long-term changes in the structure or function of the organism.

Central to the programming hypothesis was the proposition that variations in fetal nutrition were responsible for permanent changes in physiology and function, which had lifelong consequences for the individual including their risk of cardiovascular disease and type 2 diabetes in adult life (Barker 1998). While the growth of the fetus is influenced by its genes, determining its potential for growth, the intrauterine environment appears to have a greater effect on the growth achieved. The classic studies of Penrose (1954) concluded that 62% of the variation in birthweight was the result of the intrauterine environment, 20% the result of maternal genes and 18% the result of fetal genes. Support for the importance of the fetal environment has come from the study of babies born following ovum donation, since weight at birth was found to be strongly related to the weight of the recipient mother, but not to the weight of the donor mother (Brooks *et al.* 1995). However, it has also been proposed that there may be genetic factors that are linked both to low birthweight and to adult disease, which could also contribute to the association, and there is some evidence to support this (Dunger *et al.* 1998; Hattersley *et al.* 1998).

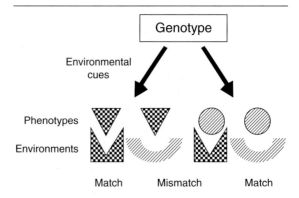

Figure 1.6 A given genotype may give rise to different phenotypes depending on the environment early in development. Cues from the environment may be used as predictors determining which of a set of alternative developmental pathways is elicited. If the environment does not change, the phenotype will be well adapted to that environment (represented in the diagram by the pattern and shape of the phenotype and the pattern and shape of the environment). However, if the environment changes between the elicitation of the particular pattern and development, then the phenotype may be mismatched to the conditions of adult life.
Reproduced from Bateson P (2007) Developmental plasticity and evolutionary biology. *Journal of Nutrition*, **137**, 1060–2, with permission from the American Society for Nutrition.

1.3.2 Developmental plasticity

In 2005, Bateson challenged the use of the term 'programming' to explain the observations that the environment, during development, has long-term effects on the offspring, and proposed that environmental induction of 'developmental plasticity' was more appropriate (Bateson 2007). Developmental plasticity describes the ability of a single genotype to produce more than one alternative form of structure, physiological state or behaviour in response to environmental conditions. Thus a range of phenotypes can arise from a single genotype in response to variations in the environment. This has evolutionary benefits, as it enables better matching of individuals to their postnatal environment than would be possible if one genotype produced the same phenotype in all environments. However, in a changing environment, the resulting phenotype may be poorly suited to its postnatal conditions because its environmental forecast was incorrect (Fig. 1.6) (Bateson *et al.* 2004; Bateson 2007). This has obvious implications for

populations undergoing rapid changes in diet and lifestyle.

The environmental cues that lead to different phenotypes are largely undiscovered, but considerable progress in understanding mechanisms has been made using animal models. In terms of the early proposition that variations in fetal nutrition were central to the associations between fetal growth and later disease (Barker, Osmond *et al.* 1989), there is now a significant body of experimental evidence that shows long-term effects of manipulations of maternal diet that are consistent with these epidemiological associations (Luther *et al.* 2005; McArdle *et al.* 2006) (see Chapters 8–14).

1.4 Nutrition of mothers and children

Despite decades of interest in maternal nutrition we know little about the long-term effects on the offspring of variations in women's diets and their

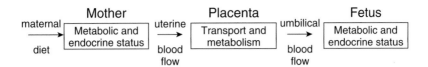

Figure 1.7 The materno–fetal supply line: factors along the fetal 'supply line' which can mediate the difference between maternal nutrition and fetal nutrition. Reproduced from Harding JE (2001) The nutritional basis of the fetal origins of adult disease. *International Journal of Epidemiology*, **30**, 15–23, copyright 2001, with permission from Oxford University Press.

nutritional status. There are also few studies of human populations that consider the adult health consequences of variations in infant and childhood nutrition.

1.4.1 Observational studies of maternal diet

Most of the information we have on the relationship between maternal nutrition and pregnancy outcomes has come from observational studies, which does not allow us to make inferences about causality in the links between early nutrition, growth and later health. Diet in pregnancy has been assessed in a number of studies and related, most commonly, to variations in size at birth and other short-term outcomes. Although individual studies have provided evidence of links between variations in maternal nutrient intake and some of these outcomes, there is little consistency in the findings across studies, and there are few nutrients for which definitive intake guidelines can be established (Jackson and Robinson 2001).

There are many methodological reasons why direct comparison of these observational studies may be difficult – not least due to differences in dietary assessment methods, timing in gestation and differences in the populations studied. The studies often rely on birthweight as the outcome, which is an incomplete statement of the success of pregnancy, and they also fail to take account of heterogeneity among women in their responses to pregnancy (Jackson and Robinson 2001). But perhaps the greatest issue is that many of the studies have looked for simple relationships between maternal intake and fetal growth – whereas the supply line that links maternal diet to fetal nutrient supply is complex (Fig. 1.7) (Harding 2001).

There are far fewer observational studies in which variations in maternal nutrition can be linked to the adult health of the offspring. Some insights have come from studies of women who were subjected to acute starvation over a short period, and in which birth outcomes can be compared for individuals born during and after a period of famine. Much of this information has come from the study of men and women who were conceived and born during the Dutch Hunger Winter. In 1944–5, food supplies to the population of western Holland were restricted such that official rations fell below 4184 kJ/day (1000 kcal/day) for a period of about 5 months (see Chapter 4, Section 4.4.2 for more details) (Lumey *et al.* 2007). The population was previously well nourished and food supplies were restored quickly after May 1945. Birthweight fell by around 300 g in babies exposed to the famine in the last trimester of pregnancy (Stein *et al.* 2004). Follow-up of the men and women who were exposed to famine in intrauterine life has shown that its effects differed according to timing in gestation. Marked effects were seen in the men and women conceived during the famine, and include a more atherogenic lipid profile, and a tripling of coronary artery disease prevalence at the age of 50 years (Painter *et al.* 2006a). Exposure to the famine in early gestation was also associated with differences in food choice at age 50 years, as these men and women were twice as likely to consume a high-fat diet (Lussana *et al.* 2008).

1.4.2 Supplementation studies

Dietary interventions to increase nutrient intake in pregnancy have largely had disappointing results, as the effects on birthweight have been small, even in marginally nourished populations (de Onis *et al.*

1998; Haider and Bhutta 2006). Taken together with the inconsistent findings of observational studies, this has added to the view that fetal growth is little affected by maternal nutrition (Harding 2001). However, many of the early studies used single-nutrient supplements, which may be of limited value, as nutrients do not operate in isolation and there are interactions between them (Jackson and Robinson 2001). Importantly, many studies have started supplementation in mid to late pregnancy. Since the fetal growth trajectory is established very early in gestation, it is possible that this is too late to be of benefit. Periconceptional nutritional status may have a greater influence on fetal growth, and ensuring adequate nutrient status before conception might be expected to be more effective.

There are a few recent studies in which the children born to women who received dietary supplements in pregnancy have been followed up as adults (Hawkesworth *et al.* 2009). The Institute of Nutrition of Central America and Panama (INCAP) trial in Guatemala conducted a randomised trial of nutritional intervention in pregnancy and early childhood between 1969 and 1977. A vegetable protein drink (Atole) or protein-free drink (Fresco) was provided for pregnant and breastfeeding women and children below the age of 7 years, in two intervention and two control villages (Stein *et al.* 2008). Follow-up of the participants in the trial has shown some differences in serum lipid levels in men and women who were born in the intervention villages, but no differences in blood pressure (Stein, Wang *et al.* 2006).

However, a follow-up study of Gambian adolescents at ages 11–17 years, born to mothers who received a protein-energy supplement in pregnancy, has not provided evidence of effects of supplementation on cardiovascular disease risk (Hawkesworth *et al.* 2011). Although maternal supplementation increased birthweight in this study, there were no differences in children's blood pressure, body composition or lipid profile when compared with children whose mothers were supplemented during lactation (Hawkesworth *et al.* 2011).

There are a number of methodological and other factors that could explain the contrasting findings of these follow-up studies when compared with the clear evidence of long-term effects of variations in maternal nutrition seen in experimental models. However, the number of studies of adult offspring born to women whose diets and nutrition were characterised

in pregnancy is currently limited, and further follow-up studies of human populations are needed.

1.4.3 Maternal body composition

Although poorer perinatal outcomes have been associated with mothers who are both underweight and overweight, the long-term consequences of variations in maternal body composition on the offspring have been little studied. Higher maternal BMI is associated with greater adiposity in the child (Gale *et al.* 2007), but the extent to which this is due to the shared postnatal environment is not known, nor whether there are persisting influences of variations in the intrauterine environment on the child's body composition. A role of prenatal experience is likely to be important. For example, women who have poor glycaemic control in pregnancy are at increased risk of having a baby large for gestational age, with greater adiposity (Catalano and Ehrenberg 2006). Importantly, even among women with normal glucose tolerance at screening, increasing maternal glycaemia has been associated with a greater risk of obesity in their children (Hillier *et al.* 2007). Set against the rapid background changes occurring in body composition in many countries (see Section 1.5 and Chapter 3, Section 3.3.1), the long-term outcomes that are associated with variation in maternal body composition need further study (see Chapter 8).

1.4.4 Postnatal nutrition

We know little about the importance of current variations in postnatal diet for long-term function. Most studies of infant diet are limited largely to comparisons of breast and formula feeding in infancy and less is known about the role of weaning practice, and whether qualitative differences in diet in late infancy affect later health. Breastfeeding is associated with a number of beneficial long-term outcomes, including effects on a number of risk factors for cardiovascular disease (Martin, Ben-Shlomo *et al.* 2005; SACN 2011b). However, the confounding effects of social gradients in breastfeeding need to be considered, and recent studies from low- and middle-income countries, where influences on infant feeding practice vary, show some differences (Brion *et al.* 2011; Fall *et al.* 2011). While further data are needed from populations that differ in confounding structures, misclassification of nutritional exposures remains a particular challenge in infancy. Important data have therefore come from randomised controlled trials of infant feeding (Singhal *et al.* 2004) and the Promotion of Breastfeeding Intervention Trial (PROBIT) in Belarus (Kramer *et al.* 2001). Further follow-up of these children will be key in providing insights into the role of infant feeding, and its effects on lifelong health, in the future (see Chapter 8, Section 8.5.2).

1.5 Nutrition of young women today

Although there have been positive changes in the diets of adults in the UK over the past decades, there are huge inequalities in diet and nutrition across the population (SACN 2008). The diets of children and young adults have become a particular concern as, not only is the prevalence of obesity rising, but it is coupled with growing evidence of low micronutrient intakes and status in these age groups (see Chapter 3, Section 3.2). Additionally there are strong social patterning influences on diet, so that poor diets are more common in disadvantaged groups in the population, such as women who are food insecure (Nelson *et al.* 2007).

Thus, for many young women, not only could their current patterns of diet impact on their own nutritional status, they may also affect their ability to meet the nutrient needs of future pregnancies. Furthermore their dietary patterns are an influence on the way that they feed their children (Fisk *et al.* 2011), suggesting that inequalities in diet and nutrition will persist in the next generation. In the context of the long-term consequences of developmental effects of poor nutrition that this report presents, inequalities in early nutrition may be expected to translate into differences in risk of adult disease in the future. Intervention strategies to lower this risk will require a very clear understanding of the influence of current variations in diet and nutrition on growth and development in early life.

1.6 Key points

- An individual's growth potential is determined by their genome, although adequate nutrient supply is required in early life to realise this growth potential.
- There is strong evidence that some nutrients have clear developmental effects, e.g. vitamin A (excess) and iodine and folate insufficiency, but the effects of more modest variations in maternal nutrition are less well understood.
- Fetal programming is defined as a process whereby a stimulus or insult acting at a critical phase of development results in long-term changes in the structure or function of the organism.
- Environmental conditions can impact on the genotype, resulting in more than one alternative form of structure, physiological state or behaviour developing. This is referred to as 'developmental plasticity'.
- Epidemiological studies show a link between early experience and adult diseases such as diabetes, cardiovascular disease and cancer.

- Some individuals may be more vulnerable to the effects of stressors in adult life as a result of poor experiences in early life, such as inadequate nutrition.
- Experimental studies provide clear evidence of developmental influences of variations in early nutrition that may be key to the links between early life and adult disease, but our current understanding of how these experimental data inform optimal patterns of maternal and infant nutrition is limited.
- The poor diets of young women observed in the UK are of concern, and may impact on their ability to meet the nutrient needs of future pregnancies.
- Intervention strategies to lower future disease risk will require a clear understanding of the influence of current variations in diet and nutrition on growth and development in early life and on lifelong health.

1.7 Key references

Barker DJP, Forsen T, Uutela A *et al.* (2001) Size at birth and resilience to the effects of poor living conditions in adult life: longitudinal study. *BMJ*, **323**, 1273–6.

Barker DJ, Osmond C, Forsén TJ *et al.* (2005) Trajectories of growth among children who have coronary events as adults. *New England Journal of Medicine*, **353**, 1802–9.

Bateson P (2007) Developmental plasticity and evolutionary biology. *Journal of Nutrition*, **137**, 1060–2.

Scientific Advisory Committee on Nutrition (SACN) (2011a) *The Influence of Maternal, Fetal and Child Nutrition on the Development of Chronic Disease in Later Life*. London, The Stationery Office.

2
Normal Growth and Development

2.1 Introduction

The period between conception and birth is an amazing period of development. Throughout this time a complex, yet highly coordinated, process guides the development and growth of a single cell, containing a complete set of genetic information, to the point at which it is an organism capable of surviving outside the womb. Given the extraordinary changes that are occurring in a relatively short period of time, it is unsurprising that external factors, such as maternal diet, may have some influence on the resultant baby. In fact, a large and growing body of evidence suggests that disturbance of growth in fetal life is a strong determinant of later disease risk in humans. If the impairment occurs during a critical stage of organ development, or if it is of sufficient severity, permanent, potentially detrimental changes can occur that cannot be compensated for after birth. This chapter describes the phases of normal human growth and development from fertilisation until the age of 2 years, to help understand these critical periods during which our disease risk is effectively programmed to some extent for life (see Table 2.1).

2.2 Prenatal development

Development that occurs before birth (prenatal development) is divided into an embryonic period and a fetal period. The embryonic period begins with fertilisation and ends 8 weeks later.

2.2.1 Embryonic period

2.2.1.1 Fertilisation, cleavage, implantation

Fertilisation of the mother's egg with the father's sperm requires about 24 hours and occurs in the fallopian tube. The genetic material from the haploid cells combines to produce a zygote with 46 chromosomes with a defined sex – either XX, which normally develops into a female, or XY, which normally develops into a male.

As the zygote passes down the fallopian tube, it undergoes rapid mitotic cell divisions. These divisions result in an increased number of smaller cells so, during this period, the size of the embryo does not change. Three days later the embryo (containing at this point roughly 12–16 cells) arrives in the uterus and approximately 7 days after fertilisation implants itself into the endometrial lining where it receives nourishment from the mother.

2.2.1.2 Formation of germ layers

Changes occur within the embryo that result in the formation of three germ layers called the endoderm, the mesoderm and the ectoderm. These three germ layers give rise to the tissues and organs as the embryo develops.

Nerve tissue is derived from ectoderm. Muscle (cardiac, skeletal and smooth) and connective tissues (such as cartilage, bone and blood vessels) are derived from mesoderm (with the exception of the head as it

Nutrition and Development: Short- and Long-Term Consequences for Health, First Edition. Edited by the British Nutrition Foundation.
© 2013 the British Nutrition Foundation. Published 2013 by Blackwell Publishing Ltd.

Table 2.1   Stages of development

	Image	Size	Complexity of the organism
Embryonic period Month 1 (0–4 weeks)		By week 4, the embryo is around 0.4 cm long	Fertilisation occurs forming a zygote cell which rapidly divides into more cells. The embryo implants into the uterine endometrium and structures that are essential for the growth of the embryo begin to develop (e.g. the placenta, umbilical cord and amniotic sac).
Month 2 (4–8 weeks)		By week 7, the embryo is around 1 cm long	The fetal-placental circulation system is established. Organ rudiments undergo growth and differentiation to form organs and organ systems. By week 4, the heart starts beating.
Fetal period Month 3 (9–12 weeks)		At 9 weeks of pregnancy, the baby is about 2.2 cm long	The end of the 8th week marks the end of the embryonic period and the start of the fetal period. The legs are short and thighs relatively small. The upper limbs have almost reached their final relative lengths. External genitalia of males and females appear similar until the end of the 9th week. Their mature fetal form is not established until the 12th week. By the 11th week, intestinal coils have formed in the abdomen. Urine formation begins between the 9th and 12th weeks and urine is discharged through the urethra into the amniotic fluid. Fetal waste products are transferred to the maternal circulation by transfer across the placental cell layer(s). Red blood cells are produced in the liver.
Month 4 (13–16 weeks)		At 14 weeks, the baby is around 8.5 cm long	Rapid growth occurs during this period. More muscle tissue and bones develop and ossification of the skeleton is active during this period (bones become harder). The liver and pancreas produce fluid secretions. The sex of the fetus can be recognised by 12–14 weeks.
Month 5 (17–20 weeks)		At 20 weeks, the baby is around 13.5 cm long	Growth slows down during this period but the length of the fetus still increases by approximately 50 mm. Muscle development increases. Eyebrows and lashes appear and nails appear on fingers and toes.
Month 6 (21–24 weeks)		At 22 weeks, the baby is around 27 cm long	At around 22 weeks, soft hair called lanugo covers the entire body (thought to help regulate the baby's temperature). Bone marrow begins to make blood cells. The lower airways of the baby's lungs develop but they do not allow gas exchange. The baby begins to store fat.

Table 2.1 (*Continued*)

	Image	Size	Complexity of the organism
Month 7 (25–28 weeks)		At 26 weeks, the baby should be around 30 cm long	Rapid brain development occurs. The nervous system is sufficiently developed to control some body functions. The respiratory system, while immature, has developed to the point where gas exchange is possible. The fetal heartbeat can be heard with a stethoscope.
Month 8 (29–32 weeks)		At 30 weeks, the baby should be around 33 cm long	A rapid increase in the amount of body fat occurs. The bones are fully developed, but still soft and pliable. The baby's body begins storing iron, calcium and phosphorus. Rhythmic breathing movements occur, but the lungs are not fully mature. Lanugo hair begins to disappear.
Month 9 (33–36 weeks)		The baby should be over 40 cm long	Body fat increases. The baby is likely to weigh over 2 kg. Fingernails reach the end of the fingertips.
BIRTH (37–40 weeks)	BIRTH	Normal birth weight in the UK is 2500–4000 g*	The respiratory and cardiovascular systems adapt immediately to the postnatal environment. The digestive system, immune system and sense organs adapt within hours or days of birth.
0–5 months		Growth should follow relevant growth curve	Immediately after birth, an infant normally loses about 5–10% of its bodyweight. By 2 weeks, the infant should start to gain weight and grow rapidly. The soft spot on the top of the head (the fontanelle) should close around 2 months. At 4–6 months, weight gain is usually around 20 g/day and the infant's weight is usually double the birthweight.
6–11 months		Growth should follow relevant growth curve	Weight is gained at a slower rate after nine months; at around 15 g/day. Increases in length are around 0.2 cm/month. Bowel and bladder evacuation become more regular.
12–17 months		Growth should follow relevant growth curve	At 12 months, the infant's weight is expected to be around triple the birthweight. The infant is growing at a slower rate and has less appetite compared with previous months.
18–24 months		At 24 months, the infant is around half their adult height	From 18 months, the infant typically is able to control the muscles used to urinate and initiate bowel movements, but may not be ready to use the toilet. By 24 months, the infant will usually have their first 16 teeth (although the number of teeth can vary).

Source: Department of Health (2009a); NHS Choices (2012).
*Regnault *et al.* (2006). Images reproduced from the NHS Choices pregnancy development slideshow, www.nhs.uk/Tools/Pages/Pregnancy.aspx

forms some of its connective tissue from a specific ectoderm derivative called the neural crest). Epithelial tissue (which is present in any organ or structure that has a lumen [a cavity or channel within a tube or tubular organ, such as a blood vessel of the intestine] or that is covered by a membrane) is derived from all three germ layers (Sweeney 1998).

2.2.2 The placenta

The extraembryonic support tissues begin to develop from week 2 and they are mainly established by week 4, although they continue to develop throughout the pregnancy to form the placenta, the umbilical cord and the amnion.

The placenta consists of a fetal and a maternal component. The fetal component is called the chorion, and remains connected to the fetus by a connecting stalk that forms the core of the umbilical cord. The maternal component is called the decidua and is formed by a layer of the endometrium (the layer that is shed during menstruation if implantation does not take place).

Before a functional fetal-placental circulation system is formed (this is in place by 4 weeks) the embryo relies on simple diffusion of nutrients and oxygen. Once the fetal-placental circulation system is established, organogenesis (the origin and development of organs) begins in earnest.

Fetal growth and development is dependent on the integrity of the maternal-placental unit (see Chapter 4, Section 4.3, for more detail on the development of the placenta). The placenta has a role in releasing hormones into the maternal circulation, which may modify maternal appetite and the mobilisation of nutrients. It also has an essential role in transferring these nutrients to the fetus (see Section 2.3 and Section 2.4.4).

2.3 Embryo development

The transformation of an embryo to a fetus is gradual, and takes place over 8 weeks. Throughout this period, rapid growth occurs and the main external features of the embryo begin to take form. This process is called differentiation and produces the varied cell types (such as blood cells, kidney cells and nerve cells). The rapid growth during the first 3 months of pregnancy (the first trimester) is one of the reasons why the embryo is especially susceptible to

the impact of external factors (such as alcohol, drugs, nutritional imbalances, X-rays and infectious agents). Once this phase has passed, the fetus can still be affected by environmental factors although, from a developmental perspective, the impact is not considered to be so extreme.

By the third week, structures that can be identified as the heart, brain and spinal cord are present and the gastrointestinal tract begins to form, although this is not the route for nutrient absorption until after birth. Throughout gestation, the embryo/fetus is dependent on the placenta to provide the nutrients and oxygen directly into the umbilical artery to support its growth, as well as providing the opportunity for waste products to be removed via the umbilical vein.

The primary role of the amniotic fluid is to protect the growing baby from any knocks or bumps the mother might encounter and to maintain a constant temperature within which the fetus can develop. The fluid also contains a solution of carbohydrates, proteins, lipids and electrolytes that will pass in and out of the fetus *in utero* by swallowing/excretion or inhalation/exhalation.

By week 4, the heart is beating and a form of blood is flowing through the main vessels of the fetus. At week 6, the neural tube closes and, by the 7th week, all organs have begun to develop to some extent. After the 8th week, the fetal period begins and it is this period that is characterised by the development of external features and the formation of limbs.

2.4 Fetal development

2.4.1 Normal fetal growth

The fetal period follows on from the embryonic period, from week 9 to birth, and is characterised by growth and elaboration of structures (see Table 2.1).

The nervous system essentially becomes fully functional with the fetus eventually being able to react to movement, sound and light and to control bodily functions (see Table 2.1). Body stores of minerals including iron, calcium and phosphorus are laid down in the third trimester, while throughout the second half of the pregnancy the fetus is laying down fat. The fetus is considered to be able to survive outside the womb from week 27, although some babies can survive from week 24. A huge level of medical intervention is required to support life at this time as the major organs are not yet fully formed and cannot function properly unaided.

Fetal growth is constrained by the capacity of the uterus towards the end of the pregnancy to allow for successful delivery. Small women tend to have lower birthweight babies. This is seen after egg donation; small women tend to have babies with lower birthweight even when the woman donating the egg was large (Brooks *et al.* 1995).

It is interesting to note that the growth of twins is fundamentally different from that of singletons, and not merely restricted by fetal space or nutrient supply in later gestation. The growth of twins will also differ depending on whether one or two placentas are present, and whether the twins are identical or non-identical. However, the mechanisms by which the growth of twins is regulated differently from singletons so early in gestation are not known (Brooks *et al.* 1995).

The male fetus grows faster and bigger than the corresponding female fetus and is more vulnerable to growth restriction due to various factors, including maternal lifestyle choices (see Chapter 5, Section 5.5).

2.4.2 Vulnerable periods: 'critical windows'

The developing fetus is entirely dependent on the mother and the maternal environment for its nutritional requirements. Therefore maternal nutrition plays a fundamental role in determining fetal health and development. As fetal tissues and organs develop, there are 'critical windows' when susceptibility to damage is elevated (see Chapter 4).

2.4.3 Mobilisation of maternal stores to protect the fetus

When maternal dietary supply does not meet fetal demand, the placenta can play an important role in mobilising some nutrients from maternal stores. The mother is able to store increased supplies of energy in adipose tissue in the first two trimesters and divert these to the fetus during the third trimester. Maternal adipose tissue storage is largely complete by the end of the second trimester and then ceases or declines in the third trimester, owing to the exponential growth of the fetus. By the third trimester, increasing insulin resistance prompts the lipolysis of stored fat and the release of free fatty acids, enabling the mother to

mobilise fatty acids to be used as an alternative source of energy for contracting muscle. Glucose is spared for maternal brain function and the increasing energy expenditure of the growing fetus (glucose is the primary fetal energy source) (Moran 2006).

After 30 weeks' gestation, a modest net loss of maternal body fat occurs (Hytten 1974) which corresponds with an exponential increase in fetal fat mass. During this period, 94% of all fat deposition in the fetus occurs (Widdowson 1968). All fatty acids can act as a source of energy but polyunsaturated fatty acids are required for particular structural and metabolic functions. The fetus has an absolute requirement for the *n*-3 and *n*-6 fatty acids and, in particular, docosahexaenoic acid (22:6 *n*-3; DHA) is needed for the development of the brain and retina. The likely rate of DHA utilisation during late pregnancy cannot be met from dietary sources alone in a significant proportion of mothers. The placenta plays an important part in mobilising fatty acids from maternal adipose tissue stores and can actively select, for example, the *n*-3 and *n*-6 fatty acids for uptake if the mother's dietary intake does not meet the demand of the growing fetus (Haggarty 2004).

Maternal hormone adaptations influence the deposition of maternal nutrients to favour fetal growth in a number of ways. Adaptations of maternal calcium metabolism enhance calcium absorption, storage and diversion to the fetus. Maternal calcium absorption and transport along with the accretion in maternal bones are enhanced in the first two trimesters. From 30 weeks' gestation, calcium resorption from maternal bone is significantly increased, presumably to meet the calcium needs of the growing fetus. As the growing fetus obtains its calcium requirements from the maternal skeleton, pregnant adolescents, particularly those who are themselves still growing, are at increased risk of bone fragility in later life (see Chapter 3, Section 3.2.1 and Chapter 15, Section 15.5.2).

2.4.4 Placental glucose transport

Fetal growth and development is dependent on an adequate supply of nutrients from the mother, in particular glucose, which is the primary energy source for the fetus. Transport of glucose across the human placenta occurs by facilitated diffusion, meaning that it goes down the concentration gradient from mother to fetus. As the fetus grows and demands for energy increase, the rate of flux goes up.

However, it is very rare that problems occur in glucose transport during pregnancy (Desoye *et al.* 2011). Glucose transport in mammalian tissues is mediated by the GLUT gene family of facilitated diffusion transporters, of which there are at least 12 members (Joost and Thorens 2001).

Glucose is transmitted in a steady stream from mother to fetus via the placenta. Glucose is produced by maternal metabolism mainly from carbohydrate in the diet and from the gluconeogenic amino acids. The hormone insulin regulates glucose levels. Some carbohydrates are absorbed more slowly than others and thus may have a weak effect on blood glucose levels. Although there is some variation between individuals, generally, foods with a lower glycaemic index give rise to a smaller blood glucose response than foods with a higher glycaemic index. During pregnancy, a mother's dietary glycaemic index is positively and significantly related to circulating blood glucose levels.

2.5 Fetal development overview

2.5.1 The heart

The cardiovascular system is the first major system to function in the embryo. Early and rapid development is necessary because the rapidly growing embryo cannot satisfy its nutritional and oxygen requirements by diffusion alone. Development begins during the middle of the third week of gestation and the heart begins to beat at 22–23 days.

The primitive heart tube is formed from the mesoderm at the end of the third week. This is followed by the formation of the heart loop which involves differential growth of the two sides of the primitive heart tube so that the right becomes longer than the left and a bend to the right occurs. The transition to the four-chamber shape begins with expansion to form the atrium and ventricle. The atrium then separates to form left and right atria receiving, respectively, the venous return from the lungs and the body. The left ventricle forms from the proximal segment of the primitive ventricle, while the right derives from the distal part.

The increase in heart size during fetal life is predominantly the result of cardiomyocyte proliferation (Soonpaa and Field 1998). The overall rate of cardiomyocyte proliferation gradually decreases during the

later stages of fetal development. This is due to the fact that, during heart development, cardiac myocytes undergo a number of phenotypic changes in order to reach the adult form. One such change is the withdrawal from the cell cycle, transitioning from the proliferative hyperplastic phenotype to a cell-growth hypertrophic phenotype. The switch from hyperplastic to hypertrophic phenotype occurs in the early neonatal period, in the rat between 3 and 4 days of age (F Li *et al.* 1996).

2.5.2 Brain development

At the beginning of the 4th week of gestation the neural folds in the cranial region form the primordium of the brain. Three distinct regions of the brain, the fore-, mid- and hindbrain, are already distinguishable. Neuronal multiplication peaks and is almost complete by the 18th week of pregnancy, and it is during the rapid phase of neural multiplication that the brain is most vulnerable. For example, exposure to X-rays during the vulnerable period of neuronal multiplication results in 'pin-headed' babies (Dobbing 1971), and severe maternal iodine deficiency results in deaf mutism (Chen and Hetzel 2010). The brain growth spurt is in the last few months of pregnancy and in the perinatal period and is accounted for mainly by grey matter growth, which includes accumulation of long-chain polyunsaturated fatty acids. Myelination continues well into the first year of life and early newborn life appears to be an important phase where there is 'hard wiring' of synaptic connections. Clearly, brain development is a complex and long-lasting process, too varied to be contained as a sub-section within one chapter. The reader is referred to Chapter 6 on neurological development.

2.5.3 The lungs

Fetal lung development from the earliest stage to the mature organ has been divided into five chronological stages: embryonic, pseudoglandular, canalicular, saccular and alveolar. During the early stages of lung growth, development of the conducting airways is prominent, whereas later in gestation the distal air spaces undergo alterations in preparation for gas exchange. The embryonic stage covers the primitive development and is generally regarded to cover the first 2 months of human development. Following formation of the primitive gut, the lungs first appears as a ventral bud off the prospective oesophagus. This lung bud elongates and forms two bronchi buds and the trachea.

During the pseudoglandular stage (8–16 weeks) the bronchial tree resembles a system of branching tubules that terminate in structures which resemble an exocrine gland. By the end of this period of development all of the major components of the lung have formed, except those involved with gas exchange.

The canalicular stage (17–27 weeks) sees the appearance of vascular channels or capillaries, which begin to approximate the potential air spaces and form a capillary network around them. By the end of this stage of development the potential air–blood barrier is thin enough to support gaseous exchange.

At the beginning of the saccular stage (26 weeks to birth) the terminal structures, saccules, are relatively smooth-walled and cylindrical. Between about 28 and 36 weeks' gestation there is continued expansion of potential air spaces, a marked decrease in interstitial tissue and development of narrower and more compact layers of lining cells.

In humans, the alveolar stage of lung development covers the late fetal period, 36 weeks' gestation, through to childhood. At the beginning of this stage, each respiratory bronchiole terminates in a cluster of thin-walled terminal subsaccules, separated from one another by loose connective tissue. It is these saccules which become the alveoli in the weeks prior to birth. Although alveolarisation is well under way at birth, only 20% of the adult number of alveoli is present in the lungs of newborn infants.

The newborn lung has to undergo marked structural changes in order to mature into an adult lung. As well as a multiplication in the number of alveoli, there is a restructuring of the microvasculature, leading to an exponential increase in the area for gaseous exchange. The microvasculature of the lung changes from the bilayered capillary network of the parenchymal septa into the single-layered network of the mature lung (Burri 1997). As seen prenatally, postnatal lung development occurs in parallel with lung growth. There are two distinguishable stages of lung growth; the first corresponds to the period of alveolar multiplication and microvasculature maturation (Zeltner *et al.* 1987). This phase of growth is characterised by a bias towards the growth of the areas of the lung involved in oxygen transport, at the expense of the parenchymal tissue compartment. During the second phase of growth, which begins around 18 months of age, there is proportionate growth of all lung compartments so that the toddler's lung is a miniaturised version of the adult lung.

The successful transition from fetus to air-breathing neonate is largely dependent on the ability of the lungs to rapidly take over the role of gas exchange from the placenta. This transition requires the clearance of liquid from the lungs to allow the entry of air. Gas exchange in the lung takes place across the lung alveoli. These are formed from type II cells, and constitute a thin barrier overlaid with surfactant. Damage to the surfactant layer may result in serious respiratory problems, as is often seen in premature infants.

Lung development during fetal life shows quite pronounced sex differences with females exhibiting earlier lung maturation than boys (see Chapter 5, Section 5.12).

2.5.4 Bone

Bone development in the human fetus begins around week 13. The bones start as mostly cartilaginous tissue, crystallising and hardening during the newborn and early childhood period. In the newborn infant, there are about 300 bones that grow and fuse to form the 206 bones of the adult.

Normal bone development is critical for health and well-being. Bone is made of a variety of cell types, both manufacturing and breaking down the bone, and a matrix of collagen and crystalline salts, primarily calcium phosphates, as hydroxyapatite crystals. As well as blood vessels, nerve cells and the cells of the bone marrow, bone also contains osteoclasts and osteoblasts. The osteoblasts are responsible for bone formation while osteoclasts are important in removing old bone. These take over the cartilage cells in the bones as development progresses, converting cartilage into bone. This process is known as ossification. It is critically dependent on an adequate supply of calcium and other salts.

Growth of the long bones (e.g. the femur and tibia) takes place at the epiphyseal plates. These are found at both ends of the bone, and are responsible for the elongation of the bones.

The mechanisms involved in regulating this process are fascinating and we are only now beginning to clarify how the process operates. Most work has been carried out in model systems such as birds, but the data seem to extrapolate well to humans. A comprehensive set of transcription factors regulate gene expression in both types of cell. As mentioned above, nutritional factors, such as calcium and vitamin D, are also essential and the whole process is under the control of hormones and growth factors.

It is well established that mechanical stress is important in developing bone strength in adults, but recent data suggest that it is also significant in the embryo. Blocking muscle contraction in chick embryos results in marked changes in the expression of collagen, and this in turn induces large alterations in bone formation. We could argue that an active baby in the womb is already preparing to have stronger bones than his or her quieter counterpart!

2.5.5 Muscle

The muscular system consists of skeletal, smooth and cardiac muscle. The muscular system develops from the mesoderm, except for the muscles of the iris in the eye, which develop from the neuroectoderm. Embryonic muscle cells, myoblasts, are derived from mesenchyme. The pattern of muscle formation is regulated by the connective tissue into which the myoblasts migrate. The myoblasts that form the skeletal muscles of the trunk are derived from the paraxial mesoderm in the myotome regions of the somites. The limb muscles develop from myogeneic precursor cells in the limb buds. Smooth muscle differentiates from the splanchnic mesenchyme surrounding the endoderm of the primordial gut. The smooth muscle in the walls of many blood and lymphatic vessels arises from the somatic mesoderm. Cardiac muscle is derived from splanchnic mesoderm surrounding the heart tube.

Myogenesis, muscle formation, begins with the elongation of the nuclei and cell bodies of the mesenchymal cells as they differentiate into myoblasts. The muscle growth during development is the result of ongoing fusion of myoblasts and myotubules. Myofilaments develop in the cytoplasm of the myotubes during or after fusion of the myoblasts. As the myotubules differentiate, they become covered with external laminae, which segregate them from the surrounding connective tissue. Most skeletal muscle develops before birth and almost all remaining muscles are formed by the end of the first year.

2.5.6 The liver

The liver, gallbladder and biliary duct system arise as a ventral outgrowth, the hepatic diverticulum, from the foregut early in the 4th week of gestation. The larger, cranial part of the hepatic diverticulum is the primordium of the liver. The proliferating endodermal cells give rise to the liver cords of hepatocytes and to the epithelial lining of the biliary apparatus. The liver cords connect around endothelium-lined spaces, the primordia of the hepatic sinusoids. The hematopoietic cells, Kupffer cells and connective tissue cells are derived from the mesoderm of the septum transversum. By late gestation the structural features of the hepatocytes are similar to those of adult hepatocytes. However, it is not until childhood that the hepatocyte plates have thinned to a single-cell thickness. During fetal life the portal circulation bypasses the liver via the ductus venosus. After birth the ductus venosus closes, with closure becoming complete by 2 weeks of age.

The liver grows rapidly and soon fills a large part of the abdominal cavity. By the 9th week, the liver accounts for approximately 10% of the total weight of the fetus. Much of the weight is due to the haematopoietic function that the liver carries out at this stage. Large groups of proliferating cells lie between the hepatic cells and walls of the vessels, which produce red and white blood cells. The liver remains the main haematopoietic organ of the developing embryo/fetus until the initiation of bone marrow haematopoiesis near birth. By the time of birth the liver makes up only 5% of the total body weight.

During fetal life the main functions of the liver are haematopoiesis and storage of essential nutrients required in the early postnatal period. It is not until the postnatal period that all the enzyme systems required for glycogenolysis, formation of bile salts and substrate elimination mature.

2.5.7 The pancreas

The pancreas develops from the dorsal and ventral pancreatic buds, which arise from the caudal part (posterior/tail) of the foregut. The dorsal bud, the first to appear, gives rise to the majority of the pancreas. The ventral pancreatic bud forms part of the head of the pancreas. The dorsal and ventral buds fuse following stages of growth and reorientation. Development of the secretory capacity of the pancreas includes increases in the enzyme content, fluid production and cell responsiveness to secretagogues. Insulin secretion begins approximately 10 weeks into gestation.

2.5.8 The kidneys

Three transitory sets of kidneys develop in the human embryo: the pronephros, mesenephros and metanephros. It is the metanephros form of the kidney, developing early in the 5th week of gestation, which gives rise to the fetal kidney. The kidney is formed of two functional components; the excretory and the collecting portion. The fetal kidneys become functional near the 12th week, with urine being excreted into the amniotic cavity. During fetal life, the kidneys are not responsible for excretion of waste products, which is carried out by the placenta. However, fetal urine is very important in the formation of amniotic fluid, and disorders of production can give rise to serious diseases such as hydramnios (the presence of an excessive amount of amniotic fluid).

The development of the kidney begins with the outgrowth of the ureteric bud from the wolffian duct and its invasion into the adjacent mesenchyme. The ureters and the collecting duct system of the kidneys differentiate from the ureteric bud. The growing ureter undergoes repeated branching, leading to the formation of the collecting duct. The metanephric mesenchyme forms the secretory components of the nephron. The formation of the epithelial part of the renal capsule, the proximal and distal tubules, involves the conversion of loose mesenchyme into epithelium, a process of tubulogenesis. After invasion of the ureteric bud, the metanephric mesenchyme condenses around its top. As the ureteric bud branches out, the condensed mesenchyme splits into two identical parts surrounding the growing tip. This continuous process leads to the formation of the renal vesicles, which grow and differentiate into the comma-shaped bodies and the S-shaped bodies that subsequently join the ureteric branches, forming nephrons. The number of nephrons formed ultimately depends on growth and branching of the ureteric bud; formation of mesenchymal condensations; and conversion to epithelial tubules.

2.5.9 Haematopoietic tissue

The yolk sac is the initial site of fetal haemopoiesis. The formation of the various types of fetal blood cells begins during the 6th week. Haematopoietic stem cells originating from the yolk sac colonise the liver. By the 10th week of gestation the liver is the major early haematopoietic organ of the embryo/fetus. This activity gradually subsides during the last 2 months of intrauterine life, and only small haematopoietic islands remain at birth. By the end of the 12th week, this activity has decreased in the liver and erythropoiesis, the formation of red blood cells, has begun in the spleen. By 28 weeks of gestation, erythropoiesis is reduced in the spleen and, by the time of birth, the bone marrow has become the major site of this process.

2.5.10 Adipose tissue

In mammals, the 'adipose organ' consists of several subcutaneous and visceral depots. The depots contain blood vessels and nerve fibres. These depots were believed to be made up of two distinct adipose cells, white (WAT) and brown adipocytes (BAT). It is now known that WAT and BAT can be present in one depot, and are able to transform from one type to the other when required (Cinti 2009). WAT store lipids to provide fuel for the organism, allowing intervals between meals, while BAT uses lipids to produce heat.

Humans, and other mammals, are exposed to their greatest temperature shock at birth, when they are immediately exposed to comparatively cool surroundings. To survive this, the newborn must have the ability to produce sufficient heat to maintain body temperature. Therefore BAT forms during weeks 17–20 of gestation and produces heat when required by oxidising fatty acids.

2.5.11 Sex hormone development

The sex hormones play a central role in fetal development and it is not useful to consider their development in the absence of the aberrations that occur as a consequence of imbalance. This aspect of fetal development, therefore, is also considered in more detail in a separate chapter (see Chapter 5).

2.5.12 Immune system development

By extrapolation of growth curves derived from cell counts from fetal thymus, spleen and bone marrow, research has implied the appearance of lymphocytes as early as 3.5 weeks' gestation (Stites and Pavia 1979). Lymphocytes derived from the yolk sac appear in the fetal liver by about 7 weeks from conception and, by 10–12 weeks, they are evident in the thymus (Stites and Pavia 1979).

At birth, the immune system is still immature and the thymus is particularly active in newborns. However, postnatal microbial exposure provides an essential source of stimulation to immunological pathways and therefore protection from allergic diseases (Schaub *et al.* 2008). At birth, the infant gut is rapidly colonised by microorganisms, leading to the development of the associated mucosal network that comprises more than 70% of the total immune system (West *et al.* 2011). Many factors may affect the development of immune tolerance, including oral and environmental exposures. However, the complex mechanisms that have evolved to promote immune tolerance are not fully understood (West *et al.* 2011).

The infant's immune system continues to develop during early feeding. Breast milk is rich in nutrients and growth factors with immunomodulatory properties as well as maternal immune cells (Rautava and Walker 2009) and antigens derived from the maternal diet (West *et al.* 2011). These factors all appear to play a role in protection from infection and promotion of oral tolerance; however, the underlying mechanisms remain unclear (West *et al.* 2011). (See Chapter 13 for discussion on allergic disease and asthma.)

2.6 Birthweight

In general, birthweight is correlated with the mother's own birthweight and with that of other female relatives (Shah and Shah 2009). The average birthweight varies between populations, as does the optimal birthweight (defined as the weight with the lowest associated perinatal mortality) (Wilcox and Russell 1986; Graafmans *et al.* 2002). Average birthweight of White infants in the UK in the nationally representative Millennium Cohort was 3.42 kg (95% CI: 3.40–3.43 kg) (Kelly *et al.* 2009). There are ethnic variations in birthweight. Average birthweight of babies born in the UK to women of Caribbean, sub-Saharan African and South Asian, particularly Indian, origin is lower than that of the babies of White European women (Office for National Statistics (ONS) 2000). Birthweight is influenced by maternal frame size and adversely affected by cigarette smoking. Even after adjusting for maternal frame size, birthweight is about 240 g lower in South Asian women who are vegetarians (Reddy *et al.* 1994). The prevalence of babies who are small for gestational age is greater in teenage pregnancy where the mother may be competing for growth with the fetus (Baker *et al.* 2009). Seasonal variation in birthweight has also been observed, with babies born in autumn being the heaviest and those born in winter the lightest (Lawlor, Leon *et al.* 2005; Watson and McDonald 2007). Suggested reasons for this include variation in vitamin D status attributable to differences in sunlight exposure or through other seasonal influences such as variation in maternal diet or insulin sensitivity. Although there is no definite mechanism to explain this, one suggested reason is that women may accrue more fat in winter which may lead to heavier babies born in the autumn.

Low birthweight is defined by the World Health Organization (WHO) as a birthweight of <2500 g at term and very low birthweight as <1500 g at term. This definition does not correct for length of gestation. A fetus or neonate described as small for gestational age (SGA) indicates a birthweight less than the 10th centile in weight expected for gestation. Other growth parameters such as estimated fetal weight, abdominal circumference or birthweight can also be used. The most commonly used centiles are the 10th, 5th and 3rd, although any centile may be used as long as it is specified (see Table 2.2).

SGA babies may be full term (born at 39 weeks) but are underweight in relation to an expected weight. SGA babies have lower energy stores (i.e. fat and glycogen) than babies of normal birthweight and are prone to hypoglycaemia. Their nutrient requirements are high and therefore most low-birthweight infants are at risk of nutritional inadequacy (Bentley *et al.* 2004).

Intrauterine growth restriction (IUGR) is a term generally applied to infants weighing less than two standard deviations below the mean of a population, born at the same estimated gestational age or for a given gestational age. These infants differ from SGA infants as they are pathologically small and at risk of poor outcomes. The causes of IUGR can include:

Table 2.2 Classification system for describing infant size at birth

Normal birthweight	2500–4000 g*
Average birthweight in UK	3420 g**
Low birthweight	Birthweight < 2500 g at term***
Very low birthweight	Birthweight < 1500 g at term***
Extremely low birthweight	Birthweight < 1000 g at term***
High birthweight	Birthweight > 4000 g at term*
Appropriate for gestational age (AGA)	Birthweight between the 10th and 90th centiles of weight expected for gestation***
Small for gestational age (SGA)	Birthweight less than the 10th centile in weight expected for gestation (small for dates)***
Intrauterine growth restriction (IUGR)	Infants who weigh less than two standard deviations below the mean of a population, born at the same estimated gestational age or for a given gestational age*
Large for gestational age (LGA)	Birthweight more than the 90th centile in weight expected for gestation***
Macrosomia	Infants who are large at birth. The cut-offs used are typically birthweight > 4000 g or a birthweight more than the 90th centile.* Macrosomia usually is a result of poorly controlled gestational diabetes.

Note: Term babies may be born between 37 and 42 completed weeks gestation.
*Regnault *et al.* (2006).
**Data from UK Millennium Cohort Study (Kelly *et al.* 2009).
***McIntosh *et al.* (2008).

- inadequate maternal nutrition, although it is unclear whether it is a lack of overall calories or a specific substrate that causes IUGR;
- fetal causes, such as chromosome abnormality or genetic causes;
- abnormalities of the fetal-maternal circulation;
- maternal causes, such as smoking, alcohol, drugs and chronic disease (e.g. congenital heart disease, chronic renal disease and hyperthyroidism).

Mild maternal diabetes and hyperglycaemia is more often associated with a large fetus (macrosomia) (see Chapter 9, Section 9.5.2.1) but the incidence of IUGR is also increased (when the maternal diabetes is more extreme) (Reece *et al.* 1998). A common risk factor for IUGR is smoking, and therefore all mothers should be encouraged to stop. Passive smoking is also harmful to the developing fetus (Department of Health 2009a).

Growth charts are available (see Section 2.8). However, it may be questioned whether a growth chart for a national or local population is most appropriate. A local population mainly consisting of ethnic women who tend to have smaller babies owing to genetic variation would favour the use of local growth charts; however, if the local population tends to have smaller babies due to deprivation and higher incidence of malnutrition, then using local growth charts would result in some babies being classified as appropriate for gestational age when in fact they were at risk of dysfunction (Chamberlain and Steer 2001). Another problem of using birth-weight curves is the estimation of gestational age. Age is normally measured in units of time, and accurate timing may not be possible in many pregnancies. Traditionally, gestational age was dated from the first day of the last normal menstrual period, which may be difficult in women who do not have regular menses. More recently, birthweight curves have been obtained from pregnancies dated by ultrasonography. These have suggested higher term birthweights and reduced flattening of the birthweight curve at term than when pregnancies are dated from menstrual history alone. These data show that ultrasound correction of gestational age leads to a more linear curve of birthweight, probably better describing the biology of human fetal growth (Sparks and Cetin 2006).

High birthweight is defined as >4000 g at term. Women who are obese (BMI > 30) during pregnancy are more likely to have a high-birthweight baby (Centre for Maternal and Child Enquiries (CMACE) and Royal College of Obstetricians and Gynaecologists (RCOG) 2010b) (see Chapter 8, Section 8.4.3).

2.7 Postnatal growth and development

Infancy (age 1–24 months) is a period of rapid growth compared to any other period of life. The relative relationships among rates of linear growth, weight gain and brain growth vary greatly during the first few years of life. Although the proportion of energy requirements for body tissue deposition decreases dramatically during infancy, brain energy demands increase markedly during the same period. Babies also do not develop at the same rate; there is a wide range of what is considered 'normal'. A baby may be more advanced in some areas and slightly behind in others.

Genetic factors are the main influence on linear growth during the first few years of life; however, infants with 'tall' genes who are born short grow more rapidly during the first few years, whereas infants with 'short' genes who are born long grow more slowly during the first few years. Indeed, genetics are the major determinants of adult height with only 20% of the variation in height estimated to be due to environmental factors, mainly nutrition and disease (Phillips and Matheny 1990; Preece 1996; Silventoinen *et al.* 2000). Both restricted growth (weight and height) and excessive growth which results in crossing the centiles can be factors in later incidence of chronic disease (see Section 2.10) (World Health Organization and Food and Agriculture Organization of the United Nations 2003).

The relative increases in length and weight during the first 2 years of life are substantially different. From birth to 2 years of age, body length increases by about 75% to a value approximately half of the final mature adult height (Feigelman 2007). Weight typically increases by more than 2.5-fold, but to only about 20% that of adult body weight. During the same time period, brain size increases to more than 80% of adult brain size and, by the age of 6 is 95% of the adult size (Clayton and Gill 2001). At birth, body weight is approximately 5% of adult weight, whereas the brain is 25% of adult weight and many other organs (e.g. reproductive organs, pancreas, liver, kidneys, lungs and heart) are 3% to 9%.

Different human tissues and organs grow at different times and rates. The weights of organs at birth vary considerably. The growth spurt of individual tissues or organs may occur earlier (e.g. the brain) or later (e.g. reproductive organs) than that of the body. The brain begins its growth spurt during the last trimester of intrauterine life and continues after birth, with most of its adult size reached by age 2–3 years. Many organs (e.g. lung, liver, kidneys heart) reach adult weight at a similar rate as the whole body. The exception to this is the reproductive organs, which grow more slowly than the body as a whole during early childhood until around puberty when rate of development is rapid (Norgan 1998).

At birth, body fat accounts for around 15% of weight. By 6 months this has increased to 25% and peaks at around 30% at 12 months. Differences between the sexes in skinfold thickness (a measure of regional fatness of subcutaneous adipose tissue) at birth are small but, on average, girls have thicker skinfold than boys (Norgan 1998).

2.8 Growth monitoring (growth charts)

Growth charts are used to monitor the growth of infants, children and adolescents to assess whether they are growing and developing as they should. In 2006, the WHO launched new child growth standards (see www.who.int/childgrowth/standards/en/). Since then, over 140 countries (including the UK in 2009) have adopted them.

In 2007, the UK Department of Health accepted recommendations made by the Scientific Advisory Committee on Nutrition and the Royal College of Paediatrics and Child Health to replace the UK 1990 reference (referred to as UK90) with the new WHO growth standards (Scientific Advisory Committee on Nutrition (SACN) and Royal College of Paediatrics and Child Health 2007). The Royal College of Paediatricians and Child Health has adopted the new WHO child growth charts that combine UK90 and WHO data (Royal College of Paediatricians and Child Health 2009). These charts were introduced in the UK in May 2009 as they represent an international standard of growth for all healthy infants and young children whether breast-fed or formula-fed.

Growth charts are used to assess the rate and pattern of growth of children over time, as it is more important to know how they are growing than to know how heavy or tall they are at a particular time. Children are expected to grow steadily, following a line curving in roughly the same way, and usually within the centile lines on the chart. However, during the first 2 years of life it is normal for the baby's weight and height measurements to occasionally cross the centiles. It is important to know that each child is growing at a steady rate along, or parallel to, the centile lines that reflect his or her own growth potential (see www.infantandtoddlerforum.org).

2.9 Secular growth trends

Secular changes refer to characteristics of populations over time. Secular growth changes are of interest as they reflect public health conditions relating to nutrition, physical activity, socioeconomic status and health, and provide insight into the link between growth and the environment.

2.9.1 Secular change in birthweight

The average birthweight varies between populations, as does the optimal birthweight (the weight associated with the least perinatal mortality). Data from the nationally representative UK Millennium Cohort Study ($n = 16\,157$) reported mean birthweight in White infants to be 3.42 kg (95% CI: 3.40–3.43 kg) (Kelly *et al.* 2009). Birthweight can be influenced not only by the mother's birthweight but also by the grandmother's birthweight. These intergenerational differences in birthweight could act as precursors for an infant being born with low birthweight, pre-term or small for gestational age if the mother herself had been born as such (Shah and Shah 2009).

On the whole, evidence of a secular trend in birthweight is not strong and, similarly, length at birth has shown no secular trend (Cole 2000). However, two factors in recent years are likely to affect such trends. First, the increase in very premature births due to medical advances has skewed the birthweight distribution to the left, as babies now have a reasonable chance of survival when born as early as 24 weeks' gestation. Second, the proportion of overweight and obese mothers has increased, which impacts directly on the birthweight on their babies (Cole 2003) (see Chapter 15, Section 15.2.1.1).

2.9.2 Secular change in height

In adults, an increasing secular trend in height has been observed in most European countries since the nineteenth century, with current advances in average height of 1 cm to 3 cm per decade (Cole 2000). Dutch and Scandinavian adults are relatively tall compared with adults from other countries; but height in the Netherlands and Scandinavia is apparently starting to plateau, while secular increases in height are still occurring in other European countries. However, these figures are mainly based on data from male conscripts. Analysis of changes in secular height among women during the twentieth century, although less clear, seems to indicate that women's height has been increasing relatively slowly compared with men's, and therefore the differences in adult height between men and women have increased.

2.10 Canalisation, catch-up and catch-down growth

Canalisation as applied to growth refers to the tendency to follow a genetically determined trajectory, given optimal health conditions and nutrient supply. Individuals, whose growth has slowed or accelerated due to disease or environmental factors such as nutrient supply, show a tendency to accelerate or decelerate once these factors are removed. The term 'catch-up growth' was introduced by Prader in 1963 to describe an increased velocity of growth which occurs after a temporary arrest of growth during infancy or early childhood. Prader defined catch-up growth as a return of the child's growth to its previous normal growth projectile (Prader *et al.* 1963), with the process normally completed by the end of the first year of life, although in some cases it may continue into the second. In other words, weight or length of the infant crosses percentiles in an upward direction. It has generally been thought that long-term beneficial effects will accrue from optimising neonatal and post-discharge nutrition to prevent growth failure and/or accelerate catch-up growth during infancy. However, there is now growing evidence that children who grow rapidly during infancy and childhood are more likely to be obese as adults and at increased risk of metabolic disturbances such as insulin resistance.

Epidemiological evidence derived mainly from term-born populations suggests that adaptations made by the fetus and young infant when undernourished induce alterations in metabolism, hormonal output and cardiac output which result in central obesity, diabetes and cardiovascular disease in middle age (Fall *et al.* 1995; Cianfarani *et al.* 1999; Forsen *et al.* 1999) (see Chapters 8, 9 and 10).

Subjects who grow rapidly (i.e. those born SGA or at a low birthweight followed by catch-up growth) are at greatest risk of these conditions (see Chapter 15, Section 15.4.3). Similar effects have been reported among pre-term survivors of neonatal intensive care (Mortaz *et al.* 2001; Singhal *et al.* 2003; Singhal *et al.* 2010). Although the above evidence suggests possible long-term deleterious health effects of catch-up growth, there is also evidence that catch-up growth may have short-term beneficial health effects, such as lower rates of hospitalisation during infancy and early childhood (Eriksson 2001; Victora *et al.* 2001). Catch-down growth refers to a relatively slow rate of postnatal growth, which may be seen in infants who have had accelerated fetal growth leading to macrosomia (e.g. the infant of a diabetic or obese mother). (Also see Chapter 12, Section 12.1.3 and Chapter 10, Section 10.3.)

2.11 Key points

- Development begins with the embryonic period, which ends 8 weeks after fertilisation. The fetal period, from week 9 to birth, is characterised by growth and elaboration of structures.
- The first 3 months of pregnancy (the first trimester) is a period of rapid growth. The main external features of the fetus begin to take form by a process of differentiation which produces various cell types (e.g. blood cells, kidney cells and nerve cells). This rapid growth results in the embryo being particularly susceptible to the impact of external factors (e.g. nutrient intake) during this time.
- The developing embryo/fetus is entirely dependent on the mother and the maternal environment for its nutritional requirements. Therefore a woman's diet during pregnancy plays a crucial role in determining fetal health and development. There are also particular periods of growth and development of tissues and organs, termed 'critical windows', when susceptibility to damage is elevated.
- The role of the placenta in development is often overlooked, but it plays a central role, as it is the conduit for nutrient and waste transfer between mother and fetus.
- The cardiovascular system is the first major system to function in the embryo. This is because the growing embryo cannot satisfy its nutritional and oxygen requirements by diffusion alone.
- The development of the lungs is a gradual process that can be divided into five stages throughout embryo and fetal life. At birth the lungs undergo marked structural changes in order to mature into the adult lungs. The lungs continue to develop up to the age of 2 years.
- Infancy (1–24 months) is a period of rapid growth compared to other periods of life. The relative relationships among rates of linear growth, weight gain and brain growth vary greatly during the first few years of life. Although the proportion of energy requirements for body tissue deposition decreases dramatically during infancy, brain energy demands increase markedly during the same period.
- The WHO launched new Child Growth Standards in 2006. The UK Department of Health accepted recommendations to replace the UK 1990 reference ('UK90') with the new WHO growth standards in 2007. Also in 2007, the Royal College of Paediatricians and Child Health adopted growth charts that combine UK90 and WHO data. These charts represent an international standard of growth for all healthy infants and young children whether breast-fed or formula-fed.
- Catch-up growth (the return of the child's growth to its previous normal projectile) may have short-term beneficial health effects, such as lower rates of hospitalisation during infancy and early childhood. However, there is now growing evidence that children who grow rapidly during infancy and childhood are more likely to be obese as adults and at greater risk of metabolic disturbances such as insulin resistance.

2.12 Recommendations for future research

- Current research suggests that catch-up growth increases risk of later disease. Further research to determine the reasons is needed.
- After birth, all sorts of growth and developmental changes occur. A better understanding is required of the regulation of the timing of development at all stages of life (from fetal life through infancy and early years, and into adolescence, adulthood and older age). Research on what upregulates or downregulates gene expression at any time from conception would be useful.

- Further research is required to identify the interplay between different organs. Investigation into whether this can be used to reduce problems associated with inappropriate growth and development would be useful.
- Further investigation of how diet and nutrients modulate growth and development is required. For example, what are the influences of phytochemicals on growth and development and could they be used therapeutically?

2.13 Key references

Department of Health (2009a) *The Pregnancy Book*. London, Department of Health.

Royal College of Paediatricians and Child Health (2009) *UK-WHO Growth Charts: Early Years* (www.rcpch.ac.uk/child-health/research-projects/uk-who-growth-charts-early-years/uk-who-growth-charts-early-years).

Scientific Advisory Committee on Nutrition (SACN) and Royal College of Paediatrics and Child Health (2007) *Application of WHO Growth Standards in the UK*. London, The Stationery Office.

Shah PS & Shah V (2009) Influence of the maternal birth status on offspring: a systematic review and meta-analysis. *Acta Obstetricia et Gynecologica Scandinavica*, **88**, 1307–18.

Ulijaszek SJ, Johnston FE & Preece MA (1998) *The Cambridge Encyclopaedia of Human Growth and Development*. Cambridge, Cambridge University Press.

3
Maternal Nutrition and Infant Feeding: Current Practice and Recommendations

3.1 Introduction

This chapter aims to set the scene regarding current practice and recommendations in relation to early life development. It begins by describing the characteristics of pregnant women in Europe today and recent trends in relation to age and ethnicity. Current recommendations relating to weight and diet alongside current practice are discussed with regard to various stages of pregnancy and early life feeding:

- pre-pregnancy;
- pregnancy;
- lactation;
- breastfeeding;
- formula feeding;
- weaning and complementary feeding.

Some of these themes are developed further in Chapter 15.

3.2 Characteristics of pregnant women in the UK

Figures from the Office of National Statistics show that the number of births in England and Wales has been increasing since a dip in 2001. During this period the number of live births has risen by 22% from 594 634 in 2001 to 723 165 in 2010 (Office for National Statistics (ONS) 2011) (Fig. 3.1). This recent rise has been attributed to several factors

including changes in maternity and paternity leave, tax and benefits for parents, the impact of recent high levels of international immigration to the UK, and women born in the 1960s and 1970s who had delayed childbearing now catching up in terms of completed family size (ONS 2011).

3.2.1 Changing age profile of mothers

A maternal age of less than 20 years and over 35 years is associated with increased risk of poor pregnancy outcome (Confidential Enquiry into Maternal and Child Health (CEMACH) 2009). Women (at all ages) giving birth for the first time have a higher risk of specific medical complications, such as pregnancy-induced hypertension and prolonged labour (EURO-PERISTAT 2008). The average age of women giving birth in England and Wales in 2010 was 29.5 years, having risen from 26.7 years in 1970 (these figures refer to all births) (Fig. 3.2) (ONS 2011). The average age of women having their first baby in 2010 was estimated to be 27.8 years. The proportion of pregnancies in women aged 35 and older is increasing in many countries (EURO-PERISTAT 2008). For example, in the UK, over the last two decades the number of live births to mothers aged 40 and over has nearly trebled from 9717 in 1990 to 27 731 in 2010.

However, there are still wide differences between European countries in the age distribution of women

Nutrition and Development: Short- and Long-Term Consequences for Health, First Edition. Edited by the British Nutrition Foundation.
© 2013 the British Nutrition Foundation. Published 2013 by Blackwell Publishing Ltd.

Children per woman

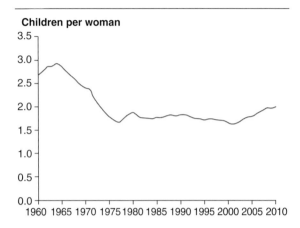

Figure 3.1   Total fertility rate in England and Wales, 1960–2010.
Source: Office for National Statistics (ONS) (2011) *Births and Deaths in England and Wales*, 2010.
Contains public sector information licensed under the Open Government Licence v1.0.

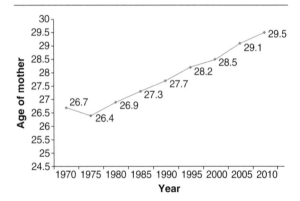

Figure 3.2   Average age of mothers giving birth in England and Wales 1970–2010.
Source: Office for National Statistics (ONS) (2011) *Births and Deaths in England and Wales*, 2010.
Contains public sector information licensed under the Open Government Licence v1.0.

at first pregnancy. For example, in 2004 less than 10% of women delivering babies in the Slovak Republic, the Czech Republic or Poland were aged 35 years or over, compared with 22% in Germany, 23% in Spain and 24% in Italy and Ireland (EURO-PERISTAT 2008) (see Fig. 3.3).

After the age of 35, women are more likely to experience pregnancy complications, as well as mul-

tiple pregnancies, and to have babies with congenital abnormalities and low birthweight, which in turn is associated with higher rates of fetal and infant mortality. Women who delay their first pregnancy may differ from younger women of equivalent education and socioeconomic status in a variety of health-related ways; for example, they are more likely to have planned their pregnancy and therefore may be more motivated to make dietary changes during pregnancy.

3.2.1.1 Teenage pregnancy

The World Health Organization (WHO) and the United Nations (UN) define adolescence as the period between 10 and 19 years of age (World Health Organization, 2013; United Nations Children's Fund, 2011). Although the general trend over the past 20 years in Europe is that of declining adolescent pregnancy, and teenagers account for a relatively small proportion of pregnancies in most European countries (EURO-PERISTAT 2008), they are associated with increased risk of obstetric complications such as pre-eclampsia, pre-term delivery, low-birthweight babies and neonatal death (Bloom and Escuro 2008). The number of teenage pregnancies in the UK has been reported to be relatively high compared with other European countries (United Nations Children's Fund (UNICEF) 2001). Nevertheless, rates have fallen slightly in recent years (ONS 2011).

Adolescence is a period of rapid physical growth, with increased nutritional needs to support growth and development. The extra energy and nutrient demands of pregnancy place adolescents at nutritional risk. In general, the closer a girl is to menarche when she becomes pregnant, the greater her need is for energy and nutrients above the normal requirements for pregnancy (Story and Alton 1995; Buschman *et al.* 2001).

The diets of teenage girls tend to differ from those of older women; for example, young women in the UK tend to eat less fruit and vegetables than older women (2.8 portions per day in 11- to 18-year-olds compared with 4.1 portions per day among adults 19–64 years) and milk consumption is less common 73% of 11- to 18-year-olds consumed semi-skimmed milk (the most commonly consumed type) compared to 83% of women aged 19–64 years during the 4-day recording period) and milk consumption has fallen among teenage girls over the past decade (Gregory

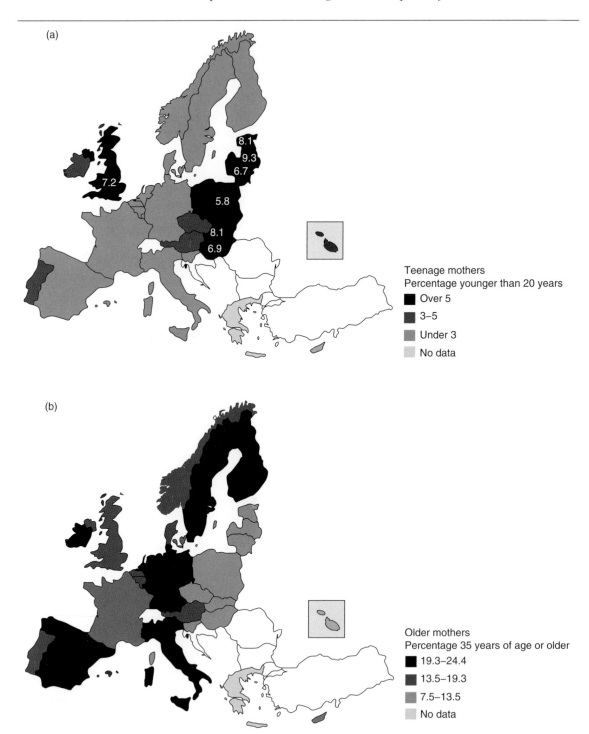

Figure 3.3 Proportion of mothers giving birth in 2004 who were (a) teenagers or (b) aged over 35 years. Source: EURO-PERISTAT (2008). Reproduced with permission from http://www.europeristat.com/images/doc/ EPHR/european-perinatal-health-report.pdf

et al. 2000; Bates *et al.* 2012). Milk is an important source of calcium and various other micronutrients. Studies suggest that intake of several nutrients recognised to be vital for fetal growth and development may be low in the diets of pregnant adolescents in industrialised countries including the US and UK. For example, a systematic review of nine studies (seven conducted in the US) found average intakes of energy, iron, folate, calcium, vitamin E and magnesium of pregnant adolescents to be below US dietary reference intakes (DRIs) (Moran 2007a), although the authors commented on the poor quality of the studies included. Another systematic review by the same author's of six papers (also mostly US studies), found evidence of anaemia and poor iron status in pregnant adolescents, particularly in the third trimester (Moran 2007b). This raises concern as iron deficiency anaemia has been associated with reduced fetal oxygenation and poor birth outcomes, such as greater risk of low birthweight, prematurity and an increased perinatal mortality rate (see Chapter 15, Section 15.3.3.5). A prospective study by Baker *et al.* (2009) drew attention to the extent of the problem in the UK. This study of 500 pregnant adolescents from two UK inner city populations, which assessed dietary intake with three 24-hour dietary recalls and micronutrient status by measurements of third trimester blood biomarkers, demonstrated a clear relationship between maternal folate and iron status and the incidence of small-for-gestational-age (SGA) birth and pre-term delivery. They also reported a high incidence of poor vitamin D status in pregnant adolescents, who derived only a small proportion of their vitamin D requirements from dietary sources. Of additional concern was the lack of a correlation between serum 25(OH)D concentration and ambient solar radiation in adolescents with melanised skin (mainly of African or African-Caribbean origin), implying that women with melanised skin may have a lower capacity to synthesise vitamin D by the action of sunlight on the skin, or that they were less exposed to sunlight because of clothing or lifestyle. Poor maternal vitamin D status may result in impaired maternal–fetal transfer of 25(OH)D and consequently reduced bone mineral content during infancy and childhood (Javaid *et al.* 2006) (see Chapter 12 and Chapter 15, Section 15.2.5). Such research highlights the urgent need to address poor nutritional status of adolescents during pregnancy and to understand better their specific nutrient needs (see Chapter 15, Section 15.5.2).

The trajectory of growth and development depends more upon underlying biological maturation than upon chronological age. The biological immaturity of an adolescent mother will therefore have a greater influence on the outcome of her pregnancy than age alone. At age 17 years, approximately half of teenage women will have reached mature stature, with the remainder still growing (Scholl 1998). Compared with non-growing teenagers and with mature women, pregnant teenagers who are still growing themselves give birth to infants weighing 150–200 g less. This occurs despite the fact that growing teenagers gain more weight during pregnancy and that greater gestational weight gain is associated with increased fetal growth and thus larger size at birth. This may be due to the fact that pregnant adolescents who are still growing themselves continue to gain fat during the third trimester when fat stores should be mobilised to support fetal growth. As a result, infant birthweight is substantially diminished. However, this finding was not confirmed in the study by Baker *et al.* (2009), a large UK study of teenage pregnancy in socioeconomically deprived groups, in which most of the mothers were 16–17 years of age. The competition between the mother and the fetus for growth may be more evident in pregnancies in younger girls aged 12–14 years when growth is rapid. Cigarette smoking during teenage pregnancy had a clear effect on birthweight (Baker *et al.* 2009), which was assessed by blood cotinine measurement, an indicator of smoking habit. Both smoking habit and maternal frame size are important determinants of birthweight. There is also some evidence to suggest that poor health outcomes of teenage pregnancy for both mother and child are more attributable to socio-demographic factors associated with pregnancy among teenagers than the woman's age per se (Smith and Pell 2001). The most consistent factors related to teenage pregnancy include socioeconomic disadvantage, disrupted family structure and limited education (Imamura *et al.* 2007).

3.2.2 Birth spacing

There is little evidence that birth interval has a large impact on maternal, perinatal and infant outcome but, in situations where food availability is limited, short birth interval could adversely affect the nutritional status of both mother and child by allowing the mother insufficient time to recover from the nutritional burden of pregnancy. After a live birth, the recommended interval before attempting the next pregnancy is at least 24 months (World Health Organization, 2005). Dewey and Cohen, in a systematic review of 34 papers, were unable to demonstrate a clear association between short birth interval and maternal anthropometric and micronutrient status but suggested that there may be an increased risk of maternal anaemia when inter-pregnancy interval is short (Dewey and Cohen 2007). However, the authors of this review claim that encouraging a longer interval between pregnancies is not likely to be an effective means to prevent adverse outcomes. Rather, nutrition support for women before, during and after pregnancy may be a more promising approach. As most of the research investigating birth interval and maternal or child nutrition has been carried out in non-industrialised countries, findings cannot be generalised more widely to industrialised countries such as the UK.

3.2.3 Ethnic minority groups

According to the census in 2001, 7.9% of the UK's population comprised non-White minority ethnic groups (4.6 million people), the largest of which were South Asians, Black African-Caribbeans and Chinese people (ONS 2005). Although the White population is 'stable', the proportion of the population of Great Britain from minority ethnic groups has been increasing over the past few decades. Data collected in 2004 showed the proportion of births to women of foreign origin, defined by country of birth, to be 21.2% in England and Wales, 7.8% in Scotland and 8.3% in Northern Ireland (EURO-PERISTAT 2008). The minority ethnic groups in the UK have a younger age profile relative to the White population. In the 2001 Census, the average age of women from minority ethnic groups was 28.8 years compared with 40.9 years for White females (ONS 2005), and the age profile varied between minority ethnic groups. The Pakistani and Bangladeshi ethnic groups are relatively youthful (mean age of women: 25.5 and 23.2 years, respectively), whereas the age profile of Indian and Black-Caribbean populations in the UK is more similar to the White population (mean age of women: 32.4 and 35.8 years, respectively), reflecting an ageing population. The Black-African population includes a large number of children, indicating that the initial migrant generation (over three-fifths of Black-Africans have come to the UK since 1990) is currently

experiencing high fertility rates (Owen 2006). The most rapidly growing population in the UK is people of mixed parentage. The risk of low birthweight is higher in South Asian pregnancies in the UK compared to White Europeans (SACN 2011a). In the UK, women of Indian ethnic origin who are Hindu (and predominantly vegetarian) have been found to have smaller babies than Muslim women of South Asian origin (McFadyen *et al.* 1984; Reddy *et al.* 1994).

3.3 Current practice and recommendations: pre-pregnancy

3.3.1 The importance of pre-pregnancy nutrient status and weight

The nutritional status of a woman before pregnancy is critical to both her baby's and her own health. It determines her well-being and that of the fetus and child, and in turn the health and reproductive capacity of the next generation's mothers (Fall 2005). It is vital that a woman has adequate nutrient stores to meet the demands of the growing baby.

Evidence suggests that underweight women have an increased risk of pre-term delivery. The reason for this increased risk is unclear but it may be due to vaginal inflammation or deficiency of certain micronutrients. For example, poor maternal folate and zinc intake and status have been associated with increased risk of pre-term delivery in many (although not all) observational studies (see Hauger *et al.* 2008 which refers to these studies) (Mahomed *et al.* 2007; Bodnar *et al.* 2010; Dunlop *et al.* 2011). There is some evidence that the second trimester may be a particularly sensitive period with regard to the effects of poor maternal weight gain on length of gestation (Sekiya *et al.* 2007).

Maternal obesity, usually defined as a body mass index (BMI) of 30 Kg/m^2 or more at the first antenatal consultation, is becoming more common (see Chapter 15, Section 15.2.1.1). For example, in 2010 in England, obesity affected an estimated 26% of adults and 19.5% of women of childbearing age (NHS Information Centre 2011). A major national study, collecting information from every maternity unit in the UK on births during March and April 2009 (≥24 weeks' gestation), estimated around 5% of the UK maternity population to be severely obese (BMI ≥ 35) (Centre for Maternal and Child Enquiries (CMACE) & Royal College of Obstetricians and Gynaecologists (RCOG)

2010b). In real terms, this equates to around 38 478 (1 in 20) pregnant women each year. Of these, 22 986 would have a BMI between 35 and 39.9 (1 in 33 pregnancies), 14 022 would have a BMI between 40 and 49.9 (1 in 55 pregnancies) and 1470 would have a BMI of ≥ 50 (1 in 524 pregnancies) (CMACE & RCOG 2010b). With growing levels of obesity in the general population, this number is expected to increase. Obesity in pregnancy is associated with an increased risk of many serious adverse outcomes, including miscarriage, fetal congenital anomaly, thromboembolism, gestational diabetes, pre-eclampsia, abnormal labour, postpartum haemorrhage, wound infections, stillbirth and neonatal death. There is a higher caesarean section rate and lower breastfeeding rate in this group of women compared with women with a healthy BMI (CMACE & RCOG 2010a). The increase in maternal obesity is resulting in an increase in macrosomia (infants with a birthweight > 4 kg) which is believed to be driven by maternal hyperglycaemia (Metzger *et al.* 2008).

3.3.2 Recommendations for pre-pregnancy

An increased intake of folic acid is recommended in early pregnancy to prevent neural tube defects (NTDs) in many countries and some have mandated folic acid fortification of flour in order to achieve this goal (see Chapter 15, Table 15.4). For example, in the US, the fortification of enriched cereal grain products with folic acid became mandatory in 1998 at a level of 140 μg/100 g and the addition of folic acid to breakfast cereals limited to 100 μg folic acid per serving (Food and Drug Administration 1996).

Countries that have mandated folic acid fortification have better folate status, as indicated by substantially higher serum folate concentrations, and NTD incidence rates have fallen. Voluntary fortification is permitted in most countries (exceptions being Sweden where it is not practised and Denmark and Norway where approval is required). In countries such as the UK, where there is voluntary folic acid fortification and the recommendation that women planning a pregnancy take 400 μg of folic acid in addition to the folate provided by diet (see Chapter 15, Section 15.3.3.2), serum folate concentrations have increased markedly over the past decade. People living in countries which have prohibited folic acid fortification, or require approval, such as Scandinavia, have markedly lower serum folate concentrations.

The risks and benefits of folic acid fortification were considered by the EU-BRAFO (Benefit-Risk Analysis of Foods) project (Verhagen *et al.* 2012). This made an estimate of the established benefits in terms of prevention of NTD and megaloblastic anaemia versus the potential risks of masking vitamin B_{12} deficiency and promoting colorectal cancer. This benefit:risk analysis supports fortification of food with folic acid up to 70 μg/100 g.

Details associated with the advice on folic acid supplementation prior to and during pregnancy, such as timing and duration, differ between European countries. The most common recommendation is to take a supplement before pregnancy until the 12th week. If folic acid is taken in a supplement that contains other vitamins, women should check that it provides 400 μg of folic acid and does not contain vitamin A or fish liver oils because excess vitamin A during pregnancy can be teratogenic (see below) (see Chapter 4, Section 4.4.1). Some groups, for example, women with coeliac disease, diabetes, obesity or women taking anti-epileptic medicines, may need a higher dose of folic acid. Those who have already had a NTD-affected pregnancy, for example, are advised in the UK to take 5 mg folic acid per day (SACN 2011a). Foods containing folate (the natural form of folic acid) such as green leafy vegetables, fruit and brown rice, should continue to be eaten, as well as folic acid fortified bread and breakfast cereals (Department of Health 2009a) (see Chapter 15, Section 15.3.3.2). Ensuring that obese pregnant women adhere to this advice may be particularly important as there is evidence of a positive association between maternal obesity and risk of NTDs (Rasmussen *et al.* 2008), as well as evidence of lower serum folate levels in obese compared to non-obese women after controlling for several factors including folate intake from food and supplementation (Mojtabai 2004). The Department of Health does not currently make any specific recommendations on folic acid supplementation for obese women wishing to become pregnant. However, the CMACE and RCOG have advised a higher intake of 5 mg folic acid per day from supplements for those with a BMI of 30 or more at first antenatal appointment (CMACE & RCOG 2010a).

Advice on periconceptional folic acid is provided alongside other dietary and lifestyle advice in the Department of Health's *The Pregnancy Book*, which provides a wealth of advice for mothers-to-be

Table 3.1   Knowledge and taking of folic acid supplements to prevent neural tube defects in the East of Ireland 1996–2002

	1996	1997	1998	1999	2000	2001	2002	
Heard of FA*	54%	76%	88%	92%	92%	94%	95%	*p* < 0.001
Knew FA can prevent NTD	21%	44%	53%	65%	67%	83%	77%	*p* < 0.001
Advised to take FA before pregnancy	13%	21%	32%	29%	30%	66%	62%	*p* < 0.001
Took FA periconceptionally	6%	16%	21%	22%	18%	24%	23%	*p* < 0.001
Took FA during pregnancy	14%	51%	68%	68%	74%	83%	83%	*p* < 0.001

*FA, folic acid.
Source: Reproduced with permission from Ward *et al.* (2004).

(Department of Health 2009a). Using *the eatwell plate* as a guide, women who are trying to become pregnant are advised to eat a variety of different foods every day in order to get the right balance of nutrients and to maintain a body weight within the healthy BMI range. Emphasis is also placed on building up iron stores before conception because poor iron status in pregnancy is common even in developed countries such as the UK (see Chapter 15, Section 15.3.3.5). Other points of advice include: the need to avoid consumption of liver, which has a high retinol (vitamin A) content, and dietary supplements containing retinol esters, especially retinyl acetate, because of the increased risk of cleft palate in the first few months of pregnancy; and avoiding consumption of long-lived fish such as shark, albacore tuna, marlin and swordfish because of the likelihood of high mercury content (Department of Health 2009a). Women should avoid consuming soft cheeses such as Camembert during pregnancy because of the risk of listeriosis. These recommendations are summarised in Table 3.4. Women who are trying to conceive are advised to stop drinking alcohol altogether. If alcohol is consumed, it should be limited to no more than one or two units of alcohol, once or twice a week, and binge drinking (more than six units a day) should be avoided (Department of Health 2009a). Women are also advised to avoid high intakes of caffeine (i.e. not to consume > 200 mg caffeine per day, which equates to two mugs of instant coffee).

3.3.3 Current dietary practices among women prior to pregnancy

National surveys, such as the National Diet and Nutrition Survey in the UK, are the main source of information about the diets of women of childbearing age. In addition, information is available from studies examining compliance with specific dietary recommendations prior to pregnancy, which have typically focused on folic acid supplement use and alcohol consumption. For example, a study from the East of Ireland suggested an increased knowledge and uptake of the message to take folic acid supplements between 1996 and 2002 (Ward *et al.* 2004) (Table 3.1) but the number of women taking folic acid supplements pre-conception remained low (<25%). In a more recent study of 296 women in Northern Ireland, 84% reported taking folic acid supplements in the first trimester, but only 19% had started before conception (McNulty *et al.* 2011). In the Southampton Women's Survey, 44% of pregnant women had taken supplements in the 3 months prior to their pregnancy but only 6% had taken the recommended daily dose of 400 μg or more (Inskip *et al.* 2009). Use during pregnancy was higher (93% at 11 weeks' gestation).

Similar findings have been reported elsewhere in the UK (e.g. Barbour *et al.* 2011; Lane 2011; McNulty *et al.* 2011). For example, in a survey of 211 mothers in Fife in Scotland, 31% indicated that they had taken supplements as recommended, 56% had taken them only during pregnancy, with 12% not taken them at all (Barbour *et al.* 2011). Morning sickness, competing priorities for concern, busy lives and poor memory were identified as the main barriers to uptake (Barbour *et al.* 2011). In most cases, health professionals did not emphasise the need to take them, and most women not taking supplements were not aware of the potential health consequences of not doing so.

Uptake has been shown to be poor in 'at risk' groups. For example, among 500 pregnant teenagers (aged 14–18 years) taking part in the About Teenage Eating

(ATE) study in London and Manchester, only 7% had taken pre-conceptional folic acid, although 44% consumed folic acid supplements in early pregnancy (<20 weeks' gestation) (Baker *et al.* 2009). In an audit of 905 obese women in the UK, only 29% reported taking supplements prior to their pregnancy and just 1.4% supplemented with 5 mg per day, the amount recommended by the CMACE and RCOG (2010b).

Studies in other countries indicate that less than half of women take folic acid supplements prior to pregnancy, with some studies showing less than 10% (Coll *et al.* 2004; Nawapun and Phupong 2007; Inskip *et al.* 2009). In Denmark, for example, where advice for women to take 400 μg folic acid per day was instituted in 1997, only 17% of the 22 000 women recruited from 2000 to 2002 had taken a supplement greater than 320 μg/day. This number increased to over 30% by week 5 of pregnancy, but demonstrates low compliance with the national recommendation (Knudsen *et al.* 2004). This study also demonstrated that advice about folic acid supplements really only affects those planning pregnancy, with little effect on women not planning to get pregnant (this is of relevance due to the high percentage of unplanned pregnancies across the world).

National surveys in countries with and without folic acid fortification suggest that the majority of women of childbearing age do not obtain 400 μg folic acid per day from food and supplements. For example, in an examination of 2617 non-pregnant women of childbearing age (15–44 years) from the 2003–4 and 2005–6 NHANES (National Health and Nutrition Examination Survey) in the US, 24% consumed the recommended intake of 400 μg/day (95% CI: 20–27%) (Tinker *et al.* 2010). The proportion achieving this intake was highest among non-Hispanic White women (30%), followed by Mexican-American (17%) and non-Hispanic Black women (9%). Among the folic acid supplement users, 72% achieved 400 μg/day. Of those not using supplements (68%), consumption of cereals fortified with folic acid was a strong determinant of whether they achieved a 400 μg/day intake.

3.4 Current practice and recommendations: during pregnancy

3.4.1 Recommendations for pregnancy

UK government advice to pregnant women, in common with most countries, is to eat a healthy and varied diet, to limit intake of foods high in fat or sugars, and to avoid excessive weight gain (although monitoring of weight during pregnancy is not currently recommended in the UK), particularly because of its association with raised blood pressure and gestational diabetes.

3.4.1.1 Recommendations on weight gain

Most women gain between 10 and 12.5 kg while pregnant. Weight gain varies widely and depends on pre-pregnancy weight. Only some of the weight gained is body fat (about 4 kg); the remainder consists of the fetus, placenta, amniotic fluid and increases in maternal blood and fluid volume (National Institute for Health and Clinical Excellence (NICE) 2010). Women weighing more than 100 kg or less than 50 kg may require specific advice about weight gain in pregnancy. It is also important for pregnant women to remain active through normal daily activity and exercise. In the UK, at present, there are no formal, evidence-based guidelines from the government or professional bodies on what constitutes appropriate weight gain during pregnancy (NICE 2010). UK recommendations on energy intake, including energy intake during pregnancy, have recently been revised (SACN 2011b), as discussed in Chapter 15, Section 15.2.1. Pregnant women are advised not to restrict energy intake and to contact their GP or midwife if they are concerned about their weight (Department of Health 2009a) (see Chapter 15, Section 15.3.1).

The US Institute of Medicine guidelines state that healthy American women who are of normal weight for their height (BMI 18.5 to 24.9) should gain 11.5–16 kg (25–35 lb) during pregnancy. Overweight women (BMI 25.9 to 29.9) should gain 7–11.5 kg (15–25 lb) and obese women (BMI ≥ 30.0) should gain only 5–9 kg (11–20 lb) (Institute of Medicine 2009) (see Table 3.2).

3.4.1.2 Recommendations: energy intake during pregnancy

The energy requirements of pregnant women are influenced by many factors, including physical activity. The FAO/WHO/UNU (Food and Agriculture Organization of the United Nations *et al.* 2004) recommend a 1.5 MJ/day increment in the second trimester, increasing to 2 MJ/day in the third trimester. In the UK, SACN has recently supported the

Table 3.2 US recommendations for total and rate of weight gain during pregnancy, by pre-pregnancy BMI

Pre-pregnancy weight	BMI (kg/m^2)	Recommended mean[a] rates of weight gain in 2nd and 3rd trimester (average range/week)		Recommended range of total weight gain[b]	
		kg/week	lb/week	kg	lb
Underweight	<18.5	0.5–0.6	1.0–1.3	12.5–18.0	28–40
Normal weight	18.5–24.9	0.4–0.5	0.8–1.0	11.5–16.0	25–35
Overweight	25.0–29.9	0.2–0.3	0.5–0.7	7.0–11.5	15–25
Obese[c]	≥30	0.2–0.3	0.4–0.6	5.0–9.0	11–20

Source: based on data from Institute of Medicine (2009) *Weight Gain During Pregnancy: Reexamining the Guidelines.* Washington, DC, National Academies Press.
[a]Rounded values.
[b]Calculations assume 0.5–2.0 kg (1.1–4.4 lb) total weight gain in the first trimester.
[c]A narrower range of weight gain may be advised for women with a BMI > 35. It is recommended these women seek individual advice.

previous UK recommendation of 0.8 MJ/day (191 kcal/day) during the third trimester only (SACN 2011b). Additionally, the Committee advised that women entering pregnancy who are overweight may not require this increment (see Chapter 15, Section 15.2.1.1). The same is true for women who become more sedentary when they are pregnant.

3.4.1.3 Recommendations: fatty acids during pregnancy

Oil-rich fish are the main dietary source of the long-chain *n*-3 (or omega 3) polyunsaturates, eicosapentaenoic acid (EPA) and docosahexaenoic (DHA). In recent years, there has been growing interest in the role of DHA in infant and child development. While considerable discussion has been undertaken to determine whether DHA should be added to infant formulas, it is only recently that the achievement of sufficient levels in breast milk has been addressed. The European Commission requested a review of this topic and two EU-funded research projects were initiated to undertake this task: PeriLip (Perinatal Lipid Nutrition) (which considered the influence of dietary fatty acids on the pathophysiology of intrauterine fetal growth and neonatal development) (www.early-nutrition.org/perilip/PeriLipPublications.html) and EARNEST (which focused on early nutrition programming) (www.project-earlynutrition.eu), and their conclusions and recommendations were reported in 2007. No evidence was identified to indicate a need for women to change the fat composition of their diets, in relation to saturates, monounsaturates or polyunsaturates composition, except for the intake of long-chain *n*-3 polyunsaturates. It was recommended that the intake of DHA in both pregnant and lactating women should be at least 200 mg/day. This would be achieved through consumption of one to two portions of oil-rich fish per week, such as herring, mackerel and salmon. Eggs can also make a significant contribution to intake of DHA. It was determined that this intake level of fish would rarely exceed the tolerable levels of environmental contaminants, such as methylmercury (Koletzko *et al.* 2007; Koletzko *et al.* 2008). The position of the American Dietetic Association and Dietitians of Canada is that adults, including pregnant and lactating women, should consume a combined intake of 500 mg/day of DHA and EPA (Kris-Etherton *et al.* 2007). In the UK, 450 mg/day of DHA and EPA combined is recommended for adults and pregnant women (SACN 2004); this equates to the consumption of two servings of fish a week, one of which is oil-rich. The European Food Safety Authority (EFSA) advice for the adult population is to have one to two portions of oil-rich fish per week or about 250 mg of EPA plus DHA per day (based mainly on evidence concerning CVD risk). EFSA recommends that 100–200 mg of preformed DHA should be added to this intake during pregnancy and lactation to compensate for oxidative losses of maternal dietary DHA and accumulation of DHA in body fat of the fetus/infant. The EFSA Panel also proposed an adequate intake of 100 mg/day of DHA for older infants (>6 months) and young children below the age of 24 months (European Food Safety Authority (EFSA) 2010). There are no specific recommendations for children above this age (FAO/WHO 2011). The Dietary Guidelines for Americans did not accept the need for preformed DHA in the diet. Currently, there is no consensus agreement on the need for pregnant women to include preformed sources of DHA in their diet, and levels advised for breast milk substitutes are based on the levels normally present in human breast milk.

3.4.1.4 Recommendations: vitamins and minerals during pregnancy

Daily vitamin D supplements containing 10 µg/day (400 IU/day) are advised for pregnant and lactating women in the UK (Department of Health 1991; SACN 2007). Supplements are also recommended elsewhere: the FAO/WHO and Australia/New Zealand suggest 5 µg/day (200 IU/day) (www.moh. govt.nz/moh.nsf/pagesmh/4678), as recommended for adult non-pregnant women aged 19–50 years. Recommendations in the US/Canada are 15 µg/day (600 IU/day), assuming minimal exposure to sunlight. Recommendations for women in Europe vary between 5 µg/day (Germany, Austria and Switzerland) and 10 µg/day (see Chapter 15, Table 15.2). The EC-funded EURRECA project has recently suggested 10 µg/day during pregnancy in Europe with an upper safe intake level of 50 µg/day (2000 IU/day) (www.serbianfood.info/eurreca).

Pregnant women may develop low iron status, so plenty of iron-rich foods should be eaten and foods containing non-haem iron should be consumed alongside foods or drinks containing vitamin C, such as fruit or vegetables, or a glass of fruit juice, to aid iron absorption. The effect of tea and coffee on iron bioavailability is no longer considered to be of major concern (SACN 2010), especially if advice on caffeine is followed (see Section 3.3.2).

Policy on iron varies around the world. In the UK, the view is that physiological adaptations during pregnancy and lactation ensure an adequate supply of iron to the fetus and developing infant, even in the presence of iron deficiency, and so an increment in iron intake is not considered necessary (Department of Health 1991). A similar position has been adopted by the recent review by the EURRECA project (www.serbianfood.info/eurreca), unlike the US, for

example (see Chapter 15, Section 15.3.3.5). However, severe iron deficiency can affect reproductive efficiency. A recent review by SACN concluded that there were not enough data to determine whether iron supplementation has any beneficial or harmful effects on low birthweight or pre-term delivery (SACN 2010). Therefore, as recommended by the National Institute for Health and Clinical Excellence (NICE) (2008), the position in the UK is that iron supplementation is not offered routinely to all pregnant women but should be considered for women identified with haemoglobin concentrations below 110 g/L in the first trimester and 105 g/L at 28 weeks (SACN 2010). In other countries, supplementation of women during pregnancy is more common than in the UK. In the US and Canada, the majority of pregnant women do not reach the recommended daily allowance of 27 mg/day (almost twice the UK recommendation, see Table 3.3) throughout pregnancy and are therefore advised to take supplements. Calculations based on Canadian intake data from pregnant women suggest that a supplement of 16 mg/day would bring women closer to the recommended daily amount (RDA) without risking reaching the upper limit of 45 mg/day (Cockell *et al.* 2009). Similarly, estimates have been made in a number of European countries about the level of supplementation which might be beneficial to achieve dietary intake recommendations but, to date, there is little evidence of systematic supplementation of pregnant women with iron in Europe, with most countries making recommendations for specific cases when anaemia is diagnosed, at which time doses of 30–50 mg/day are advised (Hess *et al.* 2001; Massot and Vanderplas 2003; Arkkola *et al.* 2006).

Calcium is also especially important because it is vital for the baby's bone and teeth formation. Foods containing calcium should be included in the diet (dairy products, fish such as sardines with edible bones, fortified breakfast cereals, dried fruit, bread, almonds, tofu and green leafy vegetables). Women on 'special' or restricted diets may require a low dose multivitamin or mineral supplement and may need advice from a dietitian (e.g. those on a restricted diet because of a food intolerance, such as coeliac disease, or for religious reasons). Calcium recommendations in the US, Australia and New Zealand during pregnancy are 1300 mg/day for those aged 14–18 years and 1000 mg/day for older women (http:// iom.edu/Reports/2010/Dietary-Reference-Intakes-

Table 3.3 Recommended intakes of protein and micronutrients during pregnancy and lactation in the UK

Nutrient per day	Women (RNI) (19–50 years)	Pregnancy	Lactation (0–4 months)	(4+ months)
Protein (g/day)	45	+ 6	+ 11	+ 8
Thiamin (mg/day)	0.8	+ 0.1*	+ 0.2	+ 0.2
Riboflavin (mg/day)	1.1	+ 0.3	+ 0.5	+ 0.5
Niacin (mg/day) (nicotinic acid equivalents)	13	–	+ 2.0	+ 2.0
Vitamin B_6 (mg/day)	1.2	–	–	–
Vitamin B_{12} (µg/day)	1.5	–	+ 0.5	+ 0.5
Folate (µg/day)	200	+ 100	+ 60	+ 60
Vitamin C (mg/day)	40	+ 10*	+ 30	+ 30
Vitamin A (µg/day)	600	+ 100	+ 350	+ 350
Vitamin D (µg/day)	**	10	10	10
Calcium (mg/day)	700	–	+ 550	+ 550
Phosphorus (mg/day)	550	–	+ 440	+ 440
Magnesium (mg/day)	270	–	+ 50	+ 50
Sodium (mg/day)	1,600	–	–	–
Potassium (mg/day)	3,500	–	–	–
Chloride (mg/day)	2,500	–	–	–
Iron (mg/day)	14.8***	–	–	–
Zinc (mg/day)	7.0	–	+ 0.3	+ 0.3
Selenium (µg/day)	60	–	+ 15	+ 15
Iodine (µg/day)	140	–	–	–

*For last trimester only.
**After age 65 the Reference Nutrient Intake (RNI) is 10 µg/day for men and women.
***Insufficient for women with high menstrual losses where the most practical way of meeting iron requirements is to take iron supplements.
– No increment.
Source: Department of Health (1991).

for-Calcium-and-Vitamin-D.aspx; www.moh.govt. nz/moh.nsf/pagesmh/4678). Recommendations for calcium intake among adult women vary widely across Europe. An intake of 700 mg/day during pregnancy was set in the European Community in 1993 (www.serbianfood.info/eurreca), and this is currently also the reference nutrient intake for women aged 19 and over in the UK (no additional amount is recommended for pregnancy) (Department of Health 1991).

3.4.1.5 Recommendations for mothers who are vegetarian and vegan

A varied and balanced vegetarian diet should generally supply sufficient nutrients during pregnancy. However, vegetarian diets that contain only small amounts of dairy products and eggs and vegan diets are likely to be lacking in vitamin B_{12} and may be low in calcium, riboflavin, iron and vitamin D, for example. In particular, women who do not consume milk or eggs or consume only small amounts of milk and eggs should be advised to take a vitamin B_{12} supplement or use foods that are fortified with vitamin B_{12}, as well as the other supplements referred to above (folic acid and vitamin D) (Department of Health 2009a).

3.4.1.6 Foods to avoid during pregnancy

In the UK, the Department of Health advises avoidance of certain foods during pregnancy, as shown in Table 3.4.

In addition, the Department of Health advises that caffeine intake should be limited to no more than 200 mg of caffeine per day (equivalent to two mugs of coffee daily) and that ideally pregnant women

Table 3.4 Foods to avoid during pregnancy

Foods to avoid	Reason
Some types of cheese: mould-ripened cheeses such as Camembert and Brie; some goats cheeses especially unpasteurised soft blue cheeses	To minimise risk of listeriosis
Pâté: all types of pâté, including vegetable	To minimise risk of listeriosis
Raw or partially cooked eggs; raw or undercooked meat; undercooked ready meals; raw shellfish	To minimise risk of food poisoning
Liver products and supplements containing vitamin A or fish liver oils	To avoid excess vitamin A intake
Some types of fish: shark, swordfish and marlin. Intake of tuna should be limited, no more than two tuna steaks a week or four medium-size cans of tuna a week	To avoid high intakes of mercury and other contaminants
Unpasteurised milk	To minimise risk of infection

should not drink alcohol. If alcohol is consumed, it should be limited to one or two units, once or twice a week (Department of Health 2009a). Additional advice from NICE is that alcohol should be avoided in the first 3 months in particular because of the increased risk of miscarriage (http://guidance. nice.org.uk/CG62/Guidance/pdf/English). However, drinking alcohol can affect the baby throughout pregnancy. Alcohol passes to the baby via the placenta. The liver is one of the last organs to develop fully and does not mature until the latter half of pregnancy, and so a baby is less able to process alcohol than its mother. A particular group of problems associated with high consumption of alcohol is known as fetal alcohol syndrome (FAS) (see Chapter 15, Section 15.3.4).

Current advice in the UK is that mothers who would like to eat peanuts or foods containing peanuts during pregnancy or breastfeeding can now choose to do so as part of a healthy, balanced diet, irrespective of whether there is a family history of allergies (see Chapter 13, Section 13.6.4 and Chapter 15, Section 15.2.6).

3.4.2 Current practice during pregnancy

Most national surveys conducted around the world do not include pregnant women, mainly because of sampling difficulties and the likelihood of insufficient numbers to enable valid comparisons with non-pregnant women. The literature on dietary intake during pregnancy is therefore limited and generally restricted to relatively small numbers of subjects and in specific locations. A number of older studies in the

1980s examined energy requirements in some detail, such as those conducted in Glasgow by Durnin and by Van Raaij and colleagues in the Netherlands (van Raaij *et al.* 1987; Durnin 1991). These provided a solid base of information about dietary energy intake during pregnancy, which have been substantiated in more recent work. Although calculations of the energy requirements for the growth of the fetus suggest that a total increase in energy intake of 70 000 kcal (293 MJ) is required throughout pregnancy (equivalent to some 250–300 kcal/day (1.05–1.26 MJ/day)), assessments of intake indicate that this is never achieved through food intake. Studies have failed to show an increase in energy intake until the last trimester of pregnancy, when intake tends to increase only by some 100 kcal (0.42 MJ) per day (Department of Health 1991). The difference between the calculated and experimental findings was suggested by Durnin and others to be accounted for by reductions in physical activity during pregnancy (Durnin 1991). More recent work has questioned this conclusion, suggesting that reductions in physical activity do not compensate for increases in basal metabolic rate and energy deposition and, based on more detailed experiments of energy expenditure during pregnancy, suggests that greater intakes are required, and although negligible in the first trimester, an additional 350 kcal/day (1.47 MJ/day) is required in the second trimester and an additional 500 kcal/day (2.1 MJ/day) in the third trimester. There therefore remains debate about the optimum energy intake in pregnancy and hence it is difficult to assess how well women are meeting recommendations in terms of total intake. See Chapter 15, Section

15.3.1 for information about the recently revised energy recommendations for the UK.

Micronutrient recommendations are somewhat clearer, although there is variability between countries in their recommendations (see Chapter 15, Table 15.2), and more emphasis has been placed in recent years on the micronutrients for which achievement of appropriate intakes is known to be challenging and where particular increases in pregnancy are recommended, such as folate, and in some countries vitamin D and iron. These nutrients have been the focus of much of the recent research on the diets and supplement intakes of pregnant women. Some of the studies described above (see Section 3.3.3) in terms of pre-pregnancy behaviours have also examined supplement taking and sometimes diet during pregnancy state as well. For example, Baker *et al.*, in the ATE study of teenagers in London and Manchester, assessed the use of folic acid, iron and multivitamin supplements in early and late pregnancy as well as before conception. While 44% took a folic acid supplement in early pregnancy, only 8% took an iron supplement. In the third trimester, while only 2% took a folic acid supplement, 14.5% took an iron supplement and 4.5% took an iron and folic acid supplement (Baker *et al.* 2009). These results corresponded to blood levels of these key nutrients, with anaemia being particularly common, especially in the third trimester, when 63.5% were assessed as anaemic, compared to 12% in early pregnancy. One-third of the teenagers had low 25-OH vitamin D (<25 nmol/L), with differences by ethnic group: 19% of White and mixed White-Caribbean adolescents had low vitamin D, compared to 49% of Black adolescents (Baker *et al.* 2009). This study found a very low use of vitamin D supplements and there was low awareness among health professionals of the Department of Health's recommendation to take vitamin D supplements.

In the 2010 Infant Feeding Survey (McAndrew *et al.* 2012), 71% of mothers knew why increasing the intake of folic acid in the early stages of pregnancy was recommended, down from 79% in the 2005 survey (Bolling *et al.* 2007). Mothers over 35 years were more aware than younger mothers. 94% said they took folic acid supplements before or during pregnancy. However, smaller surveys in different groups around the UK have suggested lower uptake (see Section 3.3.3).

In a study of pregnant women at three time points in Finland, particular attention was paid to vitamin D intakes because of the introduction of fortification of fluid milks and fat spreads in 2003. Vitamin D intakes increased following fortification but remained below optimal levels (Prasad *et al.* 2010). Finland has no specific advice on folic acid supplementation during pregnancy and relies on advice to increase consumption of folate-rich foods. This study showed mean intakes of folate to be below recommendations throughout the year (Prasad *et al.* 2010).

Also of current interest are those factors that influence the quality of the overall diet of pregnant women. A recent study from the US of diet quality, assessed using a diet quality index based on a series of food and nutrient characteristics, indicated (in 1777 women) that older pregnant women were more likely to have a better-quality diet. Those with higher BMI, with less education and with more children were more likely to have poorer diets during pregnancy (Rifas-Shiman *et al.* 2009). No difference was found between White women and those of African-American background.

In the Southampton Women's Study, a number of behaviours, such as smoking, alcohol use and eating fruits and vegetables, were assessed through pregnancy and compared to pre-pregnancy rates. While changes were seen as a result of pregnancy for alcohol use and smoking, no change was seen in fruit and vegetable consumption through pregnancy. Those with the lowest education had the lowest fruit and vegetable consumption throughout (Inskip *et al.* 2009).

In a study of diet and deprivation, in 1461 pregnant women assessed at 19 weeks' gestation in Scotland, those with greater deprivation scores, as assessed using the Scottish Index of Multiple Deprivation (SIMD), were more likely to be smokers, to be younger and to be single. Deprivation was related to pre-term birth and need for neonatal treatment. In terms of nutrients consumed, these women were more likely to have increased intakes of total and saturated fat, carbohydrate and sodium compared to those of lower deprivation scores, but lower intakes of protein, fibre and most vitamins (although not vitamin A) and minerals. This translated into those with greater deprivation having lower plasma folate and higher homocysteine concentrations. Those with greater deprivation scores were also less likely to have taken a folic acid supplement at the time of conception, although at week 12 of pregnancy there was no difference in folic acid supplement use. In terms of foods, those with greater deprivation consumed more processed meat, fried potatoes, confectionery and soft drinks and less oil-rich fish, meat, fruit, vegetables and fruit juice. Most of these relationships with deprivation were not linear, with only a modest reduction in quality of the diet with level of deprivation and the greatest differences being seen for the most disadvantaged in society (Haggarty *et al.* 2009).

3.5 Current practice and recommendations: lactation

3.5.1 Recommendations for lactation

The nutritive demands of lactation are even greater than those of pregnancy, with the milk demand over a period of 4 months being equivalent to the entire energy cost of pregnancy (Picciano 2003). While some of the energy and many of the nutrients required for the production of milk for the infant have been stored during pregnancy, there remains a need for a considerable increase in intake to meet demand. The demand and hence recommendations for lactation have been developed from the amount and composition of the milk produced during lactation, but there are few good data on whether this is appropriate, with a well-growing infant assumed to reflect adequate nutrition of the mother. The additional energy demand for lactation was calculated to be around 500 kcal/day (2.1 MJ/day) by COMA in 1991, although it was recognised to vary with the extent of breastfeeding and the age of the child (Department of Health 1991). More recently SACN has recommended the use of the US Energy DRI (Dietary Reference Intake) (Institute of Medicine 2005) based on doubly-labelled water measurements of 330 kcal/day (1.4 MJ/day) in the first 6 months of lactation, if exclusively breastfeeding. After the first 6 months, the energy intake required to support breastfeeding will be modified by maternal body composition and the breast milk intake of the infant (SACN 2011b).

Table 3.3 shows the requirements for micronutrients during lactation. In the UK, a daily vitamin D supplement (10 μg/day) is recommended (Department of Health 1991; SACN 2007). The advice on fish shown in Chapter 15, Table 15.9 and on peanuts, as described for pregnancy (see Section 3.4.1.6) also applies during lactation, and consumption of alcohol and caffeine should be only occasional. Also as described above for pregnancy (see Section 3.4.1.3),

EFSA has recommended that lactating mothers should consume a diet providing at least 200 mg of DHA per day (Koletzko *et al.* 2008). While this has been supported by the World Association of Perinatal Medicine, the Early Nutrition Academy and the Child Health Foundation, FAO/WHO suggest that women already consuming a healthy diet should obtain enough DHA and do not recommend supplementation (see Section 3.4.1.3). See Chapter 15, Table 15.9 for a summary of recommendations during lactation.

3.5.2 Current practice during lactation

As with pregnant women, lactating women are generally excluded from national surveys of the dietary intakes of the population, and hence there are few reports on the overall diets of lactating women and how these are meeting the recommendations outlined above in Section 3.5.1. Specific studies of particular aspects are available, but there is very little literature about the overall diets of lactating women and any changes that women may make because they are lactating. The particular areas of focus of papers on maternal diet tend to be either fatty acids and the supply and composition of these in breast milk, or micronutrients, particularly those micronutrients for which achievement of appropriate intakes is known to be challenging for women generally and hence may be an issue for the breast-fed infant.

In relation to fatty acids, particularly DHA, there is a wide variation in breast milk DHA content, due largely, it is believed, to variations in maternal dietary intake. Increased dietary DHA is known to result in increased concentrations in breast milk (Harris *et al.* 1984). A comprehensive review by Brenna *et al.* (2007) of the DHA and arachidonic acid (AA) content of human breast milk examined 65 studies assessing a total of 2474 women. The data indicated DHA concentration in breast milk to be lower and more variable than that of AA. The highest concentrations were primarily found in coastal populations and were associated with marine food consumption. There is evidence from the US that pregnant women have been reducing their fish intakes, because of concerns about environmental contaminants, and this has resulted in lower DHA content of breast milk over time (Carlson 2009). There is no evidence for adverse effects on visual acuity in breast-fed infants according to variations in maternal breast milk DHA.

In relation to micronutrients, information about how well lactating mothers meet recommendations is sparse, and even less is available than for pregnancy. In many longitudinal studies with detailed information about the mother during pregnancy, once the child is born, most dietary information is collected about the infant. In general, in many countries lactating women often fail to meet recommendations, although studies tend to be small and recent work is limited. In studies from the US (Mackey *et al.* 1998), Canada (Doran and Evers 1997), Italy (Giammarioli *et al.* 2002), Mexico (Caire-Juvera *et al.* 2007) and New Zealand (Todd and Parnell 1994), energy intakes of lactating women have been found to be below recommended levels; in the New Zealand study, this was particularly the case for younger women. In this study, the nutrients for which intakes were below recommendations were zinc, calcium, folate and vitamin A. In the US study, nutrient intakes met recommendations on average, except for zinc, calcium, vitamin D, vitamin E and folate. In the Canadian study, nutrient intakes were below recommendations for zinc, calcium, folate, iron, vitamin A and thiamin. No differences were seen with income for these frequencies in this study. In Mexico, intakes of zinc, calcium, vitamin C, vitamin E and folate were inadequate.

Folate is one of the nutrients commonly found to be low in the diets of lactating women. In recent years, and following fortification of the food supply in the US and Canada, new studies have been carried out to investigate the impact of fortification on the folate status of pregnant and lactating women. In a study of educated women in Toronto, 32% of the lactating women studied had folate intakes below the estimated average requirement (EAR) of 450 µg/day with fortification (Sherwood *et al.* 2006); when intake was calculated without fortified folic acid, 98% of the women would not have met their requirements for folate. Literature suggests that folate levels in breast milk are maintained at the expense of maternal folate reserves, except in the most severe cases of deficiency (Lindzon and O'Connor 2007), and while the infant is then protected, this raises concerns for the nutritional status of the mother and the impact on subsequent pregnancies. When women do not take a folic acid supplement during pregnancy or lactation, their own folate status is likely to be low during lactation.

This impacts on the concentration of homocysteine in blood which has been shown to be higher at 6 months in breastfeeding women who have not taken supplements (Mackey and Picciano 1999).

The use of supplements during lactation is encouraged in many countries. Picciano and McGuire (2009) examined supplement use by pregnant and lactating women in the US. Unfortunately supplement use during lactation is even less well documented than use in pregnancy. They quoted a study by Stultz and colleagues, who followed medication use during lactation in 46 women from giving birth until cessation of breastfeeding (or for a year). Of this small group, 73% reported taking a multivitamin supplement, but only 11% took calcium, 7% folic acid and 4% iron. Significantly more took supplements during pregnancy than during lactation (Stultz *et al.* 2007).

3.6 Infant feeding: issues relating to evidence base

Due to the changes in infant feeding practices described below (and in Chapter 15 and Appendix 3.1 in more detail), outcomes reported from long-term cohort studies where infants were fed on the artificial milks available at that time may not reflect the artificial milks currently available.

Duration of breastfeeding has changed considerably in European counties over the past few centuries, and substantial changes in infant feeding practices have occurred in the past several decades. Duration of breastfeeding reduced in the twentieth century as research in the 1930s to 1950s concluded that there were few differences between breast-fed and bottle-fed babies up to the end of the first year of life. During the twentieth century two types of infant formula were typically used as alternatives to breast milk: home-prepared formulas and commercially prepared formulas (Fomon 2001). Home-prepared formulas were popular around the 1930s to 1940s and were prepared by mixing evaporated milk or fresh cows' milk with water and a carbohydrate source (e.g. corn syrup or sucrose).

In the UK, starting in 1940 the government manufactured National Dried Milk for infant feeding, which was used during the wartime period. In the early 1970s, concern arose about the apparently high incidence of hypertonic dehydration (elevated sodium in the blood) of infants, a condition commonly induced by feeding infants excess energy and solutes because heaped scoops of milk powder were used in preparing the formula instead of the recommended level measures (Taitz and Byers 1972). In 1977, National Dried Milk was withdrawn and the use of similar formula based on unmodified dried or evaporated milk is no longer recommended (Department of Health 1980).

All infant formulas marketed in the UK now have to comply with compositional guidelines published by the Department of Health, drawn up to ensure that artificial feeds are as close in formulation as possible to human milk (Ministry of Agriculture Fisheries and Food 1995).

The nutrient composition of artificial milks has changed somewhat over recent years with increasing scientific and clinical knowledge, and regulations and revised guidance on infant formula composition. Significant improvements have been made in adapting cows' milk to bring it closer to breast milk in terms of the nutritional composition and molecular structure (Sidnell and Greenstreet 2011) and there have been major developments in understanding the effect of differences in protein content on infant growth rates, the lower protein content of breast milk being associated with slower rates (Sandstrom *et al.* 2008; Grote *et al.* 2010) (see Appendix 3.1 for more details on the historical perspective of breastfeeding and infant formula).

3.7 Current practice and recommendations: breastfeeding

3.7.1 Benefits of breastfeeding

Breast milk provides all the nutrients a baby needs during this period, in a form that is hygienic and easy to digest. The protein, carbohydrate and fat profiles are unique to human breast milk and differ in a number of ways from other mammalian milks. Breast milk also contains a range of bioactive components, including antimicrobial and anti-inflammatory factors, digestive enzymes, hormones and growth factors (Lonnerdal 2003). Antimicrobial agents include leucocytes, secretory immunoglobulin (Ig)A, IgM and IgG antibodies, oligosaccharides, lysozyme, lactoferrin, lipids, fatty acids and mucins. Growth factors present in human milk, such as IGF (Insulin-like Growth Factor) and epidermal growth factor,

are thought to be important for gut maturation (Lonnerdal 2003). Lactoferrin is one of several specific binders in human milk that greatly increases the bioavailability of iron (Lonnerdal 2003).

Both the volume and composition of breast milk vary with the stage of lactation, within each individual feed and with maternal nutritional status. Recent research in animals has shown that reduced fetal growth caused by placental insufficiency can impair the quality and quantity of breast milk (see British Medical Association 2009). Colostrum, produced during the first few days after birth, is low in volume and nutrient content but high in antimicrobial factors. Volume and nutrient content reach a peak, in mature breast milk, several weeks after birth. The feeding behaviour of the baby and the quality of the breast milk change with time in a way that may prevent overfeeding, teach the infant how to recognise satiety signals, and regulate energy intake differently from formula-fed infants (British Medical Association 2009). The mother's macronutrient intake does not have much influence on milk composition, but her diet does affect the long-chain fatty acid (see Section 3.5.2) and vitamin content of her milk.

Longer-term effects of breastfeeding are discussed in later chapters but there are benefits from the outset, summarised in a report from the British Medical Association (2009). Breast-fed babies, even in high-income countries, experience significantly fewer episodes of gastrointestinal and respiratory infection. Short-term benefits to the mother of breastfeeding include convenience, less expense, a faster return to pre-pregnant weight and delayed onset of ovulation.

3.7.2 Recommendations for breastfeeding: historical perspective and evidence base

In the latter part of the twentieth century, as evidence amassed about the benefits to both the infant and the mother of breastfeeding, policy initiatives began to appear to promote both the initiation of breastfeeding and its duration. In 1981, the WHO developed the International Code of Marketing of Breast Milk Substitutes, addressing concern about the marketing practices of infant formula manufacturers that could interfere with the promotion of breastfeeding. In 1990, the WHO and UNICEF developed the Innocenti Declaration on the Protection, Promotion and Support of Breastfeeding, co-sponsored by the US and Sweden, which was signed by more than 30 governments. The declaration included four important operational targets:

(1) By 1995, each participating country was to appoint a national breastfeeding coordinator and establish a multi-sector breastfeeding committee.
(2) Every facility providing maternity care services would fully practise the ten steps to successful breastfeeding.
(3) Each country must put into effect the principles and aim of the International Code of Marketing of Breast Milk Substitutes.
(4) Each participating country to enact legislation to protect the breastfeeding rights of working women (Thulier 2009).

In 1991, UNICEF and the WHO launched the Baby-Friendly Hospital Initiative, to ensure that facilities providing care to new mothers would be centres that supported breastfeeding. Over 10 000 centres have now earned the Baby-Friendly award (Thulier 2009).

Since the 1990s, there has been a greater emphasis not simply on breastfeeding but on exclusive breastfeeding, whereby babies are predominantly breast-fed without addition of any complementary foods, that is, no 'solid' foods or infant formula. Prior to 2001, the WHO global recommendation was that infants should be exclusively breast-fed for between 4 and 6 months before the introduction of complementary foods (World Health Organization 1995). In March 2001, an Expert Consultation met to discuss the scientific evidence on exclusive breastfeeding presented in a systematic review conducted by Kramer and Kakuma (2002). The authors identified 20 studies comparing exclusive breastfeeding for 6 months vs. 3–4 months; only two of these were randomised intervention trials of different exclusive breastfeeding durations, and both had been conducted in a developing world setting (Honduras). All the trials in developed countries were observational studies. The overall conclusion of the review was that there was no objective evidence of a 'weanling's dilemma' – 'the choice between the known protective effect of exclusive breastfeeding against infectious morbidity and the (theoretical) insufficiency of breast milk alone to satisfy the infant's energy and micronutrient requirements beyond the age of four months of age'. The evidence in the review suggested that exclusive breastfeeding for 6 months has protective effects

against gastrointestinal infection and, on this basis, the consultation recommended exclusive breastfeeding for 6 months, with introduction of complementary foods and continued breastfeeding thereafter. Kramer and Kakuma (2002) recommended the need for large randomised trials in both developed and developing world settings to rule out small adverse effects on growth and to confirm the reported health benefits of exclusive breastfeeding for 6 months. They also warned against the potential risks of iron deficiency in susceptible infants, other micronutrient deficiencies and growth faltering.

The UK, like many other countries, has adopted the WHO breastfeeding recommendations (previous advice in the UK was for introduction of complementary feeding between the ages of 4 and 6 months) (Department of Health 1980; Department of Health 1989; Department of Health 1994). Department of Health advice is that if a baby seems hungrier at any time before 6 months, they may be experiencing a growth spurt, and extra breast or formula milk will be enough to meet their needs. Trying an extra feed for a formula-fed baby can also meet their needs.

The American Academy of Paediatrics has also adopted the 6-month exclusive breastfeeding recommendation. In its 2005 report on *Breastfeeding and the Use of Human Milk*, the Academy updated its earlier 1997 report of the same title, with even stronger advice about exclusive breastfeeding for 6 months, although it does include a statement to indicate that the 'period of introduction of complementary foods may be individualised to four to eight months of age', depending on the infant's dietary requirements and feeding patterns (American Academy of Pediatrics 2005).

However, the WHO recommendation has been questioned for the developed world. Fewtrell and colleagues (Fewtrell *et al.* 2007) have questioned the evidence, raising concerns that there is insufficient research on which to base these recommendations, especially for developed countries, that exclusive breastfeeding may not meet the energy requirements of many infants at 6 months of age and that there is insufficient data about the nutrient insufficiencies that may result from exclusive breastfeeding until this age.

Another systematic review published in 2001 considered the optimal age of weaning (defined in this instance as introduction of solids) in the UK regardless of the type of milk supplied, as opposed to the most appropriate length of exclusive breastfeeding (Lanigan *et al.* 2001). This review concluded that there was no compelling evidence to support a change in the then WHO recommendation to introduce solid foods into the diet at 4–6 months of age. Furthermore, subgroups of the population were identified who might benefit from introduction of solids earlier than for the majority of the infant population, e.g. low-birthweight infants. The authors identified no studies specifically undertaken to test the appropriateness of 6 months of exclusive breastfeeding compared to 4–6 months in a randomised controlled study design with full-term infants in a developed country setting.

A Cochrane review published in 2011 investigated the benefits and harms of supplementation for full-term healthy breast-fed infants and examined the timing and type of supplementation. However, the review did not find any evidence for disagreement with the WHO recommendation (and other international health organisations) that as a general policy exclusive breastfeeding, without additional foods or fluids, should be recommended for the first 6 months after birth (Becker *et al.* 2011).

Fewtrell and colleagues concluded that 'whilst a policy of exclusive breastfeeding for 6 months is eminently sensible for countries in which clean water and safe, nutritious first solid foods are scarce, evidence supporting the same policy for the developed world is less persuasive' (Fewtrell *et al.* 2007). They also concluded that there are virtually no data available on which to generate evidence-based recommendations for the introduction of solids for infants who are receiving predominantly or exclusively infant formula. Fewtrell *et al.* (2011) highlighted data from the US that raises further concerns about whether 6 months' exclusive breastfeeding would reliably meet iron requirements. However, in one of the many responses following the publication of Fewtrell *et al.* (2011) it was pointed out that the Scientific Advisory Committee on Nutrition (SACN) endorses the adequacy of iron and energy supply during exclusive breastfeeding. SACN's advice to the UK government on the nutritional adequacy of exclusive breastfeeding for 6 months remains unchanged and the committee continues to review all new evidence; in September 2010 it started work on a detailed review of the scientific evidence underpinning infant and young child feeding policy (see www.sacn.gov. uk/meetings/sub_groups/maternal_child_nutrition/ index.html).

3.7.3 Breastfeeding: current practice

3.7.3.1 *Initiating breastfeeding*

In the UK, Infant Feeding Surveys, commissioned by the Department of Health, have been conducted every 5 years since 1975 and provide representative information about feeding practices. The 2010 Infant Feeding Survey is the eighth in the series (McAndrew *et al.* 2012). As shown in Fig. 3.4, breastfeeding rates have increased in each part of the UK between 1980 and 2010. In each of the countries within the UK, the incidence of breastfeeding is greatest among women in managerial and professional classes (see Table 3.5), in those who completed their education over the age of 18 years (Fig. 3.5) and among women over the age of 30 years (Fig. 3.6).

The Millennium Cohort, a nationally representative cohort comprising infants born between September 2003 and January 2005, has also provided valuable and relatively up-to-date information on factors influencing breastfeeding rates. In the entire cohort, 70% of mothers initiated breastfeeding, with the highest levels for England (72%) and lowest for Northern Ireland (51%). Mothers in this cohort living in advantaged or ethnic electoral wards, those with managerial or professional occupations, those educated to degree level or above and those who were non-lone mothers or primiparous were more likely to have started breastfeeding. Maternal age at first motherhood was also positively associated with breastfeeding, with a rate ratio of 1.06 for each 5-year increase in maternal age (Griffiths *et al.* 2005).

Comparing 6478 British/Irish White mothers with 2110 mothers from ethnic minority groups in the cohort, all living in England, those from ethnic minority groups were more likely to initiate breastfeeding than British/Irish White mothers (86% vs. 69%) and to continue for at least 4 months (40% vs. 27%). Highest of these groups were Black participants (95% started breastfeeding), and the ethnic group with the lowest rate was Pakistani/Bangladeshi, at 76%, which was still higher than British/Irish White mothers. Those of first- and second-generation ethnic minority groups were less likely to breastfeed than recent immigrants. For every additional 5 years spent in the UK, the likelihood of breastfeeding was reduced by 5% (Griffiths *et al.* 2007). It was also found that White mothers with a partner of different ethnicity were 14% more likely to breastfeed than those with a White partner. Lone mothers in

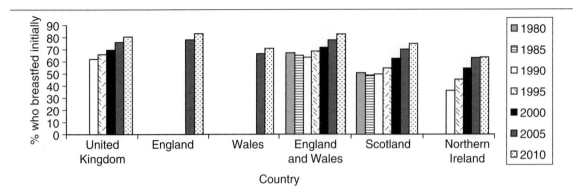

Figure 3.4 Incidence of breastfeeding by country in the UK, 1980–2010. This includes all babies who were put to the breast at all, even if this was on one occasion only, and also includes giving expressed breast milk. Source: McAndrew F, Thompson J, Fellows L *et al.* (2012) Infant Feeding Survey 2010. NHS The Information Centre. http://data.gov.uk/dataset/infant-feeding-survey-2010, copyright 2012, with permission from The Health and Social Care Information Centre. All rights reserved.

Table 3.5 Incidence of breastfeeding initiation by mother's socioeconomic classification (NS-SEC) and country (2005 and 2010)

	Total UK		Country							
			England		Wales		Scotland		Northern Ireland	
	2005	2010	2005	2010	2005	2010	2005	2010	2005	2010
% who breastfed initially	%	%	%	%	%	%	%	%	%	%
Managerial & professional	88	90	89	91	84	85	84	86	80	81
Intermediate occupations	77	80	80	81	72	73	72	72	58	59
Routine & manual	65	74	67	76	55	63	56	65	49	56
Never worked	65	71	68	74	41	47	52	56	37	30
Unclassified	71	80	73	82	62	62	53	68	64	63
All mothers	76	81	78	83	67	71	70	74	63	64

NS-SEC, National Statistics socioeconomic classification.
Source: McAndrew F, Thompson J, Fellows L *et al.* (2012) Infant Feeding Survey 2010. NHS The Information Centre. http://data.gov.uk/dataset/infant-feeding-survey-2010, copyright 2012, with permission from The Health and Social Care Information Centre. All rights reserved.

advantaged or ethnic areas were more likely to breastfeed than in disadvantaged areas, indicating that the increased rate in ethnic wards was due to mothers with a partner of different ethnicity and lone mothers breastfeeding in these wards (Griffiths *et al.* 2005).

The Millennium Cohort has also been used to examine the impact of the UNICEF Baby-Friendly programme on breastfeeding rates. The mother identified where her child was born and hence births could be categorised using information from UNICEF UK Baby-Friendly to identify accredited Baby-Friendly

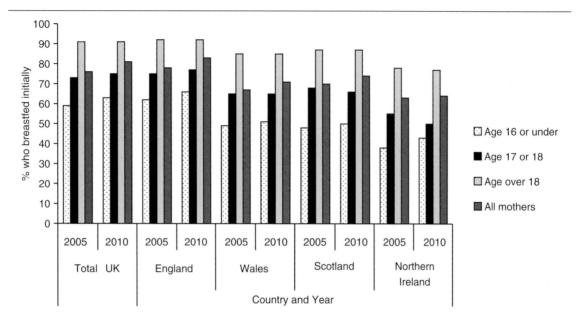

Figure 3.5   Incidence of breastfeeding by age completed full-time education and country (2005 and 2010).
Source: McAndrew F, Thompson J, Fellows L *et al.* (2012) Infant Feeding Survey 2010. NHS The Information
Centre. http://data.gov.uk/dataset/infant-feeding-survey-2010, copyright 2012, with permission from The Health
and Social Care Information Centre. All rights reserved.

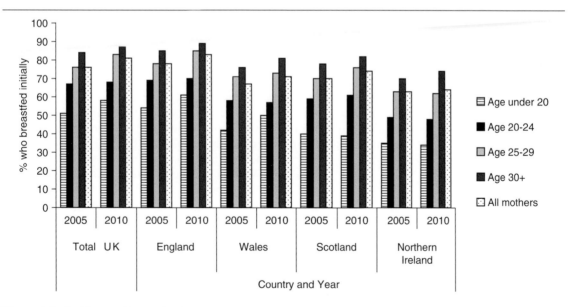

Figure 3.6   Incidence of breastfeeding initiation by mother's age and country (2005 and 2010).
Source: McAndrew F, Thompson J, Fellows L *et al.* (2012) Infant Feeding Survey 2010. NHS The Information
Centre. http://data.gov.uk/dataset/infant-feeding-survey-2010, copyright 2012, with permission from The Health
and Social Care Information Centre. All rights reserved.

hospitals, those units that were certificated (Certificate of Commitment) and those that are neither of these. Of 17 359 births in 248 maternity units, 7.4% were in accredited facilities and 31% in certificated facilities. Countries varied, with 24% of cohort births in Scotland in accredited sites, versus 3% in England. Mothers giving birth in accredited facilities were 10% more likely to start breastfeeding than in certificated or neither sites. Other factors were also found to influence initiation of breastfeeding such as UK country of residence, attendance at antenatal classes, vaginal delivery, and postpartum hospital stay > 24 hours. Accreditation was not found to affect breastfeeding at 1 month, indicating the need for provision of support for mothers once they leave the maternity unit (Bartington *et al.* 2006).

These findings were also confirmed in studies in Glasgow, where breastfeeding rates at 7 days were assessed using the Guthrie records collected on virtually 100% of infants at this stage. Using 445 623 records from 1995 to 2000, women who gave birth in a Baby Friendly accredited hospital were 28% more likely to be breastfeeding at 1 week compared to other hospitals. One of the ways to maintain support for mothers after these early days after birth is through health visitors. Investigators in Glasgow have also examined the breastfeeding rates according to the degree of specific training of health visitors to support breastfeeding. They found that infants being breast-fed at the first health visitor visit at 8–20 days were more likely to be breastfeeding at the second visit at 3–7 weeks if the health visitor had had breastfeeding training to support breastfeeding in the prior 2 years (Tappin *et al.* 2006). This study exemplifies the need, as outlined for the Millennium Cohort, for sustained support when mothers return home from hospital.

3.7.3.2 *Duration of breastfeeding*

In the 2010 Infant Feeding Survey in the UK, of all those who breast-fed initially (81%), 81% were still breastfeeding after 2 weeks, 68% after 6 weeks, 52% at 4 months and 42% at 6 months (McAndrew *et al.* 2012). Hence 42% of all mothers were still breastfeeding at 6 months, considerably higher than in 2005 (25%) (Bolling *et al.* 2007). Of those exclusively breastfeeding at birth, 58% were exclusively breastfeeding at 2 weeks, 34% at 6 weeks, 18% at 4 months and 1% at 6 months. Apart from the very first week of life, when the infant rejecting the breast was the

major reason for stopping breastfeeding, the main reason given by mothers for stopping at all other periods up to 9 months of age was insufficient milk. Rejection by the infant was also a major reason, as was painful breasts or nipples in the first few weeks. Return to work or college was given as a major reason after 4 months of age. The majority of mothers who breast-fed for less than 6 months indicated that they would have liked to have breast-fed for longer.

In the Millennium Cohort (see Section 3.7.3.1), 38% of infants were fully breast-fed for at least 1 month, 4% for at least 4 months and 1% for at least 6 months (Griffiths *et al.* 2005).

The 'Infant feeding in Asian families in England' survey, conducted between 1994 and 1996, surveyed mothers on four occasions, when the infant was 6–10 weeks old, and at 5 months, 9 months and 15 months of age (Thomas and Avery 1997). The survey was conducted in 41 local authorities which covered 95% of the Asian population at the time of the 1991 Census. Infants of Bangladeshi, Indian and Pakistani origin were included as well as White infants living in the same areas, for comparison. The incidence of breastfeeding (those who started to breastfeed) was 90% for Bangladeshi women, 82% for Indian, 76% for Pakistani and 62% for White mothers. Pakistani and Bangladeshi mothers stopped breastfeeding sooner than Indian and White mothers; the most frequent reason for stopping was 'insufficient milk' or 'the infant would not suck'. By 4 months of age, 39% of the White, 34% of the Indian, 25% of the Bangladeshi and 21% of the Pakistani mothers were still breastfeeding. Many of the Pakistani and Bangladeshi mothers who were born outside the UK indicated that they would have fed their infant differently if the child had been born outside the UK.

The Feeding Practices Study II (similar to a previous study published in 1997), conducted by the US Food and Drug Administration during 2005–7, followed women through pregnancy and the first year of the infant's life. They were surveyed at regular intervals using mail questionnaires. Of all mothers who breast-fed in hospital (83%), 74% were still breastfeeding at 1 month, 57% at 4 months and 50% at 6 months. Almost half the breast-fed infants were supplemented with infant formula while in hospital. These figures show that over 40% of all mothers surveyed were still breastfeeding at 6 months, higher than in the UK Infant Feeding Survey conducted during the same period (Grummer-Strawn *et al.* 2008). These rates

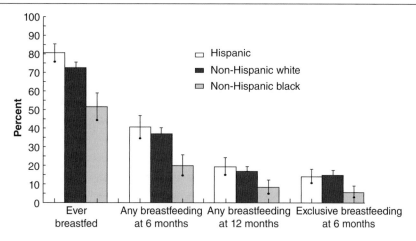

Figure 3.7 Racial/ethnic disparities in breastfeeding rates (percent and 95% CI).
Reproduced from Li R, Darling N, Maurice E et al. (2005a) Breastfeeding rates in the United States by characteristics of the child, mother, or family: the 2002 National Immunization Survey. *Pediatrics*, **115**, e31–7, copyright 2005, with permission from the American Academy of Pediatrics.

were also seen in data from another US survey, the 2002 National Immunization Survey, where 35% of infants were breast-fed at 6 months (Li *et al.* 2005a). In terms of exclusive breastfeeding, 63% initiated breastfeeding in hospital, which dropped to 57% at 1 month, and 13% at 6 months. While far off the recommendation to breastfeed exclusively for six months, these figures were substantially higher than the UK at the same period, but it is not known if they have increased, as has been seen in the UK in the most recent Infant Feeding Survey (McAndrew *et al.* 2012). The highest rates of breastfeeding in the US are seen in Hispanic groups, and the lowest in non-Hispanic Blacks, where only 20% breast-fed at all at 6 months, as shown in Fig. 3.7 (Li, Darling *et al.* 2005). Geographically, highest rates are seen on the West Coast with lowest rates in the Southern states. The youngest mothers are least likely to breastfeed and the oldest (>30 years) most likely. Higher income is also associated with increased likelihood of breastfeeding.

Ethnic differences in breastfeeding have been studied in other countries. In Singapore, it was shown that Malay mothers (28% of the sample of 2098 mothers studied) were less likely to breastfeed at 2 months after birth than their Chinese counterparts (65% of the sample), while Indian mothers were the most likely to breastfeed (8% of the sample). At 2 months, Muslim mothers were nearly seven times

more likely and Christian mothers also more likely to breastfeed than Buddhist/Taoist mothers, indicating religious differences in this society as well. Nonworking mothers were more likely to breastfeed than working mothers in this study (Foo *et al.* 2005).

Breastfeeding rates in countries in Europe are reported by the WHO's European Health for All database and are shown in Table 3.6. Rates vary widely and are not specific to certain regions, with some Western European countries having high rates and others low, and the same is true in Eastern European countries. These data indicate that rates are lower in the UK than all other countries indicated and by a substantial margin for many countries.

3.7.3.3 Exclusive breastfeeding

The most recent UK Infant Feeding Survey indicates that breastfeeding rates (includes all babies who were put to the breast, even if only on one occasion) increased from 76% in 2005 to 81% in 2010 (McAndrew *et al.* 2012) (Fig. 3.4).

3.7.3.4 Problems with breastfeeding

In the Infant Feeding Survey of 2010 (McAndrew *et al.* 2012) pregnant women who intended to breastfeed were questioned about the reasons for their

Table 3.6 Breastfeeding rates (%) in selected countries in Europe

	3 months	6 months	Year available
Albania	95	88.8	2010
Austria	72	65	2006
Belarus	82.6	58.6	2010
Czech Republic	62.4	38.6	2010
Finland	76	60	2005
Italy	59.2	40.4	2005
Netherlands	52.2	35.3	2009
Norway	88	80	2006
Sweden	83.7	66.5	2008
Turkey	98	95.9	2008
United Kingdom	42*	34	2010

Source: Reproduced from the European Health For All database (http://www.euro.who.int/en/what-we-do/data-and-evidence/european-health-for-all-database-hfa-db). Copenhagen, WHO Regional Office for Europe, 2010, © World Health Organization 2013.
*Breastfeeding rate at 4 months. UK data is from McAndrew *et al.* (2012).

decision: 83% of mothers believed that breastfeeding was best for the baby's health. Other reasons included: convenience (22%), health benefits for the mother (17%), closer bond between mother and baby (16%), breastfeeding being free, or cheaper than infant formula (15%), having breast-fed previous baby/babies (12%), breastfeeding being natural (11%) and the expectation that it would support easier weight loss (6%).

Among those women who intended to bottle feed, the reasons included: they did not like the idea of breastfeeding (20%); so other people could feed the baby (17%); they had previously fed their children with infant formula (21%); it was more convenient/due to mother's lifestyle (19%), they had breast-fed previous children and didn't get on with it (11%); medical reasons for not breastfeeding (10%); they would be embarrassed to breastfeed (10%); domestic reasons, coping with other children (3%); it allowed them to see how much the baby had consumed (5%); they expected to return to work soon (1%); feeding with infant formula less tiring (1%).

In the survey, women were also asked about their reasons for stopping breastfeeding within 1 and 2 weeks respectively. The reasons given are illustrated in Fig. 3.8.

Other breastfeeding problems mothers reported experiencing during their stay in hospital and after

leaving hospital, leading to the change of feeding approach, included poor attachment of the baby to breast; baby feeding too slowly, being distracted during feeds or not interested; a lack of support to continue breastfeeding; baby not being satisfied and requiring top-ups using formula; baby vomiting/reflux; and baby not gaining enough or having lost weight.

Evidence indicates that maternal obesity is associated with short breastfeeding duration (Robertson *et al.* 2007). The reasons may include mechanical difficulties of proper positioning of the infant, physiological differences such as lower prolactin production levels, and a high pre-pregnancy weight which is associated with a longer time before breast milk is secreted. The current increase in maternal obesity (see Section 3.3.1) is therefore likely to have a detrimental effect on breastfeeding rates.

3.8 Current practice and recommendations: formula feeding

3.8.1 Composition of infant formulas

Advances in food technology coupled with increased knowledge and understanding of the composition and molecular structure of breast milk has led to significant improvements towards the goal of making formula milk match breast milk. Although the overall protein, fat and carbohydrate content of formula milks were matched with that of breast milk quite early on, it has recently emerged that the position of the various fatty acids on the triglycerides is also important in matching that of breast milk. Technology now enables the structure of triglycerides in vegetable oil to more closely match their composition and structure in breast milk fat (Sidnell and Greenstreet 2011). Infant formulas have also, in recent years, been fortified with prebiotics which has resulted in more similarities in the gut microbiotia of breast-fed and formula-fed infants (see Chapter 7, Section 7.3.5). Innovation in formula milk development has also led to lower-protein formulas with different amino acid characteristics that have been shown, in randomised controlled trials, to slow infants' rate of weight gain (Sidnell and Greenstreet 2009) and may therefore offer health benefits (see Chapter 8, Section 8.3). New techniques are likely to continue to minimise differences between formula

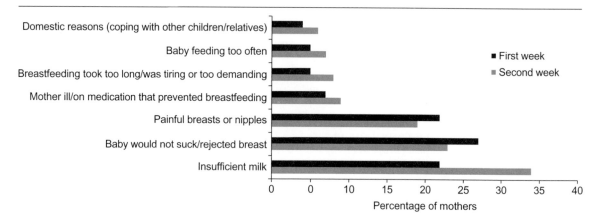

Figure 3.8 Breastfeeding problems experienced by mothers during the first and second week after birth (2010). Source: McAndrew F, Thompson J, Fellows L *et al.* (2012) Infant Feeding Survey 2010. NHS The Information Centre. http://data.gov.uk/dataset/infant-feeding-survey-2010, copyright 2012, with permission from The Health and Social Care Information Centre. All rights reserved.

and breast milk in the future; for example, they may allow the production of bioactive substances present in low concentrations in human milk but absent from bovine milk, which may have effects on nutrient utilisation or other health benefits (Hernell 2011). For a more detailed description of the composition of infant milks in the UK see Crawley and Westland (2011).

3.8.1.1 Cows' milk-based infant formulas

Infant milks based on cows' milk that can be used from birth are available, either 'whey-based' or 'casein-based'. In whey-based milks the cows' milk protein is adjusted so that the casein to whey ratio is similar to breast milk (40:60). In casein-based milks, there is more casein than whey; the ratio of casein to whey remains the same as cows' milk (80:20). Whey-based milks may also have a lower mineral content (in particular, sodium and potassium) which is important for all newborn babies, who have immature kidneys.

Whey-based milks, therefore, are the first choice of milk if a mother does not breastfeed, whereas casein-based milks are generally used if the baby appears not to be satisfied on a whey-based product. Casein-based milks can also be helpful in delaying the intro-duction of solids before the recommended age (see Section 3.9.1).

3.8.1.2 Soy-based infant formulas

Soy-based infant formulas have been available for decades in a number of countries including the UK. In the US, soy protein-based formulas were introduced in 1929 and are now estimated to contribute 20% (Bhatia and Greer 2008) or 40% (National Academy of Science (NAS) and Food and Nutrition Board (FNB)) of the formula market; in addition, a study from Israel found these to be popular, being fed to 10.4% of infants at 2 months, 20.6% at 4 months and 31.5% at 12 months (Berger-Achituv *et al.* 2005). In the UK, proportions are much lower at 1–2% of infants aged less than 14 weeks (Hamlyn *et al.* 2002) and there remains concern about the provision of soy to young infants. The major concern about soy formula is the content of phytoestrogens, a family of plant-based oestrogen-type compounds, including isoflavones, which are found in legumes generally, but in highest concentrations in soya beans. Hence the concerns are related to potentially negative effects on sexual development and repro-duction, neuro-behavioural development, immune function and thyroid function, although investigations and reviews concerning these have to date shown no differences in health outcomes at later time points (Strom *et al.* 2001; Mendez *et al.* 2002; Berger-Achituv *et al.* 2005). There is no evidence to attribute specific positive health effects to isoflavones in infants, although some positive effects have been suggested in adults (decreased risk of some cancers, lower cholesterol levels and a decreased risk of cardiovascular disease) (Vandenplas *et al.* 2011).

In the UK, soy-based infant formulas are the only choice available for those seeking non-animal sources of protein, and are the only vegan option. Current Department of Health advice is that soy infant formulas should not be the first choice for the management of infants with proven cows' milk sensitivity, lactose intolerance, galactokinase deficiency or galactosaemia, but recognise that there may be some circumstances for which soy infant formulas could be given, e.g. to infants of vegan parents who are not breastfeeding and to infants who may find the alternatives unacceptable. The total amount of carbohydrate is controlled by law (EU Directive 2006/141/EC of 22 December 2006 on infant formulae and follow-on formulae) in order to provide similar levels of sweetness to breast milk and cows' milk formulas. Glucose syrups are the most suitable alternative to lactose (present in both human and cows' milk) as they are well tolerated and easily digested by infants.

3.8.2 Feeding infant formula

The Department of Health advises that, if breastfeeding is not possible, infant formula is the only alternative until 1 year. Cows' milk-based formula is best (Department of Health 2009b). Follow-on formula can be used from 6 months as an alternative although standard formula remains appropriate. Other types of formula should be used only on medical advice: hydrolysed protein formula may be useful in cases of cows' milk allergy, and soy formula where a strict vegetarian lifestyle is being followed. Goats' milk formula, even if it has been specially formulated for babies, should not be given to babies under 1 year (see Section 3.9.5.2).

A small number of health conditions that affect the infant or the mother may justify recommending that she does not breastfeed temporarily or permanently (WHO & UNICEF 2009). WHO advises that the benefits of breastfeeding in such circumstances should be weighed against the risks posed by the specific condition.

Infants who should not receive breast milk or any other milk except specialised formula:

- Infants with classic galactosaemia: a special galactose-free formula is needed.
- Infants with maple syrup urine disease: a special formula free of leucine, isoleucine and valine is needed.
- Infants with phenylketonuria: a special phenylalanine-free formula is needed (some breastfeeding is possible, under careful monitoring).

Infants for whom breast milk remains the best feeding option but who may need other food in addition to breast milk for a limited period:

- Infants born weighing less than 1500 g (very low birthweight).
- Infants born at less than 32 weeks of gestation (pre-term).
- Newborn infants who are at risk of hypoglycaemia by virtue of impaired metabolic adaptation or increased glucose demand (such as those who are pre-term, small for gestational age or who have experienced significant intrapartum hypoxic/ischaemic stress, those who are ill and those whose mothers are diabetic) if their blood sugar fails to respond to optimal breastfeeding or breast milk feeding.

Maternal conditions that may justify permanent avoidance of breastfeeding:

- Human immunodeficiency virus (HIV) infection: if replacement feeding is acceptable, feasible, affordable, sustainable and safe.

Maternal conditions that may justify temporary avoidance of breastfeeding:

- Severe illness that prevents a mother from caring for her infant, for example sepsis.
- Herpes simplex virus type 1 (HSV-1): direct contact between lesions on the mother's breasts and the infant's mouth should be avoided until all active lesions have resolved.

- Maternal medication: for example, sedating psychotherapeutic drugs, anti-epileptic drugs and opioids and their combinations may cause side effects such as drowsiness and respiratory depression and are better avoided if a safer alternative is available; cytotoxic chemotherapy requires that a mother stops breastfeeding during therapy.

Maternal conditions during which breastfeeding can still continue, although health problems may be of concern:

- Breast abscess: breastfeeding should continue on the unaffected breast; feeding from the affected breast can resume once treatment has started.
- Hepatitis B: infants should be given hepatitis B vaccine, within the first 48 hours or as soon as possible thereafter.
- Hepatitis C.
- Mastitis: if breastfeeding is very painful, milk must be removed by expression to prevent progression of the condition.
- Tuberculosis: mother and baby should be managed according to national tuberculosis guidelines.
- Substance use: maternal use of nicotine, alcohol, ecstasy, amphetamines, cocaine and related stimulants has been demonstrated to have harmful effects on breast-fed babies; alcohol, opioids, benzodiazepines and cannabis can cause sedation in both the mother and the baby. Mothers should be encouraged not to use these substances and given opportunities and support to abstain.

3.8.3 Formula feeding: current practice

In the UK, the Infant Feeding Survey provides valuable data on current practice regarding the timing of introduction and duration of formula feeding. Table 3.7 shows that just under a third of UK babies in 2010 received infant formula from birth and, by 6 weeks of age, nearly three-quarters had received formula. Formula was introduced later by women classed as managerial/professional (Table 3.8), and by older mothers (Table 3.9).

3.9 Current practice and recommendations: weaning/complementary feeding

3.9.1 Recommendations: timing of introduction of complementary foods

In the developing world, the infant traditionally moved abruptly from exclusive breastfeeding to family foods, often when the next child arrived. In many societies, this pattern still holds, although many countries have moved to patterns closer to those of the developed world, where the infant has an elongated period of mixed feeding, passing by degrees from a diet largely of breast milk to one eventually without breast milk. The age at which solid food should be introduced to the infant has gone through many phases, with periods where very early introduction of food has been encouraged, to the current situation where solid food is recommended at 6 months and later.

Table 3.7 Age at which formula milk first introduced in the UK, by country, 2010

% of mothers who had given formula milk at	Total UK	Country			
		England	Wales	Scotland	Northern Ireland
	%	%	%	%	%
Birth	31	29	43	37	48
1 week	52	51	62	58	66
4 weeks	66	65	75	68	78
6 weeks	73	72	80	73	83
2 months	75	74	82	76	86
4 months	83	82	88	83	90
6 months	88	88	92	88	93
9 months	95	95	96	97	97

Source: McAndrew F, Thompson J, Fellows L *et al.* (2012) Infant Feeding Survey 2010. NHS The Information Centre. http://data.gov.uk/dataset/infant-feeding-survey-2010, copyright 2012, with permission from The Health and Social Care Information Centre. All rights reserved.

Table 3.8   Age at which formula milk first introduced, by mother's socio-economic classification (NS-SEC), 2010

% of mothers who had given formula milk by	Managerial & professional	Intermediate occupations	Routine & manual	Never worked	Not classified	All mothers
	%	%	%	%	%	%
Birth	20	30	39	46	32	31
1 week	42	51	61	64	54	52
4 weeks	57	67	75	73	68	66
6 weeks	65	73	81	77	74	73
2 months	67	76	82	80	76	75
4 months	78	83	88	85	83	83
6 months	85	90	92	89	87	88
9 months	94	96	96	95	94	95

NS-SEC, National Statistics socioeconomic classification.
Source: McAndrew F, Thompson J, Fellows L *et al.* (2012) Infant Feeding Survey 2010. NHS The Information Centre. http://data.gov.uk/dataset/infant-feeding-survey-2010, copyright 2012, with permission from The Health and Social Care Information Centre. All rights reserved.

Table 3.9   Age at which formula milk first introduced, by mother's age, 2005

% of mothers who had given formula milk by	Under 20	20–24	25–29	30–34	35 or over	All mothers
	%	%	%	%	%	%
Birth	54	45	28	24	24	31
1 week	71	66	50	45	46	52
4 weeks	82	80	65	61	59	66
6 weeks	84	85	71	68	67	73
2 months	87	87	73	70	70	75
4 months	90	91	82	79	80	83
6 months	95	94	87	86	86	88
9 months	100	97	95	94	94	95

Source: McAndrew F, Thompson J, Fellows L *et al.* (2012) Infant Feeding Survey 2010. NHS The Information Centre. http://data.gov.uk/dataset/infant-feeding-survey-2010, copyright 2012, with permission fromThe Health and Social Care Information Centre. All rights reserved.

Until about 1920, solid foods were rarely introduced before 1 year of age. Studies from that period onward, however, indicated a growing interest in the quantity and quality of food required by the infant (for a discussion, see Appendix 3.1). In a number of papers from the 1920s, Pritchard outlined the need for solid food and stressed both the energy needs of the infant and the need for food that requires mastication for the newly arrived teeth (Pritchard 1920; Pritchard 1928). Other studies investigated the age of introduction with data on growth, and biological measures such as iron status and risk of infections. By the mid-1930s, American paediatricians were suggesting 6 months as the proper age to introduce solid foods. The next decades saw a number of studies comparing very early introductions, within the first days or weeks of life, with later introduction. There appeared to be growing concern about the amount of protein consumed by infants, particularly in the US (Beal 1961), and often these studies investigated means to increase protein intake and hence meat was often provided as the non-milk food of interest. Glazier, for example, in

1933 compared introductions at 2–3 months, 4 months and 5–6 months and later (Glazier 1933). He found greater weight gain and earlier dentition and walking in those infants fed early, with better food habits and fewer food dislikes.

In recent decades, advice on the age at which complementary feeding (in particular, solids) should be introduced has continued to fluctuate but has typically been in the range of 3–6 months. For example, in the UK, the advice from government in 1980 was that a flexible approach was desirable and that 'it is likely that a few infants need food other than milk before 3 months of age, and that by 6–8 months nearly all babies require mixed feeding' (Department of Health 1980). At this time, the 1975 national survey of infant feeding practice in England and Wales had revealed that the introduction of solid foods was happening relatively early: 3% of babies were given food other than milk in the first 2 weeks of life, 18% within the first month, 45% by 2 months, 85% by 3 months and 97% by 4 months.

In 1989, new advice was published (Department of Health 1989). The report noted that a subsequent survey in 1980 had found a change: only 4% of babies had received solids by 4 weeks, 24% at 8 weeks and 89% at 4 months. No further change was seen in the 1985 Infant Feeding Survey. Each of the surveys had shown a strong association between bottle feeding and early introduction of solids. The 1989 report concluded that very few infants will require solid foods before the age of 3 months but the majority should be offered a mixed diet by the age of 6 months. Advice changed in 1994, the recommendation being that the majority of infants should not be given solid foods before the age of 4 months, and a mixed diet should be offered by the age of 6 months (Department of Health 1994).

Prior to 2001, the WHO advised that infants should be exclusively breastfed for 4–6 months, with the introduction of complementary foods (any fluid or food other than breast milk) not taking place before this time. The age of 4 months was identified in a prospective study in Dundee, UK, which suggested that introduction of solid foods before that age was associated with increased respiratory symptoms and greater fatness at age 7 years (Wilson *et al.* 1998). Since 2001, however, WHO's advice changed as a result of a systematic review undertaken by Kramer and Kakumo (Kramer and Kakuma 2002; WHO 2003) and exclusive breastfeeding for 6 months

is now the recommendation (see Section 3.7.2 for further discussion).

From 2003, the UK Department of Health has recommended that complementary feeding should start at around 6 months. Breastfeeding (and/or breast milk substitutes) should continue beyond the first 6 months, supplemented with appropriate types and amounts of solid foods. Mothers who do not follow these recommendations should be supported to optimise their infants' nutrition (Department of Health 2009b). Studies using focus groups suggest that those who chose not to breastfeed or discontinue before 6 months are not well supported by health professionals and look to others such as friends and family members for support (Heinig *et al.* 2006) (see Chapter 15, Sections 15.4.1.1 and 15.8.2). Solid foods should be tried when a baby can sit up, wants to chew and is putting toys and other objects in its mouth, and reaches and grabs accurately. Baby-led weaning should be combined with feeding of purees and other soft foods (see Section 3.9.4).

The Department of Health advises that if parents decide to introduce solid foods at any time before 6 months, there are some foods that should be avoided as they may cause allergies (see Section 3.9.10) or make the baby ill. These include wheat-based foods and other foods containing gluten (e.g. bread, rusks, some breakfast cereals), eggs, fish, shellfish, nuts and seeds that may provoke sensitisation in allergy-prone children; and soft and unpasteurised cheeses because of the risk of bacteria such as *Listeria monocytogenes* being present. Solid foods should never be introduced before 4 months.

The WHO advises that energy needs from complementary foods in developing countries are approximately 200 kcal/day (0.84 MJ/day) at 6–8 months of age, 300 kcal/day (1.26 MJ/day) at 9–11 months, and 550 kcal/day (2.31 kJ/day) at 12–23 months. In industrialised countries these estimates are 130, 310 and 580 kcal/day (0.55, 1.30 and 2.44 MJ/day), respectively, because of differences in average breast milk intake (Pan American Health Organisation/World Health Organization (PAHO/WHO) 2003).

3.9.2 Current practice of timing of introduction of complementary foods

In spite of the recommendation to breastfeed exclusively until 6 months or beyond, virtually all mothers

Table 3.10   Prevalence of exclusive breastfeeding at ages up to 6 months by country (2005)

	UK	England	Wales	Scotland	Northern Ireland
	%	%	%	%	%
Birth	69	71	57	63	52
1 week	46	47	36	40	33
2 weeks	40	41	32	35	27
3 weeks	35	36	28	32	23
4 weeks	30	31	23	28	19
6 weeks	23	24	17	22	13
2 months (8 weeks)	21	21	15	20	12
3 months (13 weeks)	17	18	13	17	9
4 months (17 weeks)	12	13	9	12	6
5 months (21 weeks)	5	5	3	5	3
6 months (26 weeks)	1	1	*	1	1

*Figures are negligible.
Source: Bolling *et al.* (2007).

in the UK report introducing other foods before 6 months, often because they consider their babies to be hungry and not satisfied on breast milk alone. In the UK in 2000 only 2% of mothers were breastfeeding exclusively at 6 months (Hamlyn *et al.* 2002). The corresponding figure in the US was 18% (Ryan *et al.* 2002). In the recent 2010 Infant Feeding Survey, only 1% of mothers were breastfeeding exclusively at 6 months and only 5% at 5 months, with even lower percentages in Wales and Northern Ireland (McAndrew *et al.* 2012) (see Table 3.10). This being the case, while it is important for the benefits of breastfeeding to be recognised and promoted, it is also essential that parents have access to sound advice on introduction of complementary foods should they decide to commence earlier than 6 months.

In the 2010 UK Infant Feeding Survey, women were asked about factors that influenced their decision about when to begin to feed their baby solids (McAndrew *et al.* 2012). The most common response, chosen from a prompted list, was the perception that their baby was no longer satisfied with milk feeds (52%). Other responses included: experience with a previous baby (32%), that the baby was able to sit up and hold food in hand (29%), baby waking at night (27%) and advice from a health professional (27%). Advice from friends or relatives and information in leaflets or other materials were also mentioned.

The majority (64%) of women who had already introduced solids by the age of 3 months had based their decision on a belief that the baby was no longer satisfied by milk feeds. However, this was the reason given by only 31% of women who began solids after 5 months.

Those who introduced solids later were more likely to have based their decisions on advice from health professionals (35% in those who introduced solids at 5 months compared to 20% in those who introduced solids at 3 months) or from written information sources (24% vs. 13%) as well as by the baby being able to sit up and hold food (24% vs. 13%) as well as by the baby being able to sit up and hold food (35% vs. 15%).

The Infant Feeding Surveys reveal a marked trend (between 2000 and 2010) towards mothers introducing solid food later in 2010 compared to 2000. In 2000, 85% had introduced solids by 4 months but by 2005 this had fallen to 51% (Bolling *et al.* 2007) and in 2010 was 30% (McAndrew *et al.* 2012). This decline in the practice of early weaning is evident in all countries within the UK. In each country, the proportion of mothers who had introduced solids by 3 months had more than halved between 2000 and 2005 and was further reduced in 2010 (Table 3.11). In 2000, around eight in ten mothers in each country had introduced solids by 4 months; in 2010 the equivalent levels were not reached until 5 months. Only 2% of mothers waited until 6 months of age in 2000

Table 3.11 Proportion of mothers introducing solids during different age periods by country (2005 and 2010)

	Total UK		England		Wales		Scotland		Northern Ireland	
	2005	2010	2005	2010	2005	2010	2005	2010	2005	2010
% who had introduced solids by	%	%	%	%	%	%	%	%	%	%
6 weeks	1	2	1	2	2	2	1	2	2	2
8 weeks	2	2	2	2	3	3	2	3	3	3
3 months (13 weeks)	10	5	9	5	13	9	13	6	11	7
4 months (17 weeks)	51	30	50	28	65	44	60	32	51	35
5 months (22 weeks)	82	75	81	75	88	83	85	74	78	75
6 months (26 weeks)	98	94	98	94	98	96	98	95	98	95
9 months (39 weeks)*	100	99	100	99	100	98	100	99	100	99
Base: All Stage 3 mothers	9416	10768	4563	4935	1582	1804	1666	2119	1605	1910

*Based on a reduced number of cases excluding those babies who had not reached this age by Stage 3.
Source: McAndrew F, Thompson J, Fellows L *et al.* (2012) Infant Feeding Survey 2010. NHS The Information Centre. http://data.gov.uk/dataset/infant-feeding-survey-2010, copyright 2012, with permission from The Health and Social Care Information Centre. All rights reserved.

and 2005, and this increased to 4-6% in 2010 but remained low. Mothers in Wales and began feeding solid foods earlier on average than mothers in other countries: 44% of Welsh babies had been given solids by the age of 4 months compared with 28–35% of babies in the other UK countries.

The foods being given to babies aged 4–6 months were more likely to be commercially prepared than home-prepared, but by 8–10 months home-prepared foods dominated. Compared with 2005, a higher proportion of mothers in 2010 said they avoided the use of salt and honey in their babies' diets but a lower proportion avoided nuts. The majority of mothers avoided the addition of salt completely in the diets of their 8- to 10-month-old babies but the likelihood that salt was used was greater among those mothers classified in the lower occupation groups, as well as among mothers from ethnic minority groups.

Mother's age was also a factor, there being a clear relationship between this and the timing of the introduction of solids. Whereas only 19% of mothers aged 35 or over had begun to introduce solids by 4 months, 57% of babies of teenage mothers were receiving solids by this age and, by 5 months, only 5% of babies with teenage mothers had yet to receive solids (compared to 34% of babies with mothers over 35 years). The survey reveals that between these extremes, there is a linear pattern by mother's age.

Mothers classified as having managerial or professional occupations were also less likely to introduce solids before 4 months (20%) than mothers in intermediate occupational categories (29%), mothers in routine/manual categories (38%) or mothers who had never worked (38%).

Mothers from ethnic minority groups tended to introduce solids later on average than White mothers: 62–69% compared to 77% had introduced solids by 5 months, while Chinese women were least likely to introduce solids before 4 months (19% compared with 30% for White mothers).

Although maternity leave entitlements have increased significantly over the last decade, the introduction of solids was still influenced by whether or not a mother returned to work and the timing of her return.

Robinson and colleagues studied a sample of over 1400 mothers and their infants in the Southampton area; a total of 1173 (82%) of the infants were born before the change in the recommended age of introduction of solid foods, from 4–6 months to 6 months, introduced in May 2003 (Robinson *et al.* 2007). Among the infants born before this date, 38% were introduced to solid foods before 4 months of age, and the remaining 62% by 6 months. A total of 261 infants were born between May and the end of 2003. The proportion of these infants introduced to solid foods before the age of 4 months was lower (30%; $p > 0.02$). Only three (1%) of the 261 infants born after the change in guidance were not introduced to solid food until 6 months (a similar incidence was observed in the Infant Feeding Survey of 2005; Bolling *et al.* 2007). In the study as a whole, the median age at which solid foods were introduced to the infants was 4 months (range 0.7–6 months). This study suggests that the trends seen in the recent Infant Feeding Surveys may be part of a longer-term trend, as evidenced by the findings of studies in the UK conducted during the 1990s.

In the Glasgow longitudinal infant growth study (Savage *et al.* 1998), conducted well before the change in weaning advice (see Section 3.7.2), the median age of introduction of solid food was 11 weeks (range 4–35 weeks). Only 7% of the sample had not introduced solids by age 4 months (the recommended time of weaning at the time of the study). This was similar to that reported for Scotland and the UK in the 1990 Infant Feeding Survey (White *et al.* 1992). There was no significant difference in timing of weaning between boys and girls. Younger mothers tended to introduce solids earlier, solids were introduced later in those of higher socioeconomic status (x^2 test for proportion weaned before 10 weeks and on or after 10 weeks, $p < 0.01$) and in mothers who had higher or further education (Mann-Whitney test, $p < 0.05$); 9% of mothers in social class I and II and 31% in social class III and below had introduced solids by 10 weeks. Breast-fed infants were weaned later than formula-fed infants (median 12 vs. 11 weeks, Mann-Whitney test $p < 0.001$); 8% of mothers who breast-fed introduced solids by 10 weeks compared with 33% of mothers who formula-fed. The infant's weight at 1 month was also related to timing of weaning: heavier infants were weaned earlier. Weight at 1 month was negatively correlated with age at introduction of solids ($p < 0.05$).

In the Avon Longitudinal Study of Parents and Children (ALSPAC) study (data collected in 1992–3 before the change in weaning advice), of the 933 children in the sample at 4 months, only 103 (11%) were not having any solids in their diet (Emmett *et al.* 2000). A significantly lower proportion of children drinking only breast milk were having solids (80%) compared to those having only formula milk (93%) or a combination of breast and formula (94%) ($p < 0.0001$). By 8 months of age, all children were having solids.

Also in ALSPAC, at 4 months of age 91% of the boys were given solids compared with 87% of the girls; 80% of breast-fed infants were given solids compared with 93% of infants who were formula-fed and 94% of infants who were mixed milk fed (Noble and Emmett 2006). In the three 'with solids' groups, 8% of the breast-fed infants had started solids by 3 months of age compared with 20% of the formula-fed and 16% of the mixed-fed group ($p = 0.01$).

In another study conducted in Fife, Scotland in 1999, most women (71%) had breast-fed their infants at least once after delivery, but by 3 months most (86%) had also given their infants formula milk (Alder *et al.* 2004). Only 15% breast-fed exclusively for 12 weeks. At the 12-week interview, 40% said that they had introduced solids (133/338) although 43 of these said that this had been intermittent (they had stopped and restarted). When asked at 12 weeks when they intended to give their infant solid food, most (60%) said at 16 weeks, but 23 (11%) said when their infants were ready. Seven mothers had not thought about when they might introduce solids. In the postal questionnaire follow-up at 20 weeks, 272 of the 286 respondents (95%) had given their babies solids, and in total 278 reported the age at which solids were introduced (Fig. 3.9).

3.9.3 Development of taste preferences and the importance of texture

Previous UK recommendations on introduction of weaning foods stressed the importance of experienc-

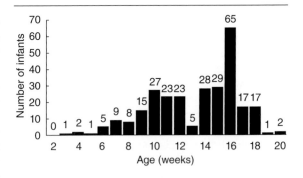

Figure 3.9 Distribution of age at which solids were introduced (combined data from 12-week interview and 20-week postal questionnaire, *n* = 278).
Reproduced from Alder EM, Williams FL, Anderson AS *et al.* (2004) What influences the timing of the introduction of solid food to infants? *British Journal of Nutrition*, **92**, 527–31, with permission from The Nutrition Society.

ing different consistencies of food and different tastes in order to develop strategies for coping with foods of different consistencies and textures – smooth purées, lumpier foods and family foods – and also to develop a repertoire of taste preferences.

The introduction of solid foods has to be in the context of neuromuscular development and the baby's willingness to experience new tastes and textures. Young infants have poor head control, and before about 3 months it is difficult to hold a baby in a position that facilitates their swallowing semi-solid food. Newborn babies suck at food, and before 3 months a baby cannot easily form a bolus of food in the mouth and move the bolus from the front to the back of the mouth. Also, at this age they are not eager to experiment with foods of different flavour, texture or consistency. By 4 months most babies can maintain posture if supported, by 5 months they can usually move soft puréed food from the front of the mouth and swallow it, and by 6 months they are able to chew (Department of Health 1994). Some argue that there are critical developmental stages when these skills are learned and, if the opportunity is missed, teaching older infants to chew can be difficult (Stevenson and Allaire 1991). A critical period for exposure to different textures during weaning has also been proposed (Illingworth and Lister 1964).

Feeding difficulties later in life have been associated with a delay in the introduction of food that contains lumps. In the ALSPAC study, children were divided into three groups based on the age at which they first received lumpy foods: 10.7% before 6 months, 71.7% between 8 and nine months and 17.6% after 10 months, using questionnaire data (Northstone *et al.* 2001). Feeding difficulties at 15 months (e.g. more definite likes and dislikes) were more likely when lumpy solids (chewy foods) were introduced at or after 10 months of age, suggesting that, once weaning onto solids starts, it needs to progress such that lumpy foods are provided by around 9 months. Furthermore, children introduced to lumpy solids after age 9 months, compared to between 6 and 9 months, had significantly more feeding problems and ate less of many of the food groups at age 7 years, in particular all ten categories of fruits and vegetables (Coulthard *et al.* 2009). The authors also reported that there was no evidence that introducing lumpy foods before 6 months, in practice around 5 months, was detrimental. Indeed, those introduced early were more likely to eat fruits and vegetables with bitter and sour tastes and to eat more vegetables more often than those who were given these foods at later ages.

Taste (sweet, sour, salty, bitter and umami, i.e. savoury) preferences have a strong innate component. Sweet, umami and salty substances are preferred, whereas bitter and many sour substances are innately rejected. These innate preferences are suggested to be influenced by pre- and postnatal experiences, via amniotic fluid and breast milk (Mennella *et al.* 2001; Beauchamp and Mennella 2009). Although data suggest that sweet taste is preferred in early infancy and later food choices, a clear association cannot be established yet (Stephen *et al.* 2012).

This research indicates that the introduction of solid foods should not be delayed beyond 6 months because the process is important in helping the baby learn to accept different tastes and textures, and to learn to move food around the mouth and to chew (British Medical Association 2009). As the introduction of solids progresses, the foods provided should gradually be increased in amount and variety so that, by 12 months, solid foods are the main part of the diet, with breast or formula milk making up the balance. Also, foods with a thicker and lumpier texture should be introduced by 9 months to encourage chewing, even before teeth emerge.

3.9.4 Baby-led weaning

The Department of Health advice is that a gradual transition is made from spoon-fed puréed foods and baby rice to foods prepared with a coarser texture, finger foods and eventually consumption of family foods by 12 months of age. In recent years in the UK, a new approach to complementary food introduction, baby-led weaning, is used by some mothers rather than standard weaning methods. The baby-led weaning approach proposes that the standard weaning practice of spoon-feeding puréed foods or baby rice is bypassed in favour of introducing foods in their whole form as finger foods rather than puréed, and that infants self-feed as opposed to being spoon-fed by adults, with reliance on breast milk until the infant has the skills to take nutritionally sufficient amounts (Rapley and Murkett 2008). A recent cross-sectional study of 655 mothers with an only child aged 6–12 months were recruited from the Swansea area in Wales. Approximately half of the study sample were categorised as using the baby-led weaning approach. The results indicated that baby-led weaning was associated with a later introduction of complementary foods, a higher number of milk feeds, increased participation in family mealtimes and fewer maternal concerns about the weaning process (Brown and Lee 2011). In an in-depth study of mothers' experiences by this same team, mothers following this method found it a natural and enjoyable way to introduce complementary food to their infants, convenient and fitting well into family mealtimes. However, they had some concerns such as initial worries about choking, and ongoing issues with mess and waste (Brown and Lee 2011). The success of baby-led weaning depends in large part on the ability of the infant to reach out, pick up and hold food, and put it into the mouth. In a small prospective study from the US, the mean age for 'eating finger foods without gagging' was found to be 8.4 months (range 6–12 months), although the mean age for 'feeds self cracker or cookie' was 7.7 months (range 4–14 months) (Carruth and Skinner 2002). Data from the Gateshead Millennium Study cohort suggest that around half the infants were reaching out for food and beginning to eat finger foods by the age of 6 months and the majority by 8 months. The recommendation of these authors was that a pragmatic approach to weaning should be adopted, based on the child's development. Baby led-weaning may be feasible for the majority of infants but might lead to nutritional problems for those relatively delayed (Wright, Cameron *et al.* 2011). Empirical research on the outcomes of baby-led weaning compared to standard weaning methods is currently sparse, but a very recent study has reported the impact of baby-led weaning compared to traditional spoon feeding on food preferences, picky eating and BMI in children aged 20–78 months. No difference in the proportion of picky eaters was found between the two groups. Those in the baby-led group were more likely to prefer carbohydrate foods. Although most children were in the average or healthy weight categories, there was an increased incidence of underweight in the baby-led group and an increased incidence of obesity in the spoon-fed group. The authors emphasised the need for a large prospective trial of different weaning styles, with greater consideration of varying parental character-

istics, and where infants having had different milk-feeding practices can be compared (Townsend and Pitchford 2012).

3.9.5 Recommendations: specific food types

3.9.5.1 *Milk and dairy products*

In the UK, current advice from the Department of Health is that whole cows' milk is not appropriate as the main drink for infants less than 1 year of age. However, it can be used in foods prepared for babies over 6 months of age. After the age of 1 year, children need less milk than they do at younger ages; smaller drinks of milk should be given in cups or beakers, not bottles. Use of beakers and cups is better for teeth and also helps in skills development. At this age, formula or follow-on milk can be replaced with cows' milk or mothers can continue to breastfeed. About three servings per day of milk, either as a drink or in the form of milk-based dishes, cheese, yogurt or fromage frais, will provide the calcium the child needs to develop strong bones and teeth.

Once the introduction of solids is under way, whole milk and full-fat dairy products (rather than lower-fat versions) are advised until the child is 2; children under 2 need the extra energy and vitamin A that these provide. Semi-skimmed milk can be introduced once the child is 2, provided the child eats well and has a varied diet. Skimmed milk is not considered suitable for children under 5 years of age (Department of Health 2009b).

3.9.5.2 *Other drinks*

The Department of Health suggests that water is the best alternative drink to milk, but that fully breast-fed babies do not need water until they start eating solid food. For babies under 6 months old, cooled boiled water from the mains tap in the kitchen is suggested.

Goats' and sheep's milk are not suitable as drinks for babies under 1 year old, as they do not contain sufficient iron. Provided they are pasteurised, they can be used once a baby is 1 year old and should not be used as a main milk before 2 years of age (www.infantandtoddlerforum.org).

Oat drinks and other plant derived drinks made from soya, pea and almond, for example, (sometimes referred to as 'milks') are not suitable for children under a year and should not be used as a main drink before 2 years of age (www.infantandtoddlerforum. org) (see Section 3.8.1.2 for information on soya formula). The Department of Health advises that rice milk is not suitable for children under 5 years to minimise exposure to inorganic arsenic (Department of Health 2009b).

Citrus fruit juices, such as orange juice or grapefruit juice, are a good source of vitamin C but also contain natural sugars and acids that can cause damage to developing teeth. The Department of Health advises that babies under 6 months should not be given fruit juices. Vitamin C may help with iron absorption, so if the baby is being fed a vegetarian diet (see Section 3.9.8) diluted fruit juice with meals after 6 months is considered acceptable. To prevent tooth decay, fruit juice should be given at mealtimes only.

The Department of Health advises that squashes, flavoured milks and juice drinks are not suitable for young infants as they contain added sugars and so can cause tooth decay even when diluted. If they are given, they should be provided at mealtimes only, diluted well with water and given in a feeder cup rather than a bottle (this is associated with less damage to teeth). It is the frequency of consumption that is of most concern and so drinking times should be kept as short as possible and the frequency restricted. Carbonated soft drinks are relatively acidic and it is thought that they can damage tooth enamel, so they should not be given to infants and toddlers. Diet drinks and 'no added sugar' drinks contain artificial sweeteners and so may be more 'tooth friendly' than other squashes, but they still encourage development of a 'sweet tooth', so are best avoided. These drinks also contain very few nutrients, so the Department of Health recommends milk and water as the preferred drinks for young children. Nevertheless, even if large amounts of dilutable soft drinks containing aspartame, acesulfame K or saccharin are consumed by young children, they would be unlikely to attain intakes that exceed the acceptable daily intake (ADI) for these sweeteners. However, as a precaution, the UK Food Standards Agency issued advice to parents to give young children no more than three beakers (about 180 mL/day) of dilutable soft drinks, or squashes containing the sweetener cyclamate (also known as E952) to avoid any risk of exceeding the ADI (Food Standards Agency (FSA) 2003). It should also be noted that sweeteners cannot be used in foods for infants and young children mentioned in the European Council Directive 89/398/EEC of 3 May 1989, including foods for infants and young children who are not in good health.

Baby and herbal drinks contain added sugars and are not recommended by the Department of Health (Department of Health 2009b).

Tea and coffee are considered unsuitable for infants or young children. Apart from being a source of caffeine, they slightly reduce iron absorption when taken with meals and, if sugar is added, may contribute to tooth decay (Department of Health 2009b).

3.9.6 Recommendations: important nutrients to include in the weaning diet

3.9.6.1 Long-chain fatty acids

Rapid brain development occurs during the last trimester of pregnancy and the first year after birth. The brain and other neural tissue, including the retina, are largely composed of phospholipids which are rich in long-chain polyunsaturated fatty acids, especially docosahexaenoic acid and arachidonic acid. The enzymes required to synthesise these long-chain *n*-3 fatty acids are inactive during fetal life and are thought to be relatively inefficient during early infancy. By the time of weaning, healthy infants are probably able to meet their needs for long-chain polyunsaturated fatty acids provided there is adequate dietary supply of essential fatty acid precursors (Department of Health 1994). Preformed long-chain *n*-3 fatty acids are found in oil-rich fish. The Department of Health's advice is to give boys up to four portions of oil-rich (such as mackerel, salmon and sardines) a week, but to limit girls to no more than two portions a week (Department of Health 2009b) (see Section 3.4.1.3 for recommendations of fatty acids during pregnancy).

3.9.6.2 Iron

Iron is essential for the child's health. Lack of iron can lead to anaemia, which can delay the child's physical and mental development. Iron comes in two forms: haem and non-haem. Haem iron is found in meat and fish and is easily absorbed by the body. Non-haem iron is found in plant foods and is absorbed less efficiently. Even a small amount of meat or fish is useful because it also helps the body to absorb iron from other food sources. Infants who do not eat meat or fish should be given other sources of iron on a frequent basis (e.g. dark green vegetables, breads, beans, lentils and dahl, and dried fruit such as apricots, figs and prunes). Although iron-fortified foods, particularly breakfast cereals, make a substantial contribution to iron intakes in the UK, evidence suggests that foods fortified with elemental iron make little practical contribution to improving iron status. This is probably due to the low solubility of elemental iron and consequently low intestinal uptake (SACN 2010). It is also a good idea to give foods or drinks that are rich in vitamin C at mealtimes, as vitamin C aids the absorption of non-haem iron from non-meat sources. See also Section 3.9.6.3 on zinc.

3.9.6.3 Zinc

Zinc has several important functions including making new cells and enzymes, healing wounds and helping the body to process carbohydrate, fat and protein in food. Zinc and iron (see Section 3.9.6.2) are two micronutrients for which the concentrations in human milk are relatively independent of maternal intake, and for which the older infant is most dependent on complementary foods to meet requirements. In practice, mothers often wean at 6 months onto food such as baby rice, fruit and vegetables and often delay giving meat until 8 or 9 months, which can adversely affect iron and zinc intakes. This is particularly true where mothers continue to breastfeed rather than give formula or follow-on milk, which is fortified with nutrients such as zinc and iron.

3.9.6.4 Vitamin D

Vitamin D occurs naturally in only a few foods such as oil-rich fish (see Chapter 15, Section 15.3.3.1). Most of our vitamin D is obtained from the action of sunlight on the skin. The Department of Health recommends that infants and children are encouraged to play outside in order to expose the skin to gentle sunlight. Human milk has little vitamin D, and supplemental vitamin D is recommended for all infants either via vitamin drops or contained in infant formula or fortified infant foods. The Department of Health recommends vitamin drops starting at 1 month of age and continuing until 5 years of age. In the UK, 'Healthy Start' vouchers and vitamin supplements are available to pregnant women under 18 years and those on low income (www.healthystart. nhs.uk). The Healthy Start children's vitamin drops contain vitamin A, vitamin C and vitamin D. Children receiving >500 mL/day (one pint) of infant formula do not need to take these vitamins (Department of Health 2009b).

3.9.7 Current practice: types of food/drink introduced

3.9.7.1 Foods

Most literature about infant feeding practices relates to the timing of the introduction of solid foods, with relatively less emphasis and hence information on the specific types of solid foods introduced and eaten by infants.

First foods introduced vary with study and country. In the Euro-Growth study, fruit (73%) and cereals (51%) were the first foods given to most infants in the 11 participating countries (Freeman *et al.* 2000). In a study investigating feeding habits in the first year of life in Italy, similar results were found, with 73% having fruit as the first solid food introduced and 64% having cereals. In the All Babies in Southwest Sweden (ABIS) study, data on over 10 000 infants provided by parents interviewed when infants were 1 year of age showed that the most common first foods in this study were vegetables, specifically potatoes, carrots and sweetcorn or products containing these (Brekke *et al.* 2005). Most of the infants in a study from Bavaria in Germany received a mash of vegetable, meat and potato as their first solid food (Rebhan *et al.* 2009).

There are few studies from the UK which report the first type of food introduced. In the Glasgow Longitudinal Infant Growth Study, commercially prepared cereals were the most commonly used first weaning foods, used by 82% of the mothers ($n = 127$). This consisted of baby rice (66%), baby cereal (9%), and rusks (5%). Only six infants (5%) were given fruit or vegetable purées as their first weaning food (Savage *et al.* 1998). In another study from Glasgow, on pre-term infants ($n = 253$), infants were also given cereals as the first food, with 85% receiving baby rice.

Only 3% had vegetables as their first food and 3% fruit (Norris *et al.* 2002).

The 2010 Infant Feeding Survey reported infant feeding practices in terms of proportion fed certain foods at specific ages. For infants aged 4–6 months, the solids given were as likely to be ready-made baby food (58%) as home-made foods (53%) and more likely to be fruit or vegetables (66%). By 8–10 months, however, mothers used commercial brands less often and offered home-prepared foods more often. In the survey, mothers were asked to record all food consumed the day before the interview. Table 3.12 shows in more detail how the nature of the infant diet changed with age. The use of home-made foods tended to increase with age, from 17% for 4–5 months to 80% for 10 months and over (McAndrew *et al.* 2012).

In terms of food types, the majority of infants aged 8 months and over were given breakfast cereals (80%), cheese, yoghurt and fromage frais (68%) and vegetables (80%) at least once a day. Meat and poultry was consumed by the majority (72%) at least once a week, as well as potatoes (65%) and rice/pasta (59%). Over half (53%) of mothers were feeding their infants fish at least once a week, but fish was rarely given on a daily basis (3%).

Foods provided varied by mother's socioeconomic group and ethnic origin. Mothers from managerial and professional occupations were more likely to provide vegetables three or more times a week (97%) compared to 90% of those in routine or manual work and 74% of those who had never worked; for these same groups, chicken was given three or more times per week by 40%, 30% and 22%; fruit by 97%, 90% and 77%; rice/pasta by 52%, 42% and 40%; and fish by 18%, 13% and 17%, respectively. On the other hand, mothers in managerial or professional occupations were less likely to give

Table 3.12 Proportion (%) of babies who had ever been given different types of food, and who had been given different types of food on the day they completed the questionnaire at Stages 2 and 3 of the Survey (UK, 2010)

	Foods ever introduced		Foods given on previous day		Foods given on previous day			
	Stage 2	Stage 3	Stage 2	Stage 3	Stage 2*		Stage 3*	
					Babies aged 4, up to 5 months	Babies aged 5, up to 7 months	Babies aged 8, up to 10 months	Babies aged more than 10 months
Ready-made baby food	58	84	38	44	31	42	45	31
Home-made foods	53	93	28	70	17	35	70	80
Baby rice	79	83	31	9	37	27	8	9
Fruit/vegetables	66	98	46	77	35	53	77	83
Fruit	58	97	34	69	25	40	69	74
Vegetables	55	97	32	58	23	38	57	67
Rusk	42	64	15	14	14	14	13	11
Other foods (*e.g.* yoghurt, fromage frais or breakfast cereal)	46	96	29	76	20	35	76	73
No solids on previous day	n/a	n/a	6	3	9	4	3	4
Base: All mothers at Stage 2/3**	9462	10769	9462	10769	3608	5565	8137	845

*Babies who fell outside these age ranges at Stage 2 and 3 have been excluded.
**The small number of babies who had not been introduced to solids by Stage 3 are treated as not given foods.
Source: Alder EM, Williams FL, Anderson AS *et al.* (2004) What influences the timing of the introduction of solid food to infants? *British Journal of Nutrition*, **92**, 527–31, copyright 2012, with permission from The Health and Social Care Information Centre. All rights reserved.

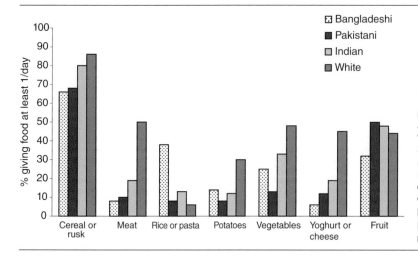

Figure 3.10 Infant feeding practices at age 9 months for Asian mothers compared to white mothers in the UK. Source: Thomas and Avery (1997) Infant Feeding in Asian Families. London. The Stationery Office, copyright 2011. Re-used with the permission of The Health and Social Care Information Centre. All rights reserved.

servings of biscuits, sweets, chocolates, or cakes three times a week (14%) compared to 27% of those in routine and manual work and 30% of those who had never worked; findings for crisps and corn snacks were 19%, 24% and 20% and eggs 6%, 7% and 14%, respectively.

There were also variations with cultural background. Mothers from ethnic minority groups were less likely to regularly give their infants cheese, yoghurt, potatoes, bread, fat spreads/butter, vegetables and fruit. However, Asian mothers were more likely than others to give pulses (beans, lentils and chickpeas) (33% compared with 15% of all mothers). Asian mothers were significantly less likely than other groups to give their infants beef regularly (5 compared with 15% overall).

A more detailed survey of infant feeding in Asian families in the UK was carried out in the 1990s (Thomas and Avery 1997). Mothers were interviewed on four occasions between 1994 and 1996, when their infants were 6 weeks old and at ages 5, 9 and 15 months. The differences between Bangladeshi, Pakistani and Indian practices (and compared to those of White mothers) are shown in Fig. 3.10 for consumption of different types of foods at age 9 months.

The results from these surveys have all been derived using questionnaires on usual practices completed by mothers. They can be compared with studies and surveys where diet has been recorded using more detailed dietary assessment instruments, such as in the ALSPAC 'Child in Focus' subgroup where a three-day diary was completed by 1131 parents for infants at the age of 8 months in 1991–2 (Noble and Emmett 2001), and also the survey of food and nutrients intake of British infants aged 6–12 months from 1986/7, published in 1992, which reported the intakes of 488 infants (Mills and Tyler 1992). Although the data are older, these surveys seem to indicate similar proportions of infants consuming many basic foods such as bread, breakfast cereals, vegetables and fruit at least three times a week, as in the 2005 Infant Feeding Survey (Table 3.13). The forthcoming Diet and Nutrition Survey of Infants and Young Children (DNSIYC) to be published in 2013, will provide up-to-date information of the diets of children of these ages.

3.9.7.2 Drinks

Vitamin C-enriched fruit drinks consumed with food may be useful to aid the absorption of iron from a meal. In the 2010 Infant Feeding Survey, 37% of the mothers had given drinks other than milk to their infants by the age of 6 weeks and 81% by 6 months, with mothers in Wales and Northern Ireland more likely than others to give other drinks, especially at younger ages (at 6 weeks, Wales 45%, Northern Ireland 55%). Younger mothers were more likely to

Table 3.13 Percentage of consumers of foods by infants at months of age in ALSPAC (Children in Focus) (Noble and Emmett 2001)[1] and Food and Nutrients Intake of British infants aged 6–12 months (Mills and Tyler 1992)[2]

	% consumers			% consumers	
	ALSPAC (8 months)	Mills & Tyler (6–9 months)		ALSPAC (8 months)	Mills & Tyler (6–9 months)
Breakfast cereals	71	66	Meat, meat products, dishes	58	61
Bread	66	65	Beef	25	NA
White	44	NA	Lamb	11	NA
Brown and wholemeal	NA	NA	Pork	7	NA
Milk	58	74	Poultry	30	NA
Whole	49	NA	Fish, fish products, dishes	25	35
Semi-skimmed	9	NA	Vegetables	75	66
Yoghurt	45	37	Potatoes	45	70
Fat spread and oils	56	57	Fruit	66	67
Eggs and egg dishes	16	55	Banana	52	NA
			Fruit juices and drinks	22	67
Commercial infant food (cans and jars)	74	74	Instant food (dried)	58	70

[1]Dietary assessment was carried out using three-day diary.
[2]Dietary assessment was carried out using a seven-day diary.
NA, not available.

give other drinks, with 64% of mothers aged under 20 giving these by 6 weeks and 94% by 6 months, compared to 24% at 6 weeks and 69% at 6 months for those aged 35 years and over (McAndrew *et al.* 2012).

The ALSPAC 'Children in Focus' study has also investigated drinks of infants specifically, at both 4 and 8 months of age (Emmett *et al.* 2000). At 4 months, the most frequently consumed drink was formula milk (69.7% had at least one formula feed over the previous 24-hour period), followed by breast milk (43% had at least one breastfeed), fruit drinks (e.g. squash/cordial, juice, diet squash) (24.2%) and herbal drinks and herbal teas (14.6%). At 8 months, 71.4% of infants had at least one formula feed over the previous 24-hour period, 55.8% had had a drink classed in the squashes/cordial group, which included commercial baby fruit drinks, and 22.9% had at least one breastfeed. The animal milk consumed by 21.8% of infants at 8 months was mainly whole cows' milk, although two infants had skimmed, five had semi-skimmed and two had goats' milk at some point during the previous 24-hour period. Infants aged under 1 year should not be given cows' milk as the

main drink, and goats' milk is not recommended in any form (Department of Health 2009b) (see Section 3.9.5).

3.9.8 Vegetarian diets

If a child is brought up on a diet without meat (vegetarian) or without any food of animal origin (vegan), they should receive two or three portions of vegetable protein every day (e.g. finely ground nuts or smooth nut butter, beans, pulses, lentils, well-cooked eggs, tofu or soya pieces) to ensure adequate protein and iron. Whole nuts should not be given to children under 5, as they could choke. Finely ground nuts or smooth nut butter are suitable alternatives. It is also important that a mixture of protein sources is provided, for example a combination of pulses and cereals, to ensure that all the essential amino acids are provided in sufficient quantities. Some vegetarian diets can be high in fibre, very bulky and so of lower energy (and possibly nutrient) density. This may make it difficult for young children to meet their nutrient needs as their appetites may prevent sufficient food

Table 3.14 Foods to avoid during the introduction of solids

Food	Advice
Salt	Salt should not be added to foods given to babies because kidney development is incomplete and hence capacity to excrete salt is limited. Babies under 1 year should have less than 1 g salt per day. For children aged 1 to 3 years, the maximum amount is 2 g of salt per day, and for children aged 4 to 6 years, the maximum is 3 g of salt per day. Addition of salt to foods especially manufactured for babies is not allowed. Some foods, such as cheese, sausages and bacon, are relatively high in salt, so should be limited in quantity. Sauces, soups, gravy and ready-made porridge can sometimes be high in salt, so it is also advised to exclude these foods from a baby's diet.
Sugar	Sweet foods and drinks can encourage a 'sweet tooth' and also have the potential to damage teeth as they emerge. Sugar should only be added to foods if it is really necessary, e.g. stewed fruit. Sweet puddings, biscuits, sweets and ice-creams are not recommended for babies under 1 year old.
Honey	Honey should not be given to babies, even for easing coughs, until they are 1 year old. Very occasionally honey can cause infant botulism. Honey is also rich in sugars, which means it can encourage a 'sweet tooth' and potentially lead to tooth decay.
Nuts	Whole nuts and roughly chopped nuts, including peanuts, should not be given to children under 5 because they may cause choking.
Low-fat, low-calorie and high-fibre foods	It is not advisable to give 'low-fat' or 'low-calorie' foods to babies because these are likely to be of low energy density. Similarly, high-fibre versions of foods (e.g. brown rice, wholemeal pasta or bran-enriched breakfast cereals) should not be given during the early stages as they are more bulky and the fibre may limit the absorption of important minerals such as calcium and iron. However, once a varied diet is accepted and provided the child has a good appetite, these foods can gradually be introduced closer to the age of 5.
Shark, swordfish and marlin	Shark, swordfish and marlin should be avoided. This is because the levels of mercury in these fish can affect a baby's nervous system. Raw shellfish should also be avoided, to reduce the risk of food poisoning.
Eggs	Raw or lightly cooked eggs should not be given to babies. Eggs can be given to babies over 6 months, but they should be thoroughly cooked until both the white and yolk are solid.

Source: Department of Health (2009b).

being consumed at mealtimes. To make sure that all the child's nutritional needs are met, they can be given smaller and more frequent main meals, with one or two snacks in between. It is also important to ensure they are getting enough calcium, vitamin B_{12} and vitamin D. Vitamin drops (containing vitamin A, vitamin C and vitamin D) are especially important up to 5 years of age. In the UK, vitamin drops that include these vitamins are available to some women through the 'Healthy Start' scheme (see Section 3.9.6.4) (www.healthystart.nhs.uk).

3.9.9 Vegan diets

Care should be taken when feeding children on a vegan diet because the challenges described above are accentuated. Supplements may be required and advice from a dietitian or doctor should be sought before starting a child on solids (Department of

Health 2009b). For mothers who are breastfeeding and eating a vegan diet, it is especially important that they take a vitamin D supplement. They may also need extra vitamin B_{12}.

3.9.10 Foods to avoid during introduction of solids

The advice on foods from the Department of Health is shown in Table 3.14. Information about drinks is given in Section 3.9.5.2.

3.9.11 Current practice: foods avoided during introduction of solids

In the 2010 Infant Feeding Survey, the foods which mothers avoided giving to their infants were consistent with health guidelines; the principal ingredients omitted being salt (54%), nuts (41%), sugar (38%), honey (19%) and eggs (12%) results that indicated that mothers were more cautious in 2010 than in 2005 about some ingredients, but less so about others, like nuts (McAndrew *et al.* 2012).

The most common reasons for avoiding giving foods were concerns about allergies (36%), belief that the food was not beneficial (27%), that it was harmful for the child (21%) or that the baby was too young (17%). In relation to specific foods, omission of sugar from the diet was not beneficial and bad for teeth; additives were considered not beneficial, with a preference to give fresh or organic food; dairy products and eggs were linked to allergies; and for honey there were concerns about food poisoning, the baby was too young and the mother had been given advice to not to give it.

The large majority of mothers avoided the use of salt completely in the diets of infants 8 months and over, although the use of salt was higher among those in lower socioeconomic groups and those from ethnic minority groups. While only 9% of White mothers never used salt, this proportion was 63% for Asian mothers, 62% for those of Chinese or other ethnic origin, 73% for Black mothers and 84% for mothers of mixed ethnic origin. However, no more than 10% of mothers from each of these ethnic groups said that they used salt 'often'.

3.10　Allergy

3.10.1　Development of allergies

Under normal circumstances, a baby rapidly becomes tolerant (non-responsive) to the many proteins that it encounters in the early days and months of its life. This process is known as the development of tolerance (see Chapter 13, Section 13.8). The mechanisms that underpin this process are not fully understood and work is underway to establish whether, for example, the timing of the introduction of foods is of importance in prompting normal tolerance. It has been suggested that there are critical windows in which presence of an allergen can induce tolerance rather than an adverse response (see Chapter 13, Section 13.8). The issue of the potential benefits of the early introduction of allergenic foods into the diet of children is currently being investigated by two major clinical intervention trials (the Learning Early About Peanut Allergy (LEAP) study [www.leapstudy.co.uk] and the Enquiring About Tolerance (EAT) study [www.eatstudy.co.uk]) (see Chapter 13, Section 13.8).

It is also unclear why most childhood allergies disappear after 12–24 months (e.g. milk or egg allergy) while others are typically present for life (e.g. peanut allergy). Another aspect that is poorly understood is the relative importance of diet in the development of allergic diseases. Although it is recognised that diet can aggravate existing conditions such as asthma and atopic dermatitis, many other factors may also be involved. Similarly, the benefit of dietary restriction in the treatment of these conditions is uncertain, particularly among adults. This is partly because it is difficult to totally exclude a food or ingredient in studies designed to investigate this.

The commonest allergies are to cows' milk protein, egg, soya, wheat, nuts and shellfish. Diagnosis is based on history, skin-prick testing, the measurement of food-specific IgE antibodies, patch tests and food challenge testing. The latter should be carried out using a blinded format, and placebo controls (British Medical Association 2009).

3.10.2　Peanut allergy

The reports of peanut-induced allergic reactions associated with the first known exposure to peanuts suggest that infants can become sensitised to peanuts early in life, perhaps through breastfeeding, via skin lesions (including via some skin ointments and oils used for atopic children), or via the respiratory system following exposure to peanut allergen in their immediate environment or as an unrecognised cross-sensitisation to similar allergens. There is also some evidence that sensitisation could happen *in utero* but a recent review commissioned by the Food Standards Agency has thrown doubt on this (Thompson *et al.* 2010) (see Section 3.4.1.6 for revised advice). Factors that can predispose an individual to peanut allergy include family and personal history of atopy, age and dietary exposure at a vulnerable stage. Atopic individuals with asthma seem to be at increased risk of developing severe food allergy reactions. See Chapter 13, Section 13.6.4 and Section 13.8 for more details on peanut allergy.

3.10.3　Coeliac disease

Coeliac disease is a permanent autoimmune condition, triggered in susceptible individuals by the presence of gluten in the diet, derived from wheat, rye or barley. Less invasive blood testing has provided a new (and increased) estimate of the prevalence of coeliac disease. It has been estimated that in the Western world, 1 in 100 people suffer from coeliac disease, many without knowing it (Rewers 2005; Mustalahti *et al.* 2010). Results from a mass screening project carried out in four European countries (Finland, Germany, Italy and UK) also showed that around 1% of the general population are affected by this disorder (Mustalahti *et al.* 2010). Most of those affected are asymptomatic or have mild signs and symptoms (Silano *et al.* 2010).

In recent years, evidence has emerged to suggest that the timing of the introduction of gluten to the diet and the pattern of breastfeeding may play a role in the development of coeliac disease in predisposed individuals. A systematic review found consistent evidence from six case–control studies that longer duration of breastfeeding, and breastfeeding at the time of introduction of gluten-containing foods, protected against the later development of coeliac disease (Akobeng *et al.* 2006).

Another contributory factor may be the amount of gluten introduced. A unique epidemic in Sweden in the 1980s, concomitant with decreases in incidence elsewhere, was found to be associated with revised feeding guidelines which stressed high intakes of breads (Silano *et al.* 2010). On the basis of the information to date, the European Society for Paediatric Gastroenterology, Hepatology and Nutrition (ESPGHAN) recommends avoidance of both early (< 4 months) and late (> 7 months) introduction of gluten and that small amounts should be introduced while the child is still being breast-fed (Silano *et al.* 2010).

This timing has been agreed by the European Food Safety Authority (EFSA) which produced a Scientific Opinion in 2009, that included a conclusion that 'presently available data on the risk of coeliac disease and type 1 diabetes mellitus support the timing of the introduction of gluten-containing food (preferably while still breastfeeding), not later than six months of age'. The timing of introduction of gluten-containing foods has been debated by the SACN subgroup on Maternal and Child Nutrition, since the recommendation of EFSA is inconsistent with the UK and

WHO recommendation to exclusively breastfeed until 6 months of age. In March 2011, the Committee on Toxicology (COT) and SACN published a joint statement following a recent examination of the available evidence to see whether the timing of introducing gluten into an infant's diet affects their risk of developing coeliac disease and also type 1 diabetes (SACN & COT 2011). The statement concluded that the currently available evidence is insufficient to support recommendations about the appropriate timing of introduction of gluten into the infant diet beyond three completed months of age, for either the general population or high-risk sub-populations. Their conclusions will inform a review to be conducted by SACN on complementary and young child feeding, which will include a critical appraisal of existing recommendations (NHS Choices 2011), regarding the appropriate timing for introduction of solids. SACN began work on this review in early 2011.

3.10.4 Cows' milk protein allergy

In comparison to feeding cows' milk formula, there is evidence that exclusive breastfeeding during the first 4–6 months of life reduces the risk of cows' milk protein allergy and most other severe allergic manifestations during early infancy (Saarinen and Kajosaari 1995).

3.11 Conclusions

The characteristics of pregnant women, such as age and ethnic group, as well as the diet and nutrient intake of women before becoming pregnant, and during pregnancy and lactation, have an important role in early life development. The timing and type of complementary foods at weaning also play key role in both the development of a wide range of tastes and textures of foods as well as physical development of the infant. It is evident that many of the food and nutrient recommendations are not being met, highlighting the need for increased nutritional education and awareness as well as providing support for women before, during and after pregnancy.

3.12 Key points

- Estimates indicate around one in five (19%) women of childbearing age in England are obese (BMI ≥ 30) and one in 20 women (5%) delivering in 2009 had a BMI ≥ 35 at any time in pregnancy. It is vital to reverse the trend in obesity in pregnancy to lessen the burden on maternity and health services and to improve the health of mothers and offspring in future generations.

- National surveys show that the majority of women of childbearing age do not obtain the recommended intake of 400 μg/day of folic acid from food and supplements. In many countries where supplementation is recommended, data indicate that less than half of the women have taken any folic acid supplements before becoming pregnant, with some studies showing less than 10%.

- Low vitamin D status is common in pregnancy. In the UK, pregnant and lactating women are advised to take daily vitamin D supplements containing 10 μg (400 IU). The awareness and compliance of women regarding vitamin D supplementation is low. This is particularly relevant for high-risk women such as women with darker skin tone or women who are housebound or cover most of their skin.

- The use of supplements during lactation is encouraged in many countries; however, information about how well lactating mothers meet recommendations is even less available than for pregnancy. Folate is one of the nutrients commonly found to be low in diets of lactating women, although zinc, calcium, iron, vitamin A, vitamin C, vitamin D, vitamin E and thiamin have also been found to be below the recommended intake.

- Prior to 2001, the WHO global recommendation was that infants should be exclusively breast-fed for between 4 and 6 months before the introduction of complementary foods. Following an Expert Consultation in March 2001 to discuss the scientific evidence on exclusive breastfeeding, the WHO recommended exclusive breastfeeding for 6 months, with introduction of complementary foods and continued breastfeeding thereafter. Like many countries, the UK has adopted this recommendation, but compliance with exclusive breastfeeding for 6 months is low.

- The timing and type of weaning foods introduced is important to help the neuromuscular development of the baby as well as influencing the baby's willingness to experience new tastes and textures. Research indicates that the introduction of solid foods should not be delayed beyond 6 months, with foods with a thicker and lumpier texture being introduced by 9 months to encourage chewing, even before teeth emerge.

3.13 Recommendations for future research

- In the UK, at present, there are no formal, evidence-based guidelines from the UK government or professional bodies on what constitutes appropriate weight gain during pregnancy. Instead, US Institute of Medicine guidelines are often used by UK health professionals as a guide. Research is needed to inform UK guidelines on the optimal weight gain during pregnancy for women in different BMI categories.
- The Department of Health advise a gradual transition from spoon-fed puréed foods and baby rice to foods prepared with a coarser texture, finger foods and eventually consumption of family foods by 12 months of age. The baby-led weaning approach proposes that the standard weaning practice of spoon-feeding puréed foods or baby rice is bypassed in favour of introducing foods in their whole form as finger foods rather than puréed, and infants self-feed as opposed to spoon-feeding. Although sparse, some research has suggested benefits of baby-led weaning compared to standard weaning practice, but further research is needed in this area. In particular, there is a need for a large prospective trial of different weaning styles, with greater consideration of varying parental characteristics, and where infants having had different milk-feeding practices can be compared (Townsend and Pitchford).

3.14 Key references

British Medical Association (2009) *Early Life Nutrition and Long Life Health*. Available at www.derbyshirelmc.org.uk/Guidance/Early%20Life%20Nutrition%20and%20Lifelong%20Health.pdf (accessed 4 January 2013).

Department of Health (1994) *Weaning and the Weaning Diet*. Report of the Working Group on the Weaning Diet of the Committee on Medical Aspects of Food Policy. Report on Health and Social Subjects No 45. London, HMSO.

Department of Health (2009b) *Birth to Five*. London, Department of Health.

McAndrew F, Thompson J, Fellows L, Large A, Speed M, Renfrew MJ (2012) Infant Feeding Survey 2010. NHS Information Centre. Available at http://data.gov.uk/dataset/infant-feeding-survey-2010 (accessed 15 January 2013).

National Institute for Health and Clinical Excellence (NICE) (2010) *NICE Public Health Guidance 27: Dietary interventions and physical activity interventions for weight management before, during and after pregnancy*. London, NICE.

Yngve and Sjostrom (2001) Breastfeeding in countries of the European Union and EFTA: current and proposed recommendations, rationale, prevalence, duration and trends. *Public Health Nutrition*, **4**, 631–45.

Appendix 3.1: Historical perspective on breastfeeding and artificial feeding

Breastfeeding

Through review of paediatric and midwifery texts between the sixteenth and eighteenth centuries, historical studies have shown that prior to the eighteenth century breastfeeding continued into the second and third years of life in European countries, as it often does in the developing world today. Towards the end of the eighteenth century, a reduction in duration of breastfeeding to about 9–12 months of age occurred, most likely a result of industrialisation and urbanisation, but also because of developments in artificial feeding in the form of better milk substitutes and improved feeding vessels. Physicians began to specialise in paediatrics and childcare and there were growing opinions that breast feeding for extended periods was unnecessary and could actually be harmful for women. At the same time, the use of wet nurses to feed children by the upper classes was reduced, shortening the period of breastfeeding in this social sector. Hence for a variety of reasons, including the availability and social acceptability of artificial feeding, the duration of breastfeeding began to be reduced, and earlier weaning also became a viable proposition (Fildes 1982).

As the twentieth century progressed, both developments in artificial formulations and increased research comparing breast and formula feeding contributed to further reductions in the duration of breastfeeding in Western populations. Studies from the 1930s to 1950s concluded that there were few differences between breast-fed and bottle-fed babies up to the end of the first year of life and, although in some cases bottle-fed babies showed somewhat greater weight gain, this was perceived positively. Indeed there was debate that breast-fed infants were undernourished, while others suggested breast-fed babies weighed less because they were more vigorous (Mackay 1957). Few differences in the prevalence of infectious diseases such as respiratory illness or gastroenteritis were seen in studies from both the US and the UK (Norval 1947; Stevenson 1949; Douglas 1950; Stewart & Westropp 1953). Neonatal mortality rates fell dramatically through this period in spite of increases in formula feeding and was attributed to improvements in hygienic standards and drugs to deal with infection (Mackay 1957).

In spite of the now accepted psychological advantages of breastfeeding for both mother and infant, artificial feeding became very popular; it required less effort for the mother, and gave her more freedom for other tasks and for employment. Following the Second World War, breastfeeding continued to decline through the 1950s and 1960s, with the lowest frequency in the late 1960s. Howie and McNeilly reported the percentage of mothers breastfeeding at the time of discharge from the maternity hospital in Edinburgh to be 50% in 1960 but about 20% by 1968/9 (Howie and McNeilly 1980). Wadsworth and colleagues also noted the declines by comparing three birth cohorts of the period, those born in 1946, 1958 and 1970 (Wadsworth *et al.* 2003), as shown in Table 3.15.

In the US, similar trends in breastfeeding rates were seen. For women born in the 1920s, two-thirds breast-fed their first infant; for women born in the late 1940s and early 1950s, only one-quarter did so. Hence over 70% of firstborn infants in the 1930s were breast-fed, while this figure was less than 30% for the late 1960s and early 1970s, with the lowest point in 1972 (Wright and Schanler 2001). Less than 10% of mothers in the 1973 National Survey of Family Growth breast-fed for 3 months or more (Hirschman and Hendershot 1979). The most precipitous declines were seen in Black women, those with less than 12 years of education and those who had never worked outside the home.

The 1970s saw a plateauing of this decline in both the UK and US. The health benefits of breastfeeding were being recognised through further research and better data in relation to infectious disease. The relationship between mode of feeding and obesity was being recognised, as was the role of breastfeeding as a natural contraceptive extending the duration of postpartum amenorrhoea. The potential protective effect of breastfeeding for later breast cancer risk was also being proposed and investigated. All these factors led to an increase in breastfeeding rates in the 1970s. While these have continued, there have been difficulties in some groups and challenges for those returning to employment, especially full-time, within months of delivery. In Sheffield, for example, there was a steady rise in the proportion of mothers successfully breastfeeding during the 1970s, but the 1980s saw a progressive and rapid decline in the number intending to breastfeed and actually breastfeeding at 1 month (Emery *et al.* 1990). While the

Table 3.15 Breastfeeding rates for cohort members in the 1946, 1958 and 1970 birth cohorts

	1946 cohort		1958 cohort		1970 cohort	
	Men	Women	Men	Women	Men	Women
	%	%	%	%	%	%
Never breast-fed	24	25	31	30	62	62
Breast-fed for < 1 month	14	12	24	25	17	16
Breast-fed for ≥ 1 month	61	63	44	44	21	22
N (100%)	5841	5426	4862	5049	4325	4557

Source: Wadsworth *et al.* (2003).

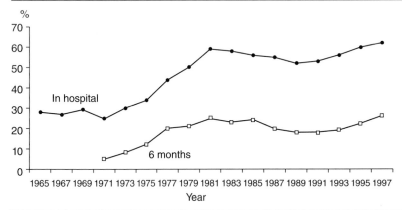

Figure 3.11 US rates of breastfeeding initiation (in hospital) and breastfeeding duration (6 months) from 1965 to 1997.
Data from Wright A & Schanler R (2001) The resurgence of breastfeeding at the end of the second millennium. *Journal of Nutrition*, **131**, 421S–5S, with permission from the American Society for Nutrition.

largest decline was seen in Asian mothers, no one factor could explain this decline. The US also saw a decline in the 1980s after rising from the 1970s, and the rate remained relatively static between the early 1980s and 1995 (Wright and Schanler 2001). In 1997, roughly 60% of US mothers initiated breastfeeding, with over 20% breastfeeding at 6 months and nearly 15% at 12 months (Wright and Schanler 2001). Data from the Ross Mothers' Surveys is shown in Fig. 3.11 (Wright and Schanler 2001).

One of the reasons given for the declines in breast-feeding rate in the 1950s and 1960s was the greater proportion of women in employment, but the increases since the 1970s have occurred in spite of substantial increases in women in the workforce with children less than 1 year of age. Hence the role of employment, while contributory, is manageable with appropriate coping systems in place. Rather than

employment, the increase in rate since the 1970s has been attributed to the growing understanding of the benefits of breastfeeding as outlined above, a growth in the movement towards 'natural' birth and feeding, and promotion of breastfeeding to low-income groups (Wright and Schanler 2001).

There is less information about breastfeeding rates in the developing world than in developed countries. For many decades, breastfeeding in the developing world has traditionally extended for many more months than in Western countries, but communications, development and availability of infant formula may have brought about reductions in breastfeeding duration. Grummer-Strawn carried out an analysis of 15 developing countries which had taken part in both the World Fertility Study in the late 1970s and the Demographic and Health Survey in the late 1980s. Between these two time points, breastfeeding rates showed increases in 11 of the 15 countries, particularly in Latin America where duration, on average about 6–14 months in the 1970s, was shorter than in the African countries assessed (averages in the 1970s of 16–20 months) and Asia and the Pacific (average duration 20–27 months) (Grummer-Strawn 1996). Hence even in developing countries, where breastfeeding duration is much longer than in the West, increases have been seen since the 1970s. Grummer-Strawn cites reduced family size and hence longer feeding duration as well as the economic downturn in the 1980s, limiting purchase of breast milk substitutes, as the main reasons for the increases seen, although the benefits of breastfeeding in these countries were also thought to have had an effect (Grummer-Strawn 1996).

Artificial infant formula

Prior to the nineteenth century, alternatives to breast milk were limited to animal milks or starchy concoctions made from bread or flour (Wickes 1953). Infant formulas were introduced in the nineteenthth century and became available in both Europe and the US. They were developed to mimic the chemical composition of breast milk, but most were based on cow's milk, either condensed or evaporated (Nestlé 1919). Dehydrated milks were first developed in about 1835 by Newton and, in 1847, Grimsdale took out a patent on evaporated milk (Wickes 1953). Chemists Justus Liebig and Henri Nestlé invented and launched patent baby foods in the 1860s, Nestlé producing the first condensed milk in 1866 (Wickes 1953; Weaver 2008). The roller process for drying milk was first introduced in Sweden, with spray drying being used in France. By 1902, both drying processes were widely used and continue to be used in the formulation of infant formula (Wickes 1953). By the early 1900s, many brands of infant feeds were available and advertised to both the medical professions and the public (Weaver 2008). One of the prominent companies in the UK, Allen & Hanbury's, developed the 'Allenbury system' in the early years of the twentieth century, with products based on human milk composition, considering cow's milk too high in casein for human infants. The system consisted of three different milks for different stages of infancy, with those for older ages having added components, such as minerals and soluble carbohydrates (Haydon 1919). As the twentieth century progressed, two types of infant formulas were typically used as alternatives to breast milk: home-prepared formulas and commercially prepared formulas (Fomon 2001).

Homemade formulas: These were popular around the 1930s to early 1940s, particularly in the US. They were prepared by mixing evaporated milk or fresh cows' milk with water and a carbohydrate source. A typical evaporated milk formula, as prepared in 1949, included evaporated milk, water and corn syrup or sucrose. A formula mix like this would provide around 67 kcal/100 mL, with proportions of energy from protein of 15%, carbohydrate of 42% and fat 43%. The evaporated milk or cows' milk was in some cases fortified with vitamin D. By the late 1960s, less than 10% of infants in the US were fed home-prepared formulas. Protein content of a number of widely used formulas ranged from 3.3 to 4.0 g/100 kcal and several formulas recommended for use in management of infants with diarrhoea provided 5.7–6.3 g/100 kcal (Fomon 2001).

Commercially prepared formulas: With the decline in breastfeeding, there was increasing use of infant formula in the UK after the Second World War. However, by the 1970s, there remained little regulation about the composition, description or labelling of infant foods. In 1974, a working group was set up by the Committee on Medical Aspects of Food Policy (COMA), to review infant feeding practice and make recommendations. Part of this work was to recommend criteria for infant food if human milk was not available. The working group report, published in 1980, determined that such milk should be able to be reconstituted easily and be acceptable to the infant. When correctly prepared, the reconstituted feed should:

(1) promote growth and development, and maintain a physical state which is as close as possible to that of the healthy breast-fed infant;

(2) be of such composition that it can be used as the sole food for young infants;

(3) be such that the nutritional needs of the growing infant are met by progressive increases in the volume of feed rather than by increases in its concentration or the addition of supplementary nutrients;

(4) contain no ingredients in amounts which are toxic;

(5) be free from harmful microorganisms;

(6) have minimal potential for allergic reactions;

(7) contain the minimum number of food additives (Committee on Medical Aspects of Food Policy (COMA) 1980).

The committee determined that such criteria were difficult to apply in practice because comprehensive knowledge on the nutritional requirements for growth and development of young infants was lacking, the relative importance of nutrition versus other factors, such as genetic and environmental factors, on growth and health was not fully understood, and because the effects of processing and storage on nutritional value of such milks was not fully known. In spite of this, the committee provided guidelines for nutrient composition in artificial milks for the first time; the levels proposed were in line with the composition of human milk, but with differences for some nutrients because of differences in bioavailability between human milk and manufactured products. It acknowledged that some of these values would likely change with increasing scientific and clinical knowledge (COMA 1996).

The European Commission Scientific Committee for Food (ECSCF) published its first report on the requirements of infant formulas based on cow's milk in 1983 (Commission of the European Communities 1983) and in 1989 a further report on formula based on soya (Commission of the European Communities 1989). Its recommendations were similar to those in the 1980 UK report, and provided the basis for EU and UK regulations. The Codex Alimetarius of the United Nations' Food and Agriculture Organization and the World Health Organization also provides guidance on infant formula composition. Its standards have been in place since 1981, and were revised in 2007 (Codex Alimentarius 2007), with considerable debate (Koletzko and Shamir 2006).

4
Mechanisms and Pathways of Critical Windows of Development

4.1 Introduction

During pregnancy, the fetus is reliant on the mother for its nutrition. It seems obvious, therefore, that maternal nutrition will alter that of the developing fetus. It also seems reasonable to assume that there are periods in development when particular organs are most sensitive to stress. We have termed these periods 'critical windows'. In this chapter, we examine briefly how development occurs and how changes in the environment can result in alterations in development.

Embryo development has been the subject of intensive study over many years in both humans and, either as models for human development or in their own right, animals. As such, it is beyond the scope of this chapter to give more than a brief overview, putting the experimental and other data relating to critical windows into context.

4.2 Embryo stages

At its initiation, the embryo is comprised of cells which have the capacity to form many different final cell types. These are often referred to as stem cells (Fig. 4.1). For convenience, embryo development has been divided into 23 different stages – the 'Carnegie stages' (O'Rahilly and Müller 1999). This classification has significant value in terms of defining development and developmental stages and will, in future,

be helpful in terms of defining how nutritional imbalances can interact with development. It is, of course, difficult to induce nutritional deficiencies with tight time windows, since the mother will mobilise stores and increase uptake of nutrients to minimise the effects. However, some studies have been carried out using both *in vivo* and *in vitro* models. These are examined in more detail below.

4.3 Development of placenta

As the embryo develops, the placenta begins to play an increasingly important role, eventually becoming the pipeline for nutrient transport and waste removal for the developing fetus. Placental development is often overlooked as a target for changing growth and health trajectories in pregnancy. Nonetheless, it is an important aspect of normal development. Not only does the placenta have the central transport function, for micronutrients as well as macronutrients (Jones *et al.* 2006a; Jones *et al.* 2006b; McArdle *et al.* 2008), it is a producer of an extremely wide range of hormones and growth factors, and aberrations of production can result in serious problems. Interestingly, many of these transporters are under the control of hormones that are implicated in the development of the fetal programming phenotype (Jones *et al.* 2006b).

Using the term 'placenta' as if all placentas are the same is a gross over-simplification. There are at least

Nutrition and Development: Short- and Long-Term Consequences for Health, First Edition. Edited by the British Nutrition Foundation.
© 2013 the British Nutrition Foundation. Published 2013 by Blackwell Publishing Ltd.

Stem cells represent natural units of embryonic development and tissue regeneration. Stem cells are defined as cells:
  (1) that can divide without limit;
  (2) that are visibly undifferentiated;
  (3) whose progeny include both further stem cells and cells destined to differentiate.

There are two types of stem cells: embryonic stem cells and tissue stem cells (often called adult stem cells). Embryonic stem cells possess the capacity for unlimited self-renewal and the potential to differentiate into virtually any cell type in the body. Tissue stem cells are found in the postnatal animal and are thought to be committed to form one particular cell type.

Figure 4.1   Description of stem cells.

four different types of placenta, classified originally by Grosser in the middle of the last century (Page 1993). These are then subdivided further into, for example, diffuse, cotyledonary or discoid. This form is not necessarily fixed throughout fetal life. For example, the human placenta varies from diffuse at early stages to discoid later in gestation. Additionally, there are differences in blood flow pattern – counter-current in some case, co-current in others. In terms of being able to understand how the placenta works, there are some problems with all the animal models used: sheep, rats or mice. However, as long as the differences are taken into account, valuable information can generally be obtained.

In a recent review, Anthony Carter examines the evolution of the placenta (Mess and Carter 2007). He concentrates on its relation to gas exchange, specifically oxygen, but a similar analysis can be carried out for most nutrients. In essence, the major differences that occur do not fundamentally alter their functional facility. However, the differences can be significant in terms of the effect that nutritional stress may have on their ability to function properly. This has to be considered carefully when carrying out experimental studies in model organisms.

Human placentas fall into the villous haemochorial placenta classification. There is one major layer of cells between the maternal and fetal circulations. This is a syncytial layer, the syncytiotrophoblast, consisting of cytotrophoblast cells that have fused together. Many of the experimental animals commonly used for programming studies, such as the rat and the mouse, also have haemochorial placentas, but others may be di- or trichorial, with two or three layers separating the two circulations.

Sheep have a different type of placenta. Theirs is an epitheliochorial placenta, which forms in cotyle-

dons. In some intriguing studies relating nutrition in pregnant adolescent sheep, Wallace and co-workers have shown that the relative amounts of fetal and maternal material in the cotyledons change (Wallace *et al.* 2002). The experimental model involves over-nourishing adolescent sheep that have been made pregnant by *in vitro* fertilisation. During the period of pregnancy, the dams continue to grow. The overfeeding results in reduced placental growth and very small lambs, who will go on to show many other abnormalities (Wallace *et al.* 2006). The data derived from these experiments show clearly that it is reduced nutrient supply and oxygen availability that cause these problems (Wallace *et al.* 2006).

The placenta, irrespective of its anatomy, must be capable of transferring gases, nutrients and other compounds from mother to fetus and of eliminating wastes to the maternal circulation. Additionally, it is also a very active endocrine organ, producing hormones, growth factors and autocrine molecules that act on both the mother and the fetus. Anything that alters the ability of the placenta to accomplish these aims will alter fetal development.

In our own studies, iron deficiency during pregnancy (in rats) results in marked changes in cytokine expression in the placenta (Gambling *et al.* 2002). In a series of studies, we reduced iron intake in the mothers to varying degrees. There was a marked change in specific gene expression and endocrine production. Tumour necrosis factor-alpha (TNFα) expression was increased in trophoblast giant cells, but not in other cell types. In the rat placenta these are thought to be involved primarily in endocrine signalling rather than transport of nutrients. In contrast, levels of the receptor (TNFαR type 1) increased in many cell types, including trophoblast giant cells, spongiotrophoblast, labyrinthine cells and cytotrophoblast cells (Gambling *et al.* 2002). Leptin levels also changed, rising in the labyrinth and marginally in trophoblast giant cells. At this stage, we cannot conclude that the changes are causally related to the postnatal hypertension that the offspring develop as a consequence of iron deficiency *in utero*, but it certainly gives a pointer as to possible directions for future research (Gambling *et al.* 2003).

Similarly, others have demonstrated that changes in the morphology of the placenta are associated with a complex series of events that increase the risk of cardiovascular disease in the offspring; see Thornburg *et al.* (2010) for a recent review.

The authors, and others, have also examined the effect of nutrient deficiency on placental transport function. This is probably its most critical role, as without adequate transport the fetus cannot survive (Cetin and Alvino 2008). Amino acid transport, in particular, seems to be affected by the nutritional and endocrine environment (Jones *et al.* 2006a; Jones *et al.* 2006b; Jones *et al.* 2007), but other transporters are also under the control of their substrates (Gambling *et al.* 2009). This is an area of growing interest, as it may be a non-invasive target for modulating and remodelling by deficiencies during fetal development.

During development, the fetus is susceptible to teratogenic influences. Depending on the stage of gestation, different organs can be affected (Fig. 4.2). For example, the central nervous system can be damaged severely up to about 16–18 weeks of gestation, while the limbs are affected primarily early on in gestation – the period when their cells are proliferating and differentiating most rapidly. Once again, it seems likely that these effects can be mimicked by inducing nutritional deficiencies. Generally, these will be more subtle than those brought on by teratogens, but this is not always the case.

For example, a series of very convincing studies have shown that folate deficiency has serious consequences for the developing embryo and fetus. Chapter 2 examines the 'normal' processes of development, which should give the reader a feeling for times when nutritional alterations may have consequences for development.

4.4 Nutritional programming: the effect of nutrition on fetal development

During pregnancy, the developing fetus is entirely dependent on the mother and the maternal environment for its nutritional requirements. It seems almost axiomatic therefore that maternal nutrition will determine fetal health and pregnancy outcome. However, it is only in the last 30 years that it has been realised that the consequences of inappropriate nutrition *in utero* can be extended into adulthood. This phenomenon was known originally as 'programming' as the fetus was programmed to show effects long after the stressor had been removed. The observations were brought together to form the 'fetal programming hypothesis' (Barker 2002). Here we discuss the fetal programming which results from a nutritional insult, from severe micronutrient deficiencies and global nutrient restriction, and put forward evidence from animal models that fetal programming may also occur when the nutritional insults are not so severe.

4.4.1 Severe effects of micronutrient deprivation in pregnancy

Deficiencies and overload of micronutrients in pregnancy can both cause teratogenic defects. Chief among these are those caused by vitamin A overload or zinc deficiency (Bhutta *et al.* 2008), diseases such as neural tube defects caused by folate deficiency and cretinism caused by iodine deficiency. Other nutritional deficiencies have more subtle effects and will be discussed separately.

Interestingly, vitamin A deficiency can also have unwanted consequences. In a recent study, Ellis-Hutchings and colleagues examined the effect of flame-retardant chemicals, polybrominated diphenyl ethers (PBDEs), on development in rats of either normal or marginal vitamin A status (Ellis-Hutchings *et al.* 2009). Marginal vitamin A status on its own had some small effects on growth and development, but these were greatly exacerbated by the chemical.

Iodine is required for normal thyroid hormone production and thyroid function. Thyroid hormone is required for normal neuronal migration, myelination and synaptic transmission and plasticity in fetal and neonatal life (de Escobar *et al.* 2007). Several studies have shown that low levels of thyroid hormone results in irreversible brain damage, with both mental retardation and neurological abnormalities (see, for example, van Wijk *et al.* 2008). Studies in a variety of low-iodine environments, using different approaches, have all shown marked effects of iodine supplementation (reviewed in Zimmermann 2009).

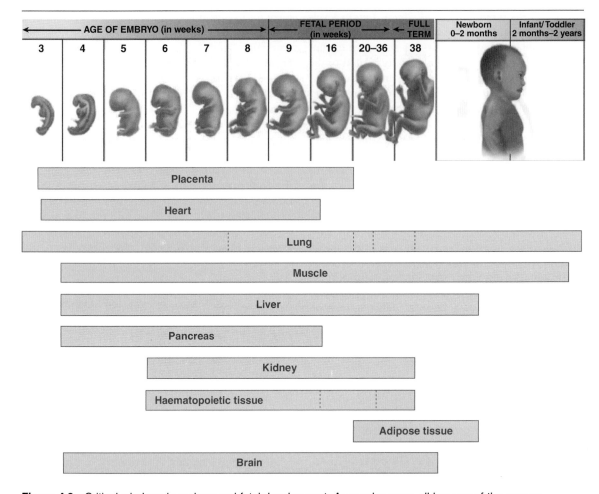

Figure 4.2 Critical windows in embryo and fetal development. As can be seen, all bar one of the organs discussed in this chapter begin their development during the critical first 8 weeks of gestation.
Note: Horizontal bars indicate time periods of development of different organs. The vertical dotted lines indicate distinct stages of organ development.
Medical illustrations: James Dowdalls. Graph production, Jane Teis Graphic Services. From the UCLA Institute of the Environment and Sustainability, Southern California Environmental Report Card, 'Air Pollution Impact on Infants and Children', Beate Ritz, MD, Ph.D. and Michelle Wilhelm, Ph.D.

Whether iodine supplementation has value in a population with an adequate intake is not so clear. Several studies in Europe have adopted different supplementation approaches during pregnancy. Summarising a considerable effort, providing supplementation can reduce the growth in thyroid size normally seen in pregnancy, but there were no significant changes in either tri-iodothyronine (T3) or thyroxine (T4) concentrations in maternal or cord blood. In one placebo-controlled double blind study, the offspring from treated groups also had smaller

thyroids than controls (Glinoer *et al.* 1995), but whether there are actually long-term effects on the children's IQ or intellectual capacity has not yet been studied (Zimmermann 2009) (see Chapter 6).

4.4.2 The effect of famine on fetal development

There are several pieces of data to support the concept that suboptimal nutrition at different times in pregnancy leads to different outcomes for the off-

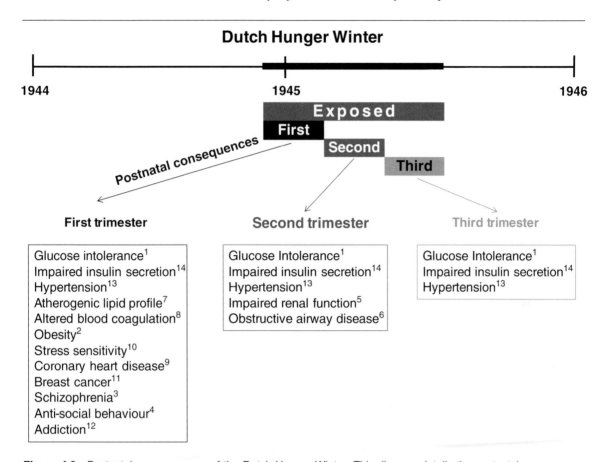

Figure 4.3 Postnatal consequences of the Dutch Hunger Winter. This diagram details the postnatal consequences of gestational specific exposure to the starvation rations. It is clear that exposure during the first trimester had the most severe effects.
[1]Ravelli *et al.* 1998; [2]Ravelli *et al.* 1999; [3]Hoek *et al.* 1996; [4]Neugebauer *et al.* 1999; [5]Painter *et al.* 2005; [6]Lopuhaa *et al.* 2000; [7]Roseboom *et al.* 2000a; [8]Roseboom *et al.* 2000b; [9]Roseboom *et al.* 2000c; [10]Painter *et al.* 2006b; [11]Painter *et al.* 2006c; [12]Franzek *et al.* 2008; [13]Stein, Zeibert *et al.* 2006; [14]de Rooij *et al.* 2006. Adapted from Roseboom *et al.* (2006) The Dutch famine and its long-term consequences for adult health. *Early Human Development*, **82**, 485–91.

spring. A major series of studies relates to the Dutch Hunger Winter (see Chapter 1, Section 1.4.1 for further details). In 1944, during the Second World War, the Dutch Government in exile called on Dutch railway workers to go on strike. In retaliation, the Germans banned food transport. The ban was lifted in November but by then the winter was too severe to allow transport of food to the west of the Netherlands. Rations were first cut to below 1000 kcal (4187 kJ) per day, then to only 400–800 kcal (1675–3349 kJ) per day for adults. Following the liberation of Holland in June 1945, the food supply was restored. Despite all the problems, however, the Dutch medical services managed to keep a record of the population and this now proves to be an invaluable resource. Because of their work it is possible to study the effect of food restriction in the first, second and third trimesters of pregnancy and to compare the data with that obtained from children born both before and after the starvation period. The timescale of the famine and the windows of exposure studies are given in Fig. 4.3.

These studies have yielded extremely valuable data, going beyond normal association studies. For more detailed information, the reader is referred to the excellent website (www.dutchfamine.nl). In summary, the effects were widespread, but differed significantly with the stage of gestation when the mother's diet was affected. Glucose tolerance in adults exposed to famine *in utero* was higher and insulin sensitivity was reduced (see Chapter 9, Section 9.4.1). This was the case irrespective of the stage of gestation. The links to blood pressure were complex. The authors found that the ratio of carbohydrate to protein was more important in terms of demonstrating a relationship than absolute levels of carbohydrate or protein (Roseboom *et al.* 1999). Airway disease was most frequent in those offspring exposed to the famine *in utero* during early and mid-gestation (Lopuhaa *et al.* 2000) (see Chapter 13, Section 13.5.1). Since this is the period when bronchial development is taking place, the data fit with the concept of nutritional imbalance having the greatest effect on those tissues that are undergoing growth and differentiation.

There are some cautionary points, however. Data from the Leningrad siege in Russia, which also occurred during the Second World War, did not produce the same results as the Dutch studies (Stanner *et al.* 1997; Stanner and Yudkin 2001). Here, there was no clear association between starvation *in utero* and postnatal hypertension. However, these authors make an important point. In the Dutch studies, there was rapid postnatal catch-up growth. This did not occur in the Russian population, which may underscore the importance of the pattern of early childhood nutrition for later health.

In summary, the effects of the famine were greatest in those exposed in early gestation. Glucose intolerance, atherogenic lipid profile and other indicators of disease were all found in the Dutch cohort (Fig. 4.3). Again, this might be predicted if one assumes that this period is the most sensitive to disorders of nutrition.

4.4.3 Experimental models for the study of poor nutrition on fetal development

A large number of animal models have been established to study the effects of unbalanced maternal nutrition on fetal development (McArdle *et al.* 2006).

Studies on single micronutrient deficiency support the hypothesis that the early stages in pregnancy are particularly vulnerable. Iron deficiency during pregnancy in the rat induces hypertension in the offspring (Crowe *et al.* 1995; Gambling *et al.* 2003). A rat embryo culture model has been used to examine the relationship between iron status early in pregnancy and growth, development and gene expression. Mothers were made iron-deficient prior to mating and embryos were removed 10.5 days later. They were cultured either in iron-deficient or in control medium for 48 hours. Following this, development and gene expression in the yolk-sac placenta and the embryo were measured. Embryos from control mothers grown in iron-deficient medium showed similar changes to those grown in an iron-deficient environment from conception (Andersen *et al.* 2006). Further, growing the embryos in an iron-sufficient medium for 48 hours (from day 10.5 to day 12.5) resulted in normal vascularisation, which would argue that this period is critical in rat vascular development.

Further evidence has been produced in other laboratories. Langley-Evans and colleagues first showed that protein deprivation during the last 7 days of pregnancy in the rat resulted in hypertension that was more severe than deprivation for other 7-day periods (Langley-Evans, Welham *et al.* 1996). In contrast, Fleming's data argues that the pre-implantation period is most important (reviewed in Watkins and Fleming 2009). In a series of studies, his group has shown that a low-protein diet during the pre-conception period results in changes in gene expression and organ size. Their data suggest this may act through alterations in genes involved in steroid metabolism, specifically the genes 11β-hydroxysteroid dehydrogenase type 1 (11β-HSD1) and phospho-enolpyruvate carboxykinase (PEPCK) (Watkins *et al.* 2007). It is, of course, possible that both are correct and that the mechanisms underpinning the changes differ as pregnancy progresses. It is also possible that postnatal changes can modulate the effects that are generated prenatally (Watkins and Fleming 2009).

4.5 Potential mechanisms of nutritional programming

The information given in this overview makes it apparent that the developing fetus is vulnerable to changes in its nutritional environment. It is also fairly clear why different organs are affected differently at different stages in pregnancy. What is not so clear is why the placenta and other homeostatic organs do not maintain the fetus against the stress of suboptimal nutrition.

Examining the literature, several possible hypotheses have been advanced to explain why programming can occur. There are some important considerations. One is that the changes represent an adaptation to a suboptimal environment which, were it to persist after birth, would have a survival advantage. This theory, known as adaptive programming (or the thrifty phenotype hypothesis) (Gluckman *et al.* 2005), has some attractive aspects, but work still needs to be done to demonstrate its accuracy. Other theories relate to a lack of nutrient supply, or endocrine imbalances (Chapman and Seckl 2008). Clearly there is much to learn about programming phenomena.

Irrespective of why the changes occur, it is still necessary to determine how they occur. Several possibilities exist. Some of these are outlined briefly below, discussed in detail in recent reviews (Langley-Evans 2009; Warner and Ozanne 2010) and are developed further in later chapters. We conclude by suggesting that there may be a common cause of much of the phenotype.

4.5.1 Disruption of organ development

The most obvious mechanism by which 'programming' could have an effect is through altering normal tissue and organ development (Brameld *et al.* 1998). Organs and tissues develop from a small set of embryonic progenitor cells; these cells follow distinct pathways of differentiation and proliferation during organogenesis. The timing of the differentiation and proliferation phases is distinct for each tissue and organ; for example, as mentioned above, the development of the heart occurs very early in gestation, while the kidney is one of the later organs to fully develop. It is clear that these periods of development will be sensitive to environmental factors and it is also apparent that the same insult at different stages of development could have different consequences. If an insult were to occur during an organ's differentiation phase then it would be expected that the organ would be of normal size but would have an altered profile of cells. While stress during the proliferative

phase would result in the normal profile of cells, the organ may be smaller, with a reduced total number of cells. The disruption to organ development during either of these phases could have significant impact on the organ's ability to function.

Evidence for such organ 'remodelling' having a direct impact on organ function has been studied most thoroughly in the kidney. Exposure of rats to low-protein diets during gestation leads to kidneys of normal size, but these kidneys possess up to 40% fewer nephrons, the main functional unit in the kidney (Langley-Evans, Welham *et al.* 1999; Vehaskari *et al.* 2001), indicating an insult that affects the differentiation phase of kidney development. This programming effect appears to be consistent across experimental models encompassing different dietary insults and species (Lisle *et al.* 2003; Gilbert *et al.* 2005; Hoppe *et al.* 2007; Tomat *et al.* 2008). Most importantly, it is also seen in human patients exhibiting symptoms of primary hypertension (Keller *et al.* 2003). Although as yet not extensively investigated, the brain (Bennis-Taleb *et al.* 1999), pancreas (Snoeck *et al.* 1990) and placenta (Gambling *et al.* 2001; Lewis *et al.* 2001; Gambling *et al.* 2002; Gambling and McArdle 2004), also show evidence of remodelling that may affect organ function.

4.5.2 Disruption of the endocrine environment

4.5.2.1 *Glucocorticoids*

Glucocorticoids are steroid hormones with a wide range of postnatal functions including regulation of stress responses, immune function and glucose metabolism. However, during fetal development they have additional functions including the promotion of tissue maturation and function. During gestation there is a large concentration gradient for glucocorticoids across the placenta. This is because the placenta controls the amount of glucocorticoids that pass from mother to fetus. It converts glucocorticoids to their inactive form by the enzyme 11β-hydroxysteroid dehydrogenase 2 (11βHSD2) (Edwards *et al.* 1996). A functioning placental 11βHSD2 ensures that fetal tissues are exposed to only low levels of glucocorticoids. The first link between nutrition and fetal glucocorticoid levels was made when it was shown that maternal under-nutrition in guinea pigs led to an increase in both maternal and fetal glucocorticoids (Dwyer and Stickland 1992).

Further studies in rats exposed to a low-protein diet during pregnancy indicated that the expression and activity of placental 11βHSD2 was reduced (Langley-Evans, Phillips *et al.* 1996). Studies went on to link lower placental 11βHSD2 levels with reduced fetal weight at birth, in both rats (Benediktsson *et al.* 1993) and humans (Shams *et al.* 1998). The direct relationship between the activity of placental 11βHSD2 and programming effects was shown by a series of experiments using pharmaceutical inhibition of the enzyme (Langley-Evans 1997) and glucocorticoids which are poor substrates for the enzyme (Dodic *et al.* 2002). Both interventions led to the offspring developing high blood pressure and renal defects. Further discussion of the endocrine environment during development can be found in Chapter 5.

4.5.2.2 Homeostatic regulation

A direct effect on the functionality of the organ, such as nephron number, is only one way in which organ remodelling could affect postnatal organ function. A second possibility is that remodelling could alter the gene expression profile of the organ, which would in turn have functional consequences for the organ (Langley-Evans 2006). For example, the response to hormones could be altered or the organ's negative feedback system could be impaired. There is now evidence from both animal and human studies that a suboptimal maternal environment can lead to permanent changes to homeostatic regulatory control of many of the body's metabolic pathways. It can clearly be seen how programming of such homeostatic mechanisms could contribute to the postnatal phenotype seen in nutritional programming.

Hypothalamo–pituitary–adrenal axis: Fetal exposure to excessive glucocorticoids is known to bring about the maturation of tissues, favouring differentiation over proliferation. This could be the mechanism behind some of the altered organ development seen in nutritional programming leading to the development of smaller organs with altered function (Seckl 2001; Dodic *et al.* 2002). However, excess fetal glucocorticoids also permanently alter the body's hormonal environment and systems. The activity of the hypothalamo–pituitary–adrenal (HPA) axis is regu-

lated by a negative feedback system where glucocorticoids released into the circulation by the adrenal gland interact with the glucocorticoid receptors of the pituitary, hypothalamus and hippocampus. Exposure to excess fetal glucocorticoids at critical periods of development can alter the set point of the HPA axis, leading both to altered basal and stress-induced glucocorticoid responses postnatally (Levitt *et al.* 1996; Matthews *et al.* 2002). This has also been suggested as the pathway that mediates the altered postnatal responses of intrauterine growth-restricted (IUGR) babies (Walker *et al.* 2002).

Any alteration in the functioning of the HPA axis could explain the range of effects seen in nutrition-induced fetal programming, such as alterations in blood pressure regulation, immune response, immune function and obesity. Further information about the role of the hypothalamo–pituitary–adrenal axis in fetal development can be found in Chapter 6.

Glucose metabolism: Type 2 diabetes is a common postnatal phenotype seen as the result of nutritional programming. There are four metabolic abnormalities that characterise type 2 diabetes: obesity, impaired insulin action, altered insulin secretion and an increase in endogenous glucose output (Leahy 2005). It is now clear that all are subject to programming during both gestational and early postnatal periods of development.

The mechanisms behind these programming effects have best been studied in rats and mice subject to a low-protein diet during gestation. The pancreas appears to be the subject of organ remodelling, reducing the number of functional beta-cells to half that of normal (Snoeck *et al.* 1990).

Maternal protein restriction during pregnancy alters the growth, morphology and activity of enzymes involved in gluconeogenesis (Burns *et al.* 1997; Desai *et al.* 1997). Glucose uptake of both muscle and adipocytes are altered (Ozanne *et al.* 1996; Ozanne *et al.* 1997), and in muscle this effect is thought to be related to the programmed increased expression of insulin receptors and altered cellular distribution of the glucose transporter GLUT4 (Ozanne *et al.* 1996).

Aspects of this programmed response are now being detected in humans (Ozanne *et al.* 2005), before any changes are detectable in glucose metabolism itself. Further discussion of glucose metabolism in development can be found in Chapter 9.

Renin–angiotensin system: Hypertension is one of the most common postnatal outcomes generated by nutritional programming. The renin–angiotensin system is a multi-organ system that regulates blood pressure. The kidney secretes the enzyme renin, which cleaves angiotensinogen, released by the liver, to produce angiotensin I (Ang I). Ang I is further cleaved by angiotensinogen-converting enzyme (ACE) leading to the formation of angiotensin II (Ang II). Ang II regulates blood pressure by both stimulating sodium transporters (Kwon *et al.* 2003) and increasing the production and release of aldosterone (Aguilera and Catt 1978).

Offspring born to mothers subject to a low-protein diet during pregnancy go on to develop high blood pressure; additional studies have shown the administration of ACE inhibitors in early postnatal life to decrease blood pressure in hypertensive animals (Langley-Evans, Sherman *et al.* 1999). If the ACE inhibitor treatment is started as early as 2 weeks postnatally, the decrease in blood pressure was maintained into adulthood, even in absence of inhibitor (Sherman and Langley-Evans 1998). These results argued that the critical step for the nutritional programming was the Ang II. Further weight was added to this hypothesis when an antagonist of the Ang II receptor was administered, giving a similar response (Sherman and Langley-Evans 2000). Studies carried out in sheep have now linked exposure to high levels of glucocorticoids to the programmed changes seen in the renin-angiotensin system (Moritz *et al.* 2002) (see Chapter 10, Section 10.6.1).

4.5.3 Epigenetics

Epigenetics describes the study of heritable changes in gene expression that are not caused by changes in the primary DNA sequence (Riggs *et al.* 1996). The epigenetic code is a series of small marks added to DNA or to histone proteins. There are currently two well-defined mechanisms by which this epigenetic code is created; the addition of methyl groups to DNA cytosine bases and the post-translational modification of histone proteins by the addition of methyl or acetyl groups (Waterland and Michels 2007). The epigenetic code can modulate how genes are expressed, which introduces significant flexibility, enabling one DNA genotype to have numerous functional genotypes.

The epigenetic code may be one way in which the fetal environment can impact life-long effects on the fetus. Although it is heritable, it is thought not to be fixed throughout the life stages. It is vulnerable to alteration during several life stages; embryogenesis, fetal and neonatal development, puberty and old age (Weaver *et al.* 2004; Dolinoy *et al.* 2007). During gestation the developing embryo/fetus is subject to both de-methlyation and re-methylation (Morgan *et al.* 2005) which leaves it susceptible to environmental interference, including that of nutrition.

The impact of nutrition on the epigenetic code was first highlighted by studies carried out in Agouti viable yellow (A^{vy}) mice. Supplementation of the maternal diet with methyl donors, such as folic acid, vitamin B_{12}, choline and betaine, altered the phenotype of the offspring, resulting in a larger proportion of the offspring being born with brown coats, compared to yellow or mottled coats (Wolff *et al.* 1998; Waterland and Jirtle 2003). Further studies have shown that maternal diets with suboptimal levels of methyl donors can lead to epigenetic-related changes in different strains of mice (Niculescu *et al.* 2006; Lillycrop *et al.* 2007) and sheep (Sinclair *et al.* 2007).

It is now well established that diets that are suboptimal in nutrients directly involved in methyl-group metabolism can significantly alter the epigenetic code. However, two mechanisms are now proposed by which all nutritional and environmental factors can alter the epigenetic code. Alterations could be caused firstly by directly interfering with the process of DNA methylation by affecting the supply of methyl donors in the diet or the activity of the enzymes responsible for DNA methylation. A second possible mechanism is by changing the amount of DNA available for methylation by altering the transcriptional activity of specific genes during times of DNA methylation (Waterland and Michels 2007).

Data supporting these hypotheses have been produced in the Dutch Hunger Winter studies (see Chapter 1, Section 1.4.1 and Chapter 4, Section 4.4.2). Heijmans *et al.* (2008) have shown epigenetic changes in the differentially methylated region (DMR) of *Igf2*, an imprinted gene, when compared to same-sex siblings born outside the Dutch Hunger Winter period. Hypomethylation of the DMR regions leads to expression of both alleles of *Igf2*. They found that there was a very significant reduction in methylation of *Igf2* in those offspring exposed early in gestation to the hunger winter. This fits well with the concept that early stages of gestation are critical in the development of postnatal disorders.

It also fits with data obtained in mice (Constancia *et al.* 2005). Using gene knockout mice, Constancia and colleagues have shown that the placental characteristics are changed and that diffusion and transport characteristics are altered markedly. Although the two sets of data are not directly comparable, the suggestions that imprinting and methylation have an important role to play are intriguing and will be explored further elsewhere in this Task Force report (e.g. Chapter 9, Section 9.5.3 and Chapter 11, Section 11.4.2).

4.5.4 Telomere length

Telomeres are nucleoproteins found at the ends of chromosomes; they consist of repetitive DNA sequences with high G-C content, two of the nucleosides needed to provide the DNA coding sequences. Telomeres protect the chromosome ends from fusion and degradation (de Lange 2005). In proliferating cells, telomere length decreases by a known amount at each cell division. Telomeres are also shortened due to oxidative stress-induced DNA damage. It is known that telomere shortening accompanies human ageing and premature ageing syndromes are often associated with short telomeres (Kappei and Londono-Vallejo 2008). This has led to the hypothesis that telomere length directly influences longevity (for example, see Cawthorn *et al.* 2003).

It has been proposed that this telomere attrition may be one mechanism which underlies fetal programming of cardiovascular disease (Demerath *et al.* 2004). The low-protein model of fetal programming shows low birthweight, vascular dysfunction and accelerated ageing in rats. Further investigations into possible mechanisms behind these symptoms have indicated that the low-protein maternal diet influences aortic telomere length through changes in DNA single-strand breaks, antioxidant capacity, and oxidative stress (Tarry-Adkins *et al.* 2008).

4.5.5 The gatekeeper hypothesis

One of the most interesting aspects of all the work carried out on experimental animals to try to understand how fetal programming may occur, is that there is actually a remarkable similarity between the

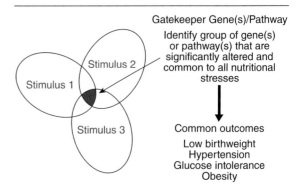

Figure 4.4   The gatekeeper hypothesis. Reprinted from McMullen S, Langley-Evans SC, Gambling L *et al.* (2012) A common cause for a common phenotype: the gatekeeper hypothesis in fetal programming. *Medical Hypotheses*, **78**, 88–94, copyright 2012, with permission from Elsevier.

symptoms that arise. For example, the low-protein model in rats, the high-fat model and the low-iron model all result in hypertension and obesity. This observation has given rise to the 'gatekeeper hypothesis' – that there are a limited number of genes or gene pathways that are altered by the nutritional insult. By performing high-throughput assays on the target tissues, followed by comparison of the genes that are changed, we hypothesise that we will be able to identify these gatekeepers (Fig. 4.4). Tying these data in with what is already known about development should allow us to develop hypotheses explaining the mechanism(s) of programming. It is too early to say yet whether we are correct, but preliminary results are encouraging.

4.6 Conclusions

This chapter has examined the process of fetal growth and development and reviewed both fetal and placental development. In the fetus we have described organ development, identifying 'critical windows' when that organ is most susceptible to damage. We have identified some of the possible mechanisms underpinning the phenomenon of fetal programming and also proposed a new theory, the gatekeeper hypothesis, which suggests that different nutritional insults can act at a common gene or gene pathway to produce a similar phenotype.

4.7 Key points

- Suboptimal nutrition can affect fetal development, in both the short and the long term.
- There are 'critical windows' in development, where the fetus is susceptible to suboptimal nutrition.
- Different organs are most vulnerable to insult during periods of growth and differentiation.
- There are many questions that remain unanswered in this area of human health and well-being. For example, it is not clear why the placenta, and indeed other homeostatic organs, do not maintain the fetus against the stress of suboptimal nutrition, and further work is needed to prove or disprove the proposed mechanisms of nutritional programming.

4.8 Recommendations for future research

- The Scientific Advisory Committee on Nutrition (SACN) or other relevant bodies should consider whether dietary recommendations during pregnancy should be modified to take into account the risk of long-term disease in the offspring in relation to pregnancy outcome.
- Further research is required to confirm or reject the adaptive programming theory as a mechanism for nutritional programming.
- Evidence indicates that the disruption of organ development (organ remodelling) in the kidney can have a direct impact on kidney function. However, research is required to determine whether the remodelling of other organs, such as the brain, pancreas and placenta, also has a direct impact on their function.
- Further research is required to determine whether a limited number of genes or gene pathways are altered by nutritional insult (the gatekeeper hypothesis).

4.9 Key references

Barker D (2002) Fetal programming of coronary heart disease. *Trends in Endocrinology and Metabolism*, **13**, 364–8.

Bhutta ZA, Ahmed T, Black RE *et al.* (2008) What works? Interventions for maternal and child undernutrition and survival. *Lancet*, **371**, 417–40.

Cetin I & Alvino G (2008) Intrauterine growth restriction: implications for placental metabolism and transport. A review. *Placenta*, **30**, 77–82.

Harding R & Bocking A (2001) *Fetal Growth and Development*. Cambridge, Cambridge University Press.

Langley-Evans SC (2009) Nutritional programming of disease: unravelling the mechanism. *Journal of Anatomy*, **215**, 36–51.

O'Rahilly R & Müller F (2000) Prenatal ages and stages: measures and errors. *Teratology*, **61**, 382–4.

5
Perinatal Effects of Sex Hormones in Programming of Susceptibility to Disease

5.1 Introduction

Nothing has a more dramatic effect on eventual body shape and composition than androgen action as part of the masculinisation process in the male fetus. This lays the foundations for transformation of the individual concerned into a phenotypic male. Not only will this result in different genitalia and reproductive tract, it also has numerous body-wide effects on fat distribution, skin, hair distribution and growth, the cardiovascular system, the kidneys, pancreas and liver, and the immune system. Dramatic effects on the brain that involve neuronal organisation, cognitive effects and reprogramming of central hormonal control systems will also occur.

Such pervasive effects reshape susceptibility to various diseases, and even life expectancy, although in general there is only superficial understanding of how this is brought about. Dramatic though these effects may sound, what they describe is not 'abnormal', but is rather just the consequences of developing as a male rather than as a female. It is nevertheless important to take account of this background, as it is increasingly recognised that disease results from interactive effects between our genes (genotype) and our environment, and the sex of the fetus is thus likely to alter the potential impact that nutritional and other factors may have in early life programming

of later disease. Moreover, recognition of these sex differences forces us to consider that disorders that stem from disruption of the masculinisation process in the male, or which involve aberrant masculinisation of the female, may bring with them altered predisposition to fat distribution (and thus body shape), altered behaviour and altered susceptibility to disease (which may be good as well as bad). Unfortunately, this touches on aspects of disease that are little studied as yet and, indeed, go largely unrecognised (Kautzky-Willer and Handisurya 2009).

The purpose of this chapter is to explore the range of the potential effects and influences of perinatal sex hormone (primarily androgen) exposure on programming of disease susceptibility, in particular whether there are interactions with growth, nutritional and/or lifestyle factors. In doing so, it should be recognised from the outset that, for most aspects, limited information is available and many of the key questions raised do not as yet have answers.

5.2 Timing of masculinisation and its body-wide effects

Female development is essentially a passive process and, although it requires specific genes to be switched

Nutrition and Development: Short- and Long-Term Consequences for Health, First Edition. Edited by the British Nutrition Foundation. © 2013 the British Nutrition Foundation. Published 2013 by Blackwell Publishing Ltd.

on, it does not involve the body-wide reprogramming that occurs in the male, nor does it require hormonal intervention. This is because female is the 'set-up' programme, the course that fetal development is set to run unless testis formation and the resultant production of hormones takes place, as in the male. Masculinisation of males as the result of hormone (primarily androgen) action occurs in fetal life, although further androgen-driven development of masculine characteristics occurs in the immediate postnatal period ('mini-puberty') and at puberty. However, the latter 'activational' effects are completely dependent on the prior 'organisational' actions of androgens in fetal life to establish a male phenotype, so it is the organisational effects that are critical. Nevertheless, it can be difficult to separate the contribution of androgen (or other hormonal) effects in fetal versus later life to disease risk in adulthood, especially if perinatal androgen action also partly determines later hormone levels, as appears likely.

Masculinisation of different organs and systems does not occur all at the same time. Thus, masculinisation of the reproductive tract/genitalia occurs very early in gestation, probably in the period 8–12 weeks gestation during what is now termed the 'masculinisation programming window' (Welsh *et al.* 2008), whereas masculinisation of the brain is a separate event and occurs late in gestation (27–35 weeks gestation); a similar disparity is evident in non-human primates and in laboratory animals (Welsh *et al.* 2008). Thus, it is possible for the reproductive system and brain to be differentially masculinised if, for example, testosterone production by the fetal testis (which drives masculinisation) was impaired just in early or late gestation; such a differential effect could account for gender dysphoria.

Androgen-driven masculinisation affects many other body organs based on limited evidence, such as the expression of androgen receptors; this includes the lungs, heart, stomach, liver, pancreas and adipose tissue. However, it is unclear exactly when masculinisation of these organs occurs, primarily because of the lack of relevant studies and the absence, for most, of any definitive markers of their 'masculinisation'. Based on limited studies in laboratory animals, it is perhaps more likely that masculinisation of these organs is a late, rather than an early, event in gestation. The absence of androgen receptor expression from some of these tissues in humans, in the first trimester of pregnancy (Sajjad *et al.* 2007), would support this view.

It should be mentioned that hormones other than androgens also play a role in masculinisation, notably anti-müllerian hormone (regression of the müllerian ducts) and insulin-like factor 3 (testis descent). However, as far as we know the effects of these hormones are restricted, mainly to the developing reproductive system, and do not affect other body systems, apart from recent evidence for effects of insulin-like factor 3 on bone (Pepe *et al.* 2009).

5.3 Disorders of masculinisation

Disorders of masculinisation such as incomplete testis descent into the scrotum (cryptorchidism) or incorrect location of the opening of the urinary tract on the penis (hypospadias) are remarkably common, affecting up to 6.9% and 0.4% of newborn boys, respectively, in the UK (Paulozzi 1999; Acerini *et al.* 2009). Although these disorders may arise for reasons unrelated to deficient androgen action, it is accepted that it is likely to be involved in some cases, especially for cryptorchidism.

Indeed, there is increasing recognition from both clinical and animal experimental studies that subtle defects in androgen-dependent masculinisation, during the masculinisation programming window, may fundamentally alter the ultimate size of all male reproductive organs (the testes, prostate, seminal vesicles and penis), and predispose to adult-onset disorders, such as low sperm counts and testicular germ cell cancer (Macleod *et al.* 2010). This being the case, it raises the possibility that other non-reproductive organ systems, including the brain, may also be affected if the subtle deficiency in androgen production or action persists later into gestation. Unfortunately, because our understanding of the developmental role of androgen action in tissues other than the brain is so sparse, it can only be speculated whether non-reproductive organs will be affected in a way that may predispose to their malfunction or to disease. One way that insight might be obtained is by examining the evidence for male–female differences in specific diseases and to ask if this difference arises because of events in perinatal life and might thus be affected, or 'programmed' by fetal androgen exposure.

5.4 Male–female differences in disease risk: the potential role of perinatal androgens

There is an extensive, but in most cases superficial, literature detailing the different risk of certain diseases in males and females. This includes cardiovascular diseases (higher in males; Liu *et al.* 2003), several autoimmune diseases such as multiple sclerosis, lupus, rheumatoid arthritis and Graves' disease (all higher in females; Fish 2008), asthma (higher in adult females; see Chapter 13), gastric ulcers (higher in males; Longstreth 1995), depressive illnesses and dementia (higher in females; Holden 2005), eating disorders and obesity (higher in females; Geary 2004), schizophrenia and autism (higher in males; Auyeung *et al.* 2009) and kidney disease (higher in males; Gilbert and Nijland 2008). Although it is recognised that these could signify the impact of differential androgen action in perinatal life, for none of these disorders is such an underlying mechanism unequivocally established. Other factors may also be important, including differential expression of X or Y chromosome-encoded genes and postpubertal (and, in women, postmenopausal) differences in circulating levels of oestrogens and androgens; these are not considered here, but they represent important confounding factors when trying to decipher if perinatal androgens may affect adult disease risk.

In contrast to androgens in the male, it is unlikely that oestrogens play any female-specific role in perinatal life in programming of disease in humans, for two reasons. First, fetal oestrogen exposure of both sexes occurs equally due to the high levels of production by the placenta and, second, steroid production by the fetal ovary is low to avoid switching on steroidogenesis, and thus the synthesis of androgens, which could lead to masculinisation. In this regard, inappropriate androgen exposure of the female fetus, most commonly as the result of congenital adrenal hyperplasia (CAH), can lead to variable masculinisation of the female fetus, and this could theoretically alter predisposition to disease as occurs in normal males. However, there is little definitive evidence for this, probably because there are numerous confounding factors related to the postnatal therapeutic management of CAH.

Inappropriate androgen exposure of the female fetus has also been advocated as a cause of polycystic ovarian syndrome (PCOS) in adulthood, based on studies in non-human primates (Abbott *et al.* 2002). However, evidence from human studies has so far failed to support this, although the possibility of fetal origins of the disease cannot be ruled out (de Zegher and Ibanez 2009). PCOS is of interest because it is remarkably common in women and has established links to risk of obesity, insulin resistance and dyslipidaemia, thus putting such individuals at greater risk of type 2 diabetes and related cardiometabolic disorders. These effects may be due to the elevated androgen and decreased oestrogen levels commonly found in PCOS, resulting in a more 'male-like' hormone profile and associated predisposition to cardiometabolic disorders (see below). Dietary changes are an important part of management of adults with PCOS, but whether perinatal nutrition plays any role in determining the course and severity of the condition is unknown and is rather dependent on resolution of the importance of perinatal factors in the aetiology of PCOS.

5.5 Fetal growth, susceptibility to intrauterine growth restriction and its long-term consequences, including timing of puberty

Intrauterine growth restriction (IUGR) is an important determinant of the risk of certain later cardiometabolic diseases, collectively termed metabolic syndrome. Perinatal factors, including both sex steroid exposure and nutrition, also influence this risk. Moreover, there is growing evidence that IUGR may also be associated with 'reprogramming' of the metabolic system in the fetus, leading to increased disease risk in adult life. Additionally, there is evidence that these risk factors may be transmissible to subsequent generations, resulting in perpetuation of elevated risk of IUGR and longer-term metabolic sequelae.

Early life programming because of IUGR is usually interpreted as an adaptation by the fetus to an anticipated low nutritional plane after birth, so that the major long-term health consequences associated with IUGR appear to occur when the affected individuals undergo 'inappropriate' catch-up growth/overgrowth in the first 6–12 months after birth. This is discussed in more detail in Chapter 2, Section 2.10. This means that the choice and amount of feeding by mothers of babies born with IUGR may be important in determining the occurrence and nature of any longer-term health consequences.

The male fetus grows faster and bigger than the corresponding female fetus. This growth difference is evident before androgen production by the fetal testis is switched on, at least in animal studies, but it has been generally presumed that androgens are at least partly responsible for the male–female growth difference. However, a recent study of androgen-insensitive male and androgen-exposed (CAH) female babies has shown that body weight, in both sexes, is comparable to normal members of their sex and appears unaffected by androgens (Miles *et al.* 2010). It is possible that androgens might still have a subtle growth-promoting effect, as this has been offered as an explanation for why the presence of a male fetus in mixed-sex twins is associated with higher growth of the female, although the effects are not huge (Luke *et al.* 2005). However, even these subtle effects may somehow alter long-term disease risk in the female co-twin, for example increasing the risk of developing breast cancer (Kaijser *et al.* 2001).

Male fetuses are more prone to pre-term birth than females, are more susceptible to IUGR than females and tend to suffer worse consequences. Detailed comparison of fetal growth curves in non-smoking, light-smoking and heavy-smoking women during pregnancy has shown that IUGR is greater in males than in females. Boys born to heavy-smoking mothers had an 8.2% reduction in body weight and a 12% reduction in fat accretion, compared with values of 4.8% and 2% in girls born to heavy-smoking mothers (Zaren *et al.* 2000). This is of interest because several large studies have shown that men whose mothers smoked heavily in pregnancy exhibit up to a 45% reduction in average testis size and sperm counts in adulthood (Sharpe 2010), and low sperm count is associated with increased overall risk of dying in adulthood (Jensen *et al.* 2009). It is suggested, but not proven, that the deficit in sperm count in this situation results from a reduced number of Sertoli cells in the testes. It is the number of these cells that determines sperm count in adulthood in men, and perinatal life is an important time of Sertoli cell proliferation (Sharpe *et al.* 2003). Additionally, in experimental animal studies, both low maternal nutrition (Alejandro *et al.* 2002) and low fetal androgen levels (Scott *et al.* 2007) can lead to reduced Sertoli cell number at birth.

Interestingly, men with low sperm counts are also more likely to exhibit low or compensated/normal blood testosterone levels, and low testosterone levels in men, especially during later age, are clearly associated with increased risk of various cardiometabolic diseases (Kupelian *et al.* 2008) and of premature death (Laughlin *et al.* 2008). Although one study has shown that IUGR is not associated with altered testosterone levels in young adulthood (Jensen *et al.* 2007), a recent, carefully controlled study has shown that birthweight is positively associated with adult testosterone levels in men across the whole birthweight spectrum (Vanbillemont *et al.* 2010). This is reminiscent of the relationship found between birthweight and hypertension in adulthood by Barker (see Chapter 10, Section 10.5), although in that instance the relationship was inverse.

High caffeine consumption (>205 mg/day) in the third trimester of pregnancy can also result in IUGR which is mainly confined to boys (Vik *et al.* 2003). Pregnant women in the UK are advised not to consume more than 200 mg of caffeine per day as intakes above this are associated with greater risk of low birthweight and miscarriage (Committee on Toxicity of Chemical in Food Consumer Products and the Environment 2008) (see Chapter 15, Section 15.3.5).

Exposure to an adverse early life environment can have profound effects on future disease susceptibility and IUGR is a marker for this. Birthweight is inversely related to blood pressure in adulthood across the full birthweight range (Barker, Hales *et al.* 1993). Therefore, aspects of maternal lifestyle (e.g. smoking) or obesity that affect fetal growth are also associated with potential lifelong health implications for the fetus. IUGR increases the risk of undescended testes (Berkowitz *et al.* 1995) and hypospadias (Akre *et al.* 2008) in male offspring, either of which may stem from deficient androgen production/action during masculinisation, and if androgen production is altered this may have wider impacts, as discussed elsewhere in this chapter.

The most important early life programming effects are those related to predisposition to metabolic syndrome and it is becoming evident that IUGR and catch-up growth, in the first 6 months after birth, may be critical in determining the degree of later health impact in this regard (see Chapter 2, Section 2.10); therefore choice of infant feeding by the mother may be of considerable importance in this context. A similar scenario may account for earlier age of puberty and increased risk of precocious puberty that occurs in girls born in developing countries who migrate or are adopted to Western countries, i.e. fetal exposure to a low nutritional plane which then switches to postnatal exposure to a much higher nutritional plane (Bourguignon *et al.* 2010).

Similarly, the advance in age of puberty in girls up until the mid-twentieth century almost certainly reflects improved nutrition and living standards, but whether more recent advances (mainly restricted to earlier age of breast development) have a similar explanation is less clear (Mouritsen *et al.* 2010). Recent discoveries concerning the kisspeptin and related systems in the brain that interlink the metabolic and reproductive systems (Castellano *et al.* 2009; see Section 5.8) may, in time, provide explanations for all of these changes, but another possibility being considered is that exposure to endocrine-disrupting environmental chemicals could play a role (Bourguignon *et al.* 2010; Mouritsen *et al.* 2010).

So far the evidence to support such a link is mainly circumstantial. If such chemicals were to play a role it seems most likely that they would do so by triggering early activation of endogenous hormone systems involved in puberty, and there is some evidence for a role for DDT (dichlorodiphenyltrichloroethane) exposure in predisposition of adopted girls from the developing world to precocious puberty (Bourguignon *et al.* 2010).

5.6 Growth hormone–insulin-like growth factor-I axis

One key pathway that regulates growth and development in fetal and postnatal life is the growth hormone–insulin-like growth factor-I (GH-IGF-I) axis. Changes in this axis have been suggested to play a role in IUGR-related programming of cardiometabolic disease (Holt 2002; Gabory *et al.* 2009). In both rodents and humans there is marked sexual dimorphism in the patterns of GH and resulting IGF-I secretion (Jaffe *et al.* 1998) that are already evident at birth (Geary *et al.* 2003). In rodents, at least, it is established that perinatal androgen action in males is responsible for programming of the male-specific pattern of GH secretion, which in turn has even more dramatic programming effects on enzyme expression and activity in the liver (Gabory *et al.* 2009). Such changes could potentially alter males' response to

dietary and other lifestyle factors (metabolism of drugs and xenobiotics), and in this way alter disposition to adult disease.

This appears to be the case with regard to certain manifestations of metabolic syndrome disorders and the predisposition of men to deposit visceral fat, as this leads to altered blood lipid profile (more atherogenic) and greater risk of fatty liver and type 2 diabetes (Regitz-Zagrosek *et al.* 2006). In turn, the accumulation of visceral fat leads to reduction in blood testosterone levels which may further promote the deposition of visceral fat. In rodents, perinatal androgen exposure converts the female pattern of GH secretion to the male pattern, although in humans it is possible that oestrogens may be as important as androgens in modulating GH and IGF-I secretion, at least in adulthood (Holt 2002).

5.7 Brain and behavioural effects

Males and females exhibit numerous behavioural and cognitive differences that may be related to the programming effects of sex steroids, notably androgens in human males, on the organisation of the developing brain. This is far too large and complex a topic for discussion here, but it is accepted that some of these behavioural differences can predispose to disease or injury (e.g. risk-taking behaviour) or may affect eating, appetite and food preferences, which may then impact secondarily on disease risk in the long term. There is a growing conviction among some that schizophrenia and autism, both of which are more common in males than in females, may stem from a relative deficiency or excess of androgen action, respectively, on the developing brain (Auyeung *et al.* 2009).

5.8 Sex differences in eating disorders, neuronal mechanisms and adipose tissue distribution

5.8.1 Eating disorders

There appear to be fundamental sex differences in the regulation of energy homeostasis and metabolism in males and females (Geary 2004; Shi *et al.* 2009). These differences reflect to an extent the different needs of the female with regard to reproduction (pregnancy, lactation) but may also have health consequences. For example, women are far more susceptible to eating disorders than are men (Geary 2004); women are nine times more likely to develop anorexia nervosa or bulimia nervosa and are more likely than men to develop extreme obesity. These variations are found in several Western countries. This is despite the generally healthier eating preferences of women compared with men (see Section 5.8.3).

Although such eating disorders are influenced by societal factors, there is general acceptance that the control of eating is sexually differentiated and that predisposition to associated disorders may therefore be established during perinatal development. Exactly how this occurs is likely to be complex, but there are numerous pieces of evidence (though much of it from experimental animal studies) which have shown differences in central mechanisms known to affect eating and appetite as well as in hormonal signalling (e.g. insulin, leptin, ghrelin) from peripheral tissues such as adipocytes, pancreas and the liver (Geary 2004).

5.8.2 Kisspeptin system

An important recent development has been the discovery of new mechanisms that appear to translate metabolic signals into hormonal effects within the brain, the so-called kisspeptin system (Oakley *et al.* 2009). This system sits directly upstream of the hypothalamic–pituitary reproductive control centres and plays a pivotal, if still incompletely understood, role in regulation of the onset and function of the reproductive system. It is also emerging that this system is of importance in mediating the modulatory effects of metabolic peripheral signals (e.g. leptin signalling from adipose tissue; Oakley *et al.* 2009) on reproduction.

Kisspeptin neurons are targets for both androgens and oestrogens and, in laboratory animals at least, exposure to androgens or oestrogens perinatally during sexual differentiation plays fundamental roles in programming of a 'male' or 'female' type kisspeptin neuron distribution (Oakley *et al.* 2009). This is still an emerging area but it is considered likely that the wider kisspeptin system could be of key importance in translating metabolic changes into reproductive disorders in conditions such as anorexia, obesity and precocious puberty (Castellano *et al.* 2009). The importance of these new mechanisms and their susceptibility to alteration (e.g. reprogramming) by sex steroids and other perinatal factors such as maternal

obesity and infant feeding (see below) remains to be elucidated, but seems likely to provide important new insights into how modern 'Western' disorders may impact on reproductive and wider health.

5.8.3 Dietary preferences

There are well-established differences in dietary preferences of men and women, the former opting for more meat, potatoes, bread and alcohol but less fruit, vegetables, fish, cheese and sweets/desserts than women. The consumption pattern in women is viewed as being healthier in general than that of men, and is likely to be an important contributor to sex differences in cardiometabolic disease (Wardle *et al.* 2004). Men require a higher energy intake, and a greater percentage of this is derived from animal products, whereas there is a greater share of products of vegetable origin in women's diets.

The extent to which these preferences are determined by programming by androgens in males is unclear, but such preferences are found across many different cultures, suggesting that there is an underlying physiological, as opposed to a cultural, basis for them (Wardle *et al.* 2004). In laboratory animals, preference for a sweet taste (saccharin preference) is sexually dimorphic and is programmed during masculinisation of the brain by sex steroids but there is no evidence that this applies simply to humans, as early parental and other influences are probably more important and, in childhood, relatively few gender differences in food preference are found.

5.8.4 Body fat distribution

Adipocyte development occurs predominantly in late fetal and early postnatal life in humans, so perinatal events, including IUGR, could affect the number and location of adipocytes. This in turn could alter the propensity to obesity and obesity-related metabolic disorders in adulthood (Muhlhausler and Smith 2009); this is covered in more detail in Chapter 8.

As body fat distribution is fundamentally different in normal males and females, with males exhibiting larger visceral fat depots than (premenopausal) women (Wajchenberg 2000), this raises the possibility that masculinisation of the fetus (or variations therein) may play a role in determining the location and possibly the size of adipose depots (Blouin *et al.* 2009). There is remarkably little information on this possibility, probably because of the major confounding effects postnatally of diet and hormones. For example, after the menopause women begin to accrue more visceral fat, a change that appears to be directly related to absence of oestrogen action. This implies that regulation of visceral fat deposition is dynamic postnatally, which obscures our understanding of the extent to which this may be permanently reshaped by perinatal hormone exposures. This is a key issue because it has become clear that visceral fat level is perhaps the most important determinant of cardiometabolic disorders ('Western disorders') in an individual and largely accounts for the difference in risk of these disorders in men versus (premenopausal) women (see Section 5.9).

5.9 Cardiovascular disease/hypertension

Men show increased susceptibility to atherosclerosis and to hypertensive and cardiovascular disease, and such effects are an important determinant of the average 5- to 10-year shorter lifespan of men than women in most countries (Liu *et al.* 2003). This difference was originally thought to reflect cardioprotective effects of oestrogens in women, but this has since been questioned in both women and in men treated with oestrogens (Liu *et al.* 2003). It is perhaps more likely that perinatal androgen exposure in males is what determines the sex difference in disease risk, although even this has not been definitively proved; rather, alternative explanations have been successively discounted (Liu *et al.* 2003). Consistent with this view, females are relatively protected from the adverse effects of fetal programming of cardiovascular disease/hypertension in association with IUGR, based on animal studies (Grigore *et al.* 2008). Thus, if placental dysfunction and resultant fetal IUGR is induced experimentally in rats, then both males and females go on to develop hypertension prepubertally (Ojeda *et al.* 2007). In this study, the hypertension in females but not in males resolved, and further experimental manipulations demonstrated that this was due to ovarian oestrogen secretion in the females and involved modulation of the renin–angiotensin system. Therefore, oestrogens can be protective in this context, which may, to an extent, explain the increased risk of cardiovascular disease that occurs in women after the menopause (Maric 2007; Ojeda *et al.* 2007), although not all studies support this view (Liu *et al.* 2003).

It has also been established that the rate of growth postnatally in IUGR babies is a critical factor in determining later risk of cardiovascular disease (see Chapter 2, Section 2.10 and Chapter 10, Section 10.3), so it can be appreciated that there may be multiple interactions between fetal androgen exposure, fetal growth (maternal nutrition and stress), postnatal nutrition/growth and postpubertal hormone exposure that ultimately determine disease risk. Indeed, this spectrum of influential factors can probably be widened to include male–female differences in liver function and metabolism (including the metabolism of lipids and steroid hormones), kidney development and disease risk and the distribution and extent of adipose tissue, which are also susceptible to nutritional and lifestyle impacts, as discussed elsewhere in this chapter. In this broader context, it can be considered that perinatal androgen exposure is simply increasing the susceptibility of males to impacts of these other factors.

5.10 Kidney disease/hypertension

Another important determinant of blood pressure and hypertension is kidney disease and this again shows clear male–female differences (Gilbert and Nijland 2008). Of particular interest is that modest maternal protein restriction in rats programmes the occurrence of later hypertension in males (Woods *et al.* 2001) but not in females (Woods *et al.* 2005) – a difference that reflects reduced nephrogenesis in the males, but not in the females, leading to a reduction in number of nephrons and associated alterations in the renin–angiotensin system in males. More severe dietary restriction in pregnancy results in equivalent effects in male and females (Woods *et al.* 2004), suggesting again that males are simply more susceptible to the adverse effects of under-nutrition and IUGR. Similar sex-specific effects of maternal undernutrition have been found in sheep (Gilbert and Nijland 2008). Exactly what underlies this sex difference in susceptibility to kidney dysfunction has been the subject of numerous studies, but is still not completely resolved (Reckelhoff 2001). There may be elevation of blood testosterone levels postpubertally in animal models of kidney-related hypertension, and suppression of androgen action at this time via castration or anti-androgen treatment can alleviate the hypertension (Reckelhoff 2001), which fits with the emergence of the sex difference in hypertension during puberty (Gilbert and Nijland 2008). However, this fails to explain why IUGR males are more prone than females to impaired nephrogenesis in fetal life. Most, but not all, studies suggest that androgen receptors are expressed in the fetal kidney, though not during the first trimester (Sajjad *et al.* 2007), but the effects of androgens on the developing kidney are unclear and there is no evidence for direct effects on nephrogenesis, which occurs mainly in the second half of pregnancy.

5.11 The immune system

In general, men get infections more frequently than do women and they tend to be more severe. These differences apply regardless of the type of infectious organism (Fish 2008). In contrast, many of the well-known autoimmune diseases (multiple sclerosis, rheumatoid arthritis, systemic lupus erythematosus and Graves' disease) are more common in women (Fish 2008). In general, adult females have greater humoral and cell-mediated immunity than males and the thymus is larger. Women mount higher titre antibodies in response to immunisation, are more susceptible to allergies and reject transplants more quickly than equivalent men (Martin 2000). It is generally accepted that these sex differences result partly from differential programming of the immune systems of males and females during perinatal development and that androgens, possibly via local conversion to oestrogens (e.g. in the thymus), play the driving role in this dimorphism (Martin 2000).

Additionally, there are further sex-specific and androgen-dependent activation effects of the immune system that come into play later in life, for example at puberty. In mouse models involving complete ablation of androgen action, due to the absence of a functioning androgen receptor, a female-type immune system develops (Martin 2000). However, whether more subtle defects in perinatal androgen action in males, or inappropriate androgen exposure of females (e.g. congenital adrenal hyperplasia), lead to significant changes in set-up of the immune system, or its function, is unknown. As females are more likely than males to develop allergies in general, it follows that differences in perinatal nutrition may be more likely to induce specific food allergies in girls than in boys.

However, some allergies are more prevalent in boys than in girls, one example being asthma, and this may reflect sex differences in lung development (see Section 5.12) as well as immune system differences. Intriguingly, this sex difference in asthma is reversed in adulthood to become more common in females than in males, the switch occurring at puberty, again suggesting the involvement of sex steroids (oestrogens). See Chapter 2, Section 2.5.12 and Chapter 13 for more discussion on the immune system.

5.12 Lung development and disease risk

Lung development during fetal life shows quite pronounced sex differences, with females exhibiting earlier lung maturation (i.e. surfactant production) than boys (see Chapter 2, Section 2.5.3) despite the latter developing larger lungs (Carey *et al.* 2007). This sex difference is an important underlying reason why boys are more susceptible to respiratory distress syndrome and risk of dying when born prematurely (Carey *et al.* 2007).

Whether differences in lung development between males and females account for the higher incidence of asthma in boys than girls prior to puberty is less clear. This could be due to immune system differences. It is well established, especially from animal studies, that both androgens and oestrogens exert effects directly on the developing lungs in fetal life, although, physiologically, this may depend more on the local synthesis of androgens rather than on effects of circulating hormones (Carey *et al.* 2007).

5.13 Effects of maternal diet/obesity and infant feeding choices

Several lines of evidence indicate that maternal diet, obesity and choice and amount of infant feeding can impact on reproductive hormone levels in the mother and/or offspring and/or on masculinisation, in ways that may have long-term health impacts. Obesity in pregnancy is associated with an increased risk of various other disorders in the offspring that are outside the scope of this chapter (see Chapter 8), and such effects may stem from the glucose intolerance or insulin resistance (and in some instances diabetes) associated with maternal obesity. This can lead to changes in placental size and function which impact on growth of the fetus (e.g. IUGR) and this may in turn affect oestrogen production by the placenta, which could alter long-term breast cancer risk in female offspring (Hilakivi-Clarke and de Assis 2006), and can also lead to other metabolic effects of IUGR/ obesity outlined elsewhere in this chapter and in Chapter 8 and Chapter 9. Conversely, in diabetic pregnancies, there can be fetal overgrowth which may lead to a similar range of consequences, but usually in the opposite direction (Hilakivi-Clarke and de Assis 2006).

With regard to masculinisation, maternal obesity is associated with a more than doubling of the risk of male offspring having undescended testes (Berkowitz *et al.* 1995) or the penile abnormality, hypospadias (Akre *et al.* 2008), at birth. The underlying mechanism is unknown, but reduced fetal testosterone or androgen production is a likely explanation (Welsh *et al.* 2008), especially as one recent study has shown a predisposition to low sperm counts in adult offspring of obese mothers (Ramlau-Hansen *et al.* 2007); perinatal androgen action is an important determinant of later sperm counts (Sharpe 2010). Furthermore, undescended testes or hypospadias are both associated with increased risk of low sperm counts in adulthood (Sharpe 2010).

Eating a vegetarian diet or a diet low in meat in pregnancy is also associated with increased risk of hypospadias in male offspring in some (Akre *et al.* 2008) but not all studies (Ormond *et al.* 2009). In view of the widespread effects of perinatal androgens outside the reproductive tract, it is possible that maternal obesity might also impact these if fetal androgen levels are truly affected.

The effects of infant feeding choice are covered in Chapter 3. However, in the context of this chapter and of male–female differences, there are additional considerations. In the first 3–4 months after birth, boys exhibit so-called 'mini puberty' or the neonatal testosterone surge, when testosterone levels increase into the adult range. The physiological role of this increase is still uncertain, although it certainly promotes penis growth and probably increases proliferation of Sertoli cells, which can impact on sperm counts in adulthood (Sharpe *et al.* 2003; Macleod *et al.* 2010); effects on other body systems, including the brain, are possible but have not yet been identified in humans.

Factors that impair the neonatal testosterone rise could therefore have health consequences, and this could happen in several ways. For example, feeding baby marmoset monkeys with soy formula milk, which contains high levels of plant oestrogens, reduces testosterone levels during the neonatal period (Sharpe *et al.* 2002), although this did not appear to have any long-lasting consequences on Sertoli cell number, sperm production or fertility in adulthood (Tan *et al.* 2006).

A recent comparison of testis size in 4-month-old boys who were breast-fed or bottle-fed with standard (cow's milk-based) or soy formula milk showed that both types of bottle-feeding were associated with significantly smaller testis volumes, but no difference according to the type of bottle-feeding (Gilchrist *et al.* 2010). It is difficult to know what to make of this apparent impact of bottle-feeding, but it is remarkable that not a single study has ever evaluated whether sperm counts or testis size in adult men are related in any way to the type of feeding that they experienced in the first 6 months of life.

This data gap has been highlighted by recent studies showing that perinatal exposure to dioxins, as a consequence of the Seveso accident in Italy in 1976, results in a substantial reduction in sperm counts in adulthood (Mocarelli *et al.* 2008). Because dioxin is lipophilic and persistent it accumulates in body fat and can then be mobilised during lactation and delivered via breast milk to the baby; this would also be the case for other persistent, lipophilic environmental chemicals such as DDT and other chlorinated compounds. Although such chemicals are now largely banned from use, they persist in the food chain and, in theory, differential exposure to such compounds via breast- or bottle-feeding might have impacted on sperm counts or testis size according to the level of *in utero* and lactational exposure (Sharpe 2010).

In this regard, it is established that maternal smoking in pregnancy (and presumably also during lactation) can profoundly lower sperm counts in offspring in adulthood (the mechanism is unknown but it could share features with dioxin effects), highlighting that the perinatal period is vital in the male for laying the foundations for future sperm counts (Sharpe 2010). The fact that one in six young men in the UK and elsewhere in Europe now have an abnormally low sperm count may therefore indicate that the lifestyle and diets of mothers during pregnancy and lactation 20–30 years ago had a major impact on this aspect of male reproductive development (Sharpe 2010).

5.14 'Fetal programming' and epigenetic mechanisms

Evidence is beginning to emerge to show that fetal programming associated with exposure to an adverse early life environment may involve epigenetic changes such as altered methylation of specific genes (Burdge and Lillycrop 2010). It is likely that some of the masculinising effects of perinatal androgens on fetal organs may involve similar processes. With this in mind, it should be remembered that dietary deficiencies in nutrients such as folate and vitamin B_{12} can potentially alter the level of gene methylation (see Chapter 4, Section 4.5.3).

Folic acid supplementation has been shown in several studies to be associated with reduced risk of hypospadias in the male offspring (Goh *et al.* 2006; Ormond *et al.* 2009), but whether there might be wider effects on the masculinisation process is, for the moment, unknown. Of major public health concern is that programming effects may be passed on to future generations via both maternal and paternal lines and this may involve epigenetic processes. The fact that the germ cells that will form the 'next' generation undergo complex epigenetic reprogramming *in utero* in both male and female fetuses emphasises the potential vulnerability of these epigenetic processes and the importance of an appropriate diet for women during pregnancy.

5.15 Conclusions

Being male or female is the most fundamental of distinctions as it largely determines our place in society and what is expected of us. As this chapter has hopefully shown, it also determines to an extent what diseases we may be prone to, although this is still a surprisingly unexplored area, especially with regard to elucidation of the underlying mechanisms for sex-specific disease risks. In some instances, hormones clearly play a determining role but overall this remains a largely unstudied area.

It is also becoming increasingly evident that maternal diet, lifestyle and body composition during pregnancy and lactation can have major impacts on sex-specific disease risks, although again our understanding of the underlying mechanisms is limited; the evidence that some such effects can be transmitted to future generations emphasises the value of gaining better understanding of these processes and what may influence them.

We all like to imagine that we are in control of our lives, but it appears increasingly likely that much of our disease predisposition is decided for us, either by our genetic make-up or via our early life experiences. Early nutrition builds on these foundations, and the better we understand how this happens the more chance we have of being able to select the optimum path for an individual that minimises the impact of disease-predisposing genes and other factors, including those that differ according to sex.

5.16 Key points

- Being male or female shapes an individual's risk of certain diseases (cardiovascular disease, autoimmune disease, asthma, depressive illnesses, eating disorders, schizophrenia, autism, gastric ulcers and kidney diseases); the basis for most of these is largely unexplored.
- Masculinisation of the (male) fetus by androgens in fetal or early postnatal life exerts effects throughout the body on non-reproductive

organs; this may partly explain male–female differences in disease predisposition.
- Subtle disorders of masculinisation in males are remarkably common, highlighting the inherent vulnerability of this process.
- Maternal body weight, diet and lifestyle choices can impact on growth of the baby before and after birth and this can exert profound effects on lifelong predisposition to the major 'Western'

Continued

diseases; these affect males and females differently.

- The male fetus grows faster and is more vulnerable to growth restriction due to various factors, including maternal lifestyle choices.
- Recent discoveries have identified some of the brain mechanisms that interlink the reproductive and metabolic systems of the body; dysfunction of these circuits may underlie disorders such as precocious puberty, eating disorders and susceptibility to obesity.
- Better understanding of the mechanistic bases for male–female differences in disease predisposition and their 'programming' in perinatal life should identify strategies for minimising their impact in later life; modulation of diet is likely to be a factor in this.

5.17 Recommendations for future research

- Further research is required of the pregnancy and lactation period to better understand how modern maternal diet and lifestyle choices may differently impact on male and female offspring, their childhood growth and development and the later impacts on well-being in adulthood.
- Further investigation is required on the fetal mechanisms that underlie male–female differences in disease risk to move them beyond their present descriptive state. In particular, resolution of the role played by hormones (mainly androgens) is needed – this will probably require experimental studies in animal models.

5.18 Key references

Geary N (2004) Is the control of fat ingestion sexually differentiated? *Physiology and Behavior*, **83**, 659–71.

Holden C (2005) Sex and the suffering brain. *Science*, **308**, 1574–7.

Kautzky-Willer A & Handisurya A (2009) Metabolic diseases and associated complications: sex and gender matter. *European Journal of Clinical Investigation*, **39**, 631–48.

Reckelhoff JF (2001) Gender differences in the regulation of blood pressure. *Hypertension*, **37**, 1199–208.

Shi H, Seeley RJ, Clegg DJ (2009) Sexual differences in the control of energy homeostasis. *Frontiers in Neuroendocrinology*, **30**, 396–404.

Vanbillemont G, Lapauw B, Bogaert V *et al.* (2010) Birthweight in relation to sex steroid status and body composition in young healthy male siblings. *Journal of Clinical Endocrinology and Metabolism*, **95**, 1587–94.

6
Neurological Development

6.1 Introduction

6.1.1 The vulnerability of the developing brain

Suboptimal development, as a consequence of nutritional insult, before and/or during the critical early years following birth can have deleterious downstream consequences for health and well-being. A range of organ systems can be involved in these processes, both at the time of the insult and during the longer term as the metabolic, physiological, behavioural and health consequences emerge. The rapid development of the human brain from the third trimester of pregnancy through to 2 years of age, the so-called 'brain growth spurt', places significant demands on nutrient supply through either maternal or infant diet in two contrasting environments. Given this dynamic state and the influence of early life nutrition on metabolic phenotype in adulthood, it would be a surprise if inadequate or unbalanced nutrition during periods of especially rapid brain development were not to compromise the structure, neuronal development and subsequent functioning of this complex organ.

Although the developing brain may be spared relative to other organs under conditions of malnutrition, it is by no means exempt. There is growing evidence to suggest that the development, and subsequent functioning, of the brain can be adversely affected by deviation from either normal growth *in utero* or normal gestation period, and can be influenced by both maternal diet during pregnancy and early diet during infant life. Brain structure may be particularly vulnerable at times of rapid growth, for example, in humans, the period immediately before normal term, which for the premature baby may be lived *ex utero*. Changes at a structural level may be visualised using contemporary imaging techniques and are likely to be permanent and hard-wired, especially if the initial nutritional insult occurs during a critical developmental period. More subtle changes may be short-term and reversible, i.e. amenable to subsequent dietary intervention, being manifest by their functional consequences, for example, through effects on cognitive performance in later life. Some changes may be resistant to direct description in human subjects but can be approached by inference through examination of appropriate animal models where deliberate nutritional interventions and more invasive technologies can be applied.

6.1.2 Mechanistic studies in animal models

For clear ethical and medical reasons, consideration of the importance of diet in neurological development in humans is largely limited to describing outcomes following unplanned and uncontrolled nutritional insults, and attempts at beneficial intervention following the diagnosis or anticipation of problems that result from these insults. Accordingly, although the implications of impaired neurological and cognitive development are obviously most important in the human context, dissection of the underlying mechanisms may only be possible by recourse to rodent or other mammalian experimental

Nutrition and Development: Short- and Long-Term Consequences for Health, First Edition. Edited by the British Nutrition Foundation.
© 2013 the British Nutrition Foundation. Published 2013 by Blackwell Publishing Ltd.

models. Consequently, the evidence base for nutritional effects on neurological development relies heavily on animal studies. This is particularly true in the case of nutritional programming effects on energy balance circuits which appear likely to be important contributors to the current obesity epidemic, and which are considered in detail below.

This raises the issue of how readily work with animal models can be extrapolated to the human situation. This discussion is relevant generically to all animal work attempting to model human health and disease, but particularly so in the area of early life nutrition where major disparities exist between species in gestation length, numbers of offspring and degree of development and independence at birth. Although clear differences exist between human and rodent brain development relative to the birth event, it is generally considered that the central nervous system (CNS) mechanisms and molecular and neuroanatomical substrates participating in processes such as the regulation of energy balance are likely to be very similar. The ability to perform a controlled nutritional manipulation during gestation or early neonatal life and then to study the effect of that manipulation on the precise neuroanatomy of the brain, the neuronal projections between key CNS sites, and the activity of these sites and their neurochemical signalling moieties will always be restricted to *in vivo* animal studies and *in vitro* analysis of post-mortem tissues from these animals.

However, these studies provide valuable insight into the equivalent processes that will be affected during so-called 'natural experiments' in human development, and their long-term outcomes. These insights will supplement developmental, structural and functional studies that can be undertaken directly in human subjects with non-invasive or minimally invasive techniques. Nevertheless, it will be difficult to translate mechanistic findings from animal model work into human interventions, and progress here will always be cautious.

6.1.3 Levels of nutritional effect

Inadequate global nutrition or specific nutrient deficiency in early life can both affect brain structure and brain function. These effects may be sustained across the life course. For example, epidemiological studies show association between early growth trajectory and human behaviours or mental illness and the evi-

dence of linkage between early environment and cognitive function, behavioural disorders such as hyperactivity and attention deficit, and certain psychiatric conditions, is now strong. The early life nutritional insults or attempted beneficial interventions that have been studied or applied in the context of neuronal development or functional outcome are varied in nature and severity. On the one hand, global energy or protein malnutrition has been examined using animal models to mimic the equivalent nutritional issues leading to growth restriction in human fetuses. In a complementary approach, other studies in animal models and, to a lesser extent, human interventions, have looked at nutrient and micronutrient deficiencies and specific dietary supplements.

In addition to energy and protein, nutrients with more substantial effects on brain development include certain fats and micronutrients including iron and zinc. In parallel with global or specific nutritional challenge during fetal or neonatal life come global or circuit-specific effects on neurological development, some of which may be assessed or visualised in the pre-term infant using contemporary neurodevelopmental approaches (Georgieff 2007). The majority of animal studies of neurological development have, as their basis, manipulations of the maternal diet during pregnancy and/or lactation. Early independent feeding in weaned rodents is rarely investigated so that the programming effect on study parameters projecting forward from the early life nutritional manipulation is not compromised.

6.1.4 Environments

The mammalian brain exhibits programmed development that is susceptible to environmental influence. Brain development in mammals takes place in two sharply contrasting physical environments, the first *in utero* and the second postnatal. As already outlined, the degree of development of different neuronal systems in these contrasting environments varies according to relative maturity of any given species at birth. Premature birth, for example in human pregnancy, will represent an additional challenge to the maturing brain due to untimely exposure to the contrasting environment and less certain nutrition. The postnatal environment is potentially very variable, and the *in utero* environment less so, but, although buffered, the developing fetus will still be sensitive to maternal nutritional signals that represent the integration of the external environment. This can lead to adaptation to the predicted postnatal environment that is designed to be advantageous but may prove to be anything but, depending on the relationship between the external environment *in utero* and the actual lifetime postnatal environment. This is the essence of the 'thrifty phenotype' hypothesis (see Chapter 4, Section 4.5).

The likely maternal signals that will influence metabolic phenotype in the offspring include hormones such as leptin and insulin, and metabolites such as glucose and fatty acids. Disadvantageous later life outcomes could result from the opposite extremes of maternal nutrition. For example, overweight and obesity, often accompanied by chronic or gestational diabetes, will generally be associated with hyperleptinaemia, and with hyperglycaemia, leading to elevated fetal insulin levels that promote growth and adiposity in the offspring. At the other end of the nutritional spectrum, malnutrition *in utero* due to inadequate maternal calorie or protein consumption may induce intrauterine growth restriction (IUGR) and give rise to a phenotype that is ill-suited to a postnatal life where calories are plentiful, thereby increasing the risk of developing obesity and insulin resistance. It is important to point out (Grayson, Kievit *et al.* 2010) that, although obesity and its metabolic and physiological consequences are primarily manifest in peripheral organs and biological processes, these functions are controlled by the brain. Whereas patterns of relative susceptibility to obesity and metabolic disorders due to early life nutrition are now well recognised, the implications for the developing brain of such perturbations and the involvement of the brain in subsequent outcomes are less well studied, but are now increasingly the focus of research effort.

6.2 The developing brain

6.2.1 Timing

There are major differences between mammalian species in the timing of developmental events in the brain relative to normal term birth. Thus in the rodent, where most developmental and mechanistic information has been obtained, hypothalamic projections, for example, are not fully developed until the third week of postnatal life. In contrast, in human

and non-human primates, the equivalent circuits are formed *in utero* during the third trimester of pregnancy.

Clearly the effect of a nutritional intervention, imposed or natural, on the brain will depend on the stage of development (e.g. neuronal generation, proliferation, migration and differentiation) and on which CNS regions are maturing most rapidly at the time of the challenge. Species differences suggest that maternal diet and health during gestation are likely to influence the development of intra-hypothalamic projections and wider brain circuitry in the primate, whereas in rodents, the postnatal nutritional environment may be equally or more important. Brain development could be influenced at either macroscopic or microscopic levels through the influence of prenatal factors on neural tube formation (neurulation) or cell migration, and by prenatal, neonatal or subsequent events during childhood or adolescence influencing myelination (ensheathment of neurons) or synapse formation (Fig. 6.1).

6.2.2 Human brain development

The adult human brain consists of 100 billion neurons, supported by 5 to 10 times that number of glial cells. The proportions of grey and white matter change as the brain matures. Primitive neurons are produced, in excess of actual requirement, at a prodigious rate, and are reduced in number by approximately 50% by programmed cell death (apoptosis) prior to birth and in the first few months following birth. Neural connections or synapses are also produced in excess in early life. The period from the start of the third trimester through to term is one of major remodelling for the human fetal brain, culminating in a structure resembling the adult brain. There is rapid structural and synaptic development in key brain regions including the hippocampus, the cortical areas responsible for sight and hearing, and the striatum. Myelination also accelerates throughout the brain during this period. The neuronal basis of learning also develops before birth.

The timing of synaptogenesis and subsequent reduction in synapse number varies by brain region, with adult densities of synapses being found in the visual cortex and angular gyrus (audition and language) by about 5 years of age, and in medial prefrontal cortex (cognition) by late adolescence (see Figs 6.1 and 6.2). This non-uniformity in brain devel-

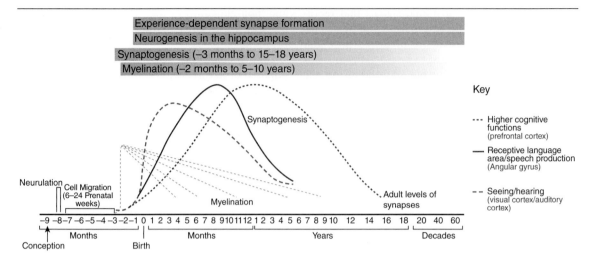

Figure 6.1 Human brain development.
Redrawn from Thompson and Nelson (2001).

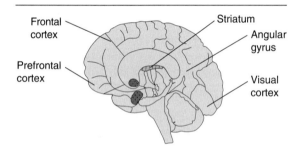

Figure 6.2 Human brain anatomy.

opment, with the frontal and prefrontal cortex and hippocampus being some of the last to mature, means that major reorganisation continues beyond puberty. The brain is about 80% of the adult weight at 2 years of age and achieves adult weight some time before the early teens. Nutritional insults early in life can limit cell proliferation and cell number, whereas later insults will affect differentiation, such as neuronal projections. In the rat, this transition from proliferation to differentiation occurs around about postnatal day 7, equivalent to late gestation in the human fetal brain. The developing brain circuitry is particularly sensitive to deficiency in the specific nutrients referred to in Section 6.4.4 during late gestation and early

neonatal life. However, this period of comparative vulnerability is also one of plasticity when repair may be able to compensate for damage inflicted by nutritional insults.

6.2.3 Pregnancy outcome

The distinguishing features and definitions of 'fetal growth restriction' (FGR) and 'small for gestational age' (SGA) are beyond the scope of this review, but these categorisations are linked by relative malnutrition, of varying cause, and consequent developmental deficit. In the brain, this developmental perturbation may involve changes in gross morphology, cell density in defined structures, connectivity between structures or neurotransmitter/receptor function. At a functional level the gross indicator of low birthweight, a proxy for under-nutrition and adverse fetal environment, may be accompanied in later life by a number of indicators of impaired cognitive and neurological development, including low intelligence quotient (IQ), hyperactivity and inattention, emotional problems, temperament and personality, stress reactivity, schizophrenia, mood disorders and suicidality.

FGR can be diagnosed by ultrasound examination during pregnancy, and FGR due to placental insufficiency is characterised by lower intracranial and cerebral cortical grey matter volumes compared to normal weight controls of similar prematurity. The consequences of these changes in later life include neurodevelopmental impairment in cognitive function, attention deficit and reduced performance in school. Interestingly, growth hormone treatment of FGR children with poor longitudinal growth also improves IQ, behaviour, self-worth and self-perception. A direct effect on cerebral functioning is suggested since improvements in IQ have been shown to be independent of height, supporting the concept of normal brain development continuing into the pre-school period. Equally, damage during this period, such as that induced by micronutrient deficiency, may have long-term consequences, particularly for still-maturing brain regions involved in reasoning (prefrontal cortex) and spatial learning (hippocampus).

Being born small for gestational age (SGA) is also associated with subsequent cognitive impairment, manifesting in IQ, academic performance, and social and behavioural problems. In one study of full-term SGA children, early evidence of slowing of head growth *in utero* was associated with greater deficit in perceptual performance, motor ability, concentration and cognitive index. This translated into poorer educational achievement. The neurodevelopmental effects may be long-lasting; magnetic resonance imaging (MRI) examination of 15-year-old children born SGA observed the persistence of lower total brain volumes.

Premature delivery in the absence of major disability is also associated with increased risk of neurological problems, including learning difficulty and attention deficit, with reduced caudate nucleus volumes and increased structural brain abnormalities. Relative malnutrition in the period between birth and term, when brain growth is most rapid, is a risk factor for many preterm infants, where feeding difficulties are common (Abernethy *et al.* 2004).

6.3 Brain energy balance circuits and peripheral feedback signals

6.3.1 Background

The *in utero* and early infancy period is critical not only in determining susceptibility to body weight problems in later life through nutritional programming (perinatally acquired predisposition), but it is also the developmental window for hypothalamic and wider central nervous system energy balance systems, suggesting a causative link. Brain circuits that contribute to the regulation of mammalian energy balance are widely distributed (Fig. 6.3). This complex neuronal network includes integratory centres in the hypothalamus and brainstem, and the hedonic circuitry of striatal and cortical regions. All these regions are sensitive to nutritional status and to peripheral metabolic signals, such as leptin and insulin, when mature and probably also during development. The developed brain monitors physiological and metabolic events in the rest of the body through feedback from peripheral hormones and metabolites, augmented by afferent nerve signalling. There is now strong evidence from the study of developing hypothalamic systems in wild-type and mutant rodents that peripheral hormones can directly influence the development of these neuronal systems and their interconnectivity, as well as evidence of similar events in other parts of the developing brain.

In rodents, these events are concentrated in the first few postnatal weeks, whereas in primates hypothalamic energy balance circuits mainly develop *in utero*. Despite this difference in timing relative to birth, cues for development are likely to be similar in all mammalian species.

6.3.2 Structures and development

6.3.2.1 Hypothalamus

It is now well established that the hypothalamus, located at the base of the forebrain, plays a key role in the regulation of energy balance. A number of identified hypothalamic structures (nuclei) or regions form an integrated network with interconnected neuronal projections and signalling to other brain areas to regulate behaviour, metabolism and physiology (Fig. 6.3). The arcuate nucleus of the hypothalamus (ARC) is home to populations of neurons which are both sensitive to blood-borne signals (such as leptin, insulin and gut hormones) and metabolites, and which express genes, the neuropeptide products of which have either orexigenic (stimulates appetite) or anorexigenic (reduces appetite) properties at downstream receptor fields. Thus the ARC acts as an integrator and transmitter for metabolic and hormonal signals into the hypothalamic circuitry that modulates feeding and energy expenditure.

Consequently, the timing of the birth of ARC neurons and their development (projections) has been studied in some detail, mainly in laboratory

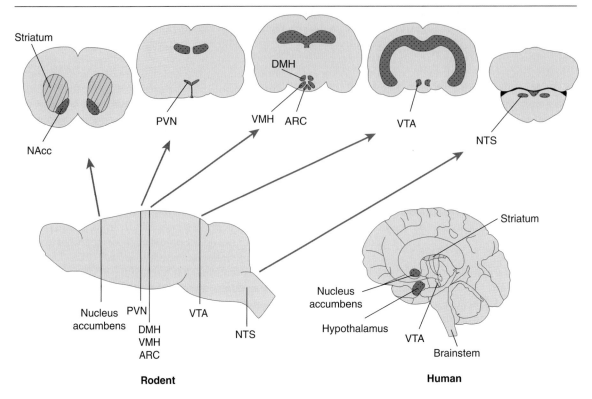

Figure 6.3 Brain circuits contributing to the regulation of mammalian energy balance.
ARC, arcuate nucleus; DMH, dorsomedial nucleus of the hypothalamus; NAcc, nucleus accumbens; NTS, nucleus of the solitary tract; PVN, paraventricular nucleus of the hypothalamus; VMH, ventromedial nucleus of the hypothalamus; VTA, ventral tegmental area.

rodents. Axonal tracer studies in mice have established the ontogeny of projections from the ARC to other hypothalamic nuclei. ARC neurones arise around embryonic days 17 and 18 (i.e. relatively late in gestation) and axonal projections successively reach hypothalamic target nuclei from the end of the first postnatal week and may take a further two weeks to complete. Adult-like distribution is achieved at around two and a half weeks of age, i.e. by weaning (Bouret and Simerly, 2007). Connections between other hypothalamic nuclei may form earlier than those originating in the ARC.

Key peptidergic neurons with cell bodies in the ARC include those that synthesise neuropeptide Y (NPY) and which co-express agouti-related peptide (AgRP), both of which are orexigenic in effect. Other key peptidergic neurons in the ARC synthesise both the family of peptides (including melanocortins) pro-

duced by post-translational processing of the pro-opiomelanocortin (POMC) precursor, and cocaine and amphetamine-regulated transcript (CART), both anorexigenic in nature. Projections from these ARC neurons extend throughout the rodent hypothalamus at maturity.

Unsurprisingly, knowledge of equivalent developmental events in higher mammals is more sparse (Grayson, Kievit *et al.* 2010). Birth of ARC neurons in human and non-human primates also occurs around mid-gestation (second trimester), but projections develop during the third trimester of pregnancy and are usually completed before birth. Detailed studies (Grayson *et al.* 2006) have described the development of the NPY and melanocortin systems in the macaque during the late second (gestational (G) day 100), early third (G130) and late third trimesters (G170). NPY gene expression was apparent in multiple hypothalamic nuclei (ARC, paraventricular [PVN] and dorsomedial nuclei [DMH]) by G100, by which time projections from the ARC to the PVN had been initiated. NPY/AgRP projections from the ARC had reached the different target sites by G170, but continued to increase in density into postnatal life. Projections from POMC neurons were slower to develop. The POMC neurons in the human brain did not co-express CART. The development of neuropeptide systems during the prenatal period in nonhuman primates places more emphasis on the maternal environment as a determinant of normal development and functioning.

6.3.2.2 Brainstem

The caudal brainstem, and especially the dorsal vagal complex that includes the nucleus of the solitary tract (NTS), links the brain and the gut via afferent and efferent neural pathways, and is an integratory centre for satiety signals produced during and after meal feeding. The NTS integrates signals from vagal nerve terminals distributed throughout the gastrointestinal tract that respond to food intake to regulate meal size. Although the NTS has an important role in short-term satiety, it also has a role in longer-term energy balance, expressing leptin receptors and prepropeptide genes, and being sensitive to leptin injections. Leptin regulates the expression of preproglucagon mRNA (the precursor to glucagon-like peptide-1 [GLP-1]) in the NTS, and can modulate the transmission of information received from vagal afferents that innervate the gut. By comparison with the hypothalamus, maturation of brainstem neurons in the rodent is relatively precocious, with efferent projections (to the hypothalamus) developing prenatally, although being subject to further development early in postnatal life. Projections from the hypothalamus arise early in postnatal life, with some being present at birth, although pathways are not mature until 3 weeks of life. This timing difference, at least in rodents, may make brainstem circuits more sensitive to nutritional insults *in utero* than hypothalamic systems although, like hypothalamic circuits, full maturity is probably not reached until weaning.

6.3.2.3 Hedonic circuitry

A number of distributed brain regions make up the hedonic circuitry, including the ventral tegmental area (VTA), nucleus accumbens (NAcc), amygdala and prefrontal cortex, and are implicated in the reward value of food. A wealth of evidence suggests that the palatability and reward value of foods that are high in fat and sugar can override the normal regulation of energy intake required to maintain homeostasis. These neural circuits encode wanting (incentive motivation) and liking (experienced pleasure) of different stimuli, including food. The NAcc integrates motivational, hedonic and cognitive tasks with the homeostatic system, i.e. the hypothalamic energy balance systems considered earlier. Inputs to the NAcc mediating motivation and reward arise in the VTA, amygdala, prefrontal cortex and lateral hypothalamus and include sensory inputs from the olfactory and gustatory systems via the caudal brainstem. The dopaminergic, GABAergic, opioid and serotonergic systems are major players in this circuitry, with the majority of studies focusing on the mid-brain dopaminergic system. This system comprises a population of dopaminergic cells in the VTA that project to the NAcc and the prefrontal cortex, among other brain areas. Despite their ability to override homeostatic regulation, the reward pathways are themselves modulated by peripheral energy status signals such as leptin.

The components of the hedonic circuitry have a maturation timetable that is more similar to the hypothalamus than the brainstem, although information relating to the development of this circuitry appears restricted to rodents. Dopamine projections from the VTA appear within the NAcc early in rodent postnatal life, but do not mature until the third postnatal week. Accordingly, it is suggested that both maternal and early postnatal nutritional influences will impact on the development of this circuitry (Grayson, Kievit *et al.* 2010).

6.3.2.4 Integration

It is likely that for each of the three interrelated systems outlined above, development will be influenced by the prevailing ambient conditions of two environments, *in utero* and after birth. The nutritional characteristics of each environment and the timing of the transition between them will be important influences on neuroanatomical and neurochemical phenotypes and their development. The potential consequences of disrupting longitudinal development and interaction between these regulatory systems could be profound, perhaps encompassing changes in food preference and drive to consume rewarding food. This may promote over-consumption of calories in later life. Evidence in support of this possibility in human populations comes from analysis of data from the Dutch Hunger Winter cohort (Lussana *et al.* 2008) (see Chapter 1, Section 1.4.1 and Chapter 4, Section 4.4.2). Individuals who were exposed to the Dutch famine in early gestation have an atherogenic blood lipid profile, which may in part be of contemporary dietary origin: they were twice as likely to consume a high-fat diet at age 58 years as individuals in a control population. There was also a trend towards lower levels of physical activity. This evidence of an effect of prenatal nutrition on subsequent dietary preference has been studied under more controlled conditions and at a mechanistic level in animal studies detailed below.

6.3.3 Hormonal feedback

6.3.3.1 Leptin

The extensive literature on the biological effects of the leptin molecule mainly centres on its anorexigenic properties in the adult, or at least the post-weaning, rodent. Studies have examined the detail of leptin's effects on physiology and behaviour, and in particular effects on energy homeostasis, its regulation *in vivo*, its integration into the CNS energy balance circuitry, and the signalling systems downstream of its receptor. The leptin–leptin receptor–POMC–melanocortin-4 receptor (MC4R) pathway is now recognised as promoting negative energy balance and as being critical for normal mammalian body weight regulation. Severe early-onset obesity mutations cluster around this axis in both rodents and humans. More recently, considerable detail has begun to emerge of the effects of leptin on the development of hypothalamic neural connections regulating energy balance (Bouret and Simerly 2007), and of wider brain structures (Udagawa *et al.* 2006). In fact, the causative mutation in leptin-deficient *ob/ob* mice was known to affect brain development more than a decade before the leptin gene was cloned. Mutant mice have a smaller brain than wild-type controls, with reduced cell density in a number of brain regions, as well as more-recently characterised hypothalamic structural abnormalities, abnormal myelination and disturbances in neuronal and glial

cell proteins (Bouret 2010a). Leptin is detected in the circulation of wild-type fetal mice from mid-gestation onwards, a stage in development when leptin receptors are also widespread in the developing CNS. In the brains of *ob/ob* mice fetuses, the same developmental stage is characterised by reduced cell number and cell proliferation activity in the cerebral cortex, which may be at least partially rescued by leptin supplementation (Udagawa *et al.* 2006), providing evidence of functional involvement in brain development.

In cultured embryonic cortical neurons leptin acts as a trophic factor, affecting growth cone size and spreading (Valerio *et al.* 2006). Involvement in brain development is also apparent in postnatal life, with administration of leptin to early postnatal *ob/ob* mice increasing brain size and normalising marker disturbances under appropriate administration regimes. Analogous changes in the human brain have been reported from MRI studies of brain structure in human congenital leptin deficiency following leptin therapy in adult life. Grey matter tissue was increased at 6 and 18 months into treatment in the anterior cingulate gyrus, the inferior parietal lobule and the cerebellum. These structural/compositional changes may be accompanied by more subtle changes in organisation and connection, and may be more far-reaching still if leptin replacement were to be commenced earlier in life (Bouret 2010a). An additional source of leptin for the developing neonate may be via maternal milk transferred during suckling (Kirk *et al.* 2009; Cottrell *et al.* 2010). Both human and rodent milk contain measurable concentrations of leptin, which can be absorbed across the neonatal gastrointestinal tract to enter the circulation. If maternal milk does prove to be a significant source of leptin for the neonate, it may contribute to both the development of energy balance circuitry and to early satiety signalling. This could be another determinant of the differential growth rates seen in breast- and formula-fed human infants.

In addition to the likely role for leptin in rodent brain development *in utero*, a developmental role in early neonatal life is suggested by the timing and characteristics of the so-called postnatal leptin 'surge'. This transient increase in circulating leptin concentration in the first 2 weeks of neonatal life is independent of any substantive change in body adiposity. The leptin surge does not appear to influence feeding behaviour and metabolic responses at this age, and there is no evidence of functional signalling to downstream energy balance pathways.

Rodent pups feed independently from around the time of weaning (approximately 3 weeks of age), and are sensitive to the metabolic effects of leptin from this point onwards. The evidence of a widespread neurotrophic role for leptin in early life neuronal development and circuit formation is now strong, and especially so in the case of the development of hypothalamic neuroendocrine systems, into which leptin will also have regulatory input in later life (Bouret and Simerly 2007).

In the absence of leptin (i.e. in *ob/ob* mice) projections from the ARC to the PVN fail to develop normally, resulting in a reduced fibre density (approximately 10-fold) within the PVN from postnatal day 12 through into adult life. Leptin is able to promote the development of these projections, increasing density and length. *In vivo*, administration of the hormone to mimic the postnatal surge seen in wild-type mice increases the density of ARC projections to the PVN in postnatal day 12 *ob/ob* mice. The deficit in density of projections between the two nuclei cannot be rescued by leptin treatment of *ob/ob* mice in adult life. *In vitro*, leptin promotes neurite outgrowth from ARC tissue dissected from the hypothalamus of postnatal day 6 neonates (Bouret and Simerly 2007).

Experimental manipulation of the leptin surge also provides support for a programming role for leptin. A leptin antagonist administered during the surge gives rise to elevated body adiposity, circulating leptin and leptin resistance, in later life. Furthermore, manipulation of leptin levels or the timing of the surge through litter size adjustments or food restriction can also affect leptin sensitivity and development of leptin-responsive hypothalamic circuits. Litter size manipulation to induce early neonatal overfeeding results in an exaggerated leptin surge and in leptin resistance in ARC neurons and inhibits development of ARC projections (Grayson, Kievit *et al.* 2010).

By contrast, food restriction during pregnancy results in a premature leptin surge and increased susceptibility to diet-induced obesity. Leptin administration to mimic this premature surge produced a similar susceptibility to weight gain on a high-fat diet in later life. Both undernourished and leptin-treated groups had an elevated density of NPY and CART nerve terminals in the adult PVN, the terminus for projections from the ARC (Yura *et al.* 2005). Whereas the evidence in support of a role for leptin in brain development, and in the development of arcuate nucleus circuitry in particular, is compelling in the rodent, equivalent evidence is lacking in higher mammals. In non-human primates, detectable leptin levels in the fetus postdate the initiation of ARC NPY/AgRP projections (Grayson, Levasseur *et al.* 2010), and there is no evidence of a surge equivalent to that seen in rodents.

6.3.3.2 Insulin

Insulin is another metabolic signal that acts as a neurotrophic factor during development and can promote neurite outgrowth (projections from the cell body of a neuron) in vitro (see Fig. 6.4). Insulin may act in concert with leptin during brain, and especially hypothalamic, development, since the intracellular signal transduction pathways of these two hormones are shared. Insulin is a periphery-brain peptide, a feature common to many gastrointestinal peptides, being produced by the pancreas and reaching the brain via the circulation, but also being synthesised locally within the brain, where gene expression and receptor expression are widespread. Peripheral insulin administration to neonatal rats gives rise to excess weight gain in later life, and also results in disrupted development of the ventromedial hypothalamic nucleus (VMH). This effect appears to be due to elevated insulin concentration within the hypothalamus since administration of insulin directly into the neonatal hypothalamus results in the same phenotype in later life and also causes morphological disruption in the VMH and other adjacent hypothalamic structures (Plagemann, Harder *et al.* 1999a).

6.3.3.3 Other gut–brain signals

The accumulating evidence that leptin, and to a lesser extent, insulin, may influence the development of hypothalamic and other CNS networks as a consequence of changes in early nutrition suggests potential roles for other energy balance-related gut-derived hormones in the development of these neuronal circuits. The food intake-stimulatory peptide, ghrelin, for example, is a likely candidate. Ghrelin is an endogenous ligand for the growth hormone secretagogue receptor (GHS-R), which is found in both brain and peripheral tissues. Ghrelin is secreted from

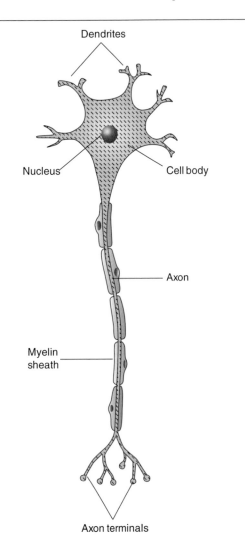

Dendrites

Nucleus

Cell body

Axon

Myelin
sheath

Axon terminals

Figure 6.4 Neuron anatomy. Adapted from Eckert R *et al* (2002) *Animal Physiology*, 5th edition, W. H. Freeman, with permission.

the empty stomach and stimulates hunger through its interaction with receptors in several hypothalamic and brainstem nuclei with established roles in body weight and food intake regulation. GHS-R mRNA is present in various rodent fetal tissues from mid-gestation onwards, and ghrelin injections during pregnancy increase birthweight, even when increased maternal food intake is prevented. Ghrelin injected into the mother enters the fetal circulation. These results indicate that maternal ghrelin regulates fetal development during the late stages of pregnancy

(Nakahara *et al.* 2006). A role in the trophic regulation of the developing fetal/neonatal hypothalamus is clearly feasible.

6.4 Nutritional influences on the developing brain

6.4.1 Risk factors

There is growing evidence that nutrition during the fetal and neonatal periods influences brain function in later life. Cognitive function, for example, increases as a function of birthweight, other than in the case of the heaviest fetuses, in both a UK child cohort and in studies of identical twins, most likely reflecting the adequacy of nutrition during the pre-birth period (Benton 2008a). This relationship draws attention to maternal nutrition and diet, the effects of which are not restricted to clinical situations of growth restriction or premature birth.

In a recent study of the relationship between IQ of Asian children at ages 8–12 and birth parameters within the normal size range, every 1 cm increase in birth length, 1 kg increase in birthweight and 1 cm increase in head circumference resulted in a corresponding IQ increase of 0.49, 2.19 and 0.62 points, respectively (Broekman *et al.* 2009), indicating that cognitive potential is influenced by antenatal factors. Besides IQ, accumulating evidence also links fetal growth with behavioural and mental health outcomes in later life (Schlotz and Phillips 2009), including hyperactivity, inattention and perhaps personality disorders and schizophrenia. Again the Dutch Hunger Winter famine (see Section 6.3.2.4) provides vital evidence of a link to early life nutrition; early prenatal exposure to famine was associated with greater risk of schizoid personality disorder and schizophrenia at age 18 (Hoek *et al.* 1996).

Although low birthweight and prematurity are risk factors from many developmental perspectives, many of these relationships which have their origin in early life nutrition are bell-shaped in form. Fetal macrosomia and being born large for gestational age (LGA) is also a risk factor for lifelong disease. High maternal BMI is an increasingly important risk factor as the prevalence of overweight and obesity exceeds 50% in women of childbearing age in a number of developed countries. Maternal obesity during pregnancy increases the risk of obesity and poor metabolic outcomes in the offspring. As a consequence of the negative influence on developmental outcomes at opposite ends of the nutritional spectrum, the search for underlying mechanisms has intensified.

A range of early life nutritional manipulations have been examined in rodent and other mammalian models for effects on the subsequent development of the brain and in particular the functioning of hypothalamic energy balance systems that directly affect feeding behaviour, energy expenditure and body phenotype in later life. These include direct dietary manipulations of mother or offspring, and litter size adjustments. The manipulations have been applied during the gestational period, during early neonatal life, or both, and have comprised global over- or under-nutrition, and diets with unbalanced macronutrient composition or micronutrient deficiency.

6.4.2 Global over-nutrition

As outlined above, predisposition of offspring to caloric over-consumption and increased body fatness as a result of maternal obesity is increasingly being recognised as an important non-genetic route of transmission of obesogenic traits across generations. The mechanisms underlying this detrimental outcome are now beginning to emerge. It is not possible to review all the studies that have adopted the maternal diet-induced obesity approach in this chapter, but some examples are given below (see also Grayson, Kievit *et al.* 2010). Cumulatively, these studies examine the effects of gestational diet on pups at or around the point of birth, and gestation/lactation diet over the first 3 weeks of life. In common with the broader literature on diet-induced obesity in the adult rodent (Mercer and Archer 2008), manipulations applied to induce maternal obesity have employed a range of species and strain combinations and diets with considerable variability in fat content, macronutrient composition, energy density and physical formulation (Ainge *et al.* 2011). Most commonly, high-fat (HF) diets are employed, but variation in experimental specifics such as duration of dietary manipulation, timing of tissue harvesting and tissue analysis all influence the phenotypic outcome and its characterisation. This complexity can lead to contrasting outcomes that make interpretation difficult. For example, in one study of term rat fetuses from dams fed a HF diet (60% energy as fat), there was hyperleptinaemia and an apparent upregulation of hypothalamic gene expression in both orexigenic (NPY, AgRP) and anorexigenic (POMC, MC4R) arms of the homeostatic system (Gupta *et al.* 2009). By contrast, day 1 postnatal offspring of rat dams fed on a cafeteria-type diet including HF (34% energy as fat) modified chow had low leptin levels and a near global downregulation of hypothalamic energy balance genes including NPY, POMC and MC4R (Morris and Chen 2009).

Although these results appear contradictory, they affirm that early life nutritional manipulations mediated through maternal obesity, in this case during gestation, have powerful influence over the activity of hypothalamic energy balance systems and the neuropeptides mediators therein.

More insight into the likely involvement of leptin in such changes comes from another recent study of the offspring of rats fed a fat- and sugar-rich diet before and during pregnancy, and on into lactation, to induce maternal obesity (Kirk *et al.* 2009). Progression of offspring through into postnatal life allows behavioural and metabolic phenotypes to be characterised more thoroughly. Offspring of obese dams were hyperphagic on a normal diet and relatively obese in adult life. However, prior to the development of hyperphagia and excessive body fat accumulation, offspring exhibit a number of potentially causative changes in energy balance signalling systems. Affected offspring have an altered neonatal leptin surge; blood concentrations of the hormone were elevated and longer-lived relative to controls. Further perturbations to the leptin signal and its hypothalamic integration were apparent. Subsequent to the leptin surge, but again before obesity develops, the animals exhibit leptin resistance, as evidenced by a failure of the injected peptide to reduce food intake, and reduced concentrations of the key neuropeptide, AgRP, within the PVN, suggestive of a restricted development of neuronal projections from the ARC.

These data suggest that the perturbation to the leptin surge before weaning affects leptin feedback to the hypothalamus and the development of ARC-PVN circuitry, i.e. permanent impairment of signalling systems related to leptin's neurotrophic properties in the hypothalamus. The effects of HF diet-induced maternal obesity are also seen in the hedonic circuitry, with evidence of changes in neurotransmitter systems in the VTA and NAcc, creating a further risk factor for a range of long-term adult behaviours and pathologies (Naef *et al.* 2008). Further evidence of the impact of maternal diet on components of the central reward system and on diet preference (towards over-consumption of palatable foods) comes from investigation of the effect of a maternal cafeteria-type, so-called 'junk food', diet (Ong and Muhlhausler 2011). Female rats were fed the modified diet for 4 weeks prior to mating and throughout gestation and lactation. Following weaning, offspring were allowed to choose between the control diet and the various components of the cafeteria diet. The cafeteria diet did not have major effects on maternal body weight, and the offspring of these dams had lower body weight at weaning and in the case of male offspring this persisted into adult life. Fat intake was elevated in the offspring of cafeteria-fed dams from weaning through into adult life. This food choice phenotype was accompanied by time-dependent changes in the expression of opioid and dopamine signalling pathway genes in the NAcc; MOR was elevated and dopamine reuptake transported (DAT) lowered in cafeteria offspring compared to controls at 6 weeks of age, whereas the opposite differences were apparent at 3 months of age.

The results from these rodent models of maternal over-nutrition add to the evidence connecting nutritional status in fetal and neonatal life to developmental phenotypes, and have clear implications for the potential for gestational overweight and obesity, and diet consumed during pregnancy, to further amplify the growing problem of obesity in the human population. Further evidence comes from higher mammalian species such as the sheep. Hypothalamic neuronal circuitry that regulates energy balance is present before birth in the sheep, as in human and non-human primates. Consequently, the period of sensitivity of these developing networks to nutrients is likely also to be shifted more into the gestational period. This is demonstrated by the effect of glucose infused into ovine fetuses shortly before term, which resulted in hyperglycaemia and hyperinsulinaemia, and elevated POMC gene expression in the ARC (Muhlhausler *et al.* 2008). The other neuropeptide mRNAs examined, NPY, AgRP and CART, were not affected by fetal infusion.

Since the hypothalamic melanocortin system develops during the third trimester in non-human primates, maternal nutrition is likely to influence the development of this system. After long-term maternal HF, high-calorie diet feeding with variable effects on adiposity and metabolic status, fetal and neonatal offspring exhibited a range of adverse metabolic symptoms. Analysis of third-trimester macaque fetuses revealed perturbations to the melanocortin system, with elevated POMC gene expression and reduced AgRP mRNA and peptide levels (Grayson, Levasseur *et al.* 2010). There was also evidence of a (possibly causative) local inflammatory response in the hypothalamus. These offspring went on to gain excess weight early in independent life. The serotonergic system in the fetal CNS also exhibits effects of maternal HF diet feeding. In newborn female offspring there was also an increased anxiety response to novel threat objects (Sullivan *et al.* 2010), suggesting that maternal diet during gestation, independent of obesity, increases the risk of developing such behavioural disorders.

Complementary to the approach of inducing maternal obesity, manipulation of litter size in rodent species provides a vehicle for altering neonatal nutrition independent of maternal nutritional status. A reduction in litter size reduces competition and gives rise to increased feeding and weight gain, and elevated leptin and insulin levels during the period when hypothalamic projections are maturing. Aspects of this phenotype are projected forward into adult life, when a range of hypothalamic maladaptations are also observed (Plagemann 2006).

6.4.3 Global under-nutrition

As for over-nutrition, the effects of under-nutrition on the developing brain can be examined either through neonatal manipulations such as maintenance of large litters, or as a consequence of maternal manipulation, in this case restriction of maternal nutrition. Paradoxically, both over-nutrition and under-nutrition predispose offspring to an overweight phenotype in later life. Maternal under-nutrition can be induced by straightforward food restriction or through manipulation of dietary macronutrients, for example, a low-protein diet. As outlined above (Yura *et al.* 2005), a 30% restriction in maternal food supply resulted in the birth of underweight pups which exhibited a premature leptin surge of greater amplitude in the early postnatal period. This was accompanied by increased susceptibility to HF diet-induced obesity and changes in nerve terminal density in the PVN, suggestive of a causative link between these observations. Maternal under-nutrition in late gestation in the sheep results in increased ARC NPY gene expression in the fetus (Muhlhausler *et al.* 2008).

Dietary protein manipulations have been studied extensively, for example by Ozanne and collaborators where 8% or 20% protein diets are fed either during gestation or from birth through to weaning. With this rat model, offspring of dams fed an 8% protein diet during pregnancy, but which are then nursed by control dams (fed a 20% protein diet) through until weaning are smaller at birth, but show catch-up growth by day 21, whereas postnatal low-protein animals (offspring of control dams fed a 20% protein diet) nursed by low-protein dams (fed an 8% protein diet) have lower body weight than control offspring at weaning (Ozanne, Lewis *et al.* 2004). Weaned recuperated pups were hypoleptinaemic compared to controls but had generally comparable hypothalamic gene expression levels.

Postnatal low-protein pups were hypoglycaemic, hypoinsulinaemic and hypoleptinaemic on day 21. Consistent with this hypoleptinaemia, the hypothalamic ARC exhibited increased gene expression for leptin receptor, NPY and AgRP, compared to controls, and reduced levels of POMC and CART mRNA. This apparent increase in overall anabolic drive in animals that remain stunted into adult life suggests that central pathways 'recognise' the early energy deficit but fail to redress this imbalance (Cripps *et al.* 2009). Analysis of a similar dietary manipulation (9% vs. 18% protein) limited to gestation revealed a preference for fatty foods in offspring exposed to a low-protein diet *in utero* (Bellinger *et al.* 2004).

Leptin administration during gestation and lactation in rats may protect against the adverse metabolic programming effect of a low-protein diet, and protect offspring of normally nourished rats from diet-induced obesity, further implicating leptin in the development of the hypothalamic energy balance circuits (Cottrell *et al.* 2010).

6.4.4 Micronutrient deficiency

A growing evidence base supports a role in fetal brain development for maternal micronutrient status during pregnancy. As with global macronutritional insults, adverse micronutrient supply *in utero* may have long-term effects on cognitive function and the likelihood of behavioural problems in later life (Schlotz and Phillips 2009).

6.4.4.1 Iron

Accumulating evidence indicates that deficiency of iron can result in abnormal brain development, with availability being critical during late fetal and early neonatal life, during the spurt in brain growth (Benton 2008b). Development of the hippocampus and frontal cortex appears to be particularly vulnerable, with the negative effects of deficiency in the first year of life extending into adulthood. Marginal and deficient intakes of iron are common in both developed and developing countries, with the deficiency disease, iron-deficit anaemia (IDA), being associated with tiredness, low mood, low IQ and difficulty with concentration, learning and memory. The mechanisms behind iron deficiency-induced impairment of normal neurological development (with motor, cognitive and behavioural outcomes) appear to include changes in the myelination of neurons, decreases in associated enzyme activity, and changes in CNS neurotransmitter systems including those involved in dopamine metabolism and signalling. Hippocampal changes may include effects at the level of gene expression, including those involved in synaptic plasticity, metabolism and electrophysiology. In addition, blood–brain barrier function may be affected by iron deficiency, allowing hormones and metabolites in the bloodstream to enter the brain in greater concentration than would otherwise be the case. Improved iron status through supplementation can enhance psychological function, depending on when deficiency is experienced. However, causality between iron deficiency during development and cognitive or behavioural function in later life remains to be definitively established (McCann and Ames 2007).

6.4.4.2 Zinc

Zinc is essential for normal fetal development and for brain development both before birth and in neonatal life. Deficiency during late pregnancy disrupts neuronal replication and synaptogenesis (Benton 2008b), and fetal deficiency decreases DNA, RNA and protein content of the brain. Human zinc deficiency is very common, affecting one in five of the world's population, and if experienced during the perinatal period may have long-term consequences for brain function and behaviour during adult life.

Zinc is found at high concentrations in the brain where, as elsewhere in the body, it is important in the activity of numerous enzymes, including those crucial to nucleic acid synthesis. Zinc deficiency in non-human primates is accompanied by reductions in activity, learning, memory and attention, while severe zinc deficiency can recapitulate the consequences of protein-energy under-nutrition. The hippocampus may again be the focus of these deleterious effects, with zinc deficiency affecting the glutamate-NMDA receptor neurotransmitter system. Zinc supplementation reduces the risk of premature birth, but not of low birthweight, and may be particularly beneficial for pre-term and low-birthweight infants in terms of overall growth and motor development.

6.4.4.3 Choline

The available evidence, mostly derived from animal studies, suggests that choline is important during fetal development, including in the determination of brain structure and function (Benton 2008b). This effect on the developing brain appears to be mediated through effects on cell proliferation and apoptosis. Animal studies of the effects of choline supplementation or deficiency in late gestation strongly support the view that choline enhances memory and cognition through its effects at the level of the hippocampus. However, although choline appears to be important in brain development and subsequent neurological function, there is no recognised deficiency in humans that would limit neural development, and no evidence that supplementation of infant formula would be beneficial.

6.4.5 Long-chain fatty acid deficiency

The long-chain polyunsaturated fatty acids and particularly the long-chain *n*-3 fatty acid docosahexaenoic acid (DHA) are found in high concentrations in phospholipid membranes in the brain. DHA is a potent neurobiologic that affects membrane structure and fluidity, synapse formation, myelination, and neurotransmitter and peptide production, and the available evidence links brain concentrations of DHA with cognitive and behavioural function (McCann and Ames 2005). Large amounts of DHA accumulate in the brain as it grows, and in the retina,

and consequently DHA is essential in normal brain development and visual function.

Since the growth spurt of the human brain takes place during the last trimester of pregnancy and during the first 18 postnatal months, the high demand for DHA must be met first directly from maternal supplies and subsequently from suckled breast or formula milk. This major structural and functional role of DHA in the developing brain, allied to the observation that induced long-chain polyunsaturate deficiency in rats is accompanied by poor learning and memory, and sensory deficits, along with reductions in the size of neurons in relevant brain areas including hippocampus, cortex and hypothalamus, makes it likely that DHA is involved in cognitive development. Breast milk is a natural source of DHA and breast-feeding is generally taken to be associated with better cognitive performance, although this is a complex and contentious subject with possible confounding effects (see Chapter 14, Section 14.3). Consumption of oil-rich fish during pregnancy is also associated with better cognitive performance in children and reduced risk of prematurity, which is itself associated with cognitive deficits and mental health problems.

6.5 Programming mechanisms

Dietary, energy balance or other manipulations or events during fetal and neonatal life can influence body phenotype, trophic hormone profiles, expression of brain transmitters and aspects of cognitive function or mental health during later life, but it is less clear how the initial adverse events are linked mechanistically to these outcomes. Fetal and neonatal glucocorticoid exposure and epigenetic alterations may be part of the mechanism linking environmental challenge with the sorts of functional and neurological changes discussed earlier.

6.5.1 Glucocorticoids

Elevated circulating levels of glucocorticoids are a likely route for signalling of poor environmental conditions, including nutritional restriction, from the mother to the fetus. However, prenatal exposure to elevated glucocorticoids can adversely programme offspring physiology since these hormones promote the maturation of tissues and organs during fetal development. Stress-induced activation of the hypothalamo–pituitary–adrenal (HPA) axis increases corticotrophin-releasing hormone (CRH) and arginine vasopressin (AVP) release from the PVN into the portal blood system. The hormones act on the anterior pituitary to stimulate adrenocorticotropic hormone (ACTH) output that then increases gluco-corticoid production by the adrenal glands. The feedback loop is completed by circulating glucocorti-coids inhibiting HPA axis activity by negative feed-back on the brain, and especially hippocampal glucocorticoid receptor-expressing neurons, and at the pituitary. Maternal dietary restriction and prena-tal stress are associated with exaggerated stress responses in offspring, indicative of reduced negative feedback of HPA axis activity.

There is growing evidence from analysis of the consequences of significant traumatic events, the most recent of which was the September 11 2001 attacks on New York's World Trade Center, that exposure to these events *in utero*, and associated consequences for the mother such as post-traumatic stress disorder (PTSD), can result in a range of adverse outcomes for the offspring including growth restriction, stress response perturbations and behavioural/psychiatric problems, e.g. temperament (Cottrell and Seckl 2009). The third trimester of human pregnancy may be the critical period for development of HPA axis abnor-malities in the offspring.

6.5.2 Epigenetics

Whereas changes in DNA sequence may have pro-found effects on major phenotypic characteristics such as food intake or body adiposity, particularly when sequence change (e.g. mutation) leads to loss of function, an additional level of complexity is pro-vided by epigenetic regulation. Epigenetic modifica-tion affects the way the genetic code is interpreted, and may be as important as the sequence itself. The epigenome controls the expression of human genes, and contributes to the regulation of metabolic response in all cells in the body. Epigenetic marking of the genome can be influenced by factors such as diet and lifestyle and has been implicated in long-term health. Both heritable and non-heritable pro-cesses contribute to brain development, and epigenetic processes are likely to be particularly prevalent in the brain, given its anatomical and physiological complexity. The hypothalamus and brainstem, for example, express a high proportion of the known imprinted genes (Kelsey 2011). That these 'hotspots'

are associated with energy homeostasis is clearly of interest in the context of perinatal programming of maladapted body phenotype and metabolic status.

Nutritionally acquired epigenetic modification during brain development has been demonstrated in the hypothalamus and in the reward circuitry. Plagemann *et al.* (2009) examined DNA methylation patterns in the promoter regions of hypothalamic energy balance genes following neonatal overfeeding achieved through litter size manipulation. Rapid neonatal weight gain and deterioration of metabolic indices were accompanied by hypermethylation of specific binding sequences in the POMC gene pro-moter that are essential for the integration of leptin and insulin signals. Coincident with these methyla-tion changes, there was no effect of the elevated leptin and insulin levels on POMC gene expression in the ARC in the overfed pups, i.e. anticipated feed-back of these key energy balance signals onto the POMC neurons was absent.

A different overfeeding model, maternal high-fat diet during pregnancy and lactation in the mouse, was used to investigate effects on dopamine and opioid gene expression within the hypothalamus and the mesocorticolimbic reward circuitry of offspring (Vucetic *et al.* 2010). Offspring of mice with diet-induced obesity (DIO) were overweight through to weaning, but this weight differential was lost in adult life, when all offspring were fed a control diet. Mater-nal DIO increased preference for palatable food (dietary sucrose and fat) in offspring. This behav-ioural change was accompanied by changes in dopamine-related and opioid-related gene expression in reward areas (VTA, NAcc, prefrontal cortex) and hypothalamus. Specifically, DAT was upregu-lated in the reward areas but downregulated in the hypothalamus, and the dopamine receptors, D1 and D2, were also downregulated on the NAcc and pre-frontal cortex. Opioid-related genes (preproenkepha-lin [PENK] and μ-opioid receptor [MOR]) were also upregulated in these brain regions in the overnour-ished offspring. The offspring of DIO female mice also had decreased global DNA methylation in all three reward centres and in the hypothalamus com-pared to control offspring, which translated into gene-specific promoter DNA hypomethylation for DAT, MOR and PENK. Both the above studies support the hypothesis that over-nutrition during early life is an epigenetic risk factor for obesity and metabolic disorders.

The hippocampus is associated with learning, memory and mood, and is one of two brain structures where neurogenesis continues into adult life. Epigenetic modification of genes in the hippocampus as a result of maternal–neonate interactions may influence cognitive, neural and behavioural phenotypes in later life. High levels of maternal care (grooming) of pups by their mother in the first postnatal week result in lower levels of anxiety and may benefit cognitive development (McGowan *et al.* 2008). Changes include increased hippocampal glucocorticoid receptor expression, decreased hypothalamic CRH expression and a reduced HPA stress response. Cross-fostering studies provide further support for an epigenetic mechanism. This mechanism centres on programmed changes in the promoter region of the glucocorticoid receptor, one of several hundred genes in the hippocampus that exhibit changes in DNA methylation and histone acetylation with contrasting investment in maternal care.

The potential for early life adversity to increase risk of mental health problems in later life through epigenetic processes is illustrated by mutations in components of the methylation process, and has wide-ranging implications. Mutations in the methylated DNA binding protein MeCp2 cause RETT syndrome (a progressive neurodevelopmental disorder), and mental retardation, and are also associated with autism. Similarly, mutation in a gene involved in the chromatin remodelling process is associated with mental retardation in the ATRX syndrome. This makes it likely that environmental exposures that impact upon these epigenetic mechanisms, although clearly less severe, will also influence susceptibility to psychiatric disorders. However, although aberrant methylation patterns may be associated with such pathologies (e.g. schizophrenia, suicidality) in later life, it is less clear when during the life course these epigenetic changes arise, and what was the causative factor. It can be speculated that the epigenetic changes that may affect mental health and psychopathology could be nutritional in origin. The evidence in support of this is reviewed by McGowan *et al.* (2008).

6.6 Nutritional interventions

Whereas dietary manipulations in either pregnancy or early postnatal life in rodent or other mammalian models can be performed under tightly controlled conditions with a subject population where genetic variability is deliberately restricted, the same control is inevitably lacking in human trials, where ethical considerations are paramount. The effect size in any nutritional intervention in human pregnancy or early life is thus subject to multiple confounding variables and consequent statistical adjustment. This has resulted in interventions that produce apparent effects of the primary manipulation, but which do not definitively demonstrate causation (see Chapter 14). Nevertheless, where a number of studies have provided evidence of a beneficial effect, systematic reviews and meta-analyses may either provide confirmation or may focus the design of future interventions. Although this chapter primarily addresses neuronal development and underlying mechanisms, it is worthwhile considering two recent examples of human interventions, one of global nutrition, the other of specific supplementation with DHA. The former strengthens the link between disruption in brain development and functional performance, whereas the latter addresses some of the deficiencies in earlier studies to add further weight to arguments that DHA supplements would benefit brain function in the newborn.

Early nutrition after pre-term birth can influence both brain structure and cognition with long-term or possibly permanent effects. Feeding a formula enriched with protein, energy, vitamins and minerals as opposed to unsupplemented banked breast milk or standard term formula for an average of one month resulted in improved cognitive performance at 7.5–8 years, most notably in boys. Subsequent MRI studies of a sample of the same cohort at 16 years of age examined the influence of this early nutritional intervention on brain structure and found larger caudate nucleus volumes in the supplemented boys. The enhanced verbal IQ observed at age 7.5–8 was sustained. This finding links transient early nutrition with long-term brain development and function, and has fundamental scientific and public health implications (Isaacs *et al.* 2008).

The results of studies using DHA supplements for cognitive benefit have been mixed. Maternal supplementation during pregnancy and lactation is associated with improved cognitive outcomes in the infant, but the outcomes of studies in which infant formula has been supplemented have been inconclusive, perhaps as a result of dosing levels, technical complications and variability in experimental design. To address some of these issues, the DIAMOND (DHA Intake and Measurement of Neural Development) study examined cognitive outcomes (Drover *et al.* 2011) and visual acuity (Birch *et al.* 2010) in infants born at term and receiving DHA supplements for 12 months from within a dose range that represents the full range of concentrations found naturally in breast milk from across the world. Infants were randomly assigned to one of four formulas that differed only in their DHA concentration. Visual acuity at 12 months was improved at each of the three supplement levels compared to controls, while cognitive function at 18 months as assessed using the Mental Development Index was higher in the pooled treatment groups than in the control group. For both outcomes there was no additional benefit beyond that obtained from the lowest dose of DHA employed (0.32%). These initial outcomes of an intervention with healthy, term, formula-fed infants link DHA, where the mechanistic basis of the benefit derived from supplementation is not understood, to visual acuity and cognitive development, in this case in the absence of adverse pregnancy outcome.

6.7 Conclusions

The human brain grows rapidly and establishes many of the structures and connections that are important for normal physiology, metabolism and behaviour during the third trimester of gestation and the first two neonatal years. The equivalent critical period is shifted towards early neonatal life in commonly employed rodent models. Adverse nutritional environments during gestational or early neonatal life that may affect birthweight or other indicators of developmental status can have a major impact on brain development, both structurally and at a more subtle level as evidenced by functional deficits such as low IQ, behavioural problems or unbalanced dietary preference. Major structural changes may be visualised in the human brain with contemporary imaging technologies such as MRI, whereas more subtle changes may only be detectable in terms of their consequence for measurable performance.

With identifiable structural abnormalities, it is possible to perform informed nutritional interventions, as outlined above, with demonstrable benefit. In the latter scenario of more subtle change, it may be possible to determine the mechanism underlying

a particular behavioural, cognitive or metabolic endpoint by assessment of equivalent animal models. Key neuronal developmental events that are sensitive to adverse nutritional environment include neurogenesis, synaptogenesis and myelination, all of which contribute eventually to the adult pattern of neuronal wiring and signalling. In the context of brain feeding and energy balance circuits, for example, it is now clear that a range of early life nutritional insults originating *in utero* or in early postnatal life can influence the activity of neuronal systems in brain regions such as the hypothalamus and striatum, and may lead to adaptations to the anticipated environment that turn out to have consequences for long-term health.

In attempting to elucidate underlying mechanisms, it is appreciated that these will be multi-step processes linking the initial nutritional challenge with what may be a complex phenotypic endpoint. Epigenetic changes may well be involved in this process.

A key question for the future is how we can best interpret and use the mechanistic information that is emerging in the areas of cognition, behaviour, mental health and feeding-related outcomes. First, for interpretation, as the evidence base emerges, some of which has been discussed here, it is apparent that to maximise the knowledge gained from experimental studies in animal models there should be more standardisation of the nutritional manipulations themselves and the outcome measures. In the former, details such as dietary composition, duration and point of manipulation commonly vary between studies and between the research groups carrying out the work. Similarly, from an analytical standpoint, interpretation would be less speculative if outcomes were verified using more than one complementary technique. For example, in an organ with the structural complexity of the brain, comparing gene expression results obtained by polymerase chain reaction-based methods with those from anatomically resolved semi-quantitative methods such as *in situ* hybridisation may be problematical. Both these considerations would allow more direct comparison of results between studies. Lack of comparability is a common problem in many research fields performing *in vivo* nutritional interventions. In terms of exploiting the information that is obtained linking insult with outcome, it will be necessary to continue to proceed with caution. What are the implications of programmed changes in neuronal circuitry for the offspring in later life? In the case of feeding/energy balance-related hypothalamic neuropeptides, for example, what does a programmed change in gene expression really mean, and how will we interpret the responses of signalling systems to subsequent challenge? There will always be a tendency to interpret changes in the context of our understanding of the functioning and interactions of the same signals in the normal animal. However, in the animal subjected to nutritional insult early in life, it is possible that any given neurotransmitter will be operating in the context of a substantially modified neuronal network, which is unlikely to have been fully characterised, and the outcome of further manipulation in later life will be uncertain. This generic issue of how to translate research findings into intervention either during or soon after pregnancy is reflected in the justifiably tentative approach to nutritional recommendations for problematic pregnancies. Nevertheless, a better understanding of the interaction between early life nutrition and neurological development using a combination of human observation and intervention and directed manipulation of appropriate animal models will facilitate future attempts to improve the outcome of both compromised pregnancies and clinical conditions or poor function in early neonatal life.

6.8 Key points

- The human brain is especially vulnerable to inadequate or inappropriate nutrition during its developmental growth spurt that broadly spans the third trimester of pregnancy and the first two postnatal years. The same period of rapid differentiation takes place in the early postnatal weeks in rodent species that are frequently employed in laboratory studies to mimic early life nutritional challenges.
- Gestational outcome, maternal nutrition and early neonatal diet can affect brain structure and developmental processes such as neurogenesis, synaptogenesis and myelination, as well as more subtle brain circuitry and transmitter signalling.
- Developmental perturbations and beneficial interventions have been studied in human subjects following exposure to adverse conditions during early life, whereas mechanistic studies of the intermediate steps between the nutritional insult and short-term or lifelong functional consequence require examination of appropriate animal models under controlled conditions.
- The extended CNS feeding and energy balance circuitry develops during late pregnancy and early neonatal life and is susceptible to nutritionally induced changes in trophic signals such as leptin, which can shape neuronal projections and connectivity between different brain regions. The potential implications of over-exposure to hormones such as leptin and insulin during gestation, such as in maternal obesity, are clear.
- Cognitive, mental health and behavioural outcomes may also be influenced by early life nutrition and pregnancy outcome, processes involving cortical areas and the hippocampus.
- Programming mechanisms linking nutritional or other challenges to functional endpoints may involve epigenetic changes and glucocorticoid exposure.
- A range of nutritional challenges of varying severity affect brain development and function, including protein/energy malnutrition, global over-nutrition (e.g. gestational diabetes, maternal obesity, over-nutrition prior to weaning), and specific micronutrient or essential fatty acid deficiencies.
- Although intervention to counter early life nutritional programming effects will be problematical in humans, more detailed knowledge of underlying mechanisms, and causation, should allow development of an evidence base to be carefully exploited to benefit outcome in compromised pregnancies.

6.9 Recommendations for future research

- Further research involving human studies and from directed manipulation of appropriate animal models is needed to gain a better understanding of the interaction between early life nutrition and neurological development.
- Further research is required to investigate the hypothesis that over-nutrition during early life is an epigenetic risk factor for obesity and metabolic disorders.
- Current evidence suggests that leptin in breast milk may contribute to the development of energy balance circuitry and to early satiety signalling, although further research is needed to determine whether leptin in breast milk is likely to contribute to the differential growth rates seen in breast-fed and formula-fed infants.

- The potential causality between iron deficiency during development and cognitive or behavioural function in later life requires further investigation.
- Breast milk is a natural source of the *n*-3 polyunsaturated fatty acid DHA, and breastfeeding is generally taken to be associated with better cognitive performance. Consumption of oil-rich fish during pregnancy is also associated with better cognitive performance in children. However, the benefit of supplementing formula milk with DHA is less clear. Further investigation of the potential benefits of DHA on neurological and cognitive development is required.

6.10 Key references

Bouret SG (2010) Neurodevelopmental actions of leptin. *Brain Research*, **1350**, 2–9.

Georgieff MK (2007) Nutrition and the developing brain: nutrient priorities and measurement. *American Journal of Clinical Nutrition*, **85**, 614S–620S.

Grayson BE, Kievit P, Smith MS & Grove KL (2010) Critical determinants of hypothalamic appetitive neuropeptide development and expression: species considerations. *Frontiers in Neuroendocrinology*, **31**, 16–31.

McGowan PO, Meaney MJ & Szyf M (2008) Diet and the epigenetic (re)programming of phenotypic differences in behavior *Brain Research*, **1237**, 12–24.

Schlotz W & Phillips DI (2009) Fetal origins of mental health: evidence and mechanisms *Brain, Behavior and Immunity*, **23**, 905–16.

7
Establishing of Gut Microbiota and Bacterial Colonisation of the Gut in Early Life

7.1 Introduction

Once considered to merely be a waste disposal system with efficient water absorption capabilities, the human colon is now recognised to be one of the most metabolically active systems in the human body. This is thanks to the actions of the colonic microbiota, which make up the greatest proportion of the human gastrointestinal (GI) or gut microbiota – a complex microbial community comprising millions and millions of bacterial cells ($>10^{12}$). Indeed, the human body contains more bacterial cells (numerically at least) than human cells, although in mass we are more human than bacterial. We not only play host to this extensive bacterial population, but (as with any ecosystem) we have evolved together with our microbial inhabitants and our health and well-being can be affected (positively or negatively) by the actions of the gut microbiota (as a whole and by individual members).

The acquisition of gut microbiota is essential, as they provide colonisation resistance (occupying adhesion sites and utilising nutrients available in the intestines or by altering the environment), thereby reducing opportunity for colonisation by harmful microorganisms; scavenge energy and enhance the bioavailability of certain nutrients and minerals for the host; stimulate epithelial development and maturation of the immune system. Certain bacterial pop-

ulations added in the diet as probiotics such as *Bifidobacterium breve* and *Lactobacillus rhamnosus* (administered maternally [during pregnancy and/or breastfeeding] or during early infancy in formula milk) have also been shown to reduce the risk of developing asthma, atopic dermatitis and other common allergies in childhood. However, certain patterns of colonisation, predominantly aerobic Gram-negative bacteria are thought to play a role in severe disorders such as necrotising enterocolitis, frequently observed in pre-term infants. Furthermore, certain bacterial species and/or microbial profiles have been associated with specific disorders (such as autism) and/or GI disorders (including ulcerative colitis, colorectal cancer and Crohn's disease).

7.1.1 Investigating gut microbiota

Before discussing the acquisition of the gut microbiota, it is important to consider the relative limitations of methods used to investigate the microbiota. There is currently no absolutely quantitative method for enumerating the faecal bacterial populations. Another issue is the reliability of using faecal samples to investigate the gut microbiota, although this is the only non-invasive way of sampling gut contents. Furthermore, protocols for obtaining samples invasively

Nutrition and Development: Short- and Long-Term Consequences for Health, First Edition. Edited by the British Nutrition Foundation.
© 2013 the British Nutrition Foundation. Published 2013 by Blackwell Publishing Ltd.

(such as biopsies) often involve bowel emptying prior to sampling – thus potentially biasing the microbiota or certain members thereof. Available methods for enumerating gut bacteria are semi-quantitative at best and subject to bias (both quantitative and qualitative). Cultivation studies rely on so-called 'selective' growth conditions, including use of 'selective' and/or 'elective' media. Stress imposed on the bacteria during cultivation may also affect which species are isolated, while presence of a bacterial symbiont (friendly neighbour) or specific host factors may be required for isolation of certain bacteria. Many bacterial species remain uncultivable and molecular-based studies have suggested that at best about 50% of the faecal microbiota can be detected by classical cultivation techniques.

Recent developments in molecular techniques have afforded a more detailed understanding of the infant gut microbiota. Clone libraries based on 16S rRNA gene sequences (16S is one of the subunits of the rRNA operon) are the most widely used qualitative method for investigating the gut microbiota, although profiling methods such as denaturing gradient gel electrophoresis (DGGE) and temperature gradient gel electrophoresis (TGGE) are becoming more popular. Terminal-restriction fragment length polymorphism (T-RFLP) analyses have also been used, to a lesser extent, in studies examining the infant faecal microbiota. Such profiling techniques are well suited for ecological studies, and enable bacterial succession to be monitored over time. Both cloning and the aforementioned profiling methods are, however, reliant on polymerase chain reaction (PCR) amplification – the limitations of which can confound results. Indeed, 'each physical, chemical and biological step involved in the molecular analysis of an environment is a source of bias which will lead to a distorted view of the "real world"' (von Wintzingerode *et al.* 1997). It is particularly pertinent to note the relative lack of bifidobacteria, and some other high G+C (content of DNA) Gram-positive organisms from cloning studies, even when these bacteria have been known to be relatively predominant members of the microbiota.

7.1.2 Human gut microbiota

The microbiota of the human GI tract forms a highly complex ecosystem. Despite a large amount of overlap in terms of the bacteria present, variation

between individuals is observed in relation to the composition of the gut microbiota. Factors such as pH, peristalsis, nutrient availability, oxidation–reduction potential within the tissue, age of host, host health, bacterial adhesion, bacterial symbiotic interactions, mucosa (including receptors and mucin secretions containing immunoglobulins), bacterial antagonism and transit time all influence the number and diversity of bacteria present in the different regions of the GI tract. In infants, factors such as gestational age, delivery mode, maternal microbiota, neonatal health and diet impact the acquisition and bacterial succession of the GI microbiota. An understanding of the bacteria making up the GI microbiota is extremely important due to its involvement in the development of the GI mucosal immune system, maintenance of a normal physiological environment and for providing essential nutrients (e.g. short-chain fatty acids and B vitamins). Understanding the acquisition and development of the GI microbiota in infants is perhaps of greatest importance, with increasing interest in the role of the microbial blueprint established in early life in relation to its impact on longitudinal host health, particularly in relation to GI disorders.

The human faecal microbiota has received the greatest attention, regarding the gut microbiota, due to the difficulty of obtaining samples from different regions of the GI tract. This is particularly true in infant studies as faeces are the only samples able to be collected from the GI tract non-invasively, and thus meet ethical guidelines for studies in neonates. Accumulated evidence from such data clearly demonstrates that each individual has their own unique faecal microbial profile, although the profiles from related individuals, such as siblings and identical twins show higher levels of similarity compared to profiles of unrelated individuals.

7.2 Acquisition of the gut microbiota

The intestinal tract of unborn infants is immature and generally considered to be sterile, with microbial exposure or acquisition during or immediately after the birthing process, depending on delivery mode. However, the traditional view of the sterility of the human gut *in utero* is now being questioned due to detection of bacteria from placenta and amniotic fluid. Indeed, the prevalence and diversity of microbes in amniotic fluid has been associated with pre-term delivery and neonatal outcomes. Martin, Langa *et al.* (2004) recovered lactic acid bacteria from the umbilical cord, placenta, amniotic fluid and meconium (the first faecal excretion) of neonates. Jimenez *et al.* (2005) collected umbilical cord blood of infants delivered by caesarean section and recovered a number of different species, including *Enterococcus faecium, Propionibacterium acnes, Staphylococcus epidermidis* and *Streptococcus sanguinis.*

Other studies have also detected the presence of lactic acid bacteria DNA in the amniotic fluid prior to birth. This suggests that the infant gut may come into contact with bacteria and/or their DNA *in utero* and that the intestinal tract may be exposed to or challenged by microorganisms during gestation. These findings have implications for the development of the fetal GI tract, as bacterial colonisation might occur earlier than previously thought. Irrespective of *in utero* exposure, microbiological studies of the meconium and neonatal faecal microbiota have unravelled a common trend in the development and maturation of the infant gut microbiota.

Traditionally, the microbial colonisation and bacterial succession of the neonatal GI tract has been divided into distinct stages. The initial stage is the birthing process and first hours of life, during which time the infant comes into contact with the maternal microbiota and environmental microorganisms. It is generally accepted that during this phase the neonatal gut microbiota largely comprises facultative anaerobes including streptococci, staphylococci, *Veillonella* spp., *Enterococcus* spp. and species from the family Enterobacteriaceae. Such organisms rapidly reduce the redox potential of the intestinal milieu, resulting in an environment more amenable to obligate anaerobes such as *Bifidobacterium* spp., *Clostridium* spp. and *Bacteroides* – which predominate the adult microbiota.

The second stage of bacterial succession is the period of exclusive milk feeding, with distinction seen in the infant microbiota based on diet (breast milk, formula milk or both). However, developments in modern formulas, including prebiotic supplementation, together with improved microbiological analysis, may explain why studies published more recently (in the last 20 years) generally demonstrate fewer differences between the faecal microbiota, particularly in relation to bifidobacterial levels, in breast-fed and formula-fed infants.

The third stage comprises the introduction of solid food into the infant's diet (i.e. weaning). This process can be very different from infant to infant, in relation to both the age at which weaning begins and the types of food and timings of introduction. This can depend on infant appetite and/or weight gain, and the parents' choice of weaning foods. Overall, it is thought that the infant microbiota stabilises around 2 years of age.

7.3 Factors affecting the infant gut microbiota (acquisition and development)

The major factors affecting early colonisation of the infant GI tract include the gestational age, mode of delivery, exposure to bacteria and host genetics. Pre-term birth and/or extremely low birthweight (ELBW) are associated with delayed colonisation, a limited complexity of the microbiota and delayed establishment of the stable microbiota. This may partially be as a result of administration of antibiotics in pre-term infants. The health, nutritional status and microbiota of the mother may also be important factors.

7.3.1 Gestational age

Pre-term neonates and those with ELBW are often transferred to neonatal intensive care units, where they are cared for in incubators and administered broad-spectrum antibiotics. As such, microbiological exposure and colonisation is generally less than that of full-term neonates, which is reflected in the simpler gut microbiota observed in these individuals. The most commonly identified members of the faecal microbiota in pre-term infants include species belonging to the family Enterobacteriaceae (particularly *E. coli* and *Klebsiella pneumoniae*), *Enterococcus, Streptococcus* and *Staphylococcus*. This may also reflect *in utero* exposure to some of these organisms, discussed previously. Necrotising enterocolitis (NEC) is a GI disease that is predominantly seen in pre-term infants and thought to have a bacterial aetiology. Bacteria belonging to the family Enterobactericeae are the most commonly found population in infants developing the disease, although no specific strain has been linked to the development of the disease. Studies comparing the microbiota of pre-term infants in relation to NEC (i.e. cohorts with or without NEC) have demonstrated that a more diverse consortium of bacteria is present in the faecal microbiota of pre-term infants without NEC compared to those with NEC (even for twin pairs).

Wang *et al.* (2009) examined the microbial profiles of 20 pre-term infants (born between 25 and 32 weeks' gestation), ten with NEC and ten matched controls without NEC. (The studied infants included four twin pairs in which one twin had NEC and the other did not.) Overall, the microbiota of all 20 infants were shown to be limited compared to that seen previously for full-term infants (as expected). The bacterial profiles of the NEC patients were, however, distinctly different from those of control infants, with significantly lower diversity and/or bacterial richness, with Proteobacteria dominant in the profiles from NEC patients. Reduced microbial diversity was also associated with significantly greater exposure to antibiotics (i.e. more days on antibiotics) prior to NEC diagnosis.

7.3.2 Mode of delivery

It is well documented that the mode of delivery affects the acquisition and development of the infant GI microbiota. Caesarean section delivery has been correlated with delayed microbiological acquisition and with lower faecal levels of clostridia. This depleted clostridial component of the GI microbiota has been seen even in children over 7 years of age who had been delivered by caesarean section, compared with vaginally delivered children. Vaginal delivery exposes the neonate to the maternal microbiota (from the birth canal, vagina and faeces). The maternal microbiota is therefore important in the initial microbial acquisition of naturally birthed neonates. The duration of vaginal delivery is also thought to affect microbial acquisition by the neonate. A number of studies have identified maternal biotypes within the faecal microbiota of vaginally delivered infants within the first few days after birth.

7.3.3 Host genetics

The faecal microbiota of genetically related individuals have consistently been shown to display greater similarity than those of unrelated individuals. This holds true even for studies of adult twins and/or siblings who no longer live in the same household. While microbiological exposure and initial acquisition of the microbiota may play a role in this, genetically determined host factors undoubtedly also have an impact, for example, mucin production and receptor sites along the epithelia. Two recent longitudinal studies in infants (both including a set of twins) demonstrated that the similarities between microbial profiles of the twins were higher than similarities between any of the other infants throughout the study (Palmer *et al.* 2007; Roger & McCartney, 2010).

An increasing number of studies associate the development of allergies with acquisition of a specific microbiota in the first year of life and the 'hygiene hypothesis' – although host genetics are also associated with allergic diseases. Bjorksten *et al.* (2001) followed 42 breast-fed infants during the first two years of life. Infants who developed allergy were less often colonised by bifidobacteria in the first year of life and *Enterococcus* spp. in the first month of life than infants who did not go on to develop allergy ($p < 0.05$). Moreover, clostridia levels were higher in allergic infants at 3 months of age ($p < 0.05$). Comparison of the faecal microbiota of 21 infants with early-onset atopic eczema, eight being highly sensitised (intolerant) and 13 sensitised (tolerant) showed significantly higher lactobacilli/enterococci counts in the highly sensitised group ($p = 0.002$). Individuals from the sensitised group were then randomly assigned to weaning with extensively hydrolysed whey formula that was supplemented with either bifidobacteria or placebo. *Bifidobacterium* supplementation during weaning significantly modulated the bacterial succession, with significantly higher *Bacteroides* numbers during weaning in the placebo group ($p = 0.04$) and significantly lower *E. coli* counts in the *Bifidobacterium*-supplemented group ($p = 0.02$), compared to pre-weaning levels. However, the clinical importance of these observations is unknown.

7.3.4 Geography and/or lifestyles

In developing countries, the majority of infants experience a more diverse intestinal microbiota and faster acquisition than in developed countries, with higher numbers of bacteroides and enterobacteria. This perhaps relates as much to living conditions (including overcrowding) as to exposure to environmental bacteria. Investigation of the enterobacterial populations of Swedish infants and Pakistani infants demonstrated that less than 50% of Swedish infants harboured *E coli* by 1 week of age, compared to virtually all Pakistani infants at the same age. Distinction between prevalence of bifidobacterial species in the infant faecal microbiota has also been shown with respect to geography. A higher prevalence of *B. longum* biovar *infantis* and *B. longum* biovar *longum* was seen in infants born in Ghana, while UK and New Zealand born infants generally harboured *B. bifidum*.

Recent work has also demonstrated that lifestyle choice may impact the gut microbiota of humans. For example, children with an anthroposophic lifestyle (restricted use of antibiotics and diets based on organic foods and higher in fermented vegetables) had significantly greater microbial diversity than control children (from same area as anthroposophic children but consuming a conventional diet; no restriction on antibiotic usage) or children living on a farm in different areas (Dicksved *et al.* 2007).

7.3.5 Diet

Perhaps the factor that has received the most coverage and research to date regarding the infant faecal microbiota is the impact of diet; specifically that during exclusive milk-feeding, namely the comparison between breast-fed and formula-fed infants. Although somewhat conflicting data have been seen between different studies, it is generally accepted that the faecal microbiota of breast- and formula-fed infants are distinguishable, with formula-fed infants generally harbouring a more complex and diverse faecal microbiota than their breast-fed counterparts. The disparity seen between some studies is most likely due to the use of different methodological procedures (sampling as well as microbiological analysis) and/or different formulas, and environmental confounders (e.g. socioeconomic group, geographical and/or ethnic cohorts). In addition, the majority of studies involve a small number of infants or cover a relatively short period of time. Relatively few studies have investigated the impact of weaning (i.e. introduction of solid food to the infant diet) on the infant microbiota.

As well as providing the nutritional requirements of the neonate, human milk delivers a range of other components important to infant health, most notably, maternal antibodies and human milk oligosaccharides, which impact the infant gut microbi-

ota, directly or indirectly. In addition, recent research has shown that breast milk contains bacterial DNA and that bacteria, including bifidobacteria and lactic acid bacteria, can be isolated from some breast milk samples. Fortification of formula milk, beyond that of the nutritional requirements of the infant, has also identified certain dietary components (e.g. α-lactalbumin, glycomacropeptides, prebiotics) which can modulate the infant gut microbiota towards a bifidobacteria predominance more similar to that of breast-fed infants.

7.4 The gut microbiota of exclusively milk-fed infants

In an effort to accurately access the microbiological findings from the numerous cultivation studies available at the time, Conway (1997) grouped the data based on the phase of microbial acquisition/succession. From her subsequent analysis and review of the data, Conway identified that the initial acquisition of the first few days of life, during the microbiota was common for all infants, breast- and formula-fed (initial colonisers being enterobacteria and streptococci, with obligate anaerobes establishing between days 4 and 5). However, anaerobic colonisation tended to occur a day earlier in formula-fed infants, compared to breast-fed infants. Subsequently, breast-fed infants tended to have higher prevalence of bifidobacteria (about 85% of breast-fed infants harboured bifidobacteria during initial stages of phase two (see Section 7.2), compared to 62% of formula-fed infants), although comparison of all data from phase two showed no significant difference in the bifidobacterial component of the infant faecal microbiota. Indeed, the prevalence and levels of other bacterial groups were more notably different between formula- and breast-fed infants during exclusive milk-feeding, in particular, higher prevalence/ levels of clostridia, enterobacteria and streptococci were found in formula-fed infants.

Compared with the relative abundance of cultivation-based studies, only a very limited number of molecular-based studies of the infant gut microbiota have been published, though this is likely to increase in the next few years. However, the overriding findings are in agreement with earlier cultivation studies, namely, that there is a clear distinction between the microbiota of breast- and formula-fed infants, with the former comprising a less diverse microbiota dominated by bifidobacteria.

Using a barrage of fluorescently labelled probes, Harmsen and colleagues (2000) demonstrated that the phase one (see Section 7.2) microbiota of infants is complex, irrespective of feeding mode – and bifidobacteria accounted for less than 40% of the microbiota. Subsequently, bifidobacterial predominance (60–91% after 1 week) was shown for the microbiota of breast-fed infants. A more complex microbiota was seen for formula-fed infants during phase two, with bifidobacteria comprising between 28% and 75% of the microbiota when detected (Bif164 counts were below the level of detection for one of the six formula-fed infants during phase two). Coriobacteriaceae, *Bacteroides* and *E. coli* proportions were notably higher in the formula-fed infants during phase two, compared to breast-fed infants. However, since the bacterial levels were only presented as proportions of the total count for each bacterial group, it is not possible to determine whether the bifidobacterial levels of breast- and formula-fed infants were significantly different. That is, did formula-fed infants harbour a numerically larger faecal microbiota that was more complex than their breast-fed counterparts (i.e. similar levels of bifidobacteria but higher *Bacteroides*, coriobacterial and enterobacterial counts [and total bacteria] in formula-fed infants)? Suffice to say, it is evident that formula feeding was not associated with the 'selective' bifidobacterial predominance in breastfeeding. Overall, the dynamics and diversity of the faecal microbiota was more substantial in the formula-fed infants during the first 20 days of life, compared to the breast-fed infants.

Favier *et al.* (2002) utilised DGGE to monitor the composition of the faecal microbiota over time for the first 10–12 months of life for two infants (both initially breast-fed, although formula milk was included in the diet of one after 2 weeks of age (i.e. mixed-fed; infant L). During phase one (see Section 7.2), the DGGE banding profiles of both infants were relatively simple. However, the complexity and diversity of the DGGE profiles progressively increased with the age of the infant. Indeed, a shift in the DGGE profiles of infant D (exclusively breast-fed prior to weaning) was observed during phase two, with bands identified as related to *Bifidobacterium breve, Enterococcus, Clostridium, Enterobacter* and *Ruminococcus*. More notable variation in the DGGE profiles and greater complexity of banding profiles were seen for infant L during phase two, with bands identified as related to *Bifidobacterium, Clostridium paraputrificum, Entero-*

bacter asburiae, Streptococcus spp. and *Ruminococcus* spp. Interestingly, the only bands seen in all samples during phase two DGGE profiles (for both infants) were related to *Bifidobacterium*.

More recently a longitudinal study monitoring the faecal microbiota of 14 infants, including a set of identical twins, breast-fed, with particular attention to the impact of weaning, demonstrated the gradual development of the infant gut microbiota with increased complexity observed after weaning and subsequent convergence towards an adult-like (climax) faecal microbiota (Roger and McCartney 2010). The main findings of this work were that the initial infant gut microbiota, and its development throughout the first 18 months of life, varies considerably among infants – with each infant harbouring their own unique microbiota. Furthermore, clear differences were seen between the faecal microbiota of breast-fed infants and formula-fed infants. In general, the breast-fed infant microbiota predominantly comprised bifidobacteria (see Fig. 7.1), while a more mixed microbiota was evident in formula-fed infants (see Fig. 7.2). During exclusive milk feeding (i.e. the pre-weaning phase) formula-fed infants were shown to harbour significantly higher levels of *Clostridium* cluster XIV (Erec 482 counts) and *Clostridium* clusters I and II (His 150 counts) and significantly lower levels of *Bifidobacterium* (Bif 164 counts) than their breast-fed counterparts. More detailed investigation of the bifidobacterial component of the faecal microbiotas in this study demonstrated that breast-fed infants generally harboured a more complex *Bifidobacterium* microbiota than their formula-fed counterparts (Roger *et al.* 2010).

Quantitative PCR (qPCR) has also been applied sparingly to investigations of the infant faecal microbiota to date. *Bifidobacterium* levels were not significantly different between 50 breast-fed and 50 formula-fed infants (at 1 month of age), while *E. coli* and clostridia levels were significantly higher in the formula-fed infants. As part of a more extensive longitudinal study (including microarray analysis and sequencing of cloned libraries) involving 14 healthy full-term infants (seven breast-fed and seven mixed-fed – including a set of fraternal twins), Palmer *et al.* (2007) performed qPCR to enumerate the total bacteria, bifidobacterial component, fungi and archaea of faecal samples. The prevalence of fungi and archaea was low, with intermittent detection by qPCR. Variation was seen in the overall bacterial

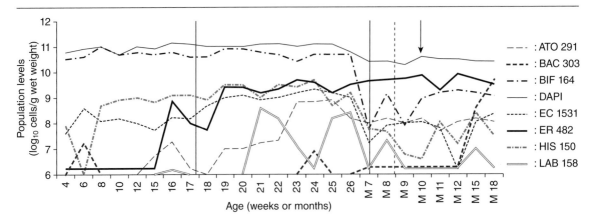

Figure 7.1 Longitudinal investigation of the faecal microbiota of a breast-fed infant, using Fluorescence *in situ* hybridization (FISH) probes, during the three dietary phases (PW, W and M).
Samples are shown in chronological order. The vertical solid black lines identify the different dietary phases. The vertical dotted line indicates administration of antibiotic therapy. The black arrow indicates the withdrawal of breast milk. PW, pre-weaning; W, initial weaning (first 10 weeks after introduction of solid food); M, monthly (after W phase). Source: Roger L (2008), Investigations into the biological succession of the infant faecal microbiota, PhD thesis, University of Reading, UK.

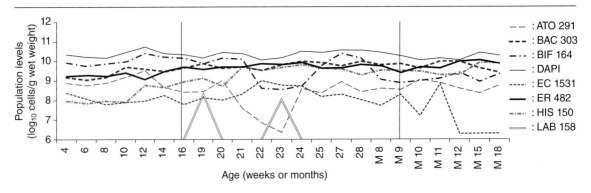

Figure 7.2 Longitudinal investigation of the faecal microbiota of a formula-fed infant, using Fluorescence *in situ* hybridization (FISH) probes, during the three dietary phases (PW, W and M).
Samples are shown in chronological order. The vertical solid black lines identify the different dietary phases. PW, pre-weaning; W, initial weaning (first 10 weeks after introduction of solid food); M, monthly (after W phase).
Source: Roger L (2008), Investigations into the biological succession of the infant faecal microbiota, PhD thesis, University of Reading, UK.

load of the infant faecal microbiota during the first year of life, with instability particularly evident during phase one. Copy numbers of bifidobacterial rRNA genes suggested that this population was a minor component of the infant microbiota – although this may be a reflection of the DNA extraction method and/or stability of DNA.

Microarray analysis of the samples from the study of Palmer *et al.* (2007) demonstrated that the profiles of faecal samples from the same infant generally clustered together (i.e. intra-individual clustering), rather than those from different infants at the same age – although the profiles from the fraternal twins tended to cluster together. A seemingly 'chaotic progression' of bacterial colonisation was noted for phase one and similarity between the initial profiles of some infants to those of vaginal swabs and/or breast-milk samples highlighted that initial acquisition was related to bacterial exposure. Overall, the microarray analysis and sequencing data (from cloned libraries) correlated well. However, the authors themselves highlighted that the broad-range PCR amplification protocol used underestimated the bifidobacterial component. Phylum-level analysis (from both microarray and sequencing data) demonstrated the infant microbiota was rather limited, dominated by *Flexibacter-Cytophaga-Bacteroides*, Proteobacteria and Gram-positive bacteria (Firmicutes and Actinobacteria).

A very limited number of studies have examined the infant faecal microbiota below the level of bacterial groups or genera and such studies have generally involved cultivation work. However, probing strategies and qPCR facilitate such investigations, although methodological detection limits can sometimes come into play – especially with regard to complex microbial ecosystems. Particular interest has been afforded to examining the *Bifidobacterium* component of infants, due to the traditional understanding that breast-fed infants harboured a predominantly *Bifidobacterium* microbiota (and the subsequent association between bifidobacteria and good health). This also elicited great interest in development of improved infant formulas (via fortification and/or supplementation) with an aim to better replicate the microbiota and health outcomes seen for breast-fed infants. Much of this work has involved prebiotic supplementation of infant formulas and the impact of such supplementation on the *Bifidobacterium* component of the microbiota.

The majority of prebiotic-supplemented formula feeding studies have involved a mixture of galacto-oligosaccharides (GOS) and fructo-oligosaccharides (FOS), in a 9:1 ratio (GOS:FOS). However, investigation of FOS supplementation has also been performed. In addition, a few studies of GOS supplementation, polydextrose (PDX) and/or PDX plus lactulose (LOS) supplementation, and supplementation with acid oligosaccharides derived from pectin hydrolysis (pectic-oligosaccharides; POS) have been published. In general these studies have involved exclusively formula-fed infants and have often included a breast-fed control cohort. However, different prebiotic dosages, study duration and age of infants at inclusion have been used. The predominant

endpoint observations of such studies have focused on the levels of bifidobacteria and stool frequency or consistency. In general, the data have been promising (Table 7.1) and consequently a number of prebiotic-supplemented infant formula are now commercially available.

A note of caution should be made, however, regarding the longitudinal effects of prebiotic-supplemented formulas (which have not been examined to date). Indeed, the relatively recent conceptualisation and development of prebiotics as dietary strategies to modulate the gut microbiota somewhat restricts the availability of such longitudinal data (even from adult feeding studies). This may be a particularly pertinent area of interest in relation to the role of the gut microbiota in energy harvest (the process by which energy is derived for the host by gut microbiota) and obesity.

7.5 The effects of weaning on the infant gut microbiota

Weaning is generally defined as the introduction of solid foods into the diet of the infant, and usually starts around 4 months of age in developed countries, although World Health Organization (WHO) weaning recommendations are to begin from 6 months of age (see Chapter 3, Section 3.9.1). The introduction of more complex foods to the infant diet has been reported to elicit major changes in the GI microbiota. It is generally thought that the microbiota essentially adapts to the wider range of nutrients available. Weaning is also associated with certain diseases, which might be triggered by an unusual microbial colonisation in response to dietary changes. Breastfeeding (and/or breast milk substitutes, if used) should continue beyond the first 6 months, supplemented with appropriate types and amounts of solid foods (Department of Health 2009b). Meals should consist mainly of milk during initial weaning, with slow introduction of vegetables and meat (to avoid food allergies and related problems) (see Chapter 3, Section 3.10). In general, investigations of the impact of weaning on the GI microbiota show a shift in bacterial species and/or strains during this period, with a more diverse microbiota elicited. The *Bifidobacterium* population is gradually superseded by a more complex ecosystem, with the predominant microbiota comprising *Bacteroides* spp., *Clostridium* spp. and *Eubacterium* spp. However, a consensus microbial pattern has not yet been identified, with the

Table 7.1 Summary of prebiotic feeding studies in pediatrics

Prebiotic(s)	Age groups	Statistically significant findings
FOS	Pre-term infants 1–6 weeks-old 12 weeks-old 7–24 months-old	↑ bifidobacteria ↑ stool frequency ↑ lactobacilli ↓ clostridia ↓ flatulence, diarrhoea, vomiting and fever
GOS	Term infants	↑ bifidobacteria ↑ stool frequency ↑ lactobacilli ↓ faecal pH ↑ faecal acetate
GOS:FOS (9:1)	Pre-term infants Newborn infants 3–12 days-old 3–20 weeks-old 3–6 months-old	↑ bifidobacteria softer stools ↑ faecal acetate ↓propionate, butyrate and iC4–5 SCFA ↓ faecal pH ↑ faecal sIgA ↓ clostridia ↑ stool frequency ↑ lactobacilli *Bifidobacterium* species profile similar to breast-fed infants
PDX:GOS (1:1) PDX:GOS:LOS (3:2:1)	13–92 days-old	harder stool consistency than breast-fed infants
POS with or without GOS:FOS	Term infants	↑ bifidobacteria ↑ lactobacilli ↑ stool frequency (POS + GOS:FOS only) ↓ faecal pH

FOS, fructo-oligosaccharides; GOS, galacto-oligosaccharides; LOS, lactulose; PDX, polydextrose; POS, acidic oligosaccharides derived from pectin hydrolysis; SCFA, short chain fatty acid.

type of diet and environment likely to be confounding factors across different studies. Overall, weaning is associated with increased complexity and dynamics of the GI microbiota of breast-fed infants, with a shift to a microbiota similar to that seen for formula-fed infants during phase two, and often reflects increased predominance of *Bacteroides*. Palmer *et al.* (2007) demonstrated that each infant had their own distinguishable microbial profile and no common developmental pattern was observed throughout the first year of life based on initial diet (i.e. common to all breast-fed or to all mixed-fed infants). Although high inter-individual diversity was evident, microbiotas of all infants tended to merge towards a common 'adult-like' microbiota after weaning, consisting of *Bacteroides* spp., Firmicutes, Proteobacteria and aerobic Gram-negative bacteria.

Roger and McCartney (2010) highlighted weaning as a transitional phase in the infant gut microbiota development, marked by greater diversity (both qualitative and quantitative) – although the bacterial shifts appeared to be greater in breast-fed infants. Principal component analysis (PCA) of the data highlighted the microbiological succession, both within each individual (Fig. 7.3a and 7.3b) and within feeding groups (Fig. 7.4). PCA of the entire dataset (from all 14 infants) also demonstrated the bacterial succession of the faecal microbiota over time. However, most interestingly, PCA of the entire dataset showed a clear distinction between the samples collected from breast-fed infants during pre-weaning and initial weaning phases compared to those from formula-fed infants and those from breast-fed infants during monthly sampling phase (i.e. after initial weaning). Samples collected after initial weaning (over 7 months of age) tended to cluster together irrespective of initial milk feeding regime (breast-fed or formula-fed). Such analysis appeared to suggest that weaning modulated the infant faecal microbiota, with greater modulation of the breast-fed infant faecal microbiota – towards one more like that of formula-fed infants (Roger and McCartney 2010).

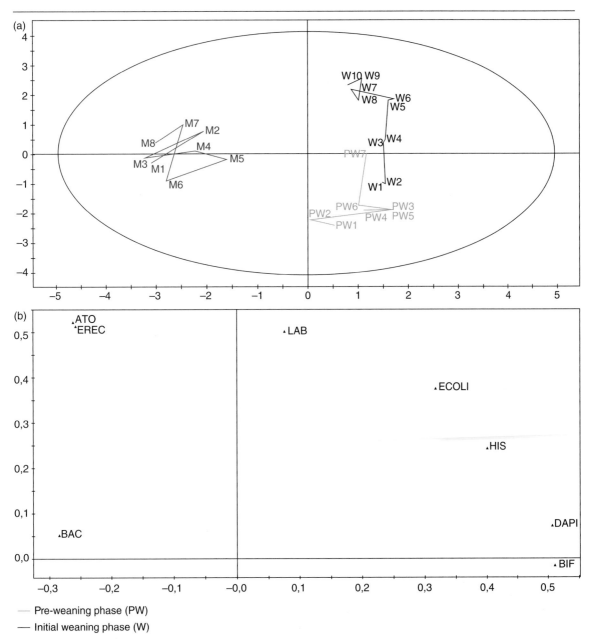

— Pre-weaning phase (PW)

— Initial weaning phase (W)

— Monthly phase (M)

Figure 7.3a Principal component analysis of the FISH data from a breast-fed infant. Score plot of the PCA model (a). Each observation is linked to the next by a line and is displayed in chronological order. Loading plot of the PCA model (b). ATO, ATO 291; BAC, BAC 303; BIF, BIF 164; DAPI, 4,6-diamidino-2-phenylindole; ECOLI, EC 1531; EREC, ER 482; HIS, HIS 150; LAB, LAB 158.

Source: Roger L (2008), Investigations into the biological succession of the infant faecal microbiota, PhD thesis, University of Reading, UK.

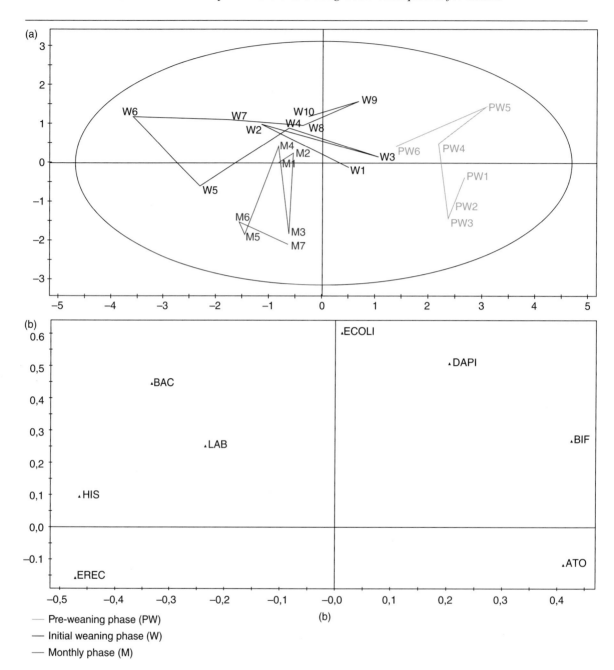

— Pre-weaning phase (PW)

— Initial weaning phase (W)

— Monthly phase (M)

Figure 7.3b   Principal component analysis of the FISH data from a formula-fed infant. Score plot of the PCA model (a). Each observation is linked to the next by a line and is displayed in chronological order. Loading plot of the PCA model (b). ATO, ATO 291; BAC, BAC 303; BIF, BIF 164; DAPI, 4,6-diamidino-2-phenylindole; ECOLI, EC 1531; EREC, ER 482; HIS, HIS 150; LAB, LAB 158.
Source: Roger L (2008), Investigations into the biological succession of the infant faecal microbiota, PhD thesis, University of Reading, UK.

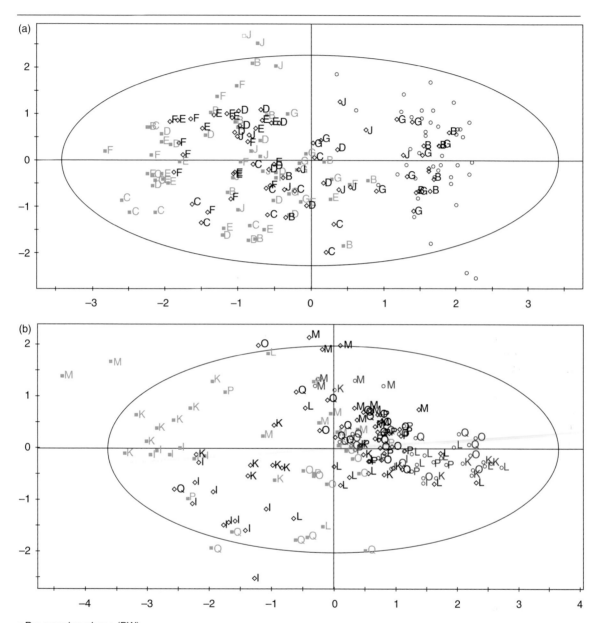

■ Pre-weaning phase (PW)

◇ Weaning phase (W)

○ Monthly phase (M)

Figure 7.4 Score plot of the PCA model for the comparison of all breast-fed infants (a) and all formula-fed infants (b).
The letter associated with each dot designates the infant (B, C, D, E, F, G, I, J, K, L, M, O, P, Q).
Source: Roger L (2008), Investigations into the biological succession of the infant faecal microbiota, PhD thesis, University of Reading, UK.

7.6 Potential long-term effects: implications for obesity

Recently, interest in the human gut microbiota and its function has increased significantly, with particular focus on the energy-harvesting capacity of members of the gut microbiota and the potential role of the gut microbiota in obesity (see Chapter 8, Section 8.7.1). Early indications are that the gut microbiota of obese individuals differs from that of lean individuals. However, caution must be exercised, as the cause-and-effect axis of this association is unknown. It is clear from pure culture (laboratory) studies and some animal studies that certain members of the gut microbiota (and/or overall composition of the gut microbiota) have greater energy harvest capacity. But one must remember that the actual harvest of energy *in vivo* is essentially restricted by what is available to the gut microbiota to degrade, and the bacteria will adapt to the environmental conditions they reside in (as evidenced by changes in the gut microbiota of obese human adults following consumption of a low carbohydrate or fat-restricted diet).

A prospective follow-up study of children from a probiotic feeding study in infants at high risk of allergy identified that those children who were overweight or obese at 7 years of age ($n = 25$; seven of whom were obese) had had significantly lower bifidobacteria levels during infancy (6 months of age) than matched normal weight children ($n = 24$) from the same study cohort. Again caution should be exercised, since no information was gathered in relation to the diet and/or lifestyle (including physical activity) of the children in this study, and the subject numbers are relatively small.

7.7 Conclusions

There have been conflicting observations in recent studies regarding the common composition of the infant intestinal microbiota during exclusive milk feeding. Most studies show that bifidobacteria is the main bacterial genus in faecal samples of 1-week-old infants and resides in high proportions until weaning. Other studies have identified bacteroides, clostridia or enterobacteria as the major bacterial constituents. Different studies utilise different techniques, which undoubtedly bias the findings.

However, it is generally accepted that the microbiota of breast-fed infants is less complex than that of formula-fed infants and consists mainly (in order of predominance) of bifidobacteria and Enterobacteriaceae. Formula-fed infants tend to be colonised by a more 'adult-like' microbiota, with higher levels and frequency of Enterobacteriaceae and enterococci – which are gradually replaced by similar levels of bifidobacteria, bacteroides, clostridia and streptococci prior to weaning. However, it is clear that each infant harbours their own unique microbiota and that the environment to which the infant is exposed is important. The global observation regarding the infant gut microbiota is that initially there is inter-individual variation, with convergence towards a more adult-like faecal microbiota seen after 1 to 2 years of age.

7.8 Key points

- The human gut microbiota comprises more cells than the rest of the human body and plays a role in the health and well-being of the host, including energy harvest (the process by which energy is derived by gut microbiota).
- The acquisition and development of the infant gut microbiota is affected by a number of factors: genetic, environmental (including diet) and health.
- Certain bacterial populations added in the diet in early life as probiotics, such as *Bifidobacterium breve* and *Lactobacillus rhamnosus*, have also been shown to reduce the risk of developing asthma, atopic dermatitis and other common allergies in later life, through infancy, early childhood and into adolescence.
- It is generally accepted that the gut microbiota of breast-fed and formula-fed infants are distinctly different, although fortification of formulas with prebiotics has partially addressed this.
- Initial weaning is associated with a transitional phase in the infant gut microbiota succession.
- Between 1 and 2 years of age the infant gut microbiota converges towards the microbiota present in an adult.

7.9 Recommendations for future research

- Further investigation of the role of the gut microbiota, or specific members thereof, in carbohydrate and fat metabolism is warranted.
- Longitudinal studies and/or prospective studies of cohorts from previous infant studies are needed to understand the impact of the neonatal microbial acquisition and development as a blueprint for gut microbiology, host health and risk of GI and/or metabolic disorders later in life.
- Relatively few studies have investigated the impact of weaning (i.e. introduction of solid food to the infant diet) on the infant microbiota. Research investigating this would be very useful

- In general, findings have shown promising results of using prebiotic-supplemented infant formulas which are now commercially available. However, the longitudinal effects of such prebiotic-supplemented formulas have not been examined. Studies with long-term follow-up are needed to determine whether using such formulas has any implication for health in later life.
- There is increasing interest in the energy-harvesting capacity of human gut microbiota and its potential role in obesity. There is some evidence to suggest that the gut microbiota in lean and obese individuals differ, although further research in this area is needed.

7.10 Key references

Fanaro S, Chierici R, Guerrini P *et al.* (2003) Intestinal microflora in early infancy: composition and development. *Acta Paediatrica Supplement*, **91**, 48–55.

Michail S & Sherman PM (2009) *Probiotics in Pediatric Medicine*. Humana Press, New Jersey.

Mountzouris KC, McCartney AL & Gibson GR (2002) Intestinal microflora of human infants and current trends for its nutritional modulation. *British Journal of Nutrition*, **87**, 405–20.

Roger LC & McCartney AL (2010) Longitudinal investigation of the faecal microbiota of healthy full-term infants using fluorescence in situ hybridization and denaturing gradient gel electrophoresis. *Microbiology*, **156**, 3317–28.

Reinhardt C, Reigstad CS & Backhed F (2009) Intestinal microbiota during infancy and its implications for obesity. *Journal of Pediatric Gastroenterology and Nutrition*, **48**, 249–56.

8
Nutrition and Development: Obesity

8.1 Introduction

In 2008, the World Health Organization (WHO) estimated that around 500 million adults were obese (BMI > 30) (World Health Organization, 2012), a figure projected to rise to 1.12 billion (if recent secular trends continue unabated) by 2030 (Kelly *et al.* 2008). In 2010, more than 40 million children under 5 years were overweight (World Health Organization 2012) and childhood obesity tracks strongly to adolescence and adulthood (Reilly *et al.* 2003; Wardle *et al.* 2006). As obese children and adults are at risk of premature adult death the world-wide epidemic of obesity could lead to a reversal in the trend of longer life expectancy (Olshansky *et al.* 2005; Franks *et al.* 2010). Genotyping studies have revealed potential 'obesity' genes, e.g. a common variant of the *FTO* gene (the fat mass and obesity-associated gene) (Frayling *et al.* 2007), but the current escalation in obesity will not be explicable on an inheritable basis; obesity is a classic example of gene–environment interaction.

The rise in obesity is most often attributed to a greater abundance of food, and reduced physical activity, but there is now good evidence for other, rather less obvious, environmental determinants. Importantly, a number of critical periods in early human development may influence an individual's risk of development of obesity in later life. As the child grows *in utero* and in early postnatal life, the mother's nutritional and metabolic status may profoundly and persistently influence fetal pathways of energy balance in a direction favouring fat accrual in later life. Indeed, it is now widely accepted that the child's nutritional status and growth trajectory in the early years of life may be determinants of obesity risk. This chapter summarises the evidence from human cohorts which underpin the theory of the 'early life' origins of obesity, highlighting strengths and inadequacies. The critical role played by animal models in the development of this theory and in providing mechanistic insight is also discussed.

8.2 Inadequate *in utero* nutrition: a risk factor for obesity in later life?

8.2.1 Evidence from human population studies

The fetus displays a remarkable facility to survive when confronted with inadequate nutrient availability. Whether the result of poor maternal nutritional status or placental insufficiency, fetal adaptive mechanisms ensure redistribution of blood flow to essential organs. This results in sustained blood flow to the brain, heart, adrenal glands and placenta, with diminished blood flow to the bone marrow, muscle, lungs, gastrointestinal (GI) tract and kidneys. This 'brain-sparing' effect may result in different fetal growth patterns. Thus, the child may be born apparently healthy but with a suboptimal weight and a low ponderal index. The fetal origins hypothesis, also referred to as the 'thrifty phenotype' hypothesis, a name coined by Hales and Barker (1992), suggested that while advantageous *in utero*, these survival strategies can confer a longer-term disadvantage when the child experiences a higher nutritional plane in later life (see Chapter 4, Section 4.5). Indeed, some have suggested that the subsequent inability to respond appropriately to a nutrient challenge in postnatal life may have contributed to the rise in obesity in the developing world, since the rapid transgenerational increase in wealth and abundance of food observed in developing countries in recent years would inevitably lead to a 'mismatch' between maternal and offspring nutritional status.

A number of investigative approaches have been applied to this hypothesis. First, it might be anticipated that low birthweight in developed countries would be associated with obesity in later life; indeed, early studies from UK cohorts showed associations between low birthweight and a raised body mass index (BMI) in adulthood (Law *et al.* 1992; Phillips *et al.* 2000; Sayer *et al.* 2004). Given that BMI is increasingly recognised as a poor index of 'fatness', others have more recently addressed relationships with low birthweight and later body composition but, in contrast, these have either shown no association or a weak association between low birthweight and fat mass (Kensara *et al.* 2005; Sachdev, Fall *et al.* 2005; Wells *et al.* 2005).

Reliance on birthweight as a surrogate for poor intrauterine growth is a potential source of error as birthweight per se provides a poor index of *in utero* growth. Birthweight does not account for genetic growth potential and does not discriminate between lean and fat mass; therefore birthweight should be considered only as a measure of convenience (Wells *et al.* 2007). This is exemplified by the observation that birthweight is reduced following growth retardation in the third trimester but not if growth retardation occurs in the first trimester (Hemachandra and Klebanoff 2006). A true estimate of suboptimal fetal growth is better provided by use of ponderal index or direct measures of fat and lean mass. Unfortunately, those studies which have addressed the hypothesised relationship between fetal growth retardation and later obesity have, to date, not considered neonatal body composition, but uniformly have relied on the measurement of birthweight, and the association remains unsubstantiated.

8.2.2 Early postnatal 'catch-up' growth and obesity risk

The majority of low-birthweight infants demonstrate rapid postnatal growth and this 'catch-up' occurs in the first 6–12 months of life. Infants born small for gestational age (SGA) who gain weight rapidly in early postnatal life are likely to later develop an increase in BMI or fatness as assessed by skinfold thickness (Parsons *et al.* 2001; Stettler *et al.* 2005; Ibanez *et al.* 2006; Ong and Loos 2006). A systematic review of 21 studies reporting significant positive associations between rapid weight gain up to 2 years and subsequent overweight or obesity has shown an overall two- to three-fold increase in overweight or obesity risk in infants whose growth trajectory crossed upwards by at least one weight centile band, equivalent to a gain in weight SD score ≥ 0.67 (Ong and Loos 2006). However, this review implied that there is no interaction with birthweight, prompting the suggestion that the effects of rapid weight gain are equally important in SGA and normal birthweight populations. Nonetheless, in the Avon Longitudinal Study of Parents and Children (ALSPAC) cohort, Ong *et al.* (2000), while showing a relationship between rapid infant growth in the first 2 years of life and later greater central adiposity, also reported that rapid infant growth was more likely when there were also indications for impaired *in utero* growth, e.g. maternal smoking or ultrasound evidence. This implies an interaction between fetal growth retardation, rapid infant growth and later obesity, as predicted by the thrifty phenotype hypothesis (Ong *et al.* 2000).

One study in term infants suggests that the period of maximal effect of rapid infant growth on later risk of obesity occurs as early as the first 8 days of life; indeed, the first few weeks postpartum represent the period when catch-up growth across the centiles is most pronounced (Stettler *et al.* 2005). This is in accord with Singhal and Lucas's proposal, from studies in pre-term infants, that growth acceleration in the first weeks postpartum comprises the primary mechanism of programming of adult diseases, including obesity (Singhal and Lucas 2004; Druet and Ong 2008).

The studies of early growth trajectories pertain to cohorts from developed countries. In non-Western populations others have reported that infant weight or BMI gain is related to later weight, height and lean mass but not fat mass. On the basis of this evidence, early catch-up growth in developing countries could be considered advantageous to later achievement of growth potential (Li *et al.* 2003a; Sachdev, Fall *et al.* 2005; Wells *et al* 2007).

8.2.3 Exposure to famine during gestation

Children born to women who were pregnant during the Dutch Hunger Winter (1944–5) (see Chapter 1, Section 1.4.1; and Chapter 4, Section 4.4.2) were subjected to under-nutrition *in utero* but in postnatal life had a relatively abundant food supply, and according to the 'thrifty phenotype' hypothesis should be at risk of developing obesity. Investigators studying offspring of the Hunger Winter found among male subjects that those exposed to the famine in early gestation were more likely to be obese in later life compared with non-exposed subjects, whereas those exposed in later pregnancy or early infancy were less obese (Ravelli *et al.* 1976).

A later, seemingly conflicting, report found a greater waist circumference in female offspring following early pregnancy famine exposure, but that this did not apply to men (Ravelli *et al.* 1999). These relationships with obesity or waist circumference were independent of birthweight which, as might be anticipated, was unaffected by famine confined to early gestation. In contrast, no such relationship between maternal semi-starvation and offspring obesity was observed in children born to women during the Leningrad Siege (see Chapter 4, Section 4.4.2), but the disparity in studies may be attributable to the lack of catch-up growth in children born to women in the Leningrad cohort compared to the Dutch Hunger Winter survivors (Stanner and Yudkin 2001).

Thus, human cohort studies provide only very modest evidence for an independent association between low birthweight and later obesity. A more robust relationship is observed when the rate of neonatal growth is considered. The obvious importance of neonatal growth trajectories has focused attention on neonatal nutritional regimes and development of interventions which may optimise the neonatal growth trajectory, with the potential for reducing the risk of obesity in later life.

8.3 Breastfeeding and risk of obesity in later life

The benefits of breastfeeding would appear to include a reduced incidence of obesity in later life, although the effect is likely to be more modest than originally proposed. In a recent review of systematic reviews of early life determinants of obesity, Monasta *et al.*

(2010) identified seven systematic reviews which examined the relationship between breastfeeding and obesity in later life, six of which were classified as 'moderate quality'. These reviews, published between 2004 and 2007, all described a reduction in overweight or obesity associated with breastfeeding with varying degree of effect, the highest estimate being a 22% reduction in childhood obesity (Arenz *et al.* 2004) and the lowest a 7% reduction in child or adulthood obesity (Owen *et al.* 2005), which was observed after correction for three major potential confounders (parental obesity, maternal smoking and social class), and with formula-fed children as a reference. The most recent analysis, published by the World Health Organization (WHO) in 2007, reported an overall 22% reduction in overweight and/or obesity in breast-fed individuals as assessed between 1 and 66 years of age (Horta *et al.* 2007). As reported by Monasta *et al.* (2010), all of the contributory studies were observational and, as in all observational studies, residual confounding cannot be excluded.

A variety of mechanistic pathways could explain an association between breastfeeding and reduction of adiposity in later life. The most likely explanation is that breast-fed infants gain weight more slowly than formula-fed infants (Ong *et al.* 2002). Some suggest that breast-fed infants are likely to imbibe less milk when dependent on more natural cues to stimulate feeding than bottle-fed infants. Proposed mechanisms include milk-borne factors such as leptin (Miralles *et al.* 2006) and insulin (Shehadeh *et al.* 2003). Others propose that the higher protein content of formula milk may be responsible (Koletzko *et al.* 2009) and this has led to the development of infant formula with lower protein content (Sidnell and Greenstreet 2009).

8.4 Maternal diabetes and obesity: early life determinants of offspring obesity?

The 'Barker hypothesis' which provoked so much interest in the developmental origins of disease was derived from studies of fetal *in utero* nutritional deprivation and later disease, and the seminal studies contributing to development of the hypothesis centred upon associations of low birthweight and adulthood disorders, leading to the interest in rapid catch-up growth, as described above. In parallel, however, numerous investigators have now addressed the opposite end of the 'energy supply' spectrum, addressing the question of whether fetal energy excess may have deleterious consequences on the developing child, and in relation to the topic of this review, whether the origins of obesity can lie in a child being exposed to a higher than optimal plane of nutrition from the earliest stages in life.

8.4.1 Association of higher birthweight with offspring adiposity

Obesity in pregnancy and gestational diabetes are associated with a high percentage of macrosomic deliveries (birthweight ≥ 90% centile), but high birthweights such as this may often be unrelated to either of these maternal conditions. A question often asked by parents is whether a child with a higher than average birthweight is predisposed to obesity in later life. Although there is some indication at the lower end of the birthweight spectrum that smaller babies may develop obesity in later life, a positive association between birthweight and later BMI is also widely reported; indeed, some authors suggest that the relationship between birthweight and later obesity follows a J- or U-shaped curve (Parsons *et al.* 2001; Rogers 2003). A systematic review published in 2006 reported a positive association between birthweight and obesity in childhood in most of the 20 studies reviewed (Martins and Carvalho 2006), and studies published since then add further evidence, as reviewed recently (Monasta *et al.* 2010). The focus on BMI rather than body composition in these reports has led many to assume that fatter infants become fatter children and adults. With the development of accurate methods of body composition analysis, the relationship between birthweight and BMI in adulthood in some cohorts has been revisited. Some authors refute the suggestion that higher birthweight leads to obesity, demonstrating an association of higher birthweight with greater adulthood lean mass, rather than fat mass, i.e. heavier babies grow into more muscular adults (Singhal, Wells *et al.* 2003; Murphy *et al.* 2006).

However, a relationship between birthweight and childhood fat mass has been reported, notably in the Avon Longitudinal Study of Parents and Children (ALSPAC) cohort of children born in the 1990s to women in the UK, where birthweight was positively related to both lean body mass and percentage fat mass in 9- and 10-year-old children, the body fat mass increasing by 2.5% per standard deviation

increase in birthweight (Rogers *et al.* 2006). The more pertinent question to be asked is whether a fatter baby, rather than a heavier baby, is predisposed to increased adiposity in later life, i.e. does excessive perinatal fat accumulation track into adulthood? Catalano and colleagues have exemplified how meaningless the measurement of birthweight may be, in observing that marginally higher birthweights among babies born to obese vs. lean women can belie highly significant increases in percentage body fat and fat mass in the child of the obese woman, when infant fat mass is measured directly by anthropometry or total body electrical conductivity (Sewell *et al.* 2006). In the ALSPAC cohort, the added observation that the ponderal index at birth was associated with higher fat mass at the age of 9 and 10 years provides some evidence that it is the fatter infant who becomes the fatter child (Rogers *et al.* 2006). Several contemporary mother–child cohorts in which offspring body composition is measured accurately have the capacity to address whether fatness at birth tracks into adulthood but, at present, there is insubstantial evidence to claim a strong relationship.

8.4.2 Maternal diabetes

Some of the earliest evidence to suggest a direct association between fetal and neonatal 'overnutritional' status and development of later obesity is derived from studies of the Pima Indians, a population with a high incidence of type 2 diabetes (Pettitt *et al.* 1983; Pettitt *et al.* 1987; Pettitt *et al.* 1991; Pettitt *et al.* 1993; Dabelea, Hanson *et al.* 2000; Dabelea, Knowler *et al.* 2000). Studies of sibling pairs discordant for *in utero* exposure to maternal diabetes demonstrated that *in utero* exposure to maternal diabetes among Pima Indians was associated with an increase in the BMI of 2.6 in adulthood (Dabelea, Knowler *et al.* 2000). In different populations, others have reported an association between pre-gestational type 1 and type 2 or gestational diabetes and increased childhood BMI (Silverman *et al.* 1998; Cho *et al.* 2000; Schaefer-Graf *et al.* 2005; Malcolm *et al.* 2006), and in a recent study Wright *et al.* report a relationship between exposure to gestational diabetes *in utero* and higher skin fold thickness at the age of 3 years (Wright *et al.* 2009). Care must be taken in interpretation of these studies because of the growing body of evidence that maternal BMI is an independent determinant of offspring BMI. Although adjustment for maternal BMI has not always been attempted (Plagemann *et al.* 1997; Hillier *et al.* 2007; Vaarasmaki *et al.* 2009), when undertaken, a positive relationship between maternal diabetes and offspring BMI or offspring adiposity sometimes persists (Pettitt *et al.* 1983; Pettitt *et al.* 1987; Clausen *et al.* 2008; Winsloe *et al.* 2009; Wright *et al.* 2009; Tam *et al.* 2010), whereas others have suggested that maternal BMI is a stronger and predominant determinant of offspring BMI (Gillman *et al.* 2003; Catalano, Farrell *et al.* 2009; Lawlor, Fraser *et al.* 2010). As noted by Lawlor (Lawlor, Fraser *et al.* 2010), adjusting the relationships between maternal diabetes and offspring BMI is likely to represent an overadjustment because of common mechanisms, but independent influences of maternal obesity imply that factors other than maternal hyperglycaemia could contribute to offspring obesity.

Undoubtedly, shared genes and environment play a role, but maternal hypertriglyceridaemia and the metabolic sequelae of maternal insulin resistance, other than hyperglycaemia per se, have been implicated (Ramsay *et al.* 2002; Catalano, Farrell *et al.* 2009). This is reinforced by a recent study in which maternal insulin resistance, independent of maternal glucose tolerance, has been associated with infant weight gain and adiposity over the first year of life (Hamilton *et al.* 2010). The Hyperglycaemia and Adverse Pregnancy Outcome study (HAPO) study has also provided important insight. This observational cohort study, which assessed pregnancy outcome in women without a diagnosis of diabetes, reported a linear correlation between maternal plasma glucose and neonatal fat mass (HAPO Study Cooperative Research Group 2009). However, this relationship did not persist at 2 years of age, when no important association was found between maternal glucose status and direct measures of infant fat mass, although maternal BMI remained a strong independent predictor of offspring BMI, Z-score and adiposity (Pettitt *et al.* 2010). This, too, adds support to the suggestion that maternal BMI per se has influences beyond those of maternal hyperglycaemia.

8.4.3 Maternal obesity: a determinant of offspring obesity?

The rapid rise in the incidence of maternal obesity worldwide has focused attention not only on the associated health risks for the mother but also the potentially longer-term sequelae for the child. In the US in 2009, the prevalence of obesity (BMI $\geq$ 30) among women aged 20 to 39 was 34% (Centers for Disease Control and Prevention 2010). Obesity among women in many developing countries is also rising (Misra and Khurana 2008) and is highly prevalent in the Middle East (Esmaillzadeh and Azadbakht 2006). Few countries have reliable data documenting the incidence of obesity in pregnant women (Guelinckx *et al.* 2008), but cohort studies in the UK show upward trajectories in parallel with those of the whole population (Heslehurst *et al.* 2010). In the US, data available from nine States showed that 20% of Americans are obese (BMI > 29) at the start of pregnancy, representing a 70% increase over a decade (Kim *et al.* 2007). In England, about half of women of childbearing age are either overweight (BMI 25–29.9) or obese (BMI $\geq$ 30) (NHS Information Centre 2008) and approximately 16% of women are obese at the start of pregnancy (Heslehurst *et al.* 2010).

As described above, several studies addressing the relationship between maternal diabetes and offspring obesity have suggested an independent association between maternal and offspring obesity. In addition, most observational studies in mother–child cohorts show an association between maternal BMI and the BMI in childhood and adulthood (Laitinen *et al.* 2001; Whitaker 2004; Li *et al.* 2005b; Reilly *et al.* 2005; Salsberry and Reagan 2005; Li *et al.* 2007; Koupil and Toivanen 2008). However, interpretation is generally confounded by the lack of accurate body compositional analysis in the mother and/or child, and dependence on BMI as an outcome. Also, the widely differing magnitude of effect observed could reflect variation in the range of BMIs in the different populations, and the different capabilities between studies to adjust for shared behaviour and potential confounders, depending on the breadth of data available.

In the few studies to have evaluated associations between maternal BMI and offspring adiposity, an independent and positive association has been reported (Burdette *et al.* 2006; Blair *et al.* 2007; Mingrone *et al.* 2008). Also, in the one investigation to have addressed relationships between directly measured adiposity in mother and child, a larger maternal mid-upper arm circumference in late pregnancy was independently associated with a higher childhood fat mass index at the age of 9 years (Gale *et al.* 2007).

Finally, if there were to be a specific added risk of obesity to the child from an *in utero* influence, a stronger association of the child's BMI with maternal obesity than with paternal obesity would be expected. Relatively few studies have both maternal and paternal weight data available but, when considered, several have shown a stronger association of maternal than paternal BMI with offspring BMI (Salsberry and Reagan 2005; Lawlor *et al.* 2007; Lawlor *et al.* 2008; Catalano, Farrell *et al.* 2009). In one of these, however, this was reported to be explicable by inheritance of the variant of the *FTO* gene association with obesity (Lawlor *et al.* 2008).

8.4.4 Gestational weight gain and offspring adiposity

The recent publication of the revised US Institute of Medicine (IoM) guidelines on gestational weight gain in pregnancy (Rasmussen and Yaktine 2009) has reawakened the worldwide debate about the value of measuring maternal weight (see Chapter 3, Table 3.2). The weight of a pregnant woman provides a poor measure of fetal weight or indeed of fat accrual, and is at best an inexact measure with which to assess pregnancy progress. In underweight women, adequate weight gain is a critical determinant of good pregnancy outcome, but in obese women pre-pregnancy BMI has generally proven to be a more important determinant of the key outcomes of pregnancy including pre-eclampsia and diabetes (Nohr *et al.* 2008). Some studies, but not all, indicate that weight gain may be a determinant of offspring obesity as assessed by BMI, but the strength of the effect is generally less than that of maternal pre-pregnancy BMI (Moreira *et al.* 2007; Oken *et al.* 2007; Oken, Rifas-Shiman *et al.* 2008; Kleiser *et al.* 2009; Mamun *et al.* 2009) and one report suggests that the association is stronger among underweight/normal weight mothers (Mamun *et al.* 2009). Others have reported no relationship between maternal weight gain and offspring BMI (Catalano *et al.* 1995; Koupil and Toivanen 2008).

Two recent studies have addressed gestational weight gain and childhood body composition; the first, from the Southampton Women's Survey (UK), assessed adiposity by dual X-ray absorptiometry (DXA) scan in 948 children. Of these, 49% were born to mothers who had gained excessive weight in pregnancy according to the Institute of Medicine (2009) guidelines. When compared to children whose mothers gained adequate weight, these children were fatter at birth, at 4 years and at 6 years, and weight gain as a continuous variable was associated with offspring fat mass in the neonates and at 6 years (Crozier *et al.* 2010). In the second, from the UK ALSPAC cohort, a similar result was found; women who exceeded the 2009 IoM recommended gestational weight gain were more likely to have offspring with greater BMI, waist circumference and fat mass (Fraser *et al.* 2010). Therefore appropriate pregnancy weight gain, as defined by 2009 IoM recommendations (Institute of Medicine 2009) may be associated with lower adiposity in the offspring although, without evidence from appropriate intervention studies, a causative relationship cannot be assumed.

8.5 Interventions to reduce offspring obesity?

This summary of the research which has contributed so much to our appreciation of the associations between the environment at the earliest stages of life and later risk of obesity can only provide a brief glimpse of the effort expended and of the many thousands of individuals studied. Despite this, these reports are all of an observational nature and subject to residual confounding. Until such time as an intervention in pregnancy or in early postnatal life has been shown unequivocally to reduce the risk of obesity in a child, there can be no evidence-based translation to improvement of public health. There are many theoretical approaches to intervention; these will now be explored and any relevant studies noted.

8.5.1 Reducing low birthweight

The evidence supporting an independent association of low birthweight and risk of obesity is not strong, but it remains theoretically possible that reduction of low birthweight could reduce the risk of obesity in the child. There is no evidence to date that any attempts to reduce the incidence of low birthweight, which is remarkably refractory to nutritional intervention, have led to a reduction in childhood obesity.

8.5.2 Reducing infant postnatal weight gain

The observation that rapid postpartum weight gain is associated with risk of obesity is more amenable to intervention, particularly because of the lower rates of infant weight gain associated with breastfeeding compared to formula-fed infants. The only randomised trial to have investigated the effect of an intervention on breastfeeding rates and duration, the Promotion of Breastfeeding and Intervention Trial (PROBIT) study from Belarus, also addressed the effects of breastfeeding on childhood obesity as a secondary outcome measure, but this did not show any effect of the intervention on adiposity in children from the breastfeeding intervention group (Kramer *et al.* 2000). Protocol design of randomised studies addressing the influence of breastfeeding holds many practical and ethical challenges, and further randomised trials are likely to be difficult to achieve. However, as breastfeeding has other unequivocal benefits, the potential for reduction of obesity adds to the rationale for promotion of breastfeeding.

A most promising intervention likely to impact upon the incidence of child and adulthood obesity lies in adoption of the International Child Growth Standards released by the WHO in 2006 (World Health Organization 2006) (see Chapter 2, Section 2.8). Key to these standards is the adoption of the breast-fed child as the normative model for growth. The growth standards were derived from studies on 8440 breast-fed children from widely differing ethnic backgrounds and, remarkably, showed that in the absence of social deprivation children born anywhere in the world have the potential to develop on a similar growth trajectory, suggesting a marked dependence of growth potential on nutritional status as opposed to genetic factors. A comparison of the WHO 2006 standards and the British 1990 Growth Reference, mainly based on formula-fed infants, has suggested that use of the new WHO standards will lead to a marked increase in the number of infants classified as overweight or obese, thus alerting parents and health professionals to the need to limit infant weight gain (Wright *et al.* 2008).

8.5.3 Formula feed composition

The European Union-funded Early Nutritional Programming Project (EARNEST) has recently reported the results of a randomised trial designed to test the hypothesis that the higher dietary protein intake in formula feed may be responsible for greater length and weight gain in infancy. In a cohort of 1138 healthy formula-fed infants, the study participants were randomised to receive cow's milk-based infant and follow-on formula with either low protein content (1.77 g and 2.2 g protein/100 kcal (419 kJ) respectively) or higher protein content (2.9 g and 4.4 g protein/100 kcal (419 kJ) respectively) for the first year of life. All children, including a group of 619 breast-fed children, were studied at intervals up to 2 years of age. At 2 years those children in the low-protein group demonstrated a lower weight/length, Z-score and BMI than those in the higher-protein group (0.20 (95% CI: 0.06–0.34) lower) and were not different in regard to this outcome from the breast-fed group (Koletzko *et al.* 2009). Because formula-fed groups at 2 years showed no difference in length, which is correlated with lean body mass, the difference in weight-for-length and in BMI was suggested to be due to decreased body fat or a difference in adiposity. According to previous studies which have tracked weight gain in infancy to later obesity, the observed increase in Z-score for weight-for-length at the age of 2 years in the higher-protein group would yield an odds ratio of 1.13 (95% CI: 1.02–1.25) for these children being obese in adolescence (Ong and Loos 2006). This study provides the first evidence that lower-protein formula feeds may be advantageous in the prevention of childhood obesity and provides an impetus for further cohort studies with longer-term follow-up.

8.6 Interventions in pregnant diabetic women

Two relevant studies in diabetic pregnancies have addressed the influence of maternal treatment of diabetes on offspring obesity. In a retrospective non-randomised study of 9439 pregnancies, Hillier *et al.* found an association between maternal glycaemia in response to a glucose challenge test and offspring obesity (at age 5–7 years), but found this attenuated towards null after treatment of women with a gestational diabetes diagnosis (Hillier *et al.* 2007). However, a follow-up study of a sub-group from the Australasian Carbohydrate Intolerance Study in Pregnant Women (ACHOIS) randomised controlled trial (RCT) of intensive treatment vs. routine care in women with mild diabetes, found no difference in childhood BMI Z-scores at age 4–5 years, despite a reduction in macrosomia between intervention and routine care groups (5.3% vs. 21.9%) (Gillman *et al.* 2010). Unfortunately, body compositional analysis was not performed. Further follow-up of children from this intervention study and a recent similar RCT in women with mild gestational diabetes (Landon *et al.* 2009) would be valuable in determining whether improved treatment of diabetes in pregnancy can reduce the risk of obesity in the child.

8.7 Interventions in obese pregnant women

While reduction of pre-pregnancy BMI would likely be advantageous in reduction of offspring adiposity, no RCT has randomised women to a weight loss regime or normal care prior to pregnancy and followed up the children to assess the effect on childhood adiposity. Pre-pregnancy weight loss might seem a straightforward intervention, but important questions should be considered, e.g. how quickly should weight be lost and is it safe for women to attempt to conceive when participating in a weight loss regime? These remain unanswered and should be investigated in a research context. Nonetheless, there is some evidence that pre-pregnancy weight loss might reduce the risk of childhood obesity.

Increasing numbers of morbidly obese women are undergoing surgical intervention to promote weight loss, and an observational study from a US cohort has suggested that, after weight loss, children born to these women have a lower risk of obesity; among 111 (aged 2.5–26 years) children born to 49 mothers who underwent maternal biliopancreatic diversion bariatric surgery for weight loss, those born after maternal weight loss ($n = 57$) demonstrated a three-fold lower prevalence of obesity than those born to the same mothers before they underwent weight loss surgery ($n = 54$) (Smith *et al.* 2009). This important observation mitigates against a genetic contribution and could infer an influence of the maternal *in utero* environment on offspring obesity risk.

Several small studies have attempted to improve pregnancy outcome through lifestyle interventions in obese women but, to date, there is no evidence for any overall benefit although a few have shown a reduction in gestational weight gain in the intervention arm. None has been sufficiently powered to address neonatal outcome and none has followed the children beyond infancy (Nelson *et al.* 2010; Ronnberg and Nilsson 2010). Several larger-scale complex intervention studies designed to change physical activity and diet in obese pregnant women are under way, but

none has yet reported on pregnancy outcomes, nor has there been any follow-up of the children for assessment of adiposity. Importantly, different dietary interventions are being tested in these intervention studies; some, including one from King's College London (UPBEAT; UK Pregnancies: Better Eating and Activity Trial), are addressing the effect of a low glycaemic index diet with a view to reducing maternal insulin resistance. This outcome was decided upon because insulin resistance is associated with some of the adverse outcomes of obese pregnancy (see Chapter 9), including pre-eclampsia as well as gestational diabetes and macrosomia, and also as described above, with childhood adiposity. Others are giving more general dietary advice with a view to reducing gestational weight gain to improve pregnancy outcome (Nelson *et al.* 2010), and as described above these observational studies suggest that this could also reduce childhood obesity risk. Again, caution must be observed in translation from observational studies to intervention; it cannot be assumed that restriction of weight gain will reduce adiposity in the child. Rapid weight loss is not recommended in pregnancy and there is real potential for harm, hence the need for carefully designed interventions.

8.7.1 Other modifiable factors which may contribute to offspring obesity

Maternal prenatal smoking has been associated with offspring obesity. As reviewed by Oken, Levitan *et al.* (2008) there is consistent evidence that children whose mothers smoked in pregnancy experienced a higher risk for overweight. These authors report an odds ratio of 1.50 (95% CI: 1.36–1.65) for the effect of maternal smoking in a total of 14 studies of offspring aged between 3 and 33 years compared with children from mothers who did not smoke, although no RCT of smoking cessation regimes has been undertaken to address the impact on childhood obesity (Oken, Levitan *et al.* 2008). Also, sleep duration in the infant or young child is emerging as a potentially important determinant of childhood weight gain (Monasta *et al.* 2010). In a recent study from the US Project Viva, a greater prevalence of overweight in 3-year-old children was reported in those who slept less than 12 hours per day during infancy than those who slept for longer periods (Taveras *et al.* 2008). Maternal smoking and sleep duration should be assessed in infants in future observational studies, and in all interventions designed to reduce childhood obesity. The intriguing suggestion that the microbiota in the gut may be associated with obesity has not been explored in the context of fetal programming, although this may offer a potential modifiable factor in relation to diet in the mother or child in early life (see Chapter 7, Section 7.6).

8.8 Mechanisms underlying the early life origins of obesity; role of animal studies

Human cohort studies have provided convincing evidence for early life origins of obesity, but the current information centred upon observational studies, together with the lack of evidence from intervention studies, presents a less than adequate evidence base to inform public health strategy. Importantly, in defining an intervention, a good scientific basis should be a fundamental prerequisite, although, unfortunately, this is not always put into practice.

Studies in experimental animals have made important contributions in this field (McMullen and Mostyn 2009). Most importantly, protocols in rodents, sheep and non-human primates have provided unequivocal evidence that maternal nutritional status can influence the risk of obesity in the offspring.

8.8.1 Maternal under-nutrition

The influence of fetal growth retardation in rodents has been extensively studied, and has generally been induced either by reduction of calorific intake or through maternal protein restriction, or in some studies by uterine artery ligation. Interpretation is not always straightforward due to differences in timing of the dietary insult and differing diets. Nonetheless, and in agreement with studies in humans, it is often cited that a combination of fetal under-nutrition followed by rapid catch-up growth in postnatal life encourages excess fat deposition in the offspring. Thus a modest reduction of calorific intake in mice by 30% leads to catch-up growth, and a high-fat diet induced obesity in the mouse (Yura *et al.* 2005); in the rat, 50% or 70% reduction in calorific intake during pregnancy but not lactation predisposes to obesity in later life (Jones and Friedman 1982; Vickers *et al.* 2003). Protein restriction protocols, which share some similarity to the dietary deprivations of the Dutch Hunger Winter (see Chapter

1, Section 1.4.1; and Chapter 4, Section 4.4.2.1), also show that transition to a higher plane of nutrition postpartum, achieved by cross fostering to a normally fed dam or by litter size reduction after delivery, leads to a higher risk of obesity in the offspring compared to controls (Ozanne, Fernandez-Twinn *et al.* 2004; Ozanne, Lewis *et al.* 2004).

Studies in pigs and sheep which, as for human infants, are born at a later stage of development than rodents, also support a major influence of fetal growth restriction on later development of obesity (Mostyn and Symonds 2009). The agricultural industry has recognised for many years that 'runt' piglets of the litter become fatter adults (Powell and Aberle 1980). In the pig, however, catch-up growth does not occur, with the smaller piglets remaining stunted, but becoming fatter adults. The deposition of fat occurs in the fat depot in the back of the animals where, unexpectedly, there is no relationship between fat mass and plasma leptin, pointing towards an important role for 'depot'-specific adipocyte function in the development of obesity (Poore and Fowden 2004).

The suggestion that the foundations of obesity are laid down in infancy has been revisited recently in humans (Spalding *et al.* 2008), in a study which has proposed that fat cell number is determined during childhood and adolescence. In the sheep, the gestational period of nutrient restriction is a determinant of later adipocyte metabolism and adiposity although the relevant studies present a complex picture (Mostyn and Symonds 2009). However, exposure to nutrient restriction during early to midgestation, the period of maximum placental growth, is associated with increased neonatal fat mass which could predispose to adiposity in later life, and thereby parallel the outcomes reported for the Dutch Hunger Winter (Bispham *et al.* 2005).

8.8.2 Maternal diabetes

To mimic type 1 diabetes in pregnancy several laboratories have employed streptozotocin (STZ) which, when administered in early gestation, destroys maternal islet function in rodents. A mild maternal STZ insult, and also maternal glucose infusion, have been shown to lead to macrosomia in the offspring. As the offspring age, insulin secretory capacity diminishes and the animals become glucose intolerant (Aerts *et al.* 1988; Gauguier *et al.* 1991). The offspring also become overweight. Since neither of these methods of inducing maternal hyperglycaemia is associated with maternal obesity, they provide clear evidence for 'programming' of offspring fat mass by maternal diabetes, independent of accompanying maternal obesity, and contrast to those observational studies in human diabetic pregnancy which have suggested a predominant influence of maternal obesity in the association with offspring obesity (Plagemann, Harder *et al.* 1999b). Also, in mice with a genetic predisposition to spontaneous development of gestational diabetes (Lep db/+) the offspring of diabetic dams, while not heavier than controls, demonstrate increased fat mass and hepatic insulin resistance (Yamashita *et al.* 2003). In all these models, offspring obesity is associated with altered glucose homeostasis. The programming of diabetes and insulin resistance by maternal diabetes is beyond the scope of this chapter, but has been reviewed recently (Poston 2010) (see Chapter 9).

8.8.3 Maternal obesity

Several laboratories, including our own, have addressed the hypothesis that maternal obesity predisposes the progeny to obesity in later life. We have developed an experimental model of maternal diet-induced obesity in rodents, in which the dams are fed a highly palatable diet rich in sugar and fat before pregnancy, and during pregnancy and lactation (Samuelsson *et al.* 2008; Nivoit *et al.* 2009). Adult offspring of obese insulin-resistant mice develop glucose intolerance, are hyperphagic and have increased fat mass (Samuelsson *et al.* 2008). Several other laboratories have similarly reported obesity in adult offspring of diet-induced obese dams (Srinivasan *et al.* 2006; Bayol *et al.* 2007; Ferezou-Viala *et al.* 2007; Chen *et al.* 2008; Shankar *et al.* 2008; Dunn and Bale 2009). Importantly, for translation to the human condition, 6-month-old offspring of Japanese macaques from fat-fed mothers also demonstrate increased adiposity (McCurdy *et al.* 2009), suggesting commonality of mechanism across species.

Many phenotypic similarities are apparent between the progeny from obese animals and experimental models of maternal diabetes in which the dams are not obese. Generally, as in many obese women, glucose intolerance and/or insulin resistance (Holemans *et al.* 2004; Samuelsson *et al.* 2008) accompanies maternal obesity, which could infer a common mechanistic role although other factors, as described below, have been implicated.

8.8.4 Neonatal overfeeding

The neonatal period is assuming a central role in the mechanistic understanding of the developmental origins of obesity. In most animal models of maternal/fetal under-nutrition, and in SGA children, it appears that postnatal catch-up growth plays a focal role in 'programming' of offspring obesity. Early overfeeding in non-human primates has also been shown to induce increased adiposity in adult males (Lewis *et al.* 1986). Furthermore, when neonatal over-nutrition in rodents is induced by small litter rearing, with each pup receiving a greater share of the maternal milk, the offspring become obese (Cryer and Jones 1980; Velkoska *et al.* 2008).

8.9 A central role for disturbance in pathways of appetite regulation

The convergence of both human and animal studies towards a window of vulnerability in early postnatal life and late development of obesity has led to an intriguing hypothesis which focuses on a central role of those hypothalamic pathways which are critical to energy balance.

8.9.1 Fetal and neonatal hyperinsulinaemia

Key to development of this hypothesis were the studies by Plagemann and co-workers which had shown that neonatal overfeeding by small litter rearing can lead to persistent changes in appetite in the offspring, as well as obesity, and that this was associated with neonatal hyperinsulinaemia (Plagemann *et al.* 1992). This laboratory also demonstrated alteration in appetite regulatory pathways at the level of the hypothalamus, as well as reduced responsiveness to the inhibitory effects of leptin and insulin, leading to reduction in the normal 'breaking' influence of these hormones on appetite (Davidowa and Plagemann 2001; Davidowa *et al.* 2003). Plagemann's laboratory used the STZ model of maternal diabetes, and also assessed the influence of neonatal injection of insulin to add convincing evidence to their theory that neonatal hyperinsulinaemia contributes to dysfunction of pathways critical to normal development of the neuronal hypothalamic networks central to energy balance, permanently changing hypothalamic function, and to persistent increases in food intake and obesity (Plagemann *et al.* 1998; Plagemann, Harder *et al.*

1999b; Plagemann, Harder *et al.* 1999c; Plagemann 2005).

8.9.2 Fetal and neonatal hyperleptinaemia

In common with insulin, leptin is likely to play a major role in development of the hypothalamus. A neurotrophic role for leptin has been demonstrated in development of the nuclei which control energy balance (Bouret *et al.* 2004; Horvath and Bruning 2006). In rodents there is a characteristic neonatal leptin surge (Ahima *et al.* 1998) unrelated to appetite regulation or growth. This is now considered to be an important 'trigger' for normal development of the hypothalamic appetite regulatory neural network (Bouret 2010b). As might be anticipated, artificial manipulation of neonatal leptin status in rodents leads to persistent change in energy balance into adulthood (Yura *et al.* 2005; Attig *et al.* 2008; Vickers *et al.* 2008). In view of widely reported disturbances in appetite and in the neonatal leptin profile in pups from different animal models, both in models of maternal under- and over-nutrition there is growing acceptance that an aberrant neonatal leptin profile may play a fundamental role in persistent changes in food intake and in the later development of obesity (Cottrell and Ozanne 2007; Morris 2009). Since rodent pups are born at a much earlier stage of development than precocial species such as humans, it should be appreciated that leptin sensitivity of the hypothalamic energy balance network may occur before birth in the human fetus.

8.9.3 Maternal obesity

Work from our laboratory has addressed the possibility that offspring of insulin-resistant obese dams may be influenced by neonatal hyperleptinaemia, as we had previously reported that these offspring were hyperphagic. In newborn rat pups we showed an exaggerated leptin surge compared with controls and, in the weanling pups, evidence of altered neural projections between the arcuate and paraventricular nuclei. We also presented evidence for hypothalamic leptin resistance and demonstrated that the young offspring of obese dams are leptin resistant, and remain leptin resistant. We proposed that this could be the central mechanism contributing to the hyperphagia observed in the adults (Kirk *et al.* 2009). Several other laboratories have similarly shown that

hyperphagia and obesity in the offspring of obese dams is associated with altered expression of several of the appetite regulatory peptides in the hypothalamus, as recently reviewed by Morris (2009). Whether these observations pertain to infants from obese women remains to be determined. However, it is theoretically possible as maternal plasma leptin concentrations are related to adiposity and cord blood leptin concentrations tend to reflect maternal fat mass (Catalano, Presley *et al.* 2009).

8.9.4 Cellular pathways of energy metabolism

The important role proposed for the central pathways of energy balance, which infers deviations from normal development in the hypothalamic neurocircuitry, has created widespread interest as a novel hypothesis which could explain associations between altered nutritional status in early life and the risk of obesity. However, other key aspects of energy balance have been implicated, suggesting important abnormalities in offspring cellular metabolism. In the sheep, altered adipocyte metabolism in offspring from nutrient-restricted ewes may facilitate fat deposition, which may occur through altered sensitivity to glucocorticoids, as a result of increasing endoplasmic reticulum stress or in association with a pronounced inflammatory response (Sharkey *et al.* 2009; Symonds *et al.* 2009). As described in the pig, and of relevance to recent studies in humans, the site of the fat depot which expands in response to early life nutritional disturbance may be all-important (Poore and Fowden 2004). Disturbances in mitochondrial function acquired early in life could also influence energy balance and have been described in sheep adipocytes including increased mRNA expression of uncoupling protein 2 (UCP2) (Symonds *et al.* 2004). We have reported abnormalities in mitochondrial function in the skeletal muscle from offspring of obese dams which may contribute to insulin resistance, but this could also have widespread implications in energy homeostasis (Shelley *et al.* 2009).

8.9.5 Mechanisms underlying persistent modification of gene expression

The precise molecular mechanisms underlying the developmental programming of disease are under intense scrutiny and are at present unclear (see Chapter 4). Persistent alteration in offspring metabolism and function arising from perturbations in the maternal environment could arise from an irreversible change during development in organ structure, as observed in the hypothalamus, with associated alteration in cell number, type or connectivity. This is intuitively a simpler concept to grasp than the persistent changes in gene expression presumed to permanently alter cellular function. These infer irreversible DNA modification by epigenetic pathways, e.g. methylation or histone deacetylation, and there are clear instances where perturbation of the maternal environment persistently alters offspring tissue gene expression through this mechanism.

This rapidly expanding field is beyond the scope of this chapter, but the reader is referred to some excellent recent reviews (Gluckman *et al.* 2008; Mathers and McKay 2009). Of relevance to the developmental origins of obesity, Plagemann's group, using the reduced litter model, reported recently increased methylation status and reduced expression of the promoter region of the anorexigenic (appetite reduc-ing) neurohormone proopiomelanocortin (POMC) in hypothalami from pre-weaning rat pups, which could lead to increased appetite, although it was not reported whether this persisted to adulthood (Plagemann *et al.* 2009). Also, decreased methylation status of the growth hormone secretagogue receptor (GHSR) in the arcuate nucleus of the hypothalamus has been reported in F2 adult offspring of obese and insulin-resistant mice (Dunn and Bale 2009).

8.10 Conclusions

In conclusion, animal models provide enormous potential to unravel the mechanisms contributing to the developmental origins of obesity, and in turn will help inform intervention strategies in humans.

There is also real potential in the near future to inform public health strategies through ongoing RCTs in obese women and follow-up of their children, through adoption of the WHO child growth standards and from interventions addressing the composition of formula feeds.

8.11 Key points

- The environmental determinants of obesity may include nutritional status in critical periods of early development.
- Growth retardation *in utero*, particularly if followed by rapid postnatal growth, may be a determinant of obesity in later life.
- Breastfeeding may protect against later obesity. The reduction in obesity in later life has been estimated to be between 7% and 22% with breastfeeding of varying degree.
- Excessive 'fuel' availability associated with maternal diabetes and obesity may predispose the developing child to enhanced risk of type 2 diabetes in later life.
- Animal studies provide unequivocal evidence for early life origins of obesity and have made a major contribution to understanding the mechanistic basis.
- The current level of evidence, in the absence of randomised controlled trials, is inadequate to support public health interventions.

8.12 Recommendations for future research

- Although the Institute of Medicine (in the US) published revised guidelines on gestational weight gain in pregnancy (Centers for Disease Control and Prevention 2010), evidence from the UK is required to enable appropriate guidelines to be developed that are relevant for implementing in a UK population. Current advice in England and Wales (National Institute for Clinical Excellence (NICE) 2010) is that pregnant women should not be weighed routinely throughout pregnancy until such time as an intervention for restriction of weight gain has been shown to safely improve pregnancy outcome.

- Recent evidence from the European Early Nutritional Programming Project (EARNEST) suggests that lower-protein formula feeds may be advantageous in the prevention of childhood obesity. Further cohort studies with longer-term follow-up are required to confirm this.
- Intervention studies are required to determine effective dietary and physical activity interventions appropriate for overweight and obese pregnant women. Some studies designed to improve physical activity or diet in overweight or obese pregnant women are currently under way, and findings are eagerly awaited.

8.13 Key references

Druet C & Ong KK (2008) Early childhood predictors of adult body composition. *Best Practice and Research Clinical Endocrinology and Metabolism*, **22**, 489–502.

Horta Bl, Bahl R, Martines JC & Victora CG (2007) *Evidence on the Long-Term Effects of Breastfeeding: Systematic Review and Meta-analyses*. Geneva, World Health Organization.

Monasta L, Batty GD, Cattaneo A *et al.* (2010) Early-life determinants of overweight and obesity: a review of systematic reviews. *Obesity Reviews*, **11**, 695–708.

Nelson SM, Matthews P & Poston L (2010) Maternal metabolism and obesity: modifiable determinants of pregnancy outcome. *Human Reproduction Update*, **16**, 255–75.

WHO Multicentre Growth Reference Study Group (2006) *Acta Paediatrica Supplement*, **450**, 76–85.

9
Nutrition and Development: Type 2 Diabetes

9.1 Introduction

Diabetes mellitus is a group of metabolic disorders characterised by persistent hyperglycaemia. There are two main forms of diabetes, termed type 1 diabetes and type 2 diabetes.

Type 1 diabetes arises through the autoimmune destruction of the pancreatic beta-cells. These are the only cells in the body capable of producing the hormone, insulin, which is required for the uptake of glucose into muscle and fat cells. Its most common age of onset is in childhood (around 11 years of age) and it is rare for it to develop in individuals over the age of 40. Type 1 diabetes accounts for around 10% of all diabetes.

Type 2 diabetes is the most common form of diabetes and accounts for almost 90% of all cases. It is associated with insulin resistance and pancreatic beta-cell dysfunction. In individuals with type 2 diabetes, the body can still produce insulin, but not in sufficient quantities (beta-cell dysfunction) and insulin-responsive tissues including muscle, fat and liver do not respond to it appropriately (insulin resistance). Beta-cell dysfunction and insulin resistance increase with age. Therefore type 2 diabetes is a progressive condition and is thought to develop when the declining beta-cell function can no longer compensate for increasing insulin resistance. Type 2 diabetes is diagnosed when fasting plasma glucose levels exceed 7 mM (millimolar) or if they exceed 11.1 mM two hours after a glucose tolerance test. However, this is a threshold for diagnosis and it is also recognised that individuals progress through a 'pre-diabetic state' which is classified as impaired glucose tolerance. Obesity is a major risk factor for insulin resistance and consequently type 2 diabetes. Therefore, although type 2 diabetes was traditionally considered to be a condition of middle age, the increasing prevalence of childhood obesity is resulting in a growing number of cases of type 2 diabetes in children.

Type 2 diabetes is of great importance to public health as it is associated with other conditions including cardiovascular disease, stroke, blindness and kidney disease. It therefore has major implications on health care costs. It is currently estimated that 10% of the National Health Service budget is spent on diabetes; in addition approximately 7% of all prescriptions are for diabetes (Diabetes UK 2010). The prevalence of type 2 diabetes continues to rise in populations worldwide, and in 2011, an estimated 366 million people worldwide had diabetes (International Diabetes Federation 2011). By 2030 it is estimated that 552 million people worldwide will have diabetes and over 90% of these will have type 2 diabetes (*ibid*). In the UK, the number of people diagnosed with diabetes has increased from 1.4 million in 1996 to an estimated 2.9 million today (Diabetes UK 2012). It is estimated that an additional 850 000 people in the UK have diabetes but have not been diagnosed. It is predicted that by 2025 this will increase to approximately 5 million (*ibid*). The rate of this rise cannot be caused by a change in genetic

Nutrition and Development: Short- and Long-Term Consequences for Health, First Edition. Edited by the British Nutrition Foundation.
© 2013 the British Nutrition Foundation. Published 2013 by Blackwell Publishing Ltd.

make-up, as a change in genes could not occur over such a short time frame. Therefore this points towards the importance of environmental factors. Diet is believed to be one such important environmental factor. Although diet at any stage of life plays a major role in metabolic health, there is accumulating evidence that diet during fetal and early postnatal life can have a major influence on long-term risk of diseases such as type 2 diabetes.

9.2 Relationships between birthweight and type 2 diabetes

9.2.1 Low birthweight and type 2 diabetes

The idea that events in early life could impact on subsequent risk of type 2 diabetes was prompted by the results of a series of epidemiological studies that link birthweight to current glucose tolerance. The first study to address this relationship was carried out by Nick Hales and David Barker on a group of men (mean age 64 years) in Hertfordshire in the UK (Hales *et al.* 1991). This revealed a continuous relationship between birthweight and presence of impaired glucose tolerance or type 2 diabetes at age 64. Those men who were smallest at birth were over six times more likely to currently have impaired glucose tolerance or type 2 diabetes than those men who were largest at birth. Since this original study in the UK, over 40 studies have confirmed these associations in populations worldwide (Newsome *et al.* 2003; Whincup *et al.* 2008).

The relationship between birthweight and type 2 diabetes has also been shown to exist in twins. A study of middle-aged twins in Denmark revealed that, in both monozygotic (identical) and dizygotic (non-identical) twin pairs who were discordant for type 2 diabetes, the diabetic twin had a significantly lower birthweight than their normoglycaemic co-twin (Poulsen *et al.* 1997). If it is assumed that the monozygotic twins are genetically identical then the difference in birthweight must be related to the fetal environment. A second study of twins in Italy, who were significantly younger (mean age 32 years) than the cohort in Demark, revealed similar findings. These studies thus provide strong evidence for the importance of a non-genetic intrauterine factor in mediating the relationship between poor fetal growth and the development of type 2 diabetes in later life.

In light of the epidemiological observations, Hales and Barker proposed that early nutrition played a key role in mediating the relationships between early growth and adult disease. They termed this the 'thrifty phenotype hypothesis' (Hales and Barker 1992) (see Chapter 4, Section 4.5). They proposed that in response to impaired nutrient supply, the growing fetus will make adaptations *in utero* in order to maximise metabolic efficiency regarding the storage and usage of fuels, to increase the chance of immediate survival postnatally. This included sparing the growth of the brain at the expense of other tissues such as the endocrine pancreas, as well as programming metabolism in a manner that promoted fuel storage. The programming of such a phenotype would continue to be beneficial if conditions of poor nutrition were extended into postnatal life. However, in the presence of adequate or plentiful nutrition, these adaptations become detrimental and predispose to the development of obesity and metabolic dysfunction.

9.2.2 High birthweight and type 2 diabetes

In some studies, notably those of native North American populations, increased risk of type 2 diabetes is also observed at the high birthweight end of the spectrum (McCance *et al.* 1994). These populations have a very high prevalence of type 2 diabetes, obesity and consequently gestational diabetes (>10% of pregnancies) (Franks *et al.* 2006). The increased risk of type 2 diabetes in individuals with high birthweight is, therefore, thought to reflect an increased risk of diabetes in the macrosomic offspring of women with gestational diabetes.

9.3 Postnatal growth

The detrimental effects of poor fetal growth on long-term metabolic health appear to be exaggerated if followed by accelerated postnatal growth and/or obesity. The initial studies in the original Hertfordshire cohort (see Section 9.2.1) observed that in 64-year-old men the worst glucose tolerance was observed in those that were in the lowest quartile of birthweight but who were currently obese (body mass index >28) (Hales *et al.* 1991). A study of 7-year-old South Africans revealed that those children with low birthweights who underwent rapid childhood weight gain had the worst glucose tolerance (Crowther *et al.* 1998). See Chapter 2, Section 2.10, for further discussion on catch-up growth.

9.4 Evidence for the role of early nutrition in humans influencing type 2 diabetes risk

9.4.1 During pregnancy

Assessing the impact of maternal nutrition on the health of the offspring in humans is difficult. However, investigations involving individuals conceived during conditions of famine have provided direct evidence of the consequential effects of maternal nutrition during gestation and lactation on the overall health of the adult offspring. The Dutch Hunger Winter (see Chapter 1, Section 1.4.1; and Chapter 4, Section 4.4.2), which occurred in the western part of the Netherlands at the end of the Second World War, was a short, defined period of famine lasting around 5 months from late November 1944 to early May 1945. Prior to the onset of the famine, the affected area of the Netherlands consisted of a reasonably well-nourished population. The occurrence of this abrupt famine therefore granted researchers a unique opportunity to retrospectively study the effect of maternal nutrition on the glucose tolerance of offspring. Compared to individuals born the year before the famine, those who were *in utero* during the famine had higher plasma glucose levels two hours after a standard oral glucose tolerance test (Ravelli *et al.* 1998). These glucose levels were highest among individuals who had been exposed to the famine during the final trimester of pregnancy and then became obese in adult life. This study therefore provided direct evidence that poor maternal nutrition leads to increased susceptibility to type 2 diabetes in the offspring. It also supports the hypothesis that the greatest risk of developing metabolic diseases exists when there is a marked conflict between the environmental conditions experienced *in utero* and that experienced in adult life.

A study in Denmark has recently demonstrated that milk consumption during pregnancy is positively associated with birthweight in a cohort of over 50 000 individuals (Olsen *et al.* 2007). However, it is not yet known if milk consumption during pregnancy is also associated with reduced risk of type 2 diabetes and insulin resistance in the offspring. A recent study in India addressed the relationship between maternal vitamin B_{12} and folate levels during pregnancy and insulin resistance in the offspring at 6 years of age (Yajnik *et al.* 2008). This revealed that low maternal vitamin B_{12} at 18 weeks of pregnancy and high maternal erythrocyte folate concentrations at 28 weeks of pregnancy were both associated with increased insulin resistance at age 6 years. Furthermore, the most insulin-resistant children were those whose mothers had low vitamin B_{12} and high folate during pregnancy.

9.4.2 During lactation

There is growing evidence to suggest that growth during the early postnatal period also has a major influence on long-term metabolic health, and that this can be independent of growth and nutrition *in utero*. Some of the strongest data relates to long-term obesity risk. There are now at least three systematic reviews demonstrating that accelerated postnatal growth increases risk of subsequent obesity (Baird, Fisher *et al.* 2005; Monteiro and Victora 2005; Ong and Loos 2006) (see Chapter 8). These reviews do not provide insight into the causes of the accelerated growth. Evidence for the effects of early nutrition on growth and long-term metabolic health has primarily come from the study of formula-fed infants compared to breast-fed infants. It is known that over the first year of life breast-fed infants gain less weight than formula-fed infants and are less likely to develop cardiovascular risk factors which are strongly associated with type 2 diabetes (Singhal 2010a).

9.5 Evidence for the role of early nutrition in animal models influencing type 2 diabetes risk

In light of the extensive data from human studies linking early growth and nutrition to risk of type 2 diabetes, a number of animal models have been established to investigate the mechanism by which this occurs.

9.5.1 Models of under-nutrition

9.5.1.1 Energy restriction

Balanced nutrient restriction has been a common strategy used to study the effects of maternal under-nutrition. In rodents, when maternal diet is severely restricted (to 30% *ad libitum*) the offspring have increased fasting plasma insulin levels in adulthood (Vickers *et al.* 2000). A less severe protocol of 50% reduction in energy intake during the last week of pregnancy and the start of lactation in the rat leads to an age-dependent loss of glucose tolerance in the offspring, which becomes apparent by 1 year of age in the male rat (Garofano *et al.* 1999). Reduced nutrition in late pregnancy in the sheep also leads to glucose intolerance in adult offspring (Gardner *et al.* 2005).

9.5.1.2 Macronutrient deficiency

The most extensively studied model of macronutrient deficiency is the maternal protein restriction model. Offspring of dams fed a diet containing 8% protein (as opposed to 20% in the controls) during pregnancy and lactation have impaired insulin secretion in adulthood (Merezak *et al.* 2004). This effect is exaggerated if the offspring are fed a high-fat diet (Wilson and Hughes 1997). Maternal protein restriction also leads to changes in glucose tolerance of the offspring. In young adult life, 'low-protein' offspring show an improved glucose tolerance compared to controls. However, they undergo a greater age-dependent loss of glucose tolerance such that they have impaired glucose tolerance at 15 months (Ozanne *et al.* 2003) and frank diabetes by 17 months of age (Petry *et al.* 2001).

9.5.1.3 Micronutrient deficiency

Iron deficiency is a common nutritional problem in humans and is especially prevalent in pregnant women. Rodent models have provided strong evidence linking maternal iron deficiency to increases in blood pressure in the offspring (Gambling *et al.* 2003). However, to date there is no evidence to suggest that these animals develop insulin resistance or type 2 diabetes.

9.5.2 Models of over-nutrition

9.5.2.1 Maternal diabetes

Diabetes during pregnancy exposes the fetus to an excess of glucose. In rodents the effects of maternal diabetes is generally studied by destruction of the maternal beta-cell using streptozotocin (Van Assche

et al. 2001). The progeny of mildly diabetic mothers are macrosomic (i.e. large at birth) and the development of their endocrine pancreas is enhanced. In adulthood, offspring of mildly diabetic mothers have a deficit in insulin secretion and have impaired glucose tolerance. When maternal diabetes is extreme, pups are born small for gestational age. Due to an over-stimulation by the excessive glucose, the offspring beta-cells are almost completely degranulated, and consequently have lower pancreatic insulin content and a reduced plasma insulin level. The offspring become insulin resistant in adulthood. See Chapter 8, Section 8.4.2, for evidence on the effect of maternal diabetes on later obesity in offspring.

9.5.2.2 Maternal high-fat feeding

Although the majority of studies on the effects of maternal diet in rodents have focused on models of under-nutrition, in light of the increased availability of fat-rich foods there are also a growing number of papers addressing the effects of maternal over-nutrition on the offspring. Feeding rats a diet rich in saturated fat during pregnancy and lactation has been demonstrated to result in insulin resistance and impaired glucose homeostasis in the offspring (Taylor *et al.* 2005). These effects are not limited to maternal diets rich in saturated fats. Studies using maternal diets rich in *n*-6 polyunsaturated fatty acids have also demonstrated effects on insulin sensitivity in the offspring (Buckley *et al.* 2005).

9.5.2.3 Maternal obesity

Obesity is a growing health problem in today's society. Of particular concern is the growing prevalence of obesity in women of childbearing age. Most of the rodent models of maternal high-fat feeding are not associated with maternal obesity as rodents are very good at regulating their energy intake in response to energy-dense foods. Therefore, recent studies have aimed at over-coming this through the use of highly palatable diets rich in simple sugars that overcome the rodents' natural satiety signals. Samuelsson *et al.* (2008) achieved this by feeding a high-fat diet supplemented with condensed milk to female mice six weeks prior to mating and through pregnancy and lactation. Male and female offspring were insulin resistant by 3 months of age and males developed impaired glucose tolerance by 6 months of age.

Similar observations were made when the protocol was applied to rats, with male offspring of the obese dams developing more pronounced glucose intolerance and insulin resistance compared to females. An alternative approach has been to feed rats a junk food diet rich in fat, sugar and salt (e.g. consisting of chocolate and doughnuts) during pregnancy and lactation. Offspring of such dams develop hyperglycaemia and hyperinsulinaemia (indicative of insulin resistance). However, in this model the phenotype is more pronounced in female than in male offspring (Bayol *et al.* 2008).

9.5.3 Underlying mechanisms

9.5.3.1 *Permanent structural changes*

One mechanism by which environmental factors at critical periods of development could have long-term phenotypic consequences is through permanent structural changes in key organs. If a certain nutrient or hormone is essential at a critical period of development for growth and differentiation of a tissue, inappropriate levels of this factor will have permanent structural consequences. For example, treatment of neonatal rat pups during the second postnatal week of life with high levels of insulin has been shown to induce permanent changes in hypothalamic morphology, in particular causing a reduction in the density of neurons within the ventromedial hypothalamus (Harder *et al.* 1998). This region of the hypothalamus has been implicated in regulation of satiety. Thus, structural alterations in this area of the brain could contribute to the excess weight gain and glucose intolerance in adult rats that were administered insulin in early life. The development of the endocrine pancreas is also very vulnerable to a suboptimal *in utero* environment (see Chapter 2, Section 2.5.7). Maternal protein restriction and maternal energy restriction lead to a reduced beta-cell mass but the mechanisms involved may be different (Dumortier *et al.* 2007). A restriction in maternal energy intake alters the differentiation of the endocrine pancreas without affecting the proliferation, while a low maternal protein intake reduces proliferation and vascularisation and increases apoptosis. High levels of glucocorticoids may be responsible for the former while low levels of taurine and growth factors such as insulin-like growth factor (IGF) and vascular endothelial growth factor (VEGF) may be involved in the latter.

9.5.3.2 *Epigenetic changes*

Identifying the fundamental molecular mechanisms by which diet influences gene expression and tissue physiology is critical. The role of epigenetic modifications in these processes is a growing area of interest. Epigenetics is the study of heritable changes in gene function that occur without alterations to the DNA sequence (Bird 2007). The best-known epigenetic modifications are DNA-methylation and histone post-transcriptional modifications, including acetylation, methylation, ubiquitination and phosphorylation. Epigenetic modification provides a form of memory that is key for the maintenance of genomic information.

It is well established that epigenetic processes are highly dependent on the dietary availability of key nutrients (e.g. methyl donors and cofactors). For example, a post-weaning diet deficient in folate, vitamin B_{12} and choline permanently affects the expression of the epigenetically sensitive imprinted insulin-like growth factor II (IGF-II) gene, with altered methylation patterns at a specific region (differentially methylated region 2: DMR-2) (Waterland *et al.* 2006). In addition to direct effects of diet on epigenetic modifications, several studies have now shown that nutritional influences in early life can induce permanent alterations in the epigenotype that could determine adult phenotype and disease susceptibility. These were initially conducted in mice that carry the epigenetically sensitive allele Agouti viable yellow (A^{vy}) that influences coat colour and obesity. When A^{vy} pregnant dams were fed a diet supplemented in methyl donors and cofactors (e.g. choline, folic acid, vitamin B_{12}) they tended to have offspring that were pseudo-agouti and lean rather than being yellow and obese as seen when the Agouti gene is ubiquitously active (Waterland and Jirtle 2003). Global changes in DNA methylation are observed in sheep that experienced alterations in vitamin B_{12} and folate and methionine during the periconceptional period (Sinclair *et al.* 2007). Maternal protein restriction has also been shown to alter the methylation status of the promoters for the glucocorticoid receptor, peroxisome proliferator-activated receptor α (Lillycrop *et al.* 2008) and the angiotensin receptor (Bogdarina *et al.* 2007), with parallel changes in gene expression. More recently it has been demonstrated that intrauterine artery ligation leads to changes in both DNA methylation and histone acetylation in the transcription factor pancreatic duodenal homeobox 1 (PDX-1) promoter of the offspring (Park *et al.* 2008).

Recent studies have also provided the first evidence that maternal diet in humans can have a long-term effect on DNA methylation in the offspring. The initial study demonstrated that individuals exposed *in utero* to the Dutch Hunger Winter (see Chapter 1, Section 1.4.1; and Chapter 4, Section 4.4.2) had lower levels of methylation in a region of the IGF-II gene in adulthood compared to their unexposed same-sex siblings (Heijmans *et al.* 2008). A second study in this same cohort identified an additional six loci that were differentially methylated after prenatal exposure to famine (Tobi *et al.* 2009). These loci were all implicated in growth and metabolic disease.

9.6 Conclusions

It is now 20 years since the original epidemiological studies revealed that there is a relationship between patterns of fetal and early postnatal growth and the subsequent risk of development of type 2 diabetes in later life. Studies in humans and animal models have provided strong evidence that the early environment and, in particular, early nutrition plays an important role in mediating this relationship. However, the mechanisms by which a phenomenon that occurs during a critical period of development can have long-term effects on the function of a cell and therefore metabolism of an organism many years later are only starting to emerge. These include: (1) Permanent structural changes in an organ, resulting from suboptimal nutrition during a critical period of development (see Chapter 4, Section 4.5.1). Such an example is the permanent reduction of beta-cell mass in the endocrine pancreas. (2) Persistent alterations in epigenetic modifications (e.g. DNA methylation and histone modifications) leading to changes in gene expression. Several transcription factors are susceptible to programmed changes in gene expression through such mechanisms. A major challenge now is to capitalise and build on this knowledge to identify individuals at risk of type 2 diabetes resulting from suboptimal early nutrition and to define suitable intervention strategies. Further advances in this field therefore have the potential to combat the burden of common diseases such as type 2 diabetes that represent major health care issues of the twenty-first century.

9.7 Key points

- Type 1 diabetes arises through the autoimmune destruction of the pancreatic beta-cells (the cells that produce insulin, which is required for the uptake of glucose into muscle and fat cells). Type 1 diabetes accounts for around 10% of all diabetes. It commonly develops in childhood and rarely in individuals aged over 40 years.
- Type 2 diabetes is far more common than type 1 diabetes (accounting for 90% of diabetes). In individuals with type 2 diabetes the body can still produce insulin but not in sufficient quantities (beta-cell dysfunction) and tissues in the body do not respond to insulin appropriately (insulin resistance).
- Obesity is a major risk factor for insulin resistance and consequently type 2 diabetes. Type 2 diabetes was traditionally thought to be a condition of middle age; however, the increasing prevalence of obesity in childhood is resulting in a growing number of cases of type 2 diabetes in children.
- Type 2 diabetes is of great importance to public health and health care costs as it is associated with other conditions including cardiovascular disease, stroke, blindness and kidney disease.
- Suboptimal nutrition during early life has a major influence on the risk of an individual developing type 2 diabetes later in life.
- Epidemiological evidence indicates both low and high birthweight is associated with increased risk of type 2 diabetes in later life.
- Over the first year of life, breast-fed infants gain less weight than formula-fed infants and are less likely to develop cardiovascular risk factors

Continued

which are strongly associated with type 2 diabetes.

- A range of different nutrient deficiencies during critical periods of development all lead to increased risk of type 2 diabetes. This is associated with both pancreatic beta-cell dysfunction and insulin resistance.

- Fundamental molecular mechanisms underlying these effects are starting to emerge. These include permanent structural changes and epigenetic programming of gene expression.
- Further understanding of these mechanisms will enable intervention and prevention strategies to be developed.

9.8 Recommendations for future research

- There is a need to establish biomarkers that could be used to identify individuals who experienced suboptimal nutrition during early life and are therefore at increased disease risk.

- There is a need to assess potential intervention strategies during pregnancy that could prevent suboptimal exposures *in utero*.

9.9 Key references

McMillen IC & Robinson JS (2005) Developmental origins of the metabolic syndrome: prediction, plasticity and programming. *Physiological Review*, **85**, 571–633.

Nathanielsz PW, Poston L & Taylor PD (2007) *In utero* exposure to maternal obesity and diabetes: animal models that identify and characterize implications for future health. *Clinics in Perinatology*, **34**, 515–26.

Pinney SE & Simmons RA (2010) Epigenetic mechanisms in the development of type 2 diabetes. *Trends in Endocrinology and Metabolism*, **21**, 223–9.

Warner MJ & Ozanne SE (2010) Mechanisms involved in the developmental programming of adulthood disease. *Biochemical Journal*, **427**, 333–4.

10
Nutrition and Development: Cardiovascular Disease

10.1 Introduction

Cardiovascular disease is the leading cause of death worldwide and its main forms are coronary heart disease (CHD) and stroke (cerebrovascular disease). Note that the term coronary heart disease is used throughout this section and has replaced ischaemic heart disease where originally cited in the source reference. Stroke can be further subdivided into two categories: haemorrhagic and occlusive. Most cardiovascular disease is caused by the presence of atherosclerosis, and clinical events (heart attack or stroke) usually result from the rupture of an atherosclerotic plaque, which triggers the formation of a blood clot, or the rupture of a blood vessel (aneurysm). These events are more likely to occur when blood pressure is high.

Human atherosclerosis is a chronic inflammatory process that develops over several decades with clinical events becoming evident in the fourth decade of life and beyond. It begins with the accumulation of fatty streaks in large or medium arteries, which progress to form fibrous plaques over time (Ross 1999). These fatty streaks consist of collections of foam cells which are derived from tissue macrophages that have taken up low-density lipoprotein (LDL) cholesterol which is rich in lipids, especially cholesteryl esters. The current view is that LDL-cholesterol becomes chemically modified or oxidised before being taken up by macrophages and it is thought that this process may be catalysed by enzyme systems such as NADPH oxidase (nicotinamide adenine dinucleotide phosphate-oxidase) (Lee et al. 2010) that play an important role in regulating endothelial cell function or lysosomal enzymes in monocytes/macrophages (Wen and Leake 2007).

Fatty streaks can disappear with time or can progress to form fibrous atherosclerotic plaques. Plaques grow over many years and develop large lipid-rich necrotic cores. Large plaques protrude into the lumen of the artery and impair the delivery of blood to the tissues (causing ischaemia), they also cause turbulence in blood flow which increases the likelihood of blood clotting. Most heart attacks result from the rupture of an atherosclerotic plaque which triggers blood clot formation and arterial occlusion, starving the heart muscle of oxygenated blood. Inflammation (e.g. smoking) or acute infections (e.g. influenza) activate white blood cells which can result in a plaque becoming unstable due to erosion of its fibrous cap and therefore prone to rupture.

Atherosclerosis and raised blood pressure develop slowly over several decades and may be determined to some extent by events in fetal and early postnatal life. This chapter considers the epidemiological evidence with regard to the effects of birthweight and early growth on risk of CHD and stroke using clinical endpoints (mortality and incidence of events rather than surrogate risk markers). It then focuses on the potential mechanisms by which programming may affect risk.

Nutrition and Development: Short- and Long-Term Consequences for Health, First Edition. Edited by the British Nutrition Foundation.
© 2013 the British Nutrition Foundation. Published 2013 by Blackwell Publishing Ltd.

10.2 Evidence-based on clinical endpoints

Counties of Norway that formerly had high rates of infant mortality between 1896 and 1925 were found to have high rates of mortality from CHD in men and women aged 40–69 years in 1964–7, when infant mortality was low in Norway (Forsdahl 1977). Forsdahl suggested that 'great poverty in childhood and adolescence followed by prosperity is a risk factor for arteriosclerotic heart disease'. This observation was systematically confirmed by Barker *et al.* in a series of ecological and longitudinal cohort studies in the UK and Finland (Barker, Winter *et al.* 1989; Barker *et al.* 1992; Barker, Hales *et al.* 1993; Barker, Osmond *et al.* 1993; Barker *et al.* 2005). Using meticulously kept birthweight and growth records of infants born in Hertfordshire between 1911 and 1930, it was possible to follow-up the causes of death of these children as adults (Barker, Winter *et al.* 1989). Risk of death from cardiovascular disease declined with increasing birthweight. Examination of the growth records of the children in the first year of life showed that infants who were heavier at 1 year had a much lower risk of CHD. Later studies in men born in Sheffield before 1925 showed risk of cardiovascular disease to be more strongly related to small head circumference and low ponderal index (weight/length^3) at birth than to birthweight (Barker, Osmond *et al.* 1993) and it was concluded that the effect was mainly due to reduced fetal growth rather than preterm birth.

Infants who are born small for gestational age (SGA) or who grow poorly during infancy are also more likely to grow up in poor communities where other environmental factors that influence cardiovascular disease risk are prevalent (e.g. poor housing, parental smoking habit, limited dietary choice). The analysis of all births in Denmark between 1981 and 2004 show poor fetal growth to still be strongly related to indices of social deprivation (Mortensen *et al.* 2009). The associations reported for poor fetal growth included non-Western ethnicity (Z-score −0.28), low education (−0.19), teenage motherhood (−0.14), single motherhood (−0.13) and poverty (−0.12) and were weakest for unemployment (−0.04). Some prospective cohort studies have been able to adjust for social deprivation in their risk estimates. A meta-analysis of 17 studies (Huxley *et al.* 2007) comprising 147 009 individuals concluded that there was a 15% (95% CI: 10–20%) reduction in relative risk of CHD with each 1 kg higher birthweight (Fig. 10.1). This estimate is much lower than those originally reported by Barker, Winter *et al.* (1989), whose participants were born between 1911 and 1930 during a period of severe economic depression. There have been marked improvement in pregnancy outcomes in economically developed countries over the past 60 years, which would be expected to reduce the strength of the association. However, maternal mortality and perinatal mortality remain high in many developing countries and thus it would be predicted that cardiovascular disease would be greater in migrants to developed countries from developing countries. This still appears to be case for the South Asian community in the UK where rates of cardiovascular disease are higher than in the White population. Birthweights remain low in South Asian pregnancies even after correcting for maternal height and gestational age.

Most of the evidence with regard to birthweight and cardiovascular disease outcomes indicates that low birthweight increases risk. However, it is possible that very high birthweight also increases risk. Blood glucose concentration is a major determinant of fetal growth and mothers who have poorly controlled gestational diabetes give birth to very heavy infants up to 8 kg (18 lb). The term macrosomia describes such large babies and is usually defined as a birthweight >4 kg (see Chapter 2, Table 2.2), although not all infants in this category would be born to mothers with gestational diabetes. It is well established that gestational diabetes increases the risk of type 2 diabetes in the offspring in adult life, and as type 2 diabetes more than doubles the risk of cardiovascular disease this in turn would be predicted to increase risk of cardiovascular disease. The prevalence of macrosomia is already high in North America and is increasing in Europe. Data from the Nurses' Health Study on 66 111 female nurses showed a significant interaction of weight gain in adult life with low birthweight, resulting in a 55% increased risk of CHD and a 74% increased risk of stroke compared with the middle quintile (Rich-Edwards *et al.* 2005). This relationship with CHD risk became stronger when infants with macrosomia were excluded from the analysis. However, the greatest risk of cardiovascular disease was seen in women who were small at birth and became obese in adult life. Although larger size in infancy is associated with increased risk of developing type 2 diabetes (see Chapter 9, Section 9.2.2) it is associated with reduced rates of CHD at least in

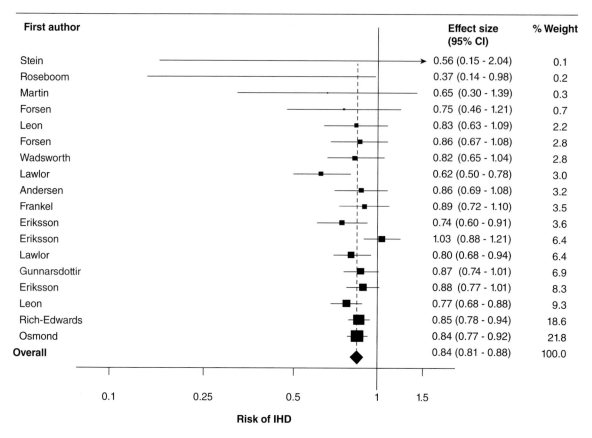

First author	Effect size (95% CI)	% Weight
Stein	0.56 (0.15 - 2.04)	0.1
Roseboom	0.37 (0.14 - 0.98)	0.2
Martin	0.65 (0.30 - 1.39)	0.3
Forsen	0.75 (0.46 - 1.21)	0.7
Leon	0.83 (0.63 - 1.09)	2.2
Forsen	0.86 (0.67 - 1.08)	2.8
Wadsworth	0.82 (0.65 - 1.04)	2.8
Lawlor	0.62 (0.50 - 0.78)	3.0
Andersen	0.86 (0.69 - 1.08)	3.2
Frankel	0.89 (0.72 - 1.10)	3.5
Eriksson	0.74 (0.60 - 0.91)	3.6
Eriksson	1.03 (0.88 - 1.21)	6.4
Lawlor	0.80 (0.68 - 0.94)	6.4
Gunnarsdottir	0.87 (0.74 - 1.01)	6.9
Eriksson	0.88 (0.77 - 1.01)	8.3
Leon	0.77 (0.68 - 0.88)	9.3
Rich-Edwards	0.85 (0.78 - 0.94)	18.6
Osmond	0.84 (0.77 - 0.92)	21.8
Overall	0.84 (0.81 - 0.88)	100.0

Risk of IHD

Figure 10.1 Relative risks and 95% confidence intervals for risk of ischaemic heart disease (IHD) associated with 1 kg higher birthweight. Reproduced from Huxley R, Owen CG, Whincup PH *et al.* (2007) Is birth weight a risk factor for ischemic heart disease in later life? *American Journal of Clinical Nutrition*, **85**, 1244–50, with permission from American Society for Nutrition.

men (Fisher *et al.* 2006). At present there is insufficient data to make any firm conclusions whether maternal obesity increases risk of cardiovascular disease in the offspring. However, the recent Jerusalem cohort study, reported that both pre-pregnancy body mass index (BMI) and gestational weight gain were independently associated with cardio-metabolic risk factors in young adult offspring, including systolic and diastolic blood pressure (Hochner *et al.* 2012).

10.3 Postnatal growth

Barker *et al.* reported that adults who had a coronary event had been, on average, small at birth and thin at 2 years of age and thereafter put on weight rapidly (Barker *et al.* 2005). A meta-analysis (Owen *et al.* 2009) relating BMI in children aged 2–19 years to later CHD risk (15 studies, 731 337 participants and

23 894 CHD events) showed a weak inverse relation between BMI in early childhood (aged 2–6 years) and later CHD risk (RR 0.94, 95% CI: 0.82–1.07). However, there was significant heterogeneity between studies. Furthermore, BMI is not a good measure of growth in children. Length or height is a better indicator of postnatal growth than BMI, especially as leg length is mainly determined by growth in the first 2 years of life. Four cohort studies (two UK, two Finnish) showed height at 1 year to be associated with a reduced rate of CHD in men but not in women (Fisher *et al.* 2006). The failure to find an effect in the women may be that a longer follow-up is required as women develop CHD some 10 years later than men. Several studies indicate that low birthweight followed by rapid postnatal weight gain ('catch-up' growth) which involves crossing growth centiles is associated with an increased risk of cardiovascular

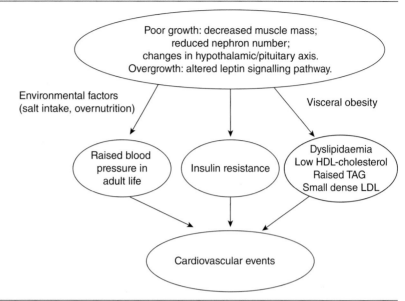

Figure 10.2 Mechanisms for programming cardiovascular disease.

HDL, high-density lipoprotein; LDL, low-densitiy lipoprotein; TAG, triacylglycerols.

disease (see Chapter 2, Section 2.10). However, what is not clear is whether the 'catch-up' is in muscle mass or fat.

Shortness in stature, which is determined by growth in early life, is consistently associated with higher blood pressure and increased risk of cardiovascular disease in later life. A meta-analysis of over 3 million people from 53 studies which compared short (<160.5 cm) with tall people (>173.9 cm) found the relative risks in the short vs. tall were 1.35 (95% CI: 1.25–1.44) for all-cause mortality, 1.55 (1.37–1.74) for cardiovascular disease mortality, 1.49 (1.33–1.67) for CHD and 1.52 (1.28–1.81) for myocardial infarction (Paajanen *et al.* 2010). Besides birthweight and nutrient intake, growth is also determined by childhood infections and other environmental stresses (e.g. poor housing) (Fig. 10.2). However, being taller as an adult is associated with a lower risk of cardiovascular disease, particularly stroke (Lee *et al.* 2009) although tall individuals may be at increased risk of cancer (see Chapter 11, Section 11.3.6).

The effect of the type of postnatal feeding on cardiovascular disease risk is less clear. A meta-analysis (Martin, Davey et al. 2004) of four studies of breastfeeding vs. formula feeding found a slightly higher cardiovascular disease death rate ratio 1.06 (95% CI: 0.94–1.20) among adults who were breast-fed. The

children in these studies (one US, three UK) were all born before 1939 when it was common practice to breastfeed to 6 months of age or longer. In contrast, the US Nurses' Health Study reported a lower risk ratio of 0.91 (95% CI: 0.83–1.01) among those who were ever breast-fed compared to those never breast-fed. The evidence published to date shows no difference in cardiovascular disease risk between ever having been breast-fed in infancy, compared to those who had not. However, more recent data are limited, most notably by the absence of prospectively gathered information on breastfeeding of a consistent type. Breast milk substitutes have changed markedly in composition over the past 50 years and nowadays are more similar in composition to breast milk, which makes past comparisons with present-day practice difficult (see Chapter 3, Section 3.8.1). Some of the earlier substitutes had higher protein content than breast milk, which may have been responsible for the accelerated growth rate observed in some studies. Nowadays in developed countries growth profiles are essentially the same in breast-fed and formula-fed infants.

10.4 Programming of atherosclerosis

Elevated total cholesterol concentration, or specifically LDL-cholesterol concentration, is well established to

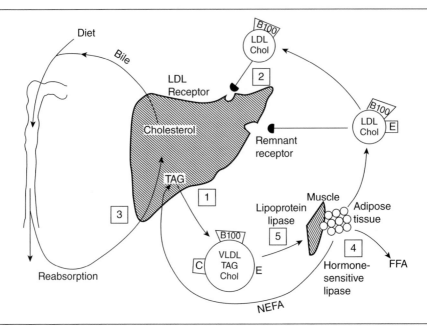

Figure 10.3 Plasma lipoprotein metabolism. (1) VLDL synthesis determined by TAG concentrations in liver which is driven by NEFA from adipose tissue and cholesterol synthesis in liver. (2) LDL receptor activity regulated by genetic and hormonal factors (cortisol, thyroid hormone, oestradiol). (3) Cholesterol reabsorption regulated by ATP cassette binding G5/8 proteins. (4) Lipolysis: stimulated by sympathetic stimulation, adrenaline, ACTH, glucagon: IL-6 inhibited by insulin, PPAE γ agonists that stimulate adiponectin. (5) Stimulated by insulin. ACTH, adrenocerticotropic hormone; ATP, adenosine triphosphate; Chol, cholesterol; FFA, free fatty acids; IL, interleukin; LDL, low density lipoprotein; NEFA, non-esterified fatty acid; PPAE γ, peroxisome proliferator-activated receptor gamma; TAG, triacylglycerols; VLDL, very low density lipoprotein.
Adapted from Sanders T and Emery P (2003) *Molecular Basis of Human Nutrition*, with permission from Taylor and Francis Ltd.

promote atherosclerosis, and a population's median cholesterol concentration is a major predictor of its risk of CHD. It is well established that LDL-cholesterol lowering therapies (by blood cholesterol-lowering drugs such as statins, plasmapheresis and diet) slow the progression of atherosclerosis and decreases the incidence of CHD. Plasma LDL-cholesterol concentrations are determined by the rate of cholesterol synthesis in the liver and the activity of the LDL receptor which is regulated by dietary, hormonal and genetic factors (Fig. 10.3). However, maternal familial hypercholesterolaemia (FH) does not programme for elevated cholesterol in the offspring that do not carry the gene for FH. More recently it has been discovered that cholesterol absorption can also be regulated by the ATP cassette binding G5/8 proteins. Insulin stimulates HMGCoA reductase (the rate-limiting enzyme in cho-

lesterol synthesis) which stimulates very low density lipoprotein (VLDL) cholesterol synthesis and secretion and lipoprotein lipase activity. Noradrenaline, adrenocorticotrophic hormone (ACTH) and glucogen downregulate receptor-mediated clearance of LDL-cholesterol, whereas oestradiol and thyroxine have the opposite effect.

Changes in the levels of these hormones can thus influence plasma LDL-cholesterol and these are potential mechanisms by which nutritional programming may influence plasma cholesterol. Plasma LDL-cholesterol levels are usually low in infancy and remain low until early adult life, after which they rise, reaching a plateau around the age of 40 in men but continuing to rise in women. LDL-cholesterol concentrations rise linearly with increasing BMI up to about 30 kg/m² (Whitlock *et al.* 2009). Cholesterol and dietary saturated fatty acids (C12–C16) have modest effects of type of fat on LDL-cholesterol (Mensink *et al.* 2003; Weggemans *et al.* 2001). There is an age-related decline in LDL receptor activity which results in increases in plasma LDL-cholesterol. This is probably due in part to the age-related decline in thyroid hormone, and oestrogen in women. Risk of cardiovascular disease is usually very low in premenopausal women, and early menopause or oophorectemy is associated with an increased risk of cardiovascular disease. It is believed that the increased risk is a consequence of the loss of the protective effect of oestradiol, which increases LDL receptor expression and thus lowers plasma LDL-cholesterol. Consequently, any early life event that influences the duration of the reproductive span in women would be predicted to reduce risk of cardiovascular disease.

There is some evidence for a secular decline in serum cholesterol concentrations (up to 0.9 mmol/L) in several countries (Rosengren *et al.* 2000; Berg *et al.* 2005; Cifkova *et al.* 2010) including the UK, which may be related to early growth and development. However, a meta-analysis reported that for each 1 kg increase in birthweight, serum cholesterol was 0.05 mmol/L lower. This is a relatively small but consistent effect which remains after adjustment for current weight (Scientific Advisory Committee on Nutrition (SACN) 2011a). A meta-analysis (Owen *et al.* 2008) concluded that total cholesterol was 0.04 mmol/L lower among adults who had ever been breast-fed infants compared with those who had not.

Several dietary intervention trials have shown that infant serum total and LDL-cholesterol can be modified by changing the fatty acid composition of breast milk or formula milk (Uauy and Dangour 2009). However, these effects are transient and do not persist into adult life. To conclude, the available evidence does not suggest any clear long-term effect of type of infant feeding on total or LDL-cholesterol.

Stronger evidence exists for a role of nutritional programming in the causation of the atherogenic lipoprotein phenotype (ALP) which is characterised by the presence of elevated plasma triacylglycerol (TAG), low HDL-cholesterol and a predominance of small dense LDL-cholesterol and is usually accompanied by visceral obesity and high plasma insulin concentrations. High-density lipoprotein (HDL) cholesterol plays a role in protecting against atherosclerosis by removing lipids from fatty streaks. The ALP is believed to result (Fig. 10.4) from

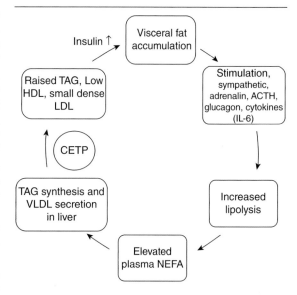

Figure 10.4 The atherogenic lipoprotein phenotype. ACTH, adrenocorticotropic hormone; CETP, cholesterol ester transfer protein; HDL, high density lipoprotein; IL, interleukin; LDL, low density lipoprotein; NEFA, non-esterified fatty acids; TAG, triacylglycerols; VLDL, very low density lipoprotein.

increased TAG synthesis in the liver, which in turn stimulates the synthesis and secretion of VLDL-cholesterol. Hepatic TAG synthesis is mainly determined by the flux of non-esterified fatty acids (NEFA) derived from adipose tissue rather than TAG synthesis from carbohydrate, which is low in humans (although VLDL secretion is enhanced on a high carbohydrate intake, presumably by the action of insulin). When plasma TAG concentrations are high (>1.7 mmol/L), VLDL donate TAG to LDL- and HDL-cholesterol in exchange for cholesteryl esters by the action of cholesterol ester transfer protein (CETP). TAG-enriched HDL-cholesterol particles and LDL-cholesterol particles, which are much smaller than VLDL-cholesterol and can pass into hepatic sinusoids, are then hydrolysed by hepatic lipase, further reducing their size. The smaller HDL-cholesterol particles are more rapidly removed from circulation by the liver, whereas the small LDL-cholesterol particles bind less well to the LDL receptor and remain in circulation for longer and have a greater capacity to promote atherosclerosis. Thus, elevated TAG carried mainly by VLDL-cholesterol promote the formation of harmful small dense LDL-cholesterol particles and reduce the concentrations of the atheroprotective HDL-cholesterol.

George Miller was among the first to recognise the association of low HDL-cholesterol and raised TAG with increased risk of CHD (Miller 1975), particularly in South Asians (Miller 1982), a finding now confirmed in many other studies. The ALP is one of the features of metabolic syndrome, a term coined by Reaven (1988) to describe the constellation of metabolic abnormalities that were associated with increased risk of cardiovascular disease (Reaven 1988). These were central obesity, insulin resistance or glucose intolerance, raised blood pressure, low HDL-cholesterol and high TAG, gout and microalbuminuria (an indicator of microvascular disease and renal dysfunction). Later research showed the metabolic syndrome to be linked to increased procoagulant activity, measured as raised fibrinogen and factor VII coagulant activity, and decreased fibrinolytic activity and impaired endothelial function. These factors cause a hypercoagulable state and a reduced capacity to break down blood clots and are associated with increased risk of coronary events.

In the landmark Hertfordshire cohort, survivors were recruited in the late 1980s (Barker, Hales *et al.* 1993; Barker *et al.* 1992; Barker, Winter *et al.* 1989) for measurements of surrogate risk markers for cardiovascular disease – blood pressure, lipid profile, fasting plasma glucose, presence of metabolic syndrome, fibrinogen, factor VII coagulant activity (Barker *et al.* 1992). The prevalence of metabolic syndrome fell from 30% in those who had weighed 2.5 kg (5.5 lb) or less to 6% in those who weighed 4 kg (9 lb) or more at birth. After adjustment for current BMI, the risk for metabolic syndrome was 18-fold greater in the lowest compared to the highest birthweight group in 50-year-old men and women. These infants also showed evidence of increased plasma fibrinogen and factor VII coagulant activity which had been shown to be a strong predictor of fatal CHD in the Northwick Park Heart Study (Meade *et al.* 1993).

The International Diabetes Federation (www. IDF.org) definition of metabolic syndrome (waist circumference greater than ethnic-specific cut-off plus at least two of the following: raised TAG, low HDL-cholesterol, raised blood pressure >130/85 mmHg or fasting glucose >5.6 mmol/L) is a pragmatic tool for identifying individuals from among the general population rather than defining the mechanisms that cause it. The development of metabolic syndrome is strongly associated with vis-

ceral adiposity as opposed to gluteal adiposity and low levels of physical activity. Rapid weight gain during the first 3 months of life has been reported to result in more central adiposity and unfavourable effects of total cholesterol:HDL-cholesterol and plasma TAG (Leunissen *et al.* 2009).

ALP and the metabolic syndrome can be corrected by loss of body fat by dieting combined with increased physical activity (Siri-Tarino *et al.* 2009) or by some types of bariatric surgery (e.g. Roux-en-Y gastric bypass) but is not corrected by insulin therapy or surgical removal of adipose tissue. Why visceral adiposity causes ALP is uncertain but it is likely to be a consequence of increased rates of lipolysis which elevate release of NEFA, and in turn, stimulate VLDL-TAG secretion. High NEFA concentrations acutely cause insulin resistance and increase the release of inflammatory cytokines. However, adipose tissue can also produce cytokines such as interleukin (IL)-6 that stimulate lipolysis as well as adipokines such as adiponectin, which besides influencing glucose homeostasis also suppresses adipose tissue lipolysis. An increased release of stress hormones or sympathetic stimulation of adipose tissue would also increase lipolysis by activating hormone-sensitive lipase in adipose tissue. ALP appears to occur when fat is stored in visceral fat depots or in the liver rather than in subcutaneous adipose tissue stores.

The rapid resolution of ALP following the Roux-en-Y procedure, which occurs before significant weight loss in morbidly obese patients (Scott 2011), is of particular interest as it suggests mechanisms involving the signalling by gut peptides such as CCK, GIP, PPY and ghrelin between the endocrine pancreas, adipose tissue and the hypothalamus (Beckman *et al.* 2010). These gut peptide hormones, along with adipokines such as adiponectin and leptin, appear to play an important role in modulating risk in lipid metabolism, insulin sensitivity and vascular function. It is possible that early development determines this capacity.

The prevalence of metabolic syndrome is three to four times greater in the South Asian ethnic minority population than in the White population in the UK, and low birthweight is more prevalent in South Asian pregnancies (Leon and Moser 2010) as is visceral adiposity and type 2 diabetes in South Asian adults. There is some evidence that the lipid changes may precede evidence of insulin resistance/impaired glucose tolerance in South Asians and these are accompanied by lower adiponectin concentrations

(Bansal *et al.* 2011). South Asians were found to have lower plasma adiponectin concentrations compared to White subjects that increase less with age (AlSaleh *et al.* 2011). The evidence to date thus suggests that low birthweight and poor growth predisposes to developing ALP, particularly when excess amounts of body fat accumulate.

Boney and colleagues in their studies of Pima Indians demonstrated how maternal obesity, especially when it resulted in gestational diabetes, increased the risk of metabolic syndrome and type 2 diabetes developing in the offspring (Boney *et al.* 2005). While these associations between maternal obesity and childhood health may be due to shared genetic obesogenic traits which influence body weight and blood pressure, converging lines of evidence suggest that susceptibility to obesity and cardiovascular disease is partly programmed in the developing fetus *in utero* or in the neonate through exposure to adverse metabolic factors during critical periods of development in early life (see Chapter 8).

10.5 Programming of blood pressure

High blood pressure is the leading risk factor for cardiovascular disease, especially stroke, particularly over the age of 50 years. The age-related increase in blood pressure is the consequence of a self-amplifying process whereby the resistance arteries become more muscular with a greater capacity to constrict as blood pressure rises. Hypertension is defined as systolic/diastolic blood pressure greater than 140/90 mmHg. However, the relationship between blood pressure and cardiovascular disease risk is not confined to hypertension, and the relationship is seen within the range of normal pressure (Lewington *et al.* 2002). Several lifestyle factors in adult life have been linked to elevated blood pressure including stress, lack of physical activity, high alcohol intake, high salt intake, obesity and low dairy, fruit and vegetable intake. However, these only explain a small fraction of the variation in blood pressure between individuals. For example, the INTERSALT study (Dyer *et al.* 1996; Elliott *et al.* 1996) concluded that an increase in sodium intake of 100 mmol/day was associated with an increase in systolic/diastolic blood pressure of 3–6/0–3 mmHg. Much attention has been focused on developmental influences on blood pressure.

There is strong and consistent evidence to show that adult height is inversely related to blood pressure and that low birthweight is associated with higher blood pressure (SACN 2011a). Secular falls in blood pressure have occurred in the UK and many other economically developed countries (Tunstall-Pedoe *et al.* 2006) which remain unexplained.

Barker *et al.* in the follow-up of birth and growth records of children born in Hertfordshire showed a strong relationship between low birthweight and low weight gain in the first year of life and adult blood pressure. Systolic blood pressure declined from 173 mmHg in the lowest birthweight group to 161 mmHg in the highest birthweight group at age 66 years and over. They went on to show that infants who have low birthweight and a low BMI at the age of 2 but who subsequently gain weight and had a high BMI at age 11 were more prone to develop hypertension (Barker *et al.* 2005). A subsequent longitudinal study of children who had been small at birth but who gained weight rapidly during early childhood (1 to 5 years) had the highest adult blood pressure at age 22 years. The Scientific Advisory Committee on Nutrition concluded that breastfeeding was associated with a 1.1 mmHg lower systolic blood pressure in later life (SACN 2011a). However, there was significant heterogeneity between studies.

The Huxley *et al.* meta-analyses conclude that each 1 kg increment in birthweight is associated with a reduction in systolic blood pressure of under 2 mmHg in later life (Huxley *et al.* 2000; Huxley *et al.* 2002). However, the US Collaborative Perinatal Project (1959–74) studied 55 908 pregnancies came to a slightly different conclusion and showed that each 1 kg increase in birthweight increased the odds by 2.19 for raised systolic blood pressure at 7 years of age (Hemachandra *et al.* 2007). Infants who were small for gestational age were not at increased risk for high blood pressure at 7 years of age but those who crossed weight percentiles upward during early childhood showed increased risk. One of the problems in interpreting this data is that there have been large improvements in pregnancy outcomes and postnatal health in most developed countries and that over-nutrition in pregnancy is becoming more common than under-nutrition.

Maternal obesity may heighten risk of elevated blood pressure and cardiovascular disease in childhood and beyond (Forsen *et al.* 1997; Lawlor *et al.* 2004; Boney *et al.* 2005; Mamun *et al.* 2009). Several studies in mother–child cohorts have reported an association between maternal BMI or gestational weight gain and childhood blood pressure (Boney *et al.* 2005; Oken, Rifas-Shiman *et al.* 2008; Mamun *et al.* 2009; Wen *et al.* 2011). Obesity in childhood tracks to adolescence and heightens the risk of early metabolic and cardiovascular diseases (Reilly and Rader 2003) including obesity-related hypertension (Rahmouni *et al.* 2005; Mamun *et al.* 2009). However, maternal obesity may have a direct effect on the developing fetal or neonatal cardiovascular system independent of offspring obesity. In a recent study, maternal pre-pregnancy obesity or overweight was shown to be significantly associated with increased systolic blood pressure in offspring at 7 years of age (Wen *et al.* 2011).

The Avon Longitudinal Study of Parents and Children is a current UK birth cohort study investigating early development on health outcome and has investigated the relationship between maternal hypertension in pregnancy and vascular health in the offspring. Maternal–offspring pairs (n = 3537–4654) were assessed at age 9–12 years. They found a higher systolic/diastolic blood pressure in the offspring at age 9 years of 2.0/1.1 mmHg (Lawlor *et al.* 2012), adjusting for BMI, salt intake and other factors known to influence blood pressure. However Lawlor *et al.* were unable to find an association between maternal hypertension in pregnancy and plasma lipid concentrations or endothelial function in the offspring.

Barker *et al.* suggest that the number of nephrons may be programmed by poor growth in infancy. Supporting this is a meta-analysis of prospective cohort studies showing that low birthweight is associated with risk of chronic kidney disease, a disease that makes a major contribution to cardiovascular disease mortality and is associated with hypertension (White *et al.* 2009). There is also evidence to suggest that low birthweight results in increased sensitivity to salt intake (de Boer *et al.* 2008; Perala *et al.* 2011). There is an intriguing possibility that the higher incidence of hypertension in people of Black African origin may be a consequence of poor fetal growth and later exposure to a high salt intake. It has been suggested that long-chain polyunsaturated fatty acids may programme for lower blood pressure in later life (Forsyth *et al.* 2003). However, another larger study reported higher blood pressure at 10 years among those who had received long-chain *n*-3 polyunsaturated fatty acids in infant formula; this difference became non-significant when changes in body weight were considered (Kennedy *et al.* 2010). In contrast to communities where maternal pregnancy outcomes are poor and

perinatal mortality is high, it would appear that in well-nourished communities the influence of differences in early diet on blood pressure are probably small.

10.6 Animal models of nutritional manipulation in early life

Various animal models have been developed to manipulate the nutritional and hormonal environment in pregnancy, ostensibly in an attempt to mimic the conditions described in the early epidemiological studies that give rise to the developmental programming of cardiovascular risk. Animal studies have several advantages over the human observational studies, which by their nature are largely associative and therefore cannot establish cause and effect. Modelling gestational environments in animals, especially rodents, can avoid many of the underlying residual confounding that can 'plague' epidemiological studies, in that genetic and social influences can be removed, experimental conditions can be tightly controlled and the underlying physiological, cellular and molecular mechanisms can be fully explored at the various 'critical windows' of development. Moreover, the relatively short life cycles, especially in rodents, means the long-term effects of early life insults can be studied in a meaningful time frame. However, the limitation of animal studies is that they do not truly mimic human cardiovascular disease and there are fundamental differences between rodents and humans in lipid metabolism in that they do not produce low-density lipoprotein containing apolipoprotein B100 and there are major differences in the cholesterol ester transfer protein activity between species. Most of the research in this area has been concerned with hypertension.

As this field has developed over the last 20 years, most animal models were designed to test the hypotheses generated by the human famine studies and the early associations described by Barker and colleagues between low birthweight or disproportionate size at birth and adult cardiovascular disease. As such there is an extensive experimental literature on protein restriction in rodents (Galler and Tonkiss 1991; Langley and Jackson 1994; Holemans *et al.* 1999; Vickers *et al.* 2001; Woods *et al.* 2001; Ozanne *et al.* 2003), although not all achieved lower birthweight (Galler and Tonkiss 1991; Langley and Jackson

1994; Langley-Evans and Jackson 1996; Holemans *et al.* 1999; Vickers *et al.* 2001; Woods *et al.* 2001). Global dietary restriction in pregnancy has also been studied extensively in both rodents (Woodall *et al.* 1996; Holemans *et al.* 1999; Ozaki *et al.* 2001; Franco *et al.* 2002; Franco *et al.* 2003) and sheep (Hawkins *et al.* 1999; Hawkins *et al.* 2000; Ozaki *et al.* 2000; Edwards and McMillen 2001). In addition there are also some surgical models involving uterine artery ligation (Brown and Vannucci 1978; Houdijk *et al.* 2000; Sanders *et al.* 2004a; Sanders *et al.* 2004b); or carunclectomy (Jones *et al.* 1988; Rees *et al.* 1998; Butler *et al.* 2002) which result in fetal growth retardation through both nutrient restriction and hypoxia in the fetus. These surgical models of placental insufficiency are relevant to human pregnancy, particularly in developed countries where the majority of fetal growth restriction is attributed to placental disease. There are also animal models of stress in pregnancy, which share a remarkable similarity in offspring phenotype with some of the nutrition models and might suggest commonality in underlying mechanisms. Exogenous treatment with synthetic glucocorticoids which cross the placental barrier (Benediktsson *et al.* 1993; Dodic *et al.* 1998; Liu *et al.* 2001; O'Regan *et al.* 2008), together with various maternal stress paradigms (Weinstock 2001; Igosheva *et al.* 2007), have been employed as a model of stress in pregnancy and give rise to the programming of altered stress reactivity and blood pressure dysregulation through the hypothalamic–pituitary–adrenal (HPA) axis. Finally, there are the animal models of micronutrient restriction, such as the iron-deficient rodent model which also produces permanent changes to cardiovascular function (Lewis, Petry *et al.* 2001). The potential mechanisms resulting from under-nutrition are shown in Fig. 10.5.

10.6.1 Mechanisms of hypertension in animal models of under-nutrition

Animal models of nutritional restriction *in utero*, together with surgical models of placental insufficiency (Sanders *et al.* 2004b), were the first to demonstrate programmed hypertension associated with marked structural and physiological alterations

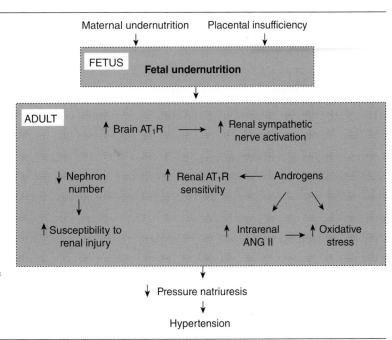

Figure 10.5 Proposed mechanisms for the development of hypertension in response to maternal under-nutrition and placental insufficiency in animal models.

ANG II, angiotensin II.

Angiotensin II receptor type 1 (AT$_1$R) has vasopressor effects and regulates aldosterone secretion controlling blood pressure and volume.

(Langley-Evans *et al.* 1994) and also highlighted the importance of critical periods in susceptibility to an environmental insult e.g. nutritional restriction during the nephrogenic period produces defecits in nephron number (Langley-Evans, Welham *et al.* 1999; Symonds *et al.* 2007). In humans, nephron number is directly correlated with birthweight and inversely correlated with blood pressure. Hence these animal models have provided mechanistic insight into the effects of low birthweight.

In addition to nutritional insult the hormonal environment in pregnancy can be critical and, in experimental studies, inappropriate exposure to testosterone during gestation results in intrauterine growth restriction (IUGR), impaired insulin sensitivity and cardiovascular dysfunction, demonstrating a critical role for sex hormones in the developmental programming of adult cardiovascular disease (Manikkam *et al.* 2004; Crespi *et al.* 2006; King *et al.* 2007) (see Chapter 5, Section 5.9).

The renin–angiotensin system (RAS) is a major candidate mechanism and maternal under-nutrition in the rat is associated with marked increases in angiotensin (Ang) type I receptor (AT_1R) expression in cardiovascular regulatory centres in the brain, upregulation of the renal AT_1R and activation of the peripheral RAS (Hall *et al.* 1999; Pladys *et al.* 2004; Grigore *et al.* 2007). The associated hypertension is reversed by blockade of the RAS (Ceravolo *et al.* 2007).

Blood pressure regulation is highly sensitive to changes in sympathetic activity and plasma catecholamine concentrations, an index of sympathetic outflow, are increased in response to fetal under-nutrition (Petry *et al.* 2000). In a rat model of IUGR, renal denervation reversed the programmed hypertension observed in adult male offspring (Alexander *et al.* 2005) which can occur as a consequence of Ang II-mediated central activation of the RAS (Dampney *et al.* 2005).

Oxidative stress may play a causative role in hypertension. Elevated blood pressure in a model of *in utero* under-nutrition is normalised by superoxide dismutase treatment (Stewart *et al.* 2005), implicating a potential redox imbalance, or antioxidant deficit, underlying the programmed hypertension observed.

Animal models highlight the mechanisms whereby nutritional insults during critical periods in development lead to suboptimal development of the normal regulatory systems involved in the long-term control of blood pressure regulation, including primary defects in the kidney or extrinsic regulatory pathways involved in sodium homeostasis (Ojeda *et al.* 2008).

10.6.2 Cardiovascular dysfunction in animal models of over-nutrition

Fewer studies have examined the effects of over-nutrition on blood pressure and the majority of work in this field has been performed in rodents (for a review see Armitage *et al.* 2005). In general, maternal over-nutrition has been found to result in increased systolic blood pressure (SBP) in the offspring (Khan *et al.* 2003; Khan *et al.* 2004; Khan *et al.* 2005; Samuelsson *et al.* 2008; Samuelsson *et al.* 2010). Maternal obesity has been induced by preconditioning rodents prior to pregnancy through the introduction of a semi-synthetic, high-fat diet in which carbohydrates are replaced by dietary fat sources such as lard. In some instances simple sugars have been added to the high-fat diet to further increase palatability and food intake, or a 'cafeteria-style' diet is employed in which highly palatable foods typical of a Western diet provide highly palatable high-fat and high-sugar intake in rodents (Bayol *et al.* 2005; Akyol *et al.* 2009). The addition of highly palatable sugars to a high-fat diet, or introduction of a cafeteria diet, appears to overcome the tight homeostatic control of calorific intake seen in rodents to effect a more rapid shift towards a more positive energy balance. Diet-induced obesity in rodent dams, similar to obese human pregnancy, appears to be associated with a degree of gestational diabetes in that maternal over-nutrition models are associated with maternal hyperinsulinaemia and glucose intolerance in pregnancy and/or lactation (Taylor *et al.* 2003; Holemans *et al.* 2004; Srinivasan *et al.* 2006; Chen *et al.* 2008; Samuelsson *et al.* 2008; Nivoit *et al.* 2009).

Adult offspring of diet-induced obese mice develop systolic and mean arterial hypertension by 3 months of age associated with resistance artery endothelial dysfunction (Samuelsson *et al.* 2008). Hypertension was also associated with increased visceral adiposity and hyperleptinaemia which might suggest obesity-related hypertension in this model. Leptin-mediated hypertension acts through central sympathetic pathways (for review see Rahmouni *et al.* 2005). However, in the rat, a larger species in which it is technically possible to measure blood pressure in younger animals, blood pressure was already elevated in juvenile offspring of obese dams prior to the development of offspring obesity and continued to increase into adulthood. Juvenile offspring of the obese dams also showed an enhanced pressor response to restraint stress, and spectral analysis of the heart rate variability derived from the blood pressure telemetry record revealed an increased ratio of low frequency to high frequency oscillations at 30 and 90 days of age, indicative of an increased sympathetic component in the autonomic regulation of blood pressure. There was also evidence of altered baroreceptor sensitivity and, taken together, these observations suggest the developmental programming of a primary hypertension of sympathetic origin in the offspring of obese dams.

Maternal obesity in rodents is associated with a marked hyperleptinaemia in the neonate during a critical period in brain development when leptin is thought to play a permissive neurotrophic role in establishing the neural circuitry of the hypothalamus, involved in both appetite and blood pressure control (Bouret *et al.* 2004). The elevation in blood pressure in early life in offspring of obese rodents may arise from perturbation of central leptin sensitivity, and dysregulation of the normal neurotrophic action of leptin. Young offspring of obese rats show behavioural and cell signalling deficits in leptin sensitivity with evidence of altered neuronal development in the hypothalamus (Kirk *et al.* 2009). Offspring of obese rats demonstrated an enhanced pressor response to leptin compared to controls of the same age (Samuelsson *et al.* 2010). Hence, increased blood pressure in juvenile offspring of obese dams may arise through a pathological leptin exposure in neonatal life and the effective 'hardwiring' of the neonatal brain towards increased central efferent sympathetic tone. The apparent paradox of 'selective leptin resistance', in which offspring were less responsive to leptin-induced appetite suppression, is similar to that observed in adult obese rodents and explicable on the basis that the cardiovascular and appetite regulatory actions of leptin may occur in regionally distinct hypothalamic neurons with differing ontogeny.

10.6.3 Developmental programming of cardiac function

The neonatal leptin surge, which appears during the early suckling period in rodents (Ahima *et al.* 1998), coincides with the critical periods for both hypothalamic (Grove *et al.* 2005) and cardiac plasticity (Anat-

skaya *et al.* 2010). Several animal studies have implied that perturbations of the nutritional or metabolic environment can influence myocardial development and function in later life (Roigas *et al.* 1996; Bae *et al.* 2003; Davis *et al.* 2003; Li *et al.* 2003b; Han *et al.* 2004; Almeida and Mandarim-de-Lacerda 2005; Battista *et al.* 2005; Cheema *et al.* 2005; Catta-Preta *et al.* 2006; Fernandez-Twinn *et al.* 2006; Xu *et al.* 2006; Elmes *et al.* 2007; Elmes *et al.* 2008; Chan *et al.* 2009; Porrello *et al.* 2009; Tappia *et al.* 2009; Xue and Zhang 2009). Experimental placental mass reduction, fetal hypertension and cortisol exposure all affect proliferation and terminal maturation of the neonatal cardiac myocytes (Giraud *et al.* 2006; Jonker *et al.* 2007; Louey *et al.* 2007). Since the number of myocytes in all species is determined *in utero* and in early postnatal life (Anatskaya *et al.* 2010), perinatal 'programming' has been proposed to be a determinant of cardiac dysfunction in adult life (Thornburg and Louey 2005; Porrello *et al.* 2009). Most of the relevant literature focuses on under-nutritional states and associated fetal growth restriction, but a recent study in obese pregnant sheep has reported markedly altered structure and function in fetal hearts in late gestation; phosphorylation of AMP-activated protein kinase, a cardioprotective signalling pathway, was reduced while the stress signalling pathway, p38 MAPK, was upregulated (Wang *et al.* 2010). In addition, fetal hearts from obese dams showed impaired cardiac insulin signalling which, if persistent into adult life, would predispose offspring to insulin resistance and cardiac dysfunction (Wang *et al.* 2010).

Cardiac development can also be compromised by increased fibrogenesis, and maternal obesity also induces fibrosis in fetal myocardium of sheep (Huang *et al.* 2010). However, to date, there has been little investigation of cardiovascular function in adult offspring of obese sheep or non-human primates. Adulthood ventricular hypertrophy has been described in adult rodents fed a high-fat diet in postnatal life (Parente *et al.* 2008), and normal (non-mutant) offspring from obese agouti mouse dams have increased susceptibility to ischaemia-reperfusion injury (Calvert *et al.* 2009).

The studies of cardiovascular function in animal models of maternal obesity have been largely confined to rodents, except for one study in the fetuses of obese ewes. Similar studies in non-human primates would be valuable in determining whether these observations were pertinent across species. Nonetheless, these reports have provided sufficient interest to prompt investigation of blood pressure and blood pressure variability in the children of obese mothers in several ongoing mother–child cohort studies.

10.7 Conclusions

Poor growth *in utero* and infancy increases risk of cardiovascular disease in adult life. Poor growth, especially if followed by unhealthy weight gain in adult life, increases risk of developing the metabolic syndrome. Low birthweight is associated with higher blood pressure in adult life and shortness in stature, which is an integrated measure of childhood growth. The incidence of cardiovascular disease has fallen over the past 30 years by as much as 20–30% in many economically developed countries including the UK. Besides a fall in smoking prevalence, the reasons for this decline remain uncertain but it is unlikely to be related to better management of hypertension or hyperlipidaemia. Increased affluence and better living conditions are likely to have been important reasons, perhaps also the widespread use of antibiotics and reduced exposure to chronic inflammation. With the global obesity epidemic, maternal obesity will increase the prevalence of macrosomia which may programme for adverse cardiovascular risk in the offspring, particularly if they become overweight in adult life.

10.8 Key points

- Poor fetal growth, especially followed by rapid postnatal growth or obesity, increases the risk of cardiovascular disease in adulthood.
- The offspring of mothers with raised blood pressure in pregnancy have increased blood pressure.
- Various animal models can replicate the effects of impaired fetal growth on the development of high blood pressure. Maternal obesity can also result in higher blood pressure in the offspring.
- The mechanism for the increase in blood pressure is uncertain but may be mediated by programming of sympathetic outflow from the central nervous system or impaired renal development, making the kidney more sensitive to salt overload.
- The risk of developing the atherogenic lipoprotein phenotype (low HDL-cholesterol, raised fasting triacylglycerol) is greater in infants with low birthweight or those who show rapid postnatal weight gain who become overweight or obese in adult life.

10.9 Recommendations for future research

- Further research is needed to ascertain whether the higher risk of stroke in people of African or Caribbean descent and coronary heart disease in South Asian people is a consequence of early life environment and whether improved pre- and postnatal growth will eradicate the differences.
- Further research is needed to understand whether there are critical windows in the differentiation of adipocytes that determine their capacity to produce adipokines.
- Further research is needed to ascertain whether high birthweight associated with maternal obesity increases risk of cardiovascular disease, using disease outcome indicators rather than surrogate risk markers.
- Several lifestyle factors, such as salt intake, have been linked to elevated blood pressure in adult life. Research has mainly focused on developmental influences on blood pressure. However, further research on whether the blood pressure raising effect of salt in adult life is determined by poor growth *in utero* would be useful.

10.10 Key references

Barker DJ, Osmond C, Forsen TJ *et al.* (2005) Trajectories of growth among children who have coronary events as adults. *New England Journal of Medicine*, **353**, 1802–9.

Ojeda NB, Grigore D & Alexander BT (2008) Developmental programming of hypertension: insight from animal models of nutritional manipulation. *Hypertension*, **52**, 44–50.

Paajanen TA, Oksala NK, Kuukasjärvi P *et al.* (2010) Short stature is associated with coronary heart disease: a systematic review of the literature and a meta-analysis. *European Heart Journal*, **31**, 1802–9.

Rinaudo P & Wang E (2012) Fetal programming and metabolic syndrome. *Annual Review of Physiology*, **74**, 107–30.

Scientific Advisory Committee on Nutrition (2011a) *The Influence of Maternal, Fetal and Child Nutrition on the Development of Chronic Disease in Later Life*. London, The Stationery Office.

11
Nutrition and Development: Cancer

11.1 Cancer incidence and trends

Cancer is a major cause of disease and mortality worldwide. Almost 11 million people are diagnosed annually with some form of cancer. There are 25 million people alive in the world who have been diagnosed with cancer within the last 5 years and the World Cancer Research Fund estimate that this will double by the year 2030 (World Cancer Research Fund/American Institute for Cancer Research 2007).

Breast cancer is the commonest cancer in women worldwide, and makes up approximately 23% of all cancers in females (lifetime risk is 1 in 8). Overall, it is the second most common cancer after lung cancer in men and women. Worldwide, almost 1 million women are diagnosed annually with breast cancer, including 45 000 in the UK (Bray *et al.* 2004; Cancer Research UK 2010a). Although it is the commonest female cancer in both developing and developed countries, there are wide differences in incidence with rates being at least three times higher in developed countries (Ferlay *et al.* 2004). The highest incidence is in North America and the lowest in Asia and Africa. There has been a marked rise in the incidence of breast cancer over the last 10 years. In European countries the incidence has been increasing by up to 2% per annum. This trend cannot be explained solely by the implementation of national breast screening programmes in some countries. Greater increases have been reported in other regions of the world without screening programmes; e.g. up to 4% per annum in Asia (Zaridze and Basieva 1990).

Prostate cancer is the second most common cancer worldwide; in developed countries it has become the commonest cancer in men, accounting for almost 20% of all malignancies (Ferlay, Bray *et al.* 2004). The incidence has been rising dramatically in more developed countries in parallel with the increasing use of PSA (prostate specific antigen) testing; no national screening programme currently exists in the UK. However, the incidence was rising prior to the increasing use of PSA tests in both developed and developing countries (Baade *et al.* 2009). Testicular cancer is a relatively rare cancer, responsible for just over 1% of all male cancers. However, it is the most common cancer in men aged 15–44 years, with incidence rates highest at around 17 or 18 per 100 000 in men aged 25–34 years (Cancer Research UK 2012). The incidence of testicular cancer is rising, particularly among White Caucasians throughout the world, for reasons as yet unknown (Cancer Research UK 2012).

Carcinoma of the bowel (colon and rectum) is the third commonest cancer worldwide with more than 1 million newly diagnosed patients per year (GLOBO-CAN 2002). In the UK, there are more than 37 500 new cases each year with approximately two-thirds occurring in the colon and the remainder in the rectum (Cancer Research UK 2010b). There are differences in incidence depending on geographical region and marked differences between different European countries. Overall, the incidence of colorectal cancer is increasing although in the US there has been a significant decrease over the last 20 years (Surveillance Epidemiology and End Results (SEER)

Nutrition and Development: Short- and Long-Term Consequences for Health, First Edition. Edited by the British Nutrition Foundation.
© 2013 the British Nutrition Foundation. Published 2013 by Blackwell Publishing Ltd.

Howlader *et al.* 2012). During the same period in the UK the increase in incidence has levelled off and there has been a slight reduction. In contrast to this, in some countries in Asia – e.g. Japan, where the incidence had been relatively low previously – there has been a substantial increase more recently (Koyama and Kotake 1997).

The incidence of stomach cancer shows a markedly differing pattern across the world. While it is the fourth commonest cancer in the world, in the UK it is the 7th commonest in men and the 14th commonest in women (Cancer Research UK 2010c). Geographically, stomach cancer is most common in eastern Asia, especially Japan, Korea and China, with the lowest rates being recorded in Africa. In Japan, gastric cancer is the most common of all cancer types. More than 880 000 people are diagnosed and 650 000 die annually from gastric cancer (Stewart and Kleihues 2003). In the UK, the incidence is lower than the average across Europe and, interestingly, there has been a 50% reduction over the last 30 years in the UK. The general reduction in mesodermal stomach cancer in developed countries is in marked contrast to the rising incidence in non-developed countries (Crew and Neugut 2006).

Oesphageal cancer is the sixth commonest cancer worldwide (almost twice as common in men) with almost half a million newly diagnosed patients each year and almost 400 000 people dying from oesphageal cancer annually (Kollarova *et al.* 2007). The two histological types of oesophageal cancer are squamous and adenocarcinoma and, although the former is more common (approximately 80%), there has been a large increase in the number of patients with adeno-carcinonomas recently (30–50% of such patients have adenocarcinomas in the West, more commonly in males (Vizcaino *et al.* 2002). There is a very marked geographical variation in distribution of this cancer with the highest incidences occurring in China, Ethiopia and Iran. Oesophageal cancer overall is more common in less well-developed countries than in developed ones (Kamangar *et al.* 2006). In addition, there are marked differences within some countries depending on factors such as race, ethnicity and deprivation (Vizcaino *et al.* 2002). For example, in the US, there is a six-fold variation in the incidence of squamous oesophageal cancer depending on ethnic background. There is also significant variation within Europe, with France having the highest incidence, followed by Hungary and the UK. However, in the UK, the incidence has been rising over the last 30 years (Cancer Research UK 2010d).

Cancer in children is relatively uncommon, with approximately 1500 newly diagnosed children per year in the UK, and it is slightly more common in boys than girls. Leukaemia is the most common type (mainly acute lymphoblastic) followed by brain and spinal tumours (astrocytomas, neuroectodermal, ependymoma), with a variety of tumour types accounting for the remainder (e.g. embryonal tumours, Ewing's sarcoma, bone and soft tissue sarcomas, germ cell and gonadal tumours) (Cancer Research UK 2010e). Overall, there has been an increase in incidence of childhood cancers of almost 1% per annum in the UK between 1962 and 1998 – with different rates of increase for different tumour types (Cancer Research UK 2010e).

11.2 Cancer biology

Cancer is a general term describing a malignant tumour. Cancers can be broadly classified into solid tumours (those arising from epithelial cells are termed 'carcinomas' and those from mesenchymal cells are 'sarcomas') and tumours arising from the lymphoreticular system (leukaemias and lymphomas). Solid cancers account for approximately 80% of all tumours. Cancers may be sub-classified according to the embryonal layer from which they originated, the organ where they developed and the variation in the way they display the architectural pattern of that tissue. However, in some cancers it may not be possible to determine the cell and tissue type of origin, due to factors such as poor differentiation of tissues, loss of architectural pattern, and loss of expression of specific tumour markers. These malignancies are termed 'anaplastic' tumours (Underwood and Cross 2009).

Cancers which remain localised by the basement membrane on which the tumour cells lie are termed 'carcinoma in situ'. However, once the cells invade through the basement membrane and into the surrounding tissues, there is then the potential for invasion of blood vessels, lymphatic vessels and perineural spaces. This gives the potential for secondary tumour deposits to arise in lymph nodes and also metastatic dissemination throughout the body. Common sites of metastatic dissemination include the liver, lungs and bone but this is dependent on tumour type, and sites anywhere in the body may be affected.

There is a growing appreciation of the importance of tumour heterogeneity in understanding the aetiology of cancer, its malignant potential and the development of effective treatments. Heterogeneity of tumour cells within the same cancer is also increasingly recognised as critical to the biology of tumour growth. Within tumours, sub-populations of cells exist which have a differing range of sensitivities to radiotherapy, chemotherapy and hormone therapy (Frank *et al.* 2010).

Recently, interest has focused on the heterogeneity of cancers with respect to the existence of putative 'cancer stem cells' which may explain some of these differences (Jones 2009). It has been suggested that cancer stem cells comprise a small number of cells which have the ability to initiate a cancer and then produce further cancer stem cells together with the malignant cells forming the greater part of the tumour. These cell types have been observed in some haematological maligancies and are characterised by the expression of specific cell surface makers (ten Cate *et al.* 2010). Potential cancer stem cells have also been described in common solid cancers (Sergeant *et al.* 2009; Luo *et al.* 2010). If the stem cell concept is correct, then this cell type should be the focus of treatment and it may explain why some tumours fail to respond to treatment or appear to respond initially only to recur subsequently.

The tumour comprises not just malignant cells but also the stroma, which includes a wide variety of different cell types including fibrous tissue, blood vessels and a lymphoreticular infiltrate including, to a variable degree, macrophages and monocytes. This microenvironment is very different from the surrounding normal tissue and is itself extremely heterogeneous. For example, there are areas of impaired vascularity which may result in hypoxia and lack of nutrient supply at the cellular level (in particular glucose), and the tissue pH may be acidic (Vaupel *et al.* 2001). These differences are important in determining how tumour cells behave. For example, under hypoxic conditions tumour cells increase in heterogeneity in a way which may increase their potential to metastasise and establish secondary tumour deposits (Heddleston *et al.* 2010).

Cancer is often described as a disease of genes, and common characteristics of cancer cells include chromosomal abnormalities, higher frequency of mutation and loss of heterozygosity. Cancer cells are also characterised by widespread epigenetic changes which include global hypomethylation coincident with hypermethylation within individual genes (e.g. tumour suppressor genes) and loss of imprinting (see Section 11.4.2.1).

11.3 Evidence linking early nutrition to cancer

There is a large body of literature, based on animal studies, which has established that early nutritional exposures can influence subsequent biology and physiology throughout life. Furthermore, these changes can be demonstrated to influence animal health in a way which appears to correspond to the aetiology of human diseases. Some of the animal data is considered here in relation to mechanisms, but the aim of this chapter is primarily to assess the evidence in humans.

The strongest evidence in humans comes from randomised controlled trials but, for obvious ethical and practical reasons, there have been very few nutritional interventions in early life specifically designed to influence later cancer risk in the offspring. Randomised controlled trials of infant feeding have been carried out but mainly in the premature infant and the numbers involved have been too small to make follow-up of cancer risk meaningful. Opportunistic analysis of adult cancer risk in the offspring of mothers exposed to famine during pregnancy (see Chapter 1, Section 1.4.1; and Chapter 4, Section 4.4.2) has also been carried out but such an intervention is very severe and its relevance to the biology of cancer in generally well-nourished individuals is not clear. Most studies in this field have been observational, relating later cancer risk to inferred nutritional exposure in early life. Most of this evidence is doubly indirect in that it involves the association of birth anthropometry and childhood growth – assumed to reflect nutritional exposure in early life – with subsequent cancer risk.

11.3.1 Interventions

Results of a randomised controlled trial in Australia suggested that folic acid and iron supplementation may reduce the incidence of acute lymphocytic leukaemia in children (Thompson, Gerald *et al.* 2001). However, subsequent studies, and meta-analyses of these, have been less convincing. These have been unable to detect a protective effect of folate in relation to acute lymphocytic leukaemia (Dockerty *et al.*

2007), while further analysis concluded that any effect 'if real' is likely to be very small (Milne *et al.* 2010).

11.3.2 Breast versus bottle feeding

Lactation is known to decrease the risk of both pre- and postmenopausal breast cancer in the mother (World Cancer Research Fund/American Institute for Cancer Research 2007) but this chapter is concerned with the effect on the offspring. Meta-analyses of case-control and cohort/nested case-control studies point to a lower risk of childhood cancer among those who had been breast-fed, with the greatest effect on the development of neuroblastoma followed by Hodgkin's lymphoma and acute lymphoblastic leukaemia (Martin, Gunnell *et al.* 2005). It has been suggested that breastfeeding may result in a small reduction in risk of pre-menopausal breast cancer but there is little evidence that it reduces overall risk of breast cancer in later life (Martin, Gunnell *et al.* 2005).

11.3.3 Famine

The offspring of women exposed to the Dutch 1944-5 famine *in utero* more frequently reported breast cancer than women unexposed to famine, with the greatest effect being observed in women who were conceived during the famine (Painter *et al.* 2006c) or when the mother was exposed to famine in early gestation (Roseboom, de Rooij *et al.* 2006c). However, it is worth noting that this effect does not appear to be mediated through the same mechanism linking birthweight to breast cancer risk (see Section 11.3.4) as the birthweights of women subsequently developing breast cancer did not differ significantly from those of women without breast cancer (Painter *et al.* 2006c).

11.3.4 Birth anthropometry

Many studies have investigated the relationship between birthweight and risk of childhood leukaemia. These studies used different birthweight categorisation and birthweight cut-off points. However, in general there appears to be an increased risk of acute lymphocytic leukaemia at higher birthweights with evidence of a graded effect throughout the birthweight range (Westergaard *et al.* 1997; Hjalgrim

et al. 2003; Hjalgrim *et al.* 2004; Paltiel *et al.* 2004). The results of studies investigating the link between birthweight and risk of acute myeloid leukaemia are more heterogeneous. A prospective study in Israel reported a positive relationship between birthweight and acute myeloid leukaemia (Paltiel *et al.* 2004) although Hjalgrim and colleagues (Hjalgrim *et al.* 2003) were unable to detect an association with acute myeloid leukaemia.

A number of very large studies and comprehensive meta-analyses and pooled analyses have demonstrated a clear positive relationship between birthweight and breast cancer risk (Ekbom *et al.* 1997; Stavola *et al.* 2000; Okasha *et al.* 2003; dos Santos Silva *et al.* 2004; de Stavola *et al.* 2005; Silva Idos *et al.* 2008) An analysis of 32 studies concluded that breast cancer risk was associated with birthweight, birth length, and head circumference, even after taking account of known breast cancer risk factors (Silva Idos *et al.* 2008). However, there may be differences between pre- and postmenopausal breast cancer, with the link with birthweight being stronger in the former and more heterogeneous in the latter (Forman *et al.* 2005); some have reported an association with breast cancer risk at any age (Ahlgren *et al.* 2003) while others have suggested that the link is specific to pre-menopausal cancer or breast cancer in younger women (Stavola *et al.* 2000; McCormack *et al.* 2005). Some groups have investigated the relationship with length at birth but it would appear that the association of higher birthweight with increased breast cancer risk is stronger.

Less work has been done on the relationship between birth anthropometry and risk of colorectal cancer and the evidence is inconclusive. There are reports of a positive link with birthweight (Sandhu, Luben *et al.* 2002; Nilsen *et al.* 2005) although the relationship is not linear as low-birthweight babies in particular appeared to have an increased risk of colorectal cancer in adulthood (Sandhu, Luben *et al.* 2002). Nilsen and colleagues reported an inverse relationship between birth length and risk of colorectal cancer in men but not in women (Nilsen *et al.* 2005).

An early report suggested that prostate cancer was five times higher in the highest quartile of birthweight than in other birthweight groups (Tibblin *et al.* 1995). A subsequent retrospective cohort study in the US (Platz *et al.* 1998) and a prospective study in Norway (Nilsen *et al.* 2005) demonstrated some trends between cancer and birth anthropometry by cancer sub-type. However, these were not linear and overall there was no significant association between birthweight and prostate cancer risk. There is a report of a possible link with ponderal index (weight in g/length in $cm^3 \times 100$) but neither this study, nor a more recent study by the same group, could detect any relationship between prostate cancer risk and birthweight or birth length (Ekbom 1998; Ekbom *et al.* 2000).

A few studies have investigated the link between birth outcome and risk of adenocarcinoma but these have found little evidence for a link with birthweight (Kaijser *et al.* 2005; Akre *et al.* 2006). Birthweight and length have been linked to cancer in all sites (Andersson *et al.* 2001), the magnitudes of the effects are generally small (McCormack *et al.* 2005). Given the heterogeneity of cancer types and their aetiology this is perhaps not surprising.

11.3.5 Childhood anthropometry and growth

The pattern of postnatal growth has been linked to risk of breast cancer. Rapid growth and falling body mass index (BMI) in childhood through to puberty, early age of peak growth, tall stature and low BMI at 14 years of age are all strongly related to later breast cancer risk (Ahlgren *et al.* 2004; de Stavola *et al.* 2005). Conversely, greater body fatness during childhood and adolescence is associated with reduced risk of pre- and postmenopausal breast cancer (Ahlgren *et al.* 2004; Weiderpass *et al.* 2004; Baer *et al.* 2006).

11.3.6 Adult stature and body composition

The evidence linking adult body fatness and attained height to cancer risk has recently been reviewed by the World Cancer Research Fund (WCRF) (World Cancer Research Fund/American Institute for Cancer Research 2007). Increased body fatness is associated with a higher risk of cancer of the colon and rectum, oesophagus, pancreas, gall bladder, kidney, ovary and postmenopausal breast cancer, but a lower risk of pre-menopausal breast cancer (WCRF & AICR 2007). Adult height is also positively related to risk of a number of cancers, and WCRF categorised the link as 'convincing' for colorectal and postmenopausal breast cancer; 'probable' for pre-menopausal breast cancer and cancer of the pancreas and ovary; and

'limited/suggestive' for endometrial cancer (WCRF & AICR 2007) (see Fig. 11.1). The associations with cancer risk seem to be stronger when leg length rather than trunk length is considered (Gunnell *et al.* 1998; Gunnell *et al.* 2001). This may be important because differences in relative dimensions of leg and trunk length, for example, may reflect dietary or other environmental effects during different phases of growth. For example, leg length increase is greater than trunk length increase during childhood growth (Hayes *et al.* 1999; Tzonou *et al.* 1999). Leg length has been particularly related to early growth, especially that occurring under 5 years of age, and the associations between cancer and height are clearest when there has been malnutrition before puberty (Vatten and Kvinnsland 1990; Moller 1993).

11.4 Possible mechanisms linking early nutrition to cancer risk

There are numerous hypothesised mechanisms through which nutrition can influence the risk of cancer. These include effects on cellular processes involving inflammation, oxidative stress, cellular differentiation, exposure to hormones, DNA damage and repair, DNA replication, gene expression and epigenetic modification (WCRF & AICR 2007). Critically, any postulated mechanism linking early nutrition to cancer risk must also explain the delay, often of decades, between the original exposure and manifestation of the disease. Likely hypotheses can be categorised into effects on genotype, epigenotype and phenotype.

11.4.1 Genotype

Genetic mutation is a hallmark of cancer and there are a number of ways in which early nutrition could result in mutation or influence the general propensity to mutation.

11.4.1.1 Embryo selection

Particular genotypes can influence the risk of cancer. Only a minority (5–10%) of cancers have been linked to specific genes, but estimates from heritability studies suggest that more genes have yet to be identified. Variations in gene sequences which are inherited are termed germline mutations. Due to the polygenic nature of cancer individuals with inherited germ-

Convincing: evidence is strong enough to support a judgement of a convincing causal relationship, which justifies goals and recommendations designed to reduce the incidence of cancer. A convincing relationship should be robust enough to be highly unlikely to be modified in the foreseeable future as new evidence accumulates.

Probable: evidence is strong enough to support a judgement of a probable causal relationship, which would generally justify goals and recommendations designed to reduce the incidence of cancer.

Limited – suggestive: evidence is too limited to permit a probable or convincing causal judgement. The evidence may have methodological flaws, or be limited in amount, but shows a generally consistent direction of effect.

Limited – no conclusion: evidence is so limited that no firm conclusion can be made.

Figure 11.1 WCRF/AICR criteria for grading evidence.
World Cancer Research Fund and American Institute for Cancer Research (2007).

line mutations will not definitely develop cancer but may have an increased risk of doing so.

Early nutrition could modulate cancer risk by selecting for embryos, or gametes, with a particular genotype which predisposes to cancer. An example of this comes from the literature on folic acid. Folic acid use before and during early pregnancy is advisable to reduce the risk of neural tube defect but concerns have been raised that its use may increase the survival of embryos with deleterious genotypes (Lucock and Yates 2005). This concern arises from a report of an increase in the frequency of mutant alleles in the folate metabolising methylene tetrahydrofolate reductase gene (MTHFR; C677T and A1298C) in babies born in Spain following the recommendation there in favour of folic acid supplement use (Munoz-Moran *et al.* 1998; Reyes-Engel *et al.* 2002). The interpretation of this finding is not that folic acid causes *de novo* mutations but that it may result in the survival of embryos carrying these mutations which would normally perish. If correct, this would be a significant public health concern as the MTHFR 677 TT genotype has been implicated in a wide range of diseases including ischaemic heart disease, deep vein thrombosis, pulmonary embolism and stroke (Klerk

et al. 2002; Wald *et al.* 2002; Casas *et al.* 2005). It has also been implicated in cancer of the breast, colon and rectum (Haggarty 2007). A subsequent study demonstrated no adverse effect of folic acid on genotype of the offspring (Haggarty *et al.* 2008) but the general concept – that maternal and paternal periconceptional nutritional status could select for embryos with genotypes which influence cancer risk in later life – remains a possibility.

11.4.1.2 Cancer stem cells

The cancer stem cell hypothesis is that cancers are driven by a cellular sub-component that has stem cell properties. However, it is not known whether the cells are derived from stem cells that have lost the ability to regulate proliferation, or from more differentiated cells that have acquired the ability to self-renew. Embryonic stem cells originate in the pre-implantation embryo and, at the earliest stages of development (see Chapter 4, Fig. 4.1), have the capacity to differentiate into all possible human cell types, including extraembryonic tissues (a property known as totipotency). As development progresses this ability is gradually lost and the range of possible cell types which can be formed is reduced. Pluripotency denotes the potential to differentiate into any of the three germ cell layers: endoderm, mesoderm or ectoderm, but not extraembryonic tissue such as the placenta. Multipotency and unipotency refer to the capacity to develop or differentiate into a limited number of cell types, or only one cell type. This is the status of adult stem cells which are found in a number of tissues where they have the capacity to differentiate into the cell types present in that tissue (Krtolica 2005). A third type of stem cell has been proposed (Ratajczak *et al.* 2009). Very small embryonic/epiblast-like stem cells have been described in bone marrow and a number of adult organs. They are thought to be deposited during early gastrulation (the process by which three germ cell layers are formed) in developing tissues and persist into adulthood where their hypothesised role is to support the turnover of tissue-committed adult stem cells (Ratajczak *et al.* 2010). If the persistence of these stems cells is confirmed, this particular type of stem cell would be a good candidate for early programming of later cancer risk.

The traditional view of cancer is that it arises from a single cell which undergoes a series of genetic alterations – e.g. human epidermal growth factor receptor 2 (HER2)/NEU in breast cancer and ERBB2 in lung cancer (Feinberg *et al.* 2006). Extensive mutation and genetic instability are thought to be necessary for subsequent development to invasive metastatic solid tumours, but in the initial stages cancer is thought to develop from benign, relatively well-differentiated, non-invasive tumours as a result of one or a small number of mutations (Feinberg *et al.* 2006). The initial 'trigger' mutations could be caused by diet or environment early in development which then persists through subsequent cell divisions within the stem cell compartment. However, if these are the same tissue stem cells involved in tissue renewal, such mutations should give rise to mosaicism within the differentiated tissue. At this stage such a mechanism can only be considered as speculative. If stem cells are on the pathway between early development and later cancer risk then the initial trigger and mechanism of propagation is more likely to be epigenetic than genetic (Feinberg *et al.* 2006).

11.4.2 Epigenotype

Epigenetics has been defined as 'heritable changes in gene function that cannot be explained by changes in DNA sequence' (Russo *et al.* 1996) but it is much more than that. Multiple layers of epigenetic modification control the expression of most human genes and this process of epigenetic control is now recognised as a fundamental regulator of the metabolic response of all cells in the body. Nucleotide sequence information within the human genome determines the function of expressed proteins while epigenetic information determines how, when and where genetic sequence data is used. Epigenetics encompasses a collection of mechanisms that define the phenotype of a cell without affecting the genotype (Sasaki and Matsui 2008). In molecular terms, it represents a range of chromatin modifications including DNA methylation, histone modifications, remodelling of nucleosomes and higher-order chromatin reorganisation and regulation by non-coding RNA (Strachan and Read 2004; Sasaki and Matsui 2008). A key characteristic of the epigenetic signal is that it is heritable through either mitosis or meiosis and therefore can be passed from somatic cell to daughter cell or across the generations. There is now considerable evidence that epigenetic status is heritable (Kaminsky *et al.* 2009) and modifiable by environment and lifestyle in humans (Jirtle and Skinner 2007).

11.4.2.1 Epigenetics and cancer

A common observation in human breast cancers and many other tumour types is epigenetic change including altered methylation of DNA (Szyf *et al.* 2004) and the histones associated with DNA (Fraga *et al.* 2005). A number of observations suggest that epigenetic change may be causal in the development of cancer and not simply a consequence of disease. Epigenetic change occurs early in the development of cancer, it is observed in even low-grade cancers (Jackson *et al.* 2004) and the pattern of methylation correlates with cancer stage. Hypomethylation in tumour cells is thought to be an early trigger which predisposes cells to genomic instability and genetic change (Robertson 2005).

A further characteristic of cancer is hypermethylation of specific genes thought to be involved in carcinogenesis and disease progression (e.g. tumour suppressor genes) in concert with global hypomethylation (Robertson 2005). The *BRCA1* gene is known to be involved in the aetiology of breast cancer and altered *BRCA1* methylation has been observed within the tumour (Umbricht *et al.* 2001; Vasilatos *et al.* 2009). More surprisingly, altered *BRCA1* methylation has also been detected in apparently normal epithelium adjacent to breast cancer (Umbricht *et al.* 2001) and in peripheral blood and buccal cells of women with the disease or at increased risk (Snell *et al.* 2008; Widschwendter *et al.* 2008). There is a growing body of evidence to suggest that tumour suppressor genes which are hypermethylated in tumour tissue are also hypermethylated in normal tissue of individuals with cancer (Feinberg *et al.* 2006). This suggests that epigenetic change is an early event, preceding cancer, rather than a consequence of the disease.

A number of lines of evidence implicate imprinted genes in particular in the development of cancer. Imprinting refers to the epigenetic marking of genes in a parent-of-origin specific manner within the germ cells such that the subsequent expression pattern depends on the parent from which the allele ultimately derived (Reik and Walter 2001). Although known imprinted genes make up only around 1% of all genes, they are thought to primarily affect embryo growth, placental function and brain function and behaviour (Reik and Walter 2001; Tycko and Morison 2002; Wilkinson *et al.* 2007). A number of imprinted genes are known tumour suppressors or oncogenes involved in cell proliferation (Allegrucci *et al.* 2005). Imprinting syndromes, such as Beckwith-Wiedemann, where the imprint is disrupted or absent, are associated with an increased risk of several cancer types (Rump *et al.* 2005) while epigenetic change and loss of imprinting – gain or loss of DNA methylation or the loss of allele-specific gene expression – are common characteristics of tumours (Yuasa 2002). Insulin-like growth factor (IGF) II is an autocrine growth factor that plays an important role in many types of cancer and loss of imprinting in IGF-II is the most commonly reported loss of imprinting event across a wide range of tumour types: it is observed in colon, liver, lung, and ovarian cancer, as well as Wilms' tumour. Again, this relaxation or loss of imprinting appears to occur in normal tissue of individuals with cancer patients and even in those at increased risk of the disease (Feinberg *et al.* 2006). Loss of imprinting in other genes has been implicated in other cancer types, e.g. MEST in breast, lung, and colon cancer.

Altered IGF-II methylation in offspring has also been reported to be related to birthweight, which is itself related to the risk of a number of cancers (Steegers-Theunissen *et al.* 2009). Altered imprinting has also been observed in the offspring of women exposed to the Dutch famine during the Second World War. These women, who had an increased risk of breast cancer, also had a lower level of DNA methylation in the imprinted IGF-II gene compared with their unexposed, same-sex siblings. This association was specific for exposure during the periconceptional and early pregnancy period (Heijmans *et al.* 2008). Further work in the same cohort suggests alteration of methylation of a number of other genes in the offspring of women exposed to famine but these changes were sex-specific and dependent on the developmental timing of exposure to food restriction (Tobi *et al.* 2009).

11.4.2.2 Diet and epigenetics

Diet and nutrition could influence human epigenetic status via:

(1) availability of methyl and acetyl groups which are used to epigenetically mark DNA and histones;
(2) direct effects on the enzymic machinery involved in setting and interpreting the epigenetic mark;
(3) direct effects on the structure and function of the genome;
(4) selection of gametes/embryos with particular epigenotypes.

The ultimate methyl donor for epigenetic methylation reactions is the folate methylation cycle, and specifically the metabolite S-adenosylmethionine (SAM). The nutritional and genetic factors which affect the activity of this cycle also appear to influence epigenetic status. Poor folate status and elevated homocysteine are associated with DNA lymphocyte hypomethylation (Jacob *et al.* 1998; Yi *et al.* 2000) and mutation in the MTHFR gene interacts with folate status to influence DNA methylation (Stern *et al.* 2000; Friso *et al.* 2002). Alcohol is also thought to influence DNA methylation in humans (Bonsch *et al.* 2004; Bonsch *et al.* 2005). Most of this work relates to global DNA methylation but, more interestingly, higher levels of methylation in the differentially methylation region (DMR) of IGF-II have been observed in the cord blood DNA of babies whose mothers had taken folic acid supplements in pregnancy (Steegers-Theunissen *et al.* 2009). However, the numbers studied were small.

There is a growing body of evidence from animal studies to suggest that the diet of the mother can influence the epigenetic status and phenotype of the offspring. Animals fed diets deficient in methyl donors such as folic acid, choline and betaine have globally hypomethylated DNA (Locker *et al.* 1986; Wainfan *et al.* 1989) and altered methylation and expression of individual genes such as axin fused (Paltiel *et al.* 2004) and the Agouti gene (A^{vy}) which is under imprinting control (Platz *et al.* 1998; Park, Kang *et al.* 2008). An effect of vitamin B_{12}, folate and methionine on methylation status has also been observed in the fetal liver in sheep (Sinclair *et al.* 2007) while protein-restriction in rats influences the methylation of peroxisome proliferator-activated receptor alpha (PPARα) and glucocorticoid receptor promoters (Burdge *et al.* 2007), with some evidence of an interaction with folic acid (Lillycrop *et al.* 2005). These nutritional effects appear to extend into the postnatal period. Feeding mice a diet lacking folic acid, vitamin B_{12}, methionine and choline in the post-weaning period altered the expression and methylation of IGF-II (Waterland *et al.* 2006) although this effect was only observed in some of the IGF-II DMR loci and was not observed in H19, for example. Dietary intake of the phytoestrogen genisten during pregnancy alters both coat colour and the methylation status of the intracistemal A particle (IAP) involved in A^{vy} regulation (Dolinoy *et al.* 2006; Jirtle and Skinner 2007). Interestingly the change in A^{vy} methylation in the offspring of mothers supplemented with genisten during pregnancy appears to confer some protection against obesity in the offspring.

Although more inconsistent there is some evidence for such nutritional effects in human pregnancy. Steegers and colleagues observed a higher level of methylation in the DMR of IGF-II in cord blood DNA in babies of mothers who took folic acid supplements (Steegers-Theunissen *et al.* 2009). In contrast, women exposed to famine during the Dutch Hunger Winter in 1944–5 (see Chapter 1, Section 1.4.1; and Chapter 4, Section 4.4.2) had a lower level of DNA methylation in the imprinted IGF-II gene compared with their unexposed, same-sex siblings (Heijmans *et al.* 2008; Tobi *et al.* 2009).

Direct effects of diet on the structure and function of the genome related to epigenetics are also possible. There are over 20 folate-sensitive fragile sites in the genome; folate-sensitive fragile sites are 'regions of chromatin that fail to compact normally during mitosis and that can be observed after culturing cells in media that is deficient in folic acid and thymidine' (Robertson 2005). They represent regions where nutrition could influence the genome directly.

11.4.3 Phenotype

The link between body fatness and cancer risk is now well established (WCRF & AICR 2007). Since obesity may itself be programmed early in life (see Chapter 8) this is another possible mechanism by which early nutrition could influence later cancer risk (Reeves *et al.* 2007; Pischon *et al.* 2008; Renehan *et al.* 2008). The relationship between obesity, hormone exposure and risk of cancer has been explored most extensively for breast cancer and in relation to menopausal status (Reeves *et al.* 2007; Pischon *et al.* 2008; Renehan *et al.* 2008). The mechanisms underlying this increased risk in breast cancer are not fully understood but the conversion of androgenic precursors to oestrogens, in adipose tissue and other tissues, by the enzyme aromatase results in increased exposure to oestrogen. In addition, an insulin-mediated decrease in sex globulin secretion also leads to an increased bioavailabilty of oestrogen. The net result is oestrogen-receptor mediated cellular proliferation and reduced apoptosis, both of which are thought to predispose to the development of breast cancer (Calle and Kaaks 2004).

Other mechanisms have been suggested which may be important in the development of a number of cancer types. A key mechanism is obesity-related hyperinsulinaemia and its sequelae. Of particular importance are changes in the bioavailablilty of IGF-I as a result of an insulin-mediated decrease in its binding proteins, 1 and 2. Increased levels of IGF-I also lead to increased cellular proliferation and reduced apoptosis (as in the case of oestrogens) and have been associated with increased risk of different cancer types such as colon and prostate cancer (Kaaks and Lukanova 2001; Sandhu, Dunger *et al.* 2002; Wu *et al.* 2002). Interestingly, IGF-I concentrations tend to be higher in men than in women, and it has been suggested that this may be important in the differences in risks of cancers between the sexes (Renehan *et al.* 2008). Other consequences of obesity relevant to cancer include insulin-mediated reductions in sex globulin secretion (increased bioavailabilty of oestrogen), and increased bioavailability of IGF-I.

It is also important to consider that adipocytes are metabolically active and produce a variety of other hormones and inflammatory and anti-inflammatory mediators with effects which may also be important in cancer development and growth. A detailed discussion is beyond the scope of this chapter but Table 11.1 highlights some of the key hormones and cytokines produced in adipose tissue (Wozniak *et al.* 2009). While many of these have roles in cancer development, growth, invasion and metastases, recent interest has focused on adipokines, adiponectin and leptin. Levels of adiponectin are inversely related to obesity and are higher in women than in men, whereas leptin levels increase in obesity and are associated with an increased risk of cancers such as prostate cancer. Their roles are incompletely understood but some of their effects relevant to cancer are show in Table 11.2 (Rose *et al.* 2004; Garofalo and Surmacz 2006).

There has been increasing interest in the relationship between inflammation and the development of cancer (Aggarwal and Gehlot 2009). It is well recognised that, in inflammatory states, metabolic activation results in the production of many regulatory molecules and growth factors. Furthermore, in certain chronic inflammatory conditions there is an increased risk of malignant disease developing, e.g. in patients with ulcerative colitis, Crohn's disease, (colon cancer) and Barrett's oesophagus (oesophageal adenocarcinoma). Arguably, the key to further understanding of the link between inflammation and malignancy was

Table 11.2 Adiponectin and leptin with relevance to cancer

Adiponectin	Leptin
Increases sensitivity to insulin	Leptin is upregulated by oestrogen and synthesis increased by insulin
Anti-inflammatory effects	Regulates food intake, fetal development and immune responses
Anti-angiogenic effects	Stimulates angiogenesis and endothelial cell growth
Direct anti-tumour effects (animal studies)	Increases levels of matrix metalloproteinases
	Stimulates proliferation of many cells, e.g. muscle and epithelial

the elucidation of the central role played by the nuclear transcription factor nuclear factor kappa B (NFkB) which is found in the cell cytoplasm in quiescent states, and also the functions of the enzyme COX-2 (cyclo-oxygenase 2). In experimental studies, NFkB and the gene products whose production it stimulates will lead to tumour formation (Aggarwal *et al.* 2009). It is central to the regulation of many cytokines including tumour necrosis factor (TNF), interleukin (IL)-1 and IL-6 molecules leading to invasion (e.g. matrix metalloproteinases), angiogenesis (e.g. vascular endothelial growth factor; VEGF), adhesion molecules, proteins controlling cellular proliferation (e.g. c-myc, cyclin D1) and anti-apoptotic proteins (e.g. B-cell lymphoma 2 (bcl-2), bcl-2 associated X (BAX) and inhibitor of apoptosis proteins (IAP)-1 and IAP-2).

The relationships with NFkB are even more complex because it may itself be regulated by many other growth factors which can also be involved directly in carcinogenesis. While experimental studies suggest a central role at the molecular level, clinical studies also support this. For example, most cancers express NFkB and its activation indicates a poorer prognosis or survival in patients with prostate cancer, oesophageal cancer, lung cancer and breast cancer.

The role of COX-2 in inflammation is also being increasingly understood, together with its implications for cancer initiation and progression. COX-2 is the inducible cyclo-oxygenase enzyme that is upregulated in inflamed tissues and leads to the synthesis

Table 11.1 Adipocyte production of hormones, inflammatory and anti-inflammatory mediators

Inflammatory cytokines	Adipokines (leptin, adiponectin)
	Interferon β and γ
	IL1 and IL6
	TNFα
	Chemokines (e.g. IL8, MCP-1)
Anti-inflammatory mediators	Adipokines (adiponectin)
	Anti-inflammatory cytokines (IL4, IL10)
	IL1 receptor antagonist
	Soluble receptors (IL1RII, sTNFR, sIL1R)

Wozniak A *et al.* (2009).
TNFα, tumour necrosis factor-alpha; IL, interleukin; IL1RII, interleukin-1 receptor II; MCP-1, monocyte chemotactic protein-1; sTNFR, soluble tumour necrosis factor receptor; sIL1R, soluble interleukin-1 receptor.

of a variety of inflammatory prostanoids, especially prostaglandin E2. However, COX-2 is also upregulated in a variety of cancers and its overexpression is associated with increased cellular proliferation, enhanced invasiveness, angiogenesis and a poorer prognosis and reduced survival in a variety of cancers including prostate, lung, oesophageal and breast cancers. The inhibition of COX-2 leads to changes which may be clinically important, e.g. the downregulation of androgen receptors (potentially important for prostate cancer treatment) and the epidermal growth factor receptor (potentially important in breast cancer treatment). In colorectal cancer COX-2 is overexpressed in 85% of cancers and up to 35% of colonic polyps, which are recognised as precursors of colon cancer. In animal studies, COX-2 inhibition causes a reduction in both the number and size of colonic polyps and will also prevent the development of colonic cancers. In human studies of patients at high risk of colorectal adenomas and carcinomas, it has been suggested that use of COX-2 inhibitors may reduce polyp formation. However, there have been concerns about toxicities and cardiovascular events attributable to these types of drugs and further work is required to understand their place in the management of such patients.

11.5 Conclusions

Much of the evidence for the programming of cancer risk and other health outcomes by early nutrition comes from studies in animals. Most of the evidence in humans to substantiate this link comes from observational data, primarily associations between birthweight and early growth and adult disease. However, there is very little evidence that the dietary intake of individual nutrients or nutrient groups have much effect on birthweight (SACN 2011a). Associations between health and birthweight are also potentially confounded by environmental and genetic effects. Low birthweight is more common in deprived communities where smoking, poor diet and other factors which themselves increase cancer risk are more prevalent (Haggarty *et al.* 2009). There is a heritable component to birthweight, adult height and a number of cancers. It is therefore possible that genetic variants involved in the regulation of birthweight and height may also be implicated in carcinogenesis or be in linkage disequilibrium with genetic variants involved in carcinogenesis.

However, there are a number of plausible mechanisms by which early nutrition could influence cancer risk in later life (see Fig. 11.2). These include effects

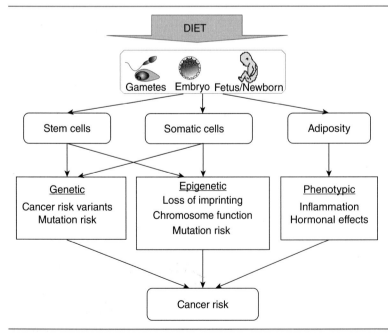

Figure 11.2 Possible mechanisms linking early diet to later cancer risk.

on body fatness in adult life (see Chapter 8), with the increase in cancer risk arising from the metabolic consequences of an increased adipose tissue mass. Alternative mechanisms include effects on stem cells which persist throughout adult life and selection of genotype. One plausible mechanism relates to epigenetic modification of the imprinted genes in particular. The epigenetic status of imprinted genes is modifiable by maternal diet before birth and loss of imprinting is a hallmark of tumours. Crucially, altered imprinting is observed in 'normal' non-tumour tissue in individuals with cancer or at elevated risk of the disease, suggesting that this may be a trigger rather a consequence of the disease. The critical developmental timing of the relevant dietary exposure depends on the mechanism and may occur in the late fetus and early postnatal life, the embryonic period when organogenesis occurs, the early preimplantation embryo, and even the gametes where the imprint is established before fertilisation (Fig. 11.2).

11.6 Key points

- The search for evidence in humans linking early nutrition to later cancer risk has largely been limited by the paucity of large randomised controlled trials of nutrient exposure in early life. While there are a number of plausible mechanisms in humans – and animal models which appear to demonstrate causality – the availability of epidemiological evidence linking early nutrition to later cancer risk in humans is patchy.
- Evidence from meta-analyses of case–control and cohort studies suggest a lower risk of childhood cancer among those who had been breast-fed.
- Evidence indicates a relationship between higher birthweight and increased breast cancer risk. Postnatal growth has also been linked to risk of breast cancer. Rapid growth and falling BMI in childhood through to puberty, early age of peak growth, tall stature and low BMI at age 14 are all strongly related to increased breast cancer risk in later life; whereas greater body fatness during childhood and adolescence are associated with reduced risk of breast cancer.
- There are numerous hypothesised mechanisms through which nutrition can influence the risk of cancer. Likely hypotheses can be categorised into effects on genotype, epigenotype and phenotype.
- It is possible that maternal and paternal periconceptional nutritional status could select for embryos with genotypes that influence cancer risk in later life.
- Diet of the mother before and during pregnancy could plausibly influence later cancer risk via effects on the epigenetic status of particular classes of genes such as the imprinted genes.
- There is some evidence that maternal diet and childhood growth may influence body fatness, which has itself been implicated in cancer risk.

11.7 Recommendations for future research

- Identification of the mechanism of action and the developmental stage(s) at which early diet and nutrition might influence later cancer risk would be of considerable practical importance.
- The search for evidence in humans linking early nutrition to later cancer risk has largely been limited by the paucity of large randomised controlled trials of nutrient exposure in early life.

While few such interventions have been carried out to investigate subsequent cancer risk specifically, there are a number of relatively large historical cohorts where nutritional interventions (e.g. folic acid, fish oils and vitamin D) have been carried out around the time of pregnancy. There are also a number of large historical observational studies where data on nutrient intake or

Continued

nutrient status in pregnancy are available. Follow-up of the offspring of these studies to assess cancer risk in adult life would be informative. Some of these cohorts have been successfully interrogated to assess links with later disease risk (e.g. the Avon Longitudinal Study of Parents and Children [ALSPAC] in the UK) but more could be done to exploit other cohorts if ethical procedures are in place to allow tracing and follow-up.

- In terms of current knowledge, one plausible mechanism linking early diet to later cancer risk involves the epigenetic status of the imprinted genes. It is important to understand the origin of heterogeneity of imprinted gene epigenetic status in normal tissues and its effects, its heritability, the modulating effect of early influences and later life exposures, and the mechanisms by which this variability might lead to the development of cancer.

- Possible mechanisms linking body fatness to cancer risk are already being studied extensively. In terms of the early dietary origins of later cancer risk it would be particularly useful to know more about the way in which early nutrition can influence later adiposity and the distribution of body fat (see Chapter 8), how any programmed pattern of adiposity might impact on cancer risk, and whether this programming can be reversed by strategies to tackle obesity in later life.

- The concept that embryonic stem cells could persist throughout life is particularly important in relation to possible mechanisms linking early diet to later cancer risk. More work is required to establish whether this phenomenon occurs, how widespread it is, and whether these cell types play a role in tumour development.

11.8 Key references

De Stavola BL, dos Santos Silva I & Wadsworth MJ (2005) Birth weight and breast cancer. *New England Journal of Medicine*, **352**, 304–6.

Feinberg AP, Ohlsson R, & Henikoff S (2006) The epigenetic progenitor origin of human cancer. *Nature Reviews Genetics*, **7**, 21–33.

Jones RJ (2009) Cancer stem cells-clinical relevance. *Journal of Molecular Medicine*, **87**, 1105–10.

Martin RM, Gunnell D, Owen CG & Smith GD (2005) Breast-feeding and childhood cancer: A systematic review with meta-analysis. *International Journal of Cancer*, **117**, 1020–31.

Park SK, Kang D, McGlynn KA *et al.* (2008) Intrauterine environments and breast cancer risk: meta-analysis and systematic review. *Breast Cancer Research*, **10**, R8.

Wozniak SE, Gee LL, Wachtel MS & Frezza EE (2009) Adipose tissue: the new endocrine organ? A review article. *Digestive Disease Science*, **54**, 1847–56.

12
Nutrition and Development: Bone Health

12.1 Early life origins of osteoporosis

12.1.1 Osteoporosis epidemiology

Osteoporosis is a skeletal disorder characterised by low bone mass and micro-architectural deterioration of bone tissue, which predisposes to fracture. These fractures typically occur at the hip, spine and wrist. It has been estimated that the remaining lifetime risk of fracture at one of these sites at age 50 years approaches 50% among women and 20% among men (van Staa *et al.* 2001). In the UK, the annual cost to the National Health Service of managing osteoporotic fracture is £1.7 billion, with about 80% attributable to hip fracture (Harvey and Cooper 2004a).

12.1.2 Normal development of bone size and volumetric density

The fetus accretes 80% of the required 30 g calcium during the last trimester in human pregnancies (Kovacs 2003), and then bone mass increases largely as a result of increase in bone size throughout childhood. During pregnancy there is a net positive calcium flux from the maternal to the fetal circulation across the placenta. A miniature version of the skeleton is laid down in the embryonic period, and primary ossification centres form in the vertebrae and long bones between the 8th and 12th weeks of gestation, but it is not until the third trimester that the bulk of mineralisation occurs (Moore and Persaud 1998) (see Chapter 2, Section 2.5.4).

The mechanism of regulation of this process is poorly understood in humans, but it is thought that both parathyroid hormone (PTH) and parathyroid hormone-related peptide (PTHrP) have important and complementary roles (Kovacs 2003). The role of vitamin D is uncertain, although 25 hydroxyvitamin D (25(OH)D) (the main circulatory form of vitamin D) does cross the placenta (Haddad *et al.* 1971). In a mouse model, lack of vitamin D receptors (VDR) did not significantly affect placental calcium transport or skeletal mineralisation (Kovacs 2003); conversely, in the rat, 1,25 hydroxyvitamin D (1,25(OH)$_2$D) did seem to influence placental calcium flux (Lester 1986). Additionally, chondrocytes are an extrarenal source of 1a-hydroxylase activity (and so convert 25(OH)D to 1,25(OH)$_2$D (the metabolically active form of vitamin D) (Anderson and Atkins 2008). This observation therefore suggests a possible mechanism by which maternal 25(OH)-vitamin D status might influence bone size in the fetus. Further evidence to support this notion comes from mouse models in which the gene for 1a-hydroxylase (Cyp27b1) was either knocked out or over-expressed in chondrocytes, leading to altered growth plate morphology (Naja *et al.* 2009). Few data exist in humans at the level of cell biology.

The main determinant of skeletal mineralisation *in utero* appears to be the fetal plasma calcium concentration (Kovacs 2003), and this is mainly influenced by fetal PTH activity, even though this is set at a low level throughout gestation. Lack of parathyroids in fetal mice leads to low fetal calcium levels and decreased skeletal mineralisation (Kovacs, Chafe *et al.* 2001). PTH does not cross the placenta, and

Nutrition and Development: Short- and Long-Term Consequences for Health, First Edition. Edited by the British Nutrition Foundation.
© 2013 the British Nutrition Foundation. Published 2013 by Blackwell Publishing Ltd.

maternal hypo- and hyperparathyroidism appear to affect the fetus via decreasing or increasing the calcium load presented to the fetal circulation. In humans maternal hyperparathyroidism may lead to stillbirth or neonatal hypocalcaemia (Kovacs 2003), secondary to suppression of fetal PTH. Maternal hypoparathyroidism leads to increased levels of fetal PTH via fetal parathyroid hyperplasia, and generalised skeletal demineralisation (Kovacs 2003).

The action of PTH seems to be by increasing calcium reabsorption from the fetal kidney, and possibly bone, to increase calcium concentration. PTH does not seem to influence placental calcium transfer, as injection of PTH into thyroparathyroidectomised fetal sheep does not increase placental calcium flux, in contrast to injection of mid-regions of PTHrP (Care *et al.* 1986). Thus there is increasing evidence that PTHrP is the major determinant of placental calcium transport in animals and that levels of PTHrP are increased in response to low fetal plasma calcium levels (Kovacs *et al.* 1996; Kovacs, Manley *et al.* 2001). PTHrP appears to be produced in the parathyroid glands in some species, but not in others, and this may explain the differing responses of mice and sheep to its removal. This procedure influences placental calcium transport in the latter but not in the former (Care *et al.* 1986; Kovacs, Manley *et al.* 2001). It is not definitely known where PTHrP is produced in human pregnancy, but it may be produced in the placenta and is present in high concentrations in breast milk (Ardawi *et al.* 1997; Kovacs 2003).

It is unclear how the actions of fetal PTH and PTHrP interact with some of the characterised molecular apparatus in the placenta. Placental calcium transfer occurs in the syncytiotrophoblast and proceeds through a sequence of events consisting of facilitated apical entry through a calcium transport channel, cytosolic diffusion of calcium bound to calbindin and, finally, basolateral extrusion of calcium ions through a plasma membrane calcium-dependent ATPase (Belkacemi *et al.* 2005) (Fig. 12.1). This last group of transport channels includes four individual isoforms (PMCA 1–4). These have been previously demonstrated in human placenta, as well as in fetal skeletal muscle and brain. PMCA 1 and 4 are present in most tissues, while PMCA 2 and 3 are found in more specialised cell types (Stauffer *et al.* 1993; Zylinska *et al.* 2002; Belkacemi *et al.* 2005).

One study in the rat has suggested that a two- to three-fold increase in PMCA gene expression is asso-

ciated with a 72-fold increase in calcium transport across the placenta during late gestation (Glazier *et al.* 1992). The regulation of this process is as yet unknown, but at least one of the isoforms of PMCA has been shown to be regulated by vitamin D (Kip and Strehler 2004), and in some animals, for example sheep, but not others such as rats, $1,25(OH)_2D$ appears necessary for maintenance of the materno-fetal calcium gradient (Lester 1986). Recent work in human subjects has shown that the level of mRNA expression of an active placental calcium transporter (PMCA 3), thought to be situated on the basal membrane of the placenta, is positively correlated with whole-body bone mineral content (BMC) in the offspring at birth (Martin *et al.* 2007). These observations may suggest a possible mechanism for the influence of maternal vitamin D status on placental calcium transport and intrauterine bone mineral accrual.

In addition to its effects on placental calcium transport, PTHrP influences linear bone growth by acting on prehypertrophic chondrocytes in the fetal growth plate to inhibit differentiation to hypertrophic chondrocytes, and both over- and under- (Weir *et al.* 1996; Calvi and Schipani 2000) expression of PTHrP or its receptor are associated with short-limbed dwarfism in animals and humans (Kato *et al.* 1990; Iwamoto *et al.* 1994; Karaplis *et al.* 1994; Lanske *et al.* 1996; Vortkamp *et al.* 1996). Additionally there is evidence that PTH and PTHrP differentially affect mineralisation of cortical and trabecular bone (Lanske *et al.* 1999; Calvi *et al.* 2001), and thus are attractive candidates for the physiological investigation of programming.

12.1.3 Tracking of growth

During the adolescent growth spurt, around a further 25% of the final peak bone mass (PBM) is achieved (Gilsanz and Nelson 2003). Peak bone mass is reached in the twenties, but the exact timing appears to vary with skeletal site and gender (Gilsanz and Nelson 2003). After the achievement of PBM, bone mass starts to decline and this is accelerated after the menopause in women.

The concept of a child remaining in the same position relative to its peers throughout growth to peak is known as 'tracking' (Tanner 1989a). This has been well described in several studies, which have sought to model the normal range of childhood growth for the purpose of clinical assessment (Tanner and

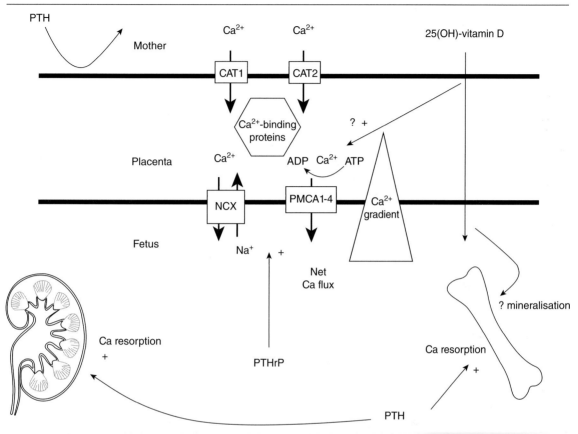

Figure 12.1 Placental calcium transport and fetal bone development.
ADP, adenosine disphosphate; ATP, adenosine triphosphate; Ca, calcium; CAT, calcium transporter; Na, sodium; NCX, sodium-calcium exchanger; PMCA1–4, plasma membrane calcium ATPase 1–4; PTH, parathyroid hormone; PTHrP, parathyroid hormone related peptide; 25(OH)-vitamin D, 25 hydroxyvitamin D.
Adapted from Williams *et al.* (2009) Maternal nutrition and bone health in the offspring. *International Journal of Clinical Rheumatology* **4**, 133–45, with permission of Future Medicine Ltd.

Whitehouse 1976; Tanner 1989a). The resulting 'centile charts' are plots of the average growth curves for healthy children, and allow identification of children who deviate from this normal pattern of growth (see Chapter 2, Section 2.8). Early attempts to formulate these charts were hampered by lack of separation of children who were breast- or bottle-fed, or of different ethnicities; therefore the World Health Organization undertook a large project to derive the optimal growth standards in normal children (World Health Organization 2006). Such charts define appropriate height and weight for age and gender; charts for bone mass have thus far not been developed.

Children who experience a temporary restriction in dietary intake respond initially with a reduced growth velocity (Tanner 1989b). Thus gain in height and weight is slowed, and noted clinically by their crossing centiles downwards. For an acute restriction, there is usually recovery of the pre-existing growth trajectory on return of adequate nutrition. This may take the form of accelerated growth and a rapid recovery of the original pattern, or of a slower, but more prolonged recovery, with subsequent delay in maturation (Tanner 1989b). This process is known as 'catch-up growth' (see Chapter 2, Section 2.10). The converse may apply after a period of nutritional excess, here known as 'catch-down growth'. These observations tend to imply that the trajectory of growth is set very early in life, either from genetic inheritance, or environmental factors *in utero*.

12.1.4 Peak bone mass and risk of fracture

The risk of osteoporotic fracture ultimately depends on two factors: the mechanical strength of bone and the forces applied to it. Bone mass (a composite measure, including contributions from bone size and from its volumetric mineral density) is an established determinant of bone strength. Bone mass in later life depends upon the peak mass attained during skeletal growth and the subsequent rate of bone loss. Longitudinal studies show that bone mass tends to track throughout growth to peak in early adulthood. Mathematical models suggest that modifying peak bone mass will have biologically relevant effects on skeletal fragility in old age (Hernandez *et al.* 2003). There is evidence that peak bone mass may be inherited, but known genetic markers explain only a small proportion of the variation in individual bone mass or fracture risk. Environmental influences during childhood and puberty have been shown to affect bone mineral accrual, but the rapid rate of bone mineral gain during fetal and early postnatal life, coupled with the plasticity of skeletal development *in utero*, offer the possibility of profound interactions between the genome and the environment at this early stage in the life course.

12.1.5 Early influences on bone development

Evidence that the risk of osteoporosis might be modified by environmental influences in early life comes from two groups of studies: first, those evaluating bone mineral and fracture risk in cohorts of adults for whom birth and/or childhood records are available; and second, those studies relating the nutrition, body build and lifestyle of pregnant women to the bone mass of their offspring (Harvey and Cooper 2004b). Cohort studies in adults from the UK, the US, Australia and Scandinavia have shown that those who were heavier at birth or in infancy have a greater bone mass (Jones *et al.* 1999; Gale *et al.* 2001; Dennison *et al.* 2003; Jones *et al.* 2004) and a reduced risk of fracture (Cooper *et al.* 2001) in later life. These associations remain after adjustment for potential confounding factors, such as physical activity, dietary

calcium intake, smoking and alcohol consumption. In a cohort of twins, intra-pair differences in birthweight were associated with bone mineral content in middle age, even among monozygous pairs (Antoniades *et al.* 2003). Mother–offspring cohort studies based in Southampton, UK, have shown that maternal smoking, poor fat stores and excessive physical activity in late pregnancy all have a detrimental effect on bone mineral accrual by the fetus, leading to reduced bone mass at birth (Godfrey *et al.* 2001; Harvey *et al.* 2010).

This review will therefore cover the importance of nutrition along the early life course, from conception to childhood. Bone is made up of a protein matrix coated with calcium hydroxyapatite crystals. Although protein nutrition is likely to be of fundamental importance in bone development, there are very few data relating to this directly. However, there is a range of evidence for the importance of calcium and vitamin D intake. This review will focus mainly on these latter two nutrients, in terms of their impact both before and after birth.

12.2 Maternal nutrition in pregnancy

12.2.1 The role of maternal vitamin D

Low levels of vitamin D are common in pregnancy (see Chapter 3, Section 3.2.1.1 and 3.4.2 and Chapter 15, Section 15.3.3.1). Traditionally, a serum 25(OH)D concentration below 25 nmol/L (10 ng/mL) has been regarded as an index of increased risk of overt bone disease and hence as vitamin D 'deficiency' (Lanham-New *et al.* 2011) (see Section 12.5). In the initial Southampton cohort, composed of White Caucasians, the prevalence of vitamin D deficiency was 31% (Javaid *et al.* 2006). In Asian cohorts the burden is even higher (Brooke *et al.* 1981; Marya *et al.* 1981; Delvin *et al.* 1986; Mallet *et al.* 1986; Marya *et al.* 1988). A study of non-pregnant South Asian women in the North of England demonstrated that 94% had circulating levels of 25(OH)D ≤ 37.4 nmol/L (15 ng/mL) and 26% had ≤ 12.5 nmol/L (5 ng/mL) (Roy *et al.* 2007); a survey of the UK population revealed 47% had levels of 25(OH)D < 40 nmol/L in winter and spring and 15% in summer and autumn (Hypponen and Power 2007). Maternal vitamin D deficiency in pregnancy has been associated with neonatal hypocalcaemia (Purvis *et al.* 1973) and other adverse birth outcomes, such as craniotabes and widened growth plates, suggestive of the changes seen in childhood rickets (Reif *et al.* 1988). Infants of mothers with low vitamin D intake may have lower calcium levels at day 4 (Paunier *et al.* 1978), as vitamin D is required for the absorption of calcium. Infant rickets is becoming more common in dark-skinned communities in the UK, due to low infant intake of vitamin D from the mother, initially via the placenta *in utero* and subsequently via breast milk after birth (Pal and Shaw 2001; Ford *et al.* 2006; Robinson, Hogler *et al.* 2006; Ginde *et al.* 2009).

A retrospective cohort study (Zamora *et al.* 1999) showing that babies who were supplemented with vitamin D (400 IU daily for a median of 12 months) had an increased radial and proximal femoral bone mass at 8 years of age gave some of the first insights into the importance of vitamin D in early life (see Section 12.2.3). Recent work in mother–offspring cohorts in Southampton has increased our understanding of the role of maternal vitamin D in pregnancy. In one such cohort, data on anthropometry, lifestyle and diet were collected from women during pregnancy and venous 25(OH)D was measured by radio-immunoassay in late pregnancy (Javaid *et al.* 2006). Whole-body, hip and lumbar spine bone area, BMC and bone mineral density (BMD) were measured in the healthy term offspring at age 9 years. Almost one-third (31%) of the mothers had reduced (insufficient or deficient) circulating concentrations of 25(OH)D in late pregnancy. Reduced maternal concentration of 25(OH)D was associated with lower whole-body ($r = 0.21$, $p = 0.01$) and lumbar spine ($r = 0.17$, $p = 0.03$) BMC in the children at age 9 years, with a suggestion of a threshold effect at 40 mmol/L. Both the estimated exposure to ultraviolet B radiation during late pregnancy and use of vitamin D supplements predicted maternal 25(OH)D concentration ($p < 0.001$ and $p = 0.01$) and childhood bone mass ($p = 0.03$). Reduced concentration of umbilical-venous calcium also predicted lower childhood bone mass ($p = 0.03$).

Similar findings, linking reduced maternal 25(OH)D concentration with lower offspring bone mass, have come from the Southampton Women's Survey, an ongoing large longitudinal cohort of women recruited for a study of nutrition and growth in pregnancy (Harvey *et al.* 2008). In this study of women aged 20–34 years, characterised before and during pregnancy, maternal 25(OH)D status was measured by radio-immunoassay in late pregnancy and 556

healthy term neonates underwent whole-body dual X-ray absorptiometry (DXA) within 20 days of birth. Offspring of mothers who were insufficient or deficient (<33 nmol/L) in vitamin D in late pregnancy had lower bone mass than those of mothers who were replete. Thus the mean whole bone area of the female offspring of deficient mothers was 112 cm^2 vs. 120 cm^2 in offspring of replete mothers ($p = 0.045$). The mean whole body BMC of offspring of deficient vs. replete mothers was 59 g vs. 64 g ($p = 0.046$) respectively. There were weaker associations in the boys and there was no association with maternal alkaline phosphatase.

12.2.2 Vitamin D intervention studies in pregnancy

There have been several, mainly small, intervention studies examining this issue (summarised in Table 12.1), but only one has so far examined bone mass at birth. Thus 506 women were supplemented at 12 weeks' gestation with 400 IU/day vitamin D and 633 women were given placebo (Cockburn *et al.* 1980). Levels of 25(OH)D were higher in maternal, umbilical cord and infant serum (day 3 and day 6) in the supplemented group. However, this was not a randomised trial, but a comparison of supplemented women from one clinic vs. those receiving placebo in another clinic. Another study compared 59 Asian women, supplemented with 1000 IU/day vitamin D from 28 to 32 weeks (Brooke *et al.* 1980) with 67 placebo controls. Plasma calcium levels were higher in the supplemented mothers, and there was a lower incidence of symptomatic neonatal hypocalcaemia and growth retardation among babies of supplemented mothers.

Again in an Asian population (Marya *et al.* 1981), 25 mothers were randomised to 1200 IU/day of 25(OH)D, 20 mothers to 600 000 IU twice (7th and 8th month), and 75 mothers to placebo. In this study there was no difference in plasma calcium and alkaline phosphatase levels between mothers taking 1200 IU/day and those taking placebo. However, those taking 600 000 IU twice had higher maternal and umbilical cord plasma calcium and lower alkaline phosphatase levels than the placebo group. In a second study (Marya *et al.* 1988) the same group supplemented 100 Asian Indian women with 600 000 IU twice during pregnancy (again at 7th and 8th

Table 12.1   Trials of vitamin D supplements in pregnancy

Setting	No.	Intervention	Outcome		Author (Date)
UK (Asian)	126	1000 IU/day or placebo	Ca maternal	↑	Brooke (1980)
			Cord	→	
			Neonatal	↑	
			Maternal weight	↑	
Scotland	1139	400 IU/day or placebo	25(OH)D maternal	↑	Cockburn (1980)
			Cord	↑	
			Infant	↑	
Asian Indian	120	600 000 IU (×2); 1200 IU/day or placebo	Ca maternal	↑	Marya (1981)
			Cord	↑	
			ALP maternal	↓	
			Cord	↓	
France	34	1000 IU/day; or no vitamin D	25(OH)D cord	↑	Delvin (1986)
			Neonatal	↑	
Asian Indian	200	600 000 IU (×2); or placebo	Ca/P maternal	↑	Marya (1988)
			Cord	↑	
			ALP maternal	↓	
			Cord	↓	
France	68	200 000 IU (×1); 1000 IU/day; or no vitamin D	25(OH)D maternal with both regimes	↑	Mallet (1986)

ALP, alkaline phosphatase; Ca, calcium; P, phosphorus; 25(OH)D, 25 hydroxyvitamin D; → no change; ↑ elevation; ↓ decrease.

months) vs. 100 controls receiving placebo and again found higher maternal and umbilical cord serum calcium and lower alkaline phosphatase levels in the former.

There have been two studies in French populations: 30 women were randomised to receive either 1000 IU/day vitamin D or placebo during the third trimester (Delvin *et al.* 1986). Day 4 neonatal calcium and 25(OH)D levels were significantly higher in the supplemented group. In the second study 21 French women received 1000 IU/day in the last trimester, 27 received 200 000 IU once during the 7th month of gestation vs. 29 placebo controls (Mallet *et al.* 1986). Neonatal calcium at day 2 and day 6 was similar in all groups, but maternal serum 25(OH)D was greater in both intervention groups than in the controls. In the one study which measured bone mineral content at birth (Congdon *et al.* 1983), there was no difference in radial BMC in the offspring of 19 Asian mothers who had taken 1000 IU/day of 25(OH)D vs. 45 controls. However, this lack of observed effect is likely to reflect both the small numbers of subjects and the poor sensitivity of single photon absorptiometry in measuring the tiny amount of bone mineral in the baby's distal radius.

12.2.3 Safety of vitamin D supplementation in pregnancy

None of the above studies has suggested that vitamin D supplementation during pregnancy carries a significant risk. Human beings have evolved to cope with as much as 25 000 IU vitamin D formation daily in the skin. Although rat studies using the equivalent of 15 000 000 IU/day have resulted in extraskeletal calcifications, there is no evidence that doses below 800 000 IU/day have any adverse effect. Two studies (Goodenday and Gordon 1971; Greer *et al.* 1984) have examined the children of hypoparathyroid women given 100 000 IU/day for the duration of pregnancy and found no morphological or physiological adverse consequences. These children were followed for up to 16 years.

Recent work has demonstrated a moderate increase in atopy in children of mothers in the highest quarter of serum vitamin D in pregnancy, where levels were greater than 30 ng/mL (Gale *et al.* 2008). However, in this study the numbers were small with only six cases of atopy (asthma, eczema) by age 9 years in the top quartile of maternal vitamin D, four each in the middle quartiles and two in the bottom quartile. These numbers, even in the highest quartile, were actually lower than the figure for the general population. Additionally, in the Southampton Women's Survey, there was no association between maternal 25(OH)D status and atopic or non-atopic eczema at age 9 months (unpublished data). The role of maternal vitamin D supplementation during pregnancy to improve offspring bone development is currently being examined in an interventional setting. MAVIDOS (Maternal Vitamin D Osteoporosis Study) is the first randomised, controlled trial to investigate whether supplementation of vitamin D during pregnancy serves to optimise skeletal development in the offspring, and commenced recruitment in 2008. The study aims to test the hypothesis that vitamin D supplementation of pregnant women who have low levels of vitamin D will result in improved neonatal BMC. Women are randomised in a double-blind design to 1000 IU/day vitamin D or a placebo and offspring bone mass is assessed by DXA at birth (Harvey *et al.* 2012).

12.2.4 Calcium nutrition in pregnancy

Vitamin D acts to increase maternal gut calcium absorption. The mechanism underlying the association between maternal 25(OH)D, umbilical cord calcium concentration and offspring bone mass is unclear, but raises the question of whether adequate calcium intake would be needed for supplemental vitamin D to be effective. A recent study has demonstrated a positive association between expression of an active calcium transporter gene in the placenta and intrauterine bone mineral accrual in humans (Martin *et al.* 2007). However, very few data exist on the influence of calcium intake on offspring bone mineral.

Trials of calcium in pregnancy have been largely focused on preventing pre-eclampsia and few studies exist with maternal or neonatal bone mass as an outcome. The World Health Organization study randomised 8325 normotensive nulliparous women with a baseline calcium intake of less than 600 mg/day to either 1500 mg/day calcium or placebo (Villar *et al.* 2006). Biochemical indices of bone metabolism were not measured, but in the calcium group pre-eclampsia was less severe and maternal and neonatal mortality reduced compared with the placebo group. A recent systematic review concluded that maternal calcium supplementation in pregnancy reduced the risk of pre-eclampsia, with no other clear benefits or harms (Hofmeyr *et al.* 2007).

The story with bone mass is less clear. Raman *et al.* (1978) supplemented mothers with placebo, 300 mg/day or 600 mg/day calcium from 20 weeks' gestation until term. Allocation was by rotation rather than randomisation. Bone density was measured at the metacarpal at enrolment and delivery in the mother, and at ulna, radius, tibia and fibula in the neonate using radiogrammetric techniques. There was a tendency to increasing bone density in the mothers and neonates with the higher dose of calcium supplementation compared to the other two groups, but differences were small (Raman *et al.* 1978). Janakiraman *et al.* (2003) found, in a cross-over design study of 31 pregnant Mexican women, that urinary N-telopeptide (NTx) (a marker of bone reabsorption) dropped during supplementation with 1200 mg/day calcium compared with supplementation with a non-calcium-containing multivitamin (Janakiraman *et al.* 2003).

The available evidence suggests that even quite large doses of calcium are safe in pregnancy. The Reference Nutrient Intake (RNI) RNI for calcium among pregnant women, like non-pregnant women, is 700 mg/day, whereas an additional 550 mg/day is recommended for women during lactation (see Table 12.2 and Chapter 3, Section 3.4.1.4). Very few of the existing studies of vitamin D supplementation in pregnancy measured dietary calcium intake, and thus it is not known whether baseline calcium intake is important in the influence of vitamin D supplementation on the fetus.

Table 12.2 RNI recommendations for calcium intake in UK

RNI (mg/day)	Age group
525	Infants 0–12 months
350	Children 1–3 years
450	Children 4–6 years
550	Children 7–10 years
800	Female teenagers (11–18 years)
1000	Male teenagers (11–18 years)
700	Adults
700	Pregnant mothers
1250 (an additional 550 mg/day)	Lactating mothers

RNI, Reference Nutrient Intake.
Source: Department of Health (1991).

12.2.5 Polyunsaturated fatty acids and bone metabolism

Recent work has suggested a role for polyunsaturated fatty acids (PUFAs) in bone metabolism. The particular compounds are long-chain *n*-3 and *n*-6 derivatives of PUFAs. Work in animals has demonstrated that dietary intake of long-chain *n*-3 PUFAs may influence bone metabolism. Supplementation with a combination of PUFAs in animals may lead to increased bone mass in the offspring (Watkins *et al.* 1996; Weiler 2000; Watkins *et al.* 2001; Blanaru *et al.* 2004). The balance of different PUFAs may be important as excess fish oil, a rich source of long-chain *n*-3 PUFA, has been shown to be detrimental to bone growth in rabbits (Judex *et al.* 2000). Feeding rat dams soyabean oil (*n*-6 and *n*-3 PUFAs in a 9:1 ratio) compared with linseed oil (predominantly *n*-3 PUFA) during late pregnancy and lactation was associated with higher bone mineral in the offspring (Korotkova *et al.* 2004).

Data from human studies also support the notion that fatty acids may influence bone development. Levels of *n*-3 PUFAs have been positively associated with peak BMD in healthy men (Hogstrom *et al.* 2007). Similar results have been found in children (Eriksson *et al.* 2009). In this study, total *n*-6 PUFA concentration and *n*-6:*n*-3 PUFA ratio was negatively associated with BMD, further supporting the idea that the proportions of different PUFAs is important. In a small study of 30 mothers and their offspring, maternal and umbilical cord red blood cell long-chain PUFA levels predicted bone mass in the offspring at birth (Weiler *et al.* 2005). The current available evidence does not allow robust recommendations to be made, and further observational and interventional studies are warranted.

12.3 Postnatal calcium and vitamin D nutrition

12.3.1 Calcium nutrition in infancy

The nature of infant feeding has been shown to influence bone mineral accrual, with a positive correlation between mineral content in the feed and infant bone mass (Specker 2004). Much of this work has been carried out in premature infants, who tend to be small and have reduced BMD. Studies of premature infants randomised to formulas of differing calcium concentrations have shown short-term increases in bone mineral accrual with the higher-calcium formulas (Bishop *et al.* 1993). However, when these children were followed up in later childhood, there was no difference in bone mass when adjusted for body size between the different feeding regimes (Fewtrell *et al.* 1999), although they were on average shorter and lighter than children born at term.

There are very few data in term infants. One of the studies, however, found that although at 6 months infants fed a high-calcium formula had greater BMD than those fed breast milk, when they were all put onto normal formula for the next 6 months, the differences disappeared (Specker *et al.* 1997), consistent with postnatal tracking along the growth trajectory. A total of 72 term infants aged 6 to 18 months were randomised to a one-year programme of either gross or fine motor activities, and calcium intake was assessed. There was no difference between the effect of the physical activity interventions when calcium intake was moderately high (mean 662 mg/day at 6 months), but among children with low calcium intakes (409 mg/day at 6 months) bone mineral accretion was lower in the gross than fine motor group (Specker *et al.* 1999). The authors suggest that if calcium intake is insufficient to match demand caused by increased loading, poorer mineralisation may result. As the collagen matrix is synthesised first and then subsequently mineralised, this may be a reasonable proposition. The UK Department of Health has issued guidance on daily intake of calcium at all ages and these recommendations are summarised in Table 12.2.

The issue of breast versus formula feeding has been explored in pre-term infants in relation to bone mass in infancy and childhood, with studies finding breast-fed infants to have lower bone mineral in infancy, but normal bones for their reduced size in older childhood (compared with term babies). These studies have suggested that there may be a short-term benefit to formula milk (Bishop *et al.* 1996), but with no difference in bone mineralisation in the longer-term (Fewtrell *et al.* 1999). The comparison between breast and bottle may also depend on the calcium content of the formula (Bishop *et al.* 1993). There is also evidence that breast-fed babies are leaner than their bottle-fed peers during childhood (Dewey 2001a) and may be at reduced risk of obesity in adult life (Demmelmair *et al.* 2006) (see Chapter 8, Section 8.3). These studies are summarised in Table 12.3.

Table 12.3 Summary of dietary calcium intervention studies in infants

Gestation	Study group	Intervention	Outcome	Persistence	Citation
Pre-term	244 preterm babies followed to 8–12 years	High calcium formula vs. breast milk	Higher neonatal BMC	No effect in childhood	Bishop *et al.* 1993; Fewtrell *et al.* 1999
Term	67 neonates	High vs. low calcium formula 6/12 then all moderate calcium formula	High calcium group higher BMC 6/12, no difference at 12/12	N/A	Specker *et al.* 1997
	72 infants, age 6–18 months, followed for 1 year	High or low calcium, high or low physical activity	High physical activity and low calcium: lower BMC	N/A	Specker *et al.* 1999

BMC, bone mineral content; N/A, not applicable.

12.3.2 Vitamin D nutrition in infancy

Vitamin D-deficiency rickets has, until recently, been thought of as an almost extinct disease. However, the lack of sunlight caused by the smog of the industrial revolution has been replaced as a risk factor by an increasing proportion of the UK population who are dark-skinned. Thus, particularly in more northern latitudes, where exposure to the necessary wavelengths of ultraviolet B (UVB) is reduced, in areas where large dark-skinned populations are clustered infantile rickets is resurgent (Lanham-New *et al.* 2011). All formula milks available in the US and UK are supplemented with a minimum of 400 IU/L (10 µg/L) of vitamin D (Greer 2008; Crawley and Westland 2011). The vitamin D content of human breast milk is related to the lactating mother's vitamin D status (Hollis and Wagner 2004; Basile *et al.* 2006; Wagner *et al.* 2006). Therefore, exclusively breast-fed infants may be at increased risk of developing vitamin D deficiency depending on the mother's vitamin D status.

A few small studies have looked at the effect of maternal vitamin D supplementation on the 25(OH)D concentrations in breast-fed infants. Vitamin D supplementation with 1000 to 2000 IU/day has been shown to have little effect on infants' 25(OH)D concentrations (Tanner and Whitehouse 1976; Ala-Houhala 1985; Ala-Houhala *et al.* 1986; Basile *et al.* 2006; Saadi *et al.* 2007). Two small studies have shown that high-dose maternal vitamin D supplementation of up to 6400 IU/day increases the infants' 25(OH)D concentrations comparable to infants receiving 300 to 400 IU of vitamin D per day (Hollis

and Wagner 2004; Wagner *et al.* 2006). However, larger studies are needed to ascertain whether such high-dose supplementations in lactating women are safe.

A few studies have examined direct vitamin D supplementation for breast-fed infants. Breast-fed infants born to Turkish mothers, whose 25(OH)D levels were below 25 nmol/L, received regular daily supplements of 400 and 800 IU of vitamin D from 2 weeks of age (Pehlivan *et al.* 2003). 25(OH)D levels were within normal range at 16 weeks in 79.5% of the infants (76.9 ± 35.4 nmol/L and 91.8 ± 61.5 nmol/L, respectively, $p = 0.873$). When comparing the infants who did not receive the recommended daily requirement of vitamin D with those who received regular doses, levels of calcium, phosphate and alkaline phosphatase did not differ significantly; however, 25(OH)D levels were considerably lower (91.3 ± 54.8 nmol/L and 42.0 ± 14.1 nmol/L, respectively, $p = 0.002$). They concluded that a daily supplement of 400 IU of vitamin D is necessary and sufficient in Turkey. Another study looked at breast-fed infants in China, receiving daily supplements of 100, 200 or 400 IU of vitamin D (Specker *et al.* 1992). They reported that daily supplements of 100 or 200 IU of vitamin D were not sufficient to maintain optimal levels of 25(OH)D in infants living in northern parts of the country where sunlight exposure is insufficient. They concluded that at least 400 IU/day of vitamin D was necessary to obtain normal levels of 25(OH)D.

Measurement of BMC in infants and young children is another functional outcome that may be useful in identifying vitamin D deficiency. The association between 25(OH)D concentration and BMC in North America has been examined in two randomised, controlled studies (Greer *et al.* 1982; Greer and Marshall 1989). In one study, the researchers randomly assigned breast-fed infants to receive 400 IU/day of vitamin D or a placebo and followed them for the first 6 months of life (Greer *et al.* 1982). They reported that 25(OH)D concentrations at both 3 and 6 months were well above 50 nmol/L and significantly higher than in the placebo group. BMC was increased significantly compared to placebo at 3 months but not at 6 months in the vitamin D group.

In the other, larger study, breast-fed infants were randomly assigned to receive 400 IU vitamin D_2/day or a placebo and followed for 6 months (Greer and Marshall 1989). The results showed that total 25(OH)D concentrations were also well above 50 nmol/L in the vitamin D group and nearly twice as high as the concentration in the placebo group at 6 weeks, 3 months and 6 months of age. However, BMC was higher in the placebo group than in the vitamin D group at 6 months. The results of these studies examining the relationship between 25(OH)D concentrations and BMC in US infants are inconsistent. They do not currently support using BMC or PTH concentrations in infants and young children as functional outcomes to define deficient or sufficient levels of 25(OH)D (Greer 2008).

Based on the above, and previous evidence that suggests maintaining serum 25(OH)D concentrations higher than 50 nmol/L prevents rickets in infants and young children (Greer 2008), the American Academy of Pediatrics (AAP) currently recommends daily vitamin D supplements of 400 IU/L (10 μg/L) for breast-fed infants, which should continue throughout childhood to maintain serum 25(OH)D concentrations ≥50 nmol/L (Wagner and Greer 2008).

In one of the few long-term examinations of infant supplementation, Zamora and colleagues (Zamora *et al.* 1999) performed a retrospective cohort study of 149 healthy pre-pubertal Caucasian girls (age 7–9 years). The aim was to determine whether vitamin D supplementation of breast-fed infants during the first year of life is associated with greater BMC and/or areal BMD in later childhood. The supplemented group had received 400 IU/day vitamin D for a median supplementation period of 12 months. Areal BMD was significantly higher in the supplemented group at the level of the distal forearm (0.301 vs. 0.283 g/cm^2; $p = 0.03$) and proximal femoral neck

(0.638 vs. 0.584 g/cm^2; $p = 0.007$). However, several potential confounding factors were noted (Zamora *et al.* 1999). Calcium consumption and sunlight exposure in infancy were impossible to appraise and may have contributed to the observed difference between the two groups. The information on vitamin D was evaluated several years after the supplementation, and misclassification of this variable may have occurred. Table 12.4 summarises the available study data.

12.4 Calcium and vitamin D nutrition in older children

There is much evidence to suggest that calcium and vitamin D are necessary for adequate bone development through childhood and adolescence. Rickets is an extreme example of the consequences of calcium, phosphate or vitamin D deficiency. Observational studies have suggested that children with greater calcium intake or vitamin D levels have greater BMD (Black *et al.* 2002; Cheng *et al.* 2003) and intervention studies have similarly demonstrated increases in BMD, at least in the short-term, with additional supplementation with either of these two minerals (Bonjour *et al.* 1997; Bonjour *et al.* 2001). What is not clear is how long the benefits of a period of supplementation will last, as very few of these studies followed the subjects for more than a year or so. There are few data pertaining to the long-term effects of vitamin D supplementation, but Zamora *et al.* (1999) did find higher hip BMD in 8-year-old children who had been supplemented with vitamin D in the first year of life, compared with those children who had not. There is some suggestion that calcium intake from milk sources (which might also include growth factors such as IGF-I) may lead to longer-term benefits over three years post supplementation (Bonjour *et al.* 2001).

12.5 Vitamin D: problems with defining normality

Most intervention studies have shown that vitamin D supplementation has a positive effect on BMD or BMC in childhood and maintains 25(OH)D concentrations at higher levels (Lamberg-Allardt and Viljakainen 2008). However, there is still no real consensus on what a normal vitamin D level should be. Histori-

Table 12.4 Summary of studies of vitamin D supplementation in infants

Study group	Intervention	Outcome	Persistence	Citation
40 infants from 2 weeks old	Breast-fed infants given 400 or 800 IU vitamin D/day if maternal 25(OH)D levels ≤25 nmol/L	25(OH)D levels in normal range at 16 weeks in 79.5% of the infants	N/A	Pehlivan *et al.* 2003
256 term infants up to 6 months age	Breast-fed infants given 100, 200 or 400 IU vitamin D/day	400 IU vitamin D needed to obtain normal 25(OH)D levels	N/A	Specker *et al.* 1992
18 term infants 1 year follow-up	Breast-fed infants given 400 IU vitamin D/day vs. placebo	25(OH)D > 50 nmol/L in treatment group. BMC increased significantly at 3 months in treatment group	N/A	Greer *et al.* 1982
46 term infants followed up to 6 months age	Breast-fed infants given 400 IU vitamin D_2 vs. placebo	25(OH)D > 50 nmol/L in treatment group. BMC higher in placebo group at 6 months	N/A	Greer & Marshall 1989

BMC, bone mineral content; N/A, not applicable; 25(OH)D, 25 hydroxyvitamin D.

cally, serum levels of 25(OH)D have been classed as deficient, insufficient or replete, and in the UK, the corresponding values have been defined as deficient: <25 nmol/L (<10 ng/mL), insufficient: <50 nmol/L but >25 nmol/L (<20 ng but >10 ng/mL) and replete: >50 nmol/L (>20 ng/mL). The distinction between replete and insufficient has been made on the basis of a level when a secondary rise in PTH would be expected, and deficient as a cut-off below this level. Previously studies have looked at the level of 25(OH)D in populations where a rise in PTH is seen, and this cut-off has been around 50 nmol/L (20 ng/mL) (El-Hajj Fuleihan *et al.* 2006). However, a proportion of the population do not show a rise in PTH with decreasing 25(OH)D levels, possibly as a result of concomitant magnesium deficiency (Sahota *et al.* 2006), making the assumption of a threshold relationship unreliable.

An alternative approach is to explore the relationship between fractional calcium absorption in the bowel and level of 25(OH)D. Using this technique there appears to be a threshold where absorption reaches a plateau at levels of around 80 nmol/L (32 ng/mL) of 25(OH)D (Heaney *et al.* 2003; Heaney 2006). As a result of these data, the prevailing view currently in much of the US has been that the minimum healthy level of 25(OH)D is 75–80 nmol/L (30–32 ng/mL). The normal level in pregnancy is difficult to define as there is a rise in diastolic blood pressure (DBP) and also haemodilution. However,

the current US view is that the standard adult level of 75–80 nmol/L should apply in pregnancy as well, in the absence of any specific data (Heaney 2006). This is a higher level than historically used in Europe and although there is a move in some areas of Europe towards adopting these higher levels, a more conservative appraisal of the risk/benefit balance has led many to maintain the lower thresholds, particularly in UK.

Thus at a recent meeting of the RANK Foundation (Lanham-New *et al.* 2011), where vitamin D deficiency and supplementation were discussed in some detail, the consensus was that population levels should certainly be above 25 nmol/L (10 ng/mL) to minimise risk of adverse bone-related consequences but that the available data do not allow a reliable judgement to be made regarding a higher cut-off for deficiency, particularly with regard to other health outcomes. The rationale here was that in the absence of definitive data it is safer to opt for lower doses to reduce risk of side-effects, in contrast to the US view, where in the absence of data showing harm, it has been considered better to aim for higher levels. However, the US view appears to be changing, with the recent publication of reference intakes by the Institute of Medicine, suggesting a serum threshold of 50 nmol/L (Institute of Medicine 2011). Clearly further work, which needs to be interventional in nature, will be required to elucidate these issues further. In the UK, a working group on vitamin D has been established by the Scientific Advisory Committee on Nutrition. This group aims to review the Dietary Reference Values for vitamin D and make recommendations (www.sacn.gov.uk/).

There are very few data relating dose of supplementation required to reach a particular level of circulating 25(OH)D over a particular time span. Recommended daily amount (RDA) figures have been based on expert opinion rather than on dose–response studies, so it is difficult to know whether current guidelines are correct. The studies cited above suggest that supplementation with 400 IU/day (10 μg/day) might have beneficial effects on bone, but these may also depend on baseline level. For those subjects who have profoundly low circulating levels of 25(OH)D, a large bolus dose may be required to rapidly replenish stores. Indeed, Heaney (2004) and Vieth *et al.* (2001) examined the influence of giving adults daily doses of cholecalciferol from 200 IU/day (5 μg/day) to 10 000 IU/day (250 μg/day) over 5 months. In these studies, 200 IU/day was associated with a small drop in circulating 25(OH)D levels, 1000 IU/day led to a rise of around 25 nmol/L (10 ng/mL) and 5000 IU/day was associated with a rise of 92 nmol/L (37 ng/mL). The optimal levels of 25(OH)D in pregnancy and lactation are even more uncertain. Current UK guidance on vitamin D supplementation across the life course is summarised in Table 12.5.

Again, there are few dosing studies for calcium intake, particularly in pregnancy and early postnatal life. However, gut absorption of calcium is saturable and the few data that do exist would be consistent with there being a threshold above which further increases yield no additional benefit. Table 12.5 summarises current UK recommendations.

12.6 Physical activity and bone health in childhood

Several reports in children and adolescents involved in competitive sport or ballet indicate that intense physical activity is associated with an increase in bone mineral accrual at weight-bearing skeletal sites (Kannus *et al.* 1995; Karlsson *et al.* 1995; Bass *et al.* 1998; Zamora *et al.* 1999). In some of these investigations, intense physical activity seems to be associated with a greater gain in bone size than volumetric BMD. However, the more relevant issue for public health programmes is the effect of moderate physical activity on bone mineral accrual. Some prospective studies have indicated that physical activity programmes undertaken in schools may have a positive effect on this outcome (Morris *et al.* 1997; Bradney *et al.* 1998). There have been several studies on the impact of physical activity programmes on bone mass in late childhood. Bass *et al.* (1998) found that mean BMD at weight-bearing sites was higher in 45 pre-pubertal gymnasts (mean age 10.4 years) than in sedentary controls. Bone mass was also higher in retired gymnasts than in age-matched controls (Bass *et al.* 1998). An increase in bone mineral at the femoral neck and lumbar spine was found in a group of 9- and 10-year-olds, allocated to either control, or to 10-month exercise programme (Morris *et al.* 1997). A moderate physical activity programme of 30-minute sessions, three times a week for 8 months was associated with a significantly greater increase in BMD at the lumbar spine and femoral neck, compared with controls, in one randomised controlled trial in 10-year-old boys (Bradney *et al.* 1998). A persisting association between bone mass and childhood physical activity was found in one study of female American college students.

Table 12.5 RNI recommendations for vitamin D intake in UK

RNI (μg/day)	IU/day	Group	Supplementation
8.5	340	Infants 0 to 6 months	
7.0	280	Children 7 months to 3 years	From weaning to 2 years
0	0	4 years to 50 years	High-risk groups
10	400	50+ years	65+ years
10	400	Pregnant and lactating adults	Yes
Higher dose		Pregnant and lactating mothers	

RNI, Reference Nutrient Intake.
Source: Department of Health (1991).

Those who did not participate in high school sports were seven times more likely to have low bone mass in early adulthood than those who did (Ford *et al.* 2004).

However, much less is known about the influence of physical activity on bone mass in younger children, and in particular, whether bone mineral accrual varies significantly within the normal range of activity for a healthy population. One study to address this issue examined the association between physical activity measured by accelerometry, and BMD measured by DXA in 368 children aged 4–6 years. Statistically significant positive associations were found between physical activity and BMD at each of whole-body, hip and lumbar spine; hours of television viewing per day inversely predicted hip BMD in girls ($r = -0.15$, $p < 0.01$) (Janz *et al.* 2001). Additionally in this cohort, the femoral neck cross-sectional area was positively associated with physical activity (Janz *et al.* 2004). A more recent study of 4-year-old children born to the Southampton Women's Survey (UK) found positive relationships between mean time spent in moderate to vigorous physical activity (assessed over 7 days by accelerometer) and proximal femoral bone mass (assessed by DXA). In this study the relationships were stronger where daily calcium intake was above, compared with below, the median (Harvey *et al.* 2012).

The relationship between everyday activity and bone mineral is an important issue, as levels of physical activity may be amenable to modification by public health interventions. It remains uncertain to what extent the greater gains in areal BMD observed in intervention studies translate into long-term increases in bone strength and a reduction in later fracture risk.

Thus the data suggest that children with habitually greater levels of physical activity have higher bone mineral accrual, and that programmes of increased physical activity may increase bone mass temporarily. However, whether these observations translate into long-term benefits or a reduction in fracture risk, either in childhood, or in later adulthood, remains to be seen.

12.7 Conclusions

Evidence suggests that bone health is amenable to modulation by environmental factors throughout the life course, and that this process begins *in utero*. The fetal period is likely to be a critical time for the origin of long-term influences on skeletal growth. Epidemiological studies described above suggest that maternal factors, such as vitamin D status, may have a permanent impact on bone health in the offspring. The reduced peak bone mass resulting from an adverse intrauterine environment is likely to increase risk of osteoporotic fracture in older age. In contrast to the lifetime influence of intrauterine factors, postnatal nutrition has not been shown to have effects longer than a few years. Putting these data together gives the hypothesis that gene–environment interactions *in utero* set up the skeletal growth trajectory to peak bone mass, and postnatal factors may then temporarily modulate this pattern. This suggests the importance of good long-term postnatal nutrition to fulfil the potential growth started before birth. Finally, these data may give rise to novel public health interventions, such as maternal vitamin D supplementation in pregnancy, to improve bone health in the offspring and reduce osteoporotic fractures in future generations.

12.8 Key points

- Reduced peak bone mass in early adulthood is associated with increased risk of osteoporosis and fractures in later life.
- Maternal smoking, poor fat stores and excessive physical activity in late pregnancy all have a detrimental effect on bone mineral accrual by the fetus, leading to reduced bone mass at birth.
- Maternal vitamin D status may be critical to bone development in the offspring. All pregnant and lactating women are advised to take a vitamin D supplement of 10 μg/day (400 IU/day). Dark-skinned ethnic minorities are of particular risk of low vitamin D and, in the UK, all Asian children and women are advised to take supplementary vitamin D. The RNI for calcium among pregnant women, like non-pregnant women, is 700 mg/day, whereas an additional 550 mg/day is recommended for women during lactation.

Continued

- Long-term skeletal growth trajectory may be programmed by gene–environment interactions *in utero*. Skeletal growth is particularly important in the last trimester.
- Postnatal modulation of calcium and vitamin D intake may, at least transiently, influence bone mass, but there is a lack of evidence to support any longer-term influence.
- Fatty acid intake also seems to influence bone development; in particular, levels of *n*-3 PUFAs have been positively associated with peak BMD in adults and children. One study has also suggested a positive link between maternal cord blood levels of long-chain *n*-3 fatty acids and bone mass in offspring.
- Exclusively breast-fed babies may be at increased risk of vitamin D deficiency if the mother is vitamin D-deficient and they have minimal effective exposure to sunlight (for example, pigmented skin). Infant supplementation with vitamin D should be considered in these situations.
- As bone is made up of a protein matrix, protein nutrition is likely to be of fundamental importance in bone development. However, there are very few data relating to this directly.
- Several studies have shown beneficial effects of physical activity on bone mass in late childhood. However, the evidence is less clear on the influence of physical activity on bone mass in younger children and, in particular, whether bone mineral accrual varies significantly within the normal range of activity for a healthy population. Children with habitually greater levels of physical activity have higher bone mineral accrual; however, whether these observations translate into long-term benefits or a reduction in fracture risk, either in childhood, or in later adulthood, remains to be seen.

12.9 Recommendations for future research

- Investigation of novel public health interventions, such as supplementation of pregnant women with vitamin D, is warranted.
- Many of the trials of calcium intake during pregnancy have focused on preventing pre-eclampsia, with very few studies investigating maternal or neonatal bone mass as an outcome. Research into the effect of maternal calcium intake on the bone mineral density of offspring would be useful.
- It is unclear whether maternal baseline calcium intake is important in the influence of vitamin D supplementation on the fetus. There are also very few data available on the influence of calcium intake on the bone mineral density of offspring.
- There are few dosing studies for calcium intake, particularly in pregnancy and early postnatal life. Gut absorption of calcium is saturable, and the few data that do exist would be consistent with there being a threshold above which further increases yield no additional benefit. However, the optimal levels of 25(OH)D in pregnancy and lactation are currently uncertain.

12.10 Key references

Gale CR, Robinson SM, Harvey NC *et al.* (2008) Maternal vitamin D status during pregnancy and child outcomes. *European Journal of Clinical Nutrition*, **62**, 68–77.

Godfrey K, Walker-Bone K, Robinson S *et al.* (2001) Neonatal bone mass: influence of parental birthweight, maternal smoking, body composition, and activity during pregnancy. *Journal of Bone Mineral Research*, **16**, 1694–1703.

Harvey NC, Javaid MK, Arden NK *et al.* (2010) Maternal predictors of neonatal bone size and geometry: the Southampton Women's Survey. *Journal of Developmental Origins of Adult Health and Disease*, **1**, 35–41.

Javaid MK, Crozier SR, Harvey NC *et al.* (2006) Maternal vitamin D status during pregnancy and childhood bone mass at age 9 years: a longitudinal study. *Lancet*, **367**, 36–43.

Kovacs CS (2003) Skeletal physiology: fetus and neonate. In: *Primer on the Metabolic Bone Diseases and Disorders of Mineral Metabolism*. Ed. Favus MJ. Washington, DC, American Society for Bone and Mineral Research: 65–71.

13
Nutrition and Development: Asthma and Allergic Disease

13.1 Introduction

Asthma and the allergic diseases of atopic dermatitis (eczema), allergic rhinitis (hayfever) and immunoglobulin (Ig)E-mediated food allergy are closely associated inflammatory conditions that share a common immunological aetiology. The presence of a family history of asthma and allergic disease increases the likelihood of developing asthma and allergic disease and the presence of one allergic condition increases the likelihood of developing others.

Asthma is a chronic inflammatory disorder of the lung airways associated with increased airway responsiveness and variable airflow obstruction. Typical symptoms include periodic wheezing, breathlessness, paroxysmal cough and chest tightness, with severity ranging from occasional minor symptoms to disabling persistent severe symptoms and/or frequent life-threatening exacerbations (Holgate *et al.* 2006). Atopic dermatitis is a chronic relapsing inflammatory skin disorder that is characterised by itching, inherently dry skin and typical excoriated, ulcerated eczematous skin lesions with a characteristic distribution (face, flexures of the elbows, knees, wrists, ankles and sides of neck). Atopic dermatitis usually starts in early infancy, with 60% of patients presenting in the first year of life and 90% by the age of 5 years (Holgate *et al.* 2006). Allergic rhinitis is an inflammatory disorder of the nasal mucosa that has been defined for clinical purposes as symptoms of

nasal itching, sneezing, discharge, or nasal blockage lasting for at least one hour a day on most days (Holgate *et al.* 2006). IgE-mediated food allergy is an abnormal state of heightened IgE-based immune responsiveness to specific food constituents (usually glycoproteins) resulting in symptoms after ingestion of the foods containing the specific food constituents. The symptoms of IgE-mediated food allergy range from mild tingling in the mouth, to swelling of lips, abdominal pain and diarrhoea through to life-threatening anaphylaxis with oropharyngeal swelling, airway compromise, hypovolaemic shock and bronchospasm (Holgate *et al.* 2006).

13.2 Pathogenesis

Asthma and allergic diseases are characterised by inflammatory processes in the involved tissues (airways, skin, nasal mucosa, intestinal system), with effector CD4+ T-helper (Th) cells of the predominantly Th2 phenotype being considered crucial for the initiation and perpetuation of asthmatic and allergic inflammation (Holgate *et al.* 2006). Activated Th2 cells secrete cytokines such as interleukin (IL)-4, IL-5 and IL-13 that are considered to be important mediators in asthmatic and allergic inflammatory processes (see Fig. 13.1). IL-4 promotes the isotype switching of B-cells to the secretion of IgE that subsequently binds to IgE receptors present on the surface of tissue mast cells. The cross-linking of

Nutrition and Development: Short- and Long-Term Consequences for Health, First Edition. Edited by the British Nutrition Foundation.
© 2013 the British Nutrition Foundation. Published 2013 by Blackwell Publishing Ltd.

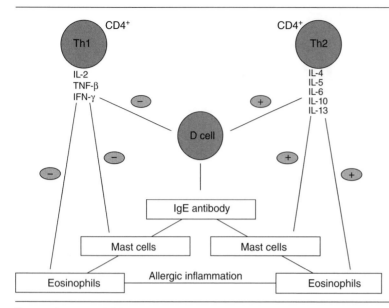

Figure 13.1 Cellular and molecular. Reproduced from Buttriss, J., Ed. (2002). *Adverse Reactions to Food: The Report of the British Nutrition Foundation Task Force.* Wiley-Blackwell Publishing Ltd, Oxford.

Two main types of CD4⁺T helper cell are recognised and these are designated Th1 and Th2. IFN-γ, interferon γ; IgE, immunoglobulin E; IL, interleukin; TNF-β, tumour necrosis factor β.

allergen-specific mast cell-bound IgE by allergen stimulates the release and synthesis of mast cell-derived mediators that are responsible for many features of acute allergic reactions (e.g. bronchospasm, nasal discharge, anaphylaxis). IL-5 stimulates bone marrow to produce and release eosinophils and in addition plays a major role in the localisation of eosinophils to sites of inflammation. In addition to having important effector functions, Th2 cytokines have important regulatory properties, promoting Th2 differentiation and inhibiting development of the other major functional Th-cell subset known as Th1. The Th1 cytokine interferon (IFN)-γ promotes Th1 differentiation and inhibits Th2 differentiation. A consequence of the self-amplification and the mutual antagonism of the reciprocal phenotype is that once a Th-cell-mediated immune response deviates towards either the Th1 or Th2 phenotype then the Th-cell response becomes increasingly polarised towards that phenotype. There is increasing interest in the role of regulatory T(Tr)-cells in the pathogenesis of asthma and allergic disease because of their ability to directly inhibit both Th1 and Th2 responses. Studies of Tr-cells suggest that asthma and allergic disease are associated with reduced numbers and/or reduced activity of IL-10 producing Tr1 cells, and CD25+ Tr-cells that appear to suppress via cell–cell

contact. In some studies reduced Tr-cell numbers pre-date the development of disease.

Until recently, asthma and allergic diseases were considered to be primarily immunological diseases; however, it seems increasingly likely that these conditions are a consequence of the combination of an aberrant immune response in the context of a tissue-specific defect. In asthma it would appear that the airway epithelium is intrinsically structurally and functionally abnormal and critically contributes to the inflammatory response and long-term remodelling of asthmatic airways (Holgate *et al.* 2000). The airway epithelial cells are more susceptible to environmental stressors (e.g. viruses or pollution) and the epithelium has an impaired ability to repair itself. This combination of increased susceptibility to injury with impaired capacity to repair appears to be a potent pro-inflammatory stimulus that, when combined with the parallel development of a Th2-biased immune response, results in asthmatic airway inflammation. Recent studies have also highlighted the importance of Th2 differentiation in the presence of an intrinsic tissue-specific deficit in the pathogenesis of atopic dermatitis. Mutations in the gene coding for the epidermal barrier protein filaggrin have been strongly associated with the development of atopic dermatitis and it has been suggested that atopic dermatitis is a consequence of Th2 immune differentiation in the presence of an epithelial barrier defect.

13.3 Increasing prevalence of asthma and allergic disease

Since the early 1960s there has been a marked increase in the prevalence of asthma and allergic disease throughout the world, but particularly in affluent westernised countries. In the UK, the lifetime prevalence of parentally reported asthma in schoolchildren living in Aberdeen was approximately 4% in 1964, whereas by 2004 it had increased to around 26% (Devenny *et al.* 2004) (see Fig. 13.2). Similarly, the lifetime prevalence of eczema increased from about 5% in 1964 to 26% in 2004, and hayfever increased from about 3% to 19% in the same period. In the US, the prevalence of self-reported asthma increased from 3.1% in 1980 to 5.6% in 1995, being more marked in children (an increase from 3.5% to 7.5%) than adults (an increase from 2.9% to 5.0%) and associated with increased asthma-related activity in primary and secondary care settings, e.g. physician office visits for asthma increasing from 5.9 million in 1980 to 13.6 million in 2004 (Moorman *et al.* 2007). Although in most countries the prevalence of asthma, atopic dermatitis and allergic rhinitis continues to increase, recent studies (Asher *et al.* 2006) suggest that in some countries the prevalence of asthma, and to a lesser extent atopic dermatitis and allergic rhinitis, has plateaued and might even be declining. Given the close association between IgE-mediated food allergy and the other allergic diseases, it is likely that the prevalence of food allergy has increased in recent years. Analysis of allergic reactions severe enough to warrant hospital admission in England suggested that the prevalence of such severe reactions increased 5.8-fold between 1990 and 2000 (Gupta *et al.* 2004). Follow-up of serial birth cohorts from the Isle of Wight in the UK suggests that the prevalence of IgE sensitisation to peanut in 3- and 4-year-old children was higher (3.3%) in those born in 1994–6 than in those born in 1989 (1.1%) (Grundy *et al.* 2002). Follow-up of a more recent birth cohort suggests that the rate of increase may have plateaued or indeed decreased, with a reported prevalence of 2.0% (Venter *et al.* 2008). The rapid increase in asthma and allergic disease in recent decades is almost certainly a consequence of changing environment and/or lifestyle and there is increasing evidence that exposure to such factors during fetal development and the first few years of life play a particularly important role in modifying the likelihood of asthma and allergic disease in later life.

13.4 Impact of asthma and allergic disease

Asthma is now one of the world's most common chronic diseases with approximately 300 million people suffering from it. It has been estimated that by 2025 there could be an additional 100 million people with the disease. Asthma is a common and costly disease globally as it accounts for the loss of approximately 15 million disability-adjusted life years (DALYs), similar to that for diabetes, cirrhosis, or schizophrenia (Masoli *et al.* 2004). In the UK, there are an estimated 5.2 million people with asthma, 1.1 million being children, and the total annual direct and indirect costs to the UK economy are about £2.5 billion (Asthma UK 2004). In the US, 20 million people have asthma, 6.2 million being children, and the total direct and indirect costs to the US economy are about $20 billion annually (Moorman *et al.* 2007). In affluent countries, atopic dermatitis is common, affecting up to 30% of pre-school children, 15–20% of schoolchildren and 7% of adults, with estimated direct and indirect economic costs similar to those for asthma (Jenner *et al.* 2004). It has been estimated that

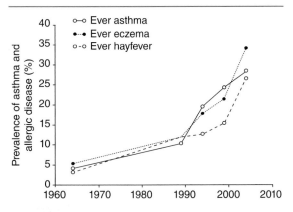

Figure 13.2 The increasing prevalence of asthma and allergic diseases in serial cross-sectional surveys of Aberdeen schoolchildren aged 9–12 years between 1964 and 2004.
Adapted from McNeill *et al.* (2009) Changes in the prevalence of asthma, eczema and hayfever in pre-pubertal children: a 40-year perspective. *Paediatric and Perinatal Epidemiology*, **23**: 506–12, with permission from Wiley-Blackwell Publishing, Oxford.

10–15% of the UK population has allergic rhinitis, with significant and unappreciated adverse effects on quality of life, schooling and employment. In the UK and the US the prevalence of IgE-mediated food allergies in children is about 5–6%, but in young children less than 3 years old food allergies are more common, affecting approximately 6–8% with a predominance of allergic reactions to cows' milk and hens' egg. In adults the prevalence of food allergies is approximately 3–4% (Buttriss 2002). Food allergies are associated with a significant reduction in the quality of life of food-allergic patients and their families because of the restrictions imposed by food allergen avoidance, the difficulty in avoiding food allergens and the potential for sudden, life-threatening anaphylactic reactions.

13.5 Importance of antenatal and early life influences on asthma and allergic disease

It now seems increasingly likely that early life factors play a critical role in the development of asthma and allergic disease and that exposures during fetal life can influence the development of these conditions. Furthermore, some of the reported associations suggest that fetal nutritional status has long-term consequences for the development of asthma and allergic disease in children and adults.

13.5.1 Birth anthropometry

The first indications of the importance of antenatal factors in the development of asthma and allergic disease were reports of associations between anthropometric measurements made at birth (e.g. head circumference, length and weight) and the subsequent development of asthma and allergic disease. One of the first studies reported that IgE concentrations were elevated in 50-year-old adults who, at birth, had relatively larger head circumferences (0.30 inches or 0.8 cm) relative to their trunk and limbs (Godfrey *et al.* 1994). It was suggested that disproportionate fetal growth of the head relative to the trunk and limbs reflected relative fetal malnutrition with consequent diversion of fetal blood and nutrients to the brain at the expense of the trunk and limbs. The relative under-nutrition of the trunk was surmised to adversely impact on thymic development, leading to the development of Th2-biased immune responses.

Overt maternal malnutrition during pregnancy is rare in westernised countries with a high prevalence of asthma; however, Dutch adults aged about 50 years were more likely to have an elevated IgE to pollen, and to suffer from obstructive airways disease (a term covering asthma, chronic bronchitis and emphysema) if they were exposed *in utero* to the Dutch famine in early and mid-gestation (Lopuhaa *et al.* 2000) (see Chapter 1, Section 1.4.1; and Chapter 4, Section 4.4.2). Reports from many birth cohort and cross-sectional studies suggest that reduced birthweight is associated with an increased likelihood of asthma, and that increased birthweight and birth head circumference are associated with an increased likelihood of allergic rhinitis, atopic dermatitis and elevated serum IgE. There are very few studies investigating associations between birth measurements and food allergy, one reporting increased birthweight associated with an increased risk (Hikino *et al.* 2001) and one reporting no associations (Liem *et al.* 2007). While it would appear that birth measurements are associated with the subsequent development of asthma and allergic disease, the exact mechanisms underlying these associations are unknown. The suggestion that relative fetal under-nutrition, by preserving brain development, adversely affects thymic development now seems unlikely. This hypothesis predicts that an increased ratio of head circumference to birthweight should be associated with an increased risk of allergic disease such as hayfever. However, a well-conducted study has reported hayfever to be associated with a reduced ratio of birth head circumference to birthweight (Katz *et al.* 2003). Moreover, birth head circumference has been reported to be positively associated with thymic size as assessed by ultrasound one week after birth. The demonstration of associations between birth measurements and asthma and allergic disease support the concept of fetal programming contributing to these conditions, and fetal nutrition is generally considered to be relevant to these associations.

13.5.2 Neonatal lung function and asthma

Long-term follow-up of several birth cohorts has demonstrated that fetal lung and airway development tracks throughout life, with reduced lung function at birth being mirrored by reduced lung function during child and adulthood (Turner *et al.* 2004; Haland *et al.* 2006). Suboptimal fetal airway development appears to be one mechanism by which ante-natal factors can increase the likelihood of childhood asthma, particularly if there is parallel Th2 differentiation as evidenced by the development of allergic diseases. This is supported by cohort studies that have reported the likelihood of childhood asthma and wheezing illness to be associated with reduced lung function at birth (Haland *et al.* 2006). Recent tracking of postnatal lung function has been shown to commence *in utero*, with a reduced fetal growth trajectory being associated with reduced lung function and an increased likelihood of asthma at the age of 5. Moreover, there is some indication that the rate of fetal growth is associated with first-trimester maternal plasma α-tocopherol (Turner *et al.* 2010).

13.5.3 Neonatal immunology

Further evidence for the importance of antenatal factors in the development of asthma and allergic disease comes from work with cord blood mononuclear cells (CBMC) isolated from the umbilical cords of neonates. CBMC samples contain Th-cells and antigen-presenting cells. *In vitro*, allergen-specific neonatal CBMC proliferative and cytokine responses have been reported to be not only associated with the subsequent development of allergic disease (Warner *et al.* 1994), but also with reported antenatal risk factors for asthma and allergic disease, e.g. maternal allergic disease, maternal diet and maternal smoking (Devereux *et al.* 2002). In the broadest sense, the associations with CBMC suggest that antenatal factors influence the developing fetal immune system and subsequent asthma and allergic disease. CBMC responses and their associations have contributed in some countries to shaping public health advice to pregnant women and will be discussed below.

Speculation persists as to the possible influence of nutrition on the development of asthma and allergic disease and the mechanisms involved. Two components of the diet have been investigated: food allergens in the diet, and the nutrient content of the foods consumed.

13.6 Maternal dietary food allergen intake during pregnancy and breastfeeding

The potential for early life exposure to common food allergens such as cows' milk, hens' eggs and peanuts

to programme the immune system towards the development of food allergy has attracted much scientific and popular interest. In the early 1990s, several lines of evidence led to the belief that maternal consumption of food allergens during pregnancy and lactation increased the likelihood of susceptible children developing food allergies:

(1) Reports of allergic reactions after the first known consumption of a food allergen (e.g. egg, milk or peanut) by young children suggested prior occult exposure and allergic sensitisation to food allergens (van Asperen *et al.* 1983). These reports were in keeping with an adverse effect of maternally ingested food allergens being transmitted to children either during fetal development or during breastfeeding.

(2) A number of mechanisms have been identified that prevent the maternal immune system mounting a lethal immune response against the paternal antigens expressed by the fetus. The microenvironment of the placental materno–fetal interface is heavily biased against Th1 differentiation, with placental trophoblast secreting progesterone and cytokines such as IL-4, IL-10, IL-13, TGF-β that inhibit Th1 differentiation and Th1 effector function within the uterus. The success of a pregnancy is critically dependent on an intrauterine cytokine microenvironment biased against the Th1 phenotype. This led to the idea that fetal allergen exposure in the context of the intrauterine environment biased against the Th1 phenotype increases the likelihood of a Th2-biased fetal immune response to allergens, and a subsequent increase in the likelihood of childhood allergic disease.

(3) Reports of *in vitro* allergen-specific proliferative and cytokine CBMC responses after stimulation by aeroallergens (e.g. house dust mite, cat) and food allergens (typically β-lactoglobulin and ovalbumin) were interpreted as evidence of fetal exposure to, and immunological sensitisation by, maternally sourced allergens (Miles *et al.* 1996). Moreover, reports that such CBMC responses are associated with the subsequent development of childhood allergic disease supported the hypothesis that fetal exposure to maternally ingested food allergens increased the risk of food allergy in children (Warner *et al.* 1994).

In 1998, based on the available data the United Kingdom Committee on Toxicity of Chemicals in

Food, Consumer Products and the Environment (COT) (Committee on Toxicity of Chemicals in Food Consumer Products and the Environment 1998) whilst acknowledging that studies relating peanut consumption by pregnant and lactating women to allergy in their offspring were inconclusive, concluded that 'There is some support for the suggestions that peanut allergy in an infant can result from exposure *in utero* or during lactation' and that 'with regard to the mechanism of sensitisation and allergy such a link is, however, possible. It was decided therefore that it would be unwise to discount sensitisation of offspring resulting from exposure of the mother.' The COT recommended that, for pregnancies where the mother, father or sibling had allergic disease, the pregnant woman may wish to avoid eating peanuts and peanut products during pregnancy, and subsequently while breastfeeding. The COT recommendation was accepted by the UK Department of Health and issued as advice in 1998 to pregnant women (see Section 13.6.4). The New Zealand Medicines and Medical Devices Safety Authority also reached similar conclusions and issued the same advice as the UK COT (Hannah 2000). The American Academy of Pediatrics recommended that no maternal dietary restrictions during pregnancy were necessary, with the possible exception of excluding peanuts, and that breastfeeding women should not consume peanuts and tree nuts (American Academy of Pediatrics 2000). Research since this advice was issued suggests that, while the fetus is exposed to allergens, the relationship (if any) between such allergen exposure and CBMC responses and food allergy is not straightforward and is discussed below.

13.6.1 Fetal allergen exposure

Artificial perfusion of fresh human placentas from term and pre-term deliveries has shown the food allergens β-lactoglobulin and ovalbumin rapidly cross the placenta from mother to fetus, and that this occurs in nearly all placentas (Szepfalusi, Loibichler *et al.* 2000; Edelbauer *et al.* 2004). In contrast, transfer of the inhaled allergen Bet v1 was shown to occur in only 20% of placentas. Further work using this model suggests that approximately 1 in 10 000 molecules of β-lactoglobulin and ovalbumin in the maternal circulation cross the placenta into the fetal circulation. This experimental work is supported by the detection of β-lactoglobulin and ovalbumin in umbilical cord blood at birth. The house dust mite allergen, der p1, has been detected in cord blood (60% of births) and amniotic fluid (10% of pregnancies) suggesting diamniotic transfer of allergens in addition to transplacental transfer. These studies suggest that the fetus is exposed to tiny amounts of ubiquitous nutrient allergens derived from the mother. However, the placental transfer of inhaled allergens appears to be less efficient and much less frequent.

13.6.2 Cord blood mononuclear cell responses and maternal exposure to allergen

The relationship between CBMC responses and maternal exposure to allergens during pregnancy has been clarified by studies of inhaled allergens. Nearly all studies relating maternal allergen exposure during pregnancy to neonatal CBMC responses have demonstrated that CBMC responses are not necessarily a consequence of maternal allergen exposure. In an allergen avoidance study in Manchester, UK, with a 21 000-fold difference between highest and lowest maternal exposures to der p1, there was no association between measured der p1 levels in the maternal mattress during pregnancy and CBMC proliferative responses after stimulation with der p1. Studies of seasonal allergens such as birch pollen and timothy grass pollen, which are only present in the air for well-defined periods of the year, have shown that CBMC responses after stimulation with these allergens are absent in a sizeable proportion of cord blood samples from children born to mothers exposed during pregnancy, and conversely, CBMC responses are present in children born to mothers who could not have been exposed during pregnancy (Szepfalusi, Pichler *et al.* 2000). Further work has used the CD45 isoform of Th-cells to identify whether CBMC responses are mediated by 'naive' or 'memory' Th-cells, and have shown that, while some CBMC responses after stimulation with timothy grass are mediated by 'memory' Th-cells (presumably stimulated *in utero*), some are mediated by 'naive' Th-cells that have never been stimulated before (Devereux *et al.* 2001). Taken as a whole, this work suggests that the association between antenatal allergen exposure and CBMC responses is complex, and that CBMC responses after stimulation with inhaled allergens do not necessarily reflect *in utero* exposure to the allergens.

13.6.3 Cord blood mononuclear cell responses and subsequent allergic disease

Although neonatal CBMC responses are associated with subsequent allergic disease, detailed investigation of such responses, and the timing of allergen sensitisation, suggest that the associations probably do not represent causality. CBMC and neonatal T-cell responses to allergens appear to differ markedly from those occurring later in life, and the CBMC/neonatal T-cells that respond are not those that subsequently underlie allergic disease. Responding neonatal T-cells have been reported to be naive immature thymic emigrants with modified antigen receptors which interact non-specifically with protein antigens, providing short-lived cellular immunity that does not generate conventional T-cell memory. It has also been demonstrated that stable IgE-associated Th2-cell memory to house dust mite and peanut occurs entirely postnatally and does not appear until after 6 months of age (Rowe *et al.* 2007).

13.6.4 Observational and intervention studies of maternal diet during pregnancy and lactation

The numerous observational and intervention studies investigating the association between childhood allergic disease and maternal dietary intake of food allergens during pregnancy and lactation have been systematically reviewed. These reviews have all highlighted the need for further trials because of the methodological shortcomings of the available data, but nevertheless the reviews have contributed to changes in the precautionary advice issued in the late 1990s.

In a position statement, the Australasian Society of Clinical Immunology and Allergy concluded that randomised controlled trials had not convincingly shown that dietary avoidance of multiple potential food allergens during pregnancy reduces the risk of allergic disease in children (Prescott and Tang 2005). Moreover, although several studies reported that maternal avoidance of potential food allergens while breastfeeding may reduce the risk of atopic dermatitis in the first few years of life, this was not a consistent finding. The recommendation of the Society was that pregnant and breastfeeding women should not avoid foods containing potential food allergens, and that the practice of avoiding potential food allergens

should be discouraged because of potential adverse nutritional consequences for the mother and fetus.

In 2008, the American Academy of Pediatrics revised its position statement on peanut avoidance during pregnancy and lactation by mothers of children at high risk of developing allergic disease (Greer *et al.* 2008). The overall conclusion of the Academy was that current evidence did not support a major role for maternal dietary restriction during pregnancy and while breastfeeding. A review of the available evidence concluded that, in general, maternal exclusion of potential food allergens during pregnancy had not been shown to reduce the risk of allergic disease in children. The Academy highlighted the methodological shortcomings in the studies that had related maternal food allergen avoidance during breastfeeding to childhood allergic disease, and that there was some disparity between the conclusions of systematic reviews. Most systematic reviews had concluded that there was no convincing evidence that maternal food allergen avoidance while breastfeeding had any long-term (>4 years) benefit on childhood allergic disease. However, one review concluded that while there was insufficient evidence that food allergen avoidance during breastfeeding reduced the risk of allergic disease in children, this may not be the case for atopic dermatitis and that further trials were required, particularly for atopic dermatitis.

In 2009, after a systematic review of the literature, the UK COT revised its 1998 precautionary advice that pregnant and breastfeeding women should avoid peanuts if there was a history of allergic disease in first-degree relatives of the child (Committee on Toxicity of Chemicals in Food 2009). The overall conclusion of this review was that the available evidence does not suggest an adverse or beneficial effect of maternal peanut consumption during pregnancy and lactation on the development of peanut allergy in children. However, because of the lack of high-quality studies, it is still possible that maternal peanut intake has no effect on the likelihood of childhood peanut allergy.

The COT also addressed the issue of allergic reactions after the first known consumption of a food allergen, by highlighting the potential importance of non-oral routes of peanut exposure, for example through inflamed skin, in the development of childhood peanut allergy. This route of exposure and sensitisation was highlighted by a report of an observational study that the use of peanut (arachis oil)-containing skin creams to treat inflamed eczematous skin is a risk factor for the development of peanut allergy in children (Lack *et al.* 2003). This finding is supported by work in animal models where the application of relatively small amounts of peanut extract or ovalbumin to eczematous skin can induce IgE-mediated immune responses to the allergens. Furthermore IgE sensitisation by this non-oral route appears to prevent induction of the tolerance that would normally develop after oral ingestion of the allergen. In the UK, all arachis oil-containing creams and ointments for use on the skin are now clearly labelled. The COT review also highlighted the reports in animal models that oral administration of ovalbumin to pregnant and lactating rodents reduced the development of IgE-mediated sensitisation to ovalbumin in offspring. Further animal studies have demonstrated that oral exposure to either ovalbumin or peanut extract in low doses may induce IgE sensitisation, whereas oral exposure to higher doses of the allergens may result in oral tolerance to the same allergen. Clearly the applicability of the animal data to humans is limited and should be interpreted with caution. However, if applicable to humans, these animal data suggest that attempts to avoid food allergens by women that result in 'low dose' exposure of children may increase the likelihood of allergic disease. Therefore further research is needed.

13.7 Breastfeeding and childhood atopic dermatitis and asthma

While breastfeeding of infants is recommended because of well-documented benefits for mother and child, the effects of breastfeeding on the subsequent development of atopic dermatitis, wheezing disease and asthma are not so clear. Many studies have investigated this issue, and these have been subject to several systematic reviews, most of which highlight the limitations and difficulties in conducting and interpreting such studies (e.g. confounding, recruitment bias, reporting bias, reverse causation, variation in breastfeeding patterns and an inability to randomise and 'blind'). The systematic reviews have themselves been reviewed in consensus documents (Prescott and Tang 2005; Greer *et al.* 2008). Overall, it would appear that the exclusive breastfeeding of infants at high risk of developing atopic disease (because of a positive first-degree family history of atopic disease) for 3–4 months reduces the likelihood of atopic dermatitis. Breastfeeding beyond 3–4 months appears to confer no additional benefit. The available evidence suggests that the breastfeeding of infants at low risk of developing atopic disease does not reduce the incidence of atopic dermatitis. The evidence for a protective effect of breastfeeding on the development of respiratory disease is controversial. While breastfeeding appears to reduce the incidence of viral-associated wheezing episodes in young children (<4 years), the evidence for an effect of breastfeeding on the development of asthma is conflicting. Systematic reviews suggest that exclusive breastfeeding for 3–4 months is associated with a reduced risk of asthma in children aged 2–5 years, but this beneficial effect is limited to infants at high risk of atopic disease. The 2008 American Academy of Pediatrics consensus report highlighted a number of studies that had reported breastfeeding to be associated with an increased likelihood of asthma in older children (>9 years), and that this increased risk was not necessarily related to the asthma/atopic risk status of the mother and child. The consensus report concluded that 'it is not possible to conclude that exclusive breastfeeding protects young infants who are at risk of developing atopic disease from developing asthma in the long-term (>6 years of age), and it may even have a detrimental effect'.

13.8 Infant dietary food allergen intake

The timing of the introduction of foods containing food allergens to the immature immune systems of infants, and the possible consequences for the development of allergic disease, especially food allergy, has attracted much scientific and popular attention. Of particular concern has been the timing of the introduction of cows' milk and cows' milk-based formula feeds. In the 2000 position statement, the American Academy of Pediatrics reflected these concerns by recommending that children at high risk of developing allergic disease should avoid eggs until the age of 2, and peanuts, tree nuts and fish until the age of 3. The most recent position statements on the introduction of complementary feeds from the American Academy of Pediatrics and the Australasian Society of Clinical Immunology and Allergy, while very similar, differ from previous advice (Prescott and Tang 2005; Greer *et al.* 2008). In line with WHO advice, exclusive breastfeeding is recommended for at least the first 4–6 months of life.

Numerous studies have investigated the role of partially and extensively hydrolysed formulas in reducing the risk of childhood allergic disease. However, most of the studies have focused on infants at high risk of allergic disease because of a family history of allergic disease in a first-degree relative. Follow-up of children in these trials has generally been relatively short and there is a need for trials to ascertain whether any beneficial effects on allergic disease are sustained into later childhood and adolescence. None of the studies of partially or extensively hydrolysed formulas reported any adverse effects. The review (Greer *et al.* 2008) concluded that in infants at high risk of allergic disease who are not exclusively breast-fed for 4–6 months, or who are formula-fed, there is modest evidence that atopic dermatitis may be delayed or prevented by the use of extensively or partially hydrolysed formulas rather than cows' milk-based formula. There is no evidence to suggest that partially and extensively hydrolysed formulas are any better than breast milk in the prevention of allergic disease, and such formulas should not be used in preference to breast milk. Based on the results of a meta-analysis, Greer *et al.* (2008) also concluded that there is no convincing evidence for the use of soy-based infant formula in the prevention of allergic disease.

Both the American and Australasian position statements recommend that solid foods should not be introduced before 4–6 months of age, and both reviews conclude that there is no convincing evidence that delaying the introduction of allergenic foods beyond this age reduces the likelihood of food allergy and allergic disease. However, even in the absence of evidence, the Australasian Society of Clinical Immunology suggests that peanut, tree nut and shellfish may be avoided for the first 2–4 years in high-risk children on the basis that it is unlikely to cause harm. However, as discussed above and below, this assertion could be contested.

A recent large cross-sectional study of Jewish schoolchildren living in the UK and Israel raises the possibility that the emphasis on delaying the introduction of food allergens, and the avoidance of food allergens, may be flawed. The prevalence of peanut allergy among UK children was 1.85% and in the Israeli children 0.17%, with the UK children being 9.8 times more likely to be allergic to peanuts (Du Toit *et al.* 2008). One of the many differences between Israel and the UK is in weaning practices; in Israel peanuts are introduced into the diet early and they are eaten more frequently and in larger amounts. It was suggested by the authors of this study that perhaps the early introduction of peanut-containing foods induced oral tolerance to the allergen. While this study is of scientific interest, it is insufficient evidence upon which to make recommendations. The issue of the potential benefits of the early introduction of allergenic foods into the diet of children is currently being investigated by two major clinical intervention trials, one focusing on peanuts in high-risk children (Learning Early About Peanut Allergy (LEAP); www.leapstudy.co.uk), the other on six allergenic foods in the general infant population (a randomised controlled trial of early introduction of allergenic foods to induce tolerance in infants; www.eatstudy.co.uk). The results of these studies are likely to influence advice given to parents of young children in the near future.

13.9 Early life nutrient intake

Although scientific and popular interest has mainly focused on the potential association between childhood allergic disease and early life food allergen exposure, there is increasing interest in the potential for the non-allergenic nutrient content of the maternal and infant diet to influence the development of childhood asthma, and to a lesser extent allergic disease. The basis for this work are hypotheses proposing that changing diet in westernised countries has contributed to the increase in asthma and allergic disease in the last decades of the twentieth century. When compared with the evidence pertaining to early life food allergen exposure, the evidence relating nutrients to asthma and allergic disease is very limited and speculative, but is included in this chapter because it is an area of active research with the potential to influence dietary advice to pregnant women (see Fig. 13.3).

13.9.1 Antioxidant hypothesis

The hypothesis that the recent increase in asthma has been, in part, a consequence of declining dietary antioxidant intake was based on the observation that, in the UK, asthma had increased concurrently with marked changes in the diet from a traditional diet comprising foods produced and marketed locally and eaten shortly after harvesting, to the modern

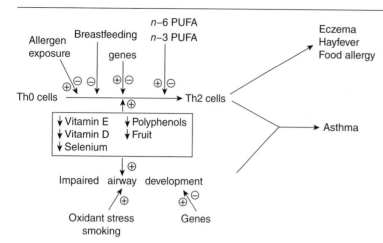

Figure 13.3 Potential mechanisms by which early life dietary exposures may influence the development of childhood asthma and allergy. Maternal nutrient status during pregnancy, as well as genetic and other environmental factors, has the potential to promote Th-cell responses towards the Th2 phenotype. This bias increases the likelihood of developing asthma, eczema and hayfever in childhood. Nutrient intake by mothers during pregnancy also has the potential to impair the development of the fetal airways, increasing the risk of development of asthma in childhood.

diet dominated by foods that have been processed, stored and transported great distances (Seaton *et al.* 1994). Limited evidence suggests that the dietary intake of some antioxidant nutrients (e.g. selenium and vitamin E) has declined, whereas for some antioxidants average intake has increased (e.g. vitamin C).

13.9.2 Polyunsaturated fatty acids hypothesis

In westernised countries the change from a traditional to a modern diet has been associated with changes in dietary fat intake, principally, increasing intake of *n-6* polyunsaturated fatty acid (PUFA) present in spreads and oils sourced from plant sources, and decreasing intakes of saturated fats (e.g., butter, lard) and long chain *n-3* PUFA such as eicosapentaenoic acid (EPA) and docosahexaenoic acid (DHA) that are present in oil-rich fish (e.g. herring, mackerel, trout, salmon) or derived fish oil products (cod liver oil). The 'lipid' hypothesis proposes that the combination of decreasing *n-3* and increasing *n-6* PUFA intakes has contributed to the increase in allergic disease and consequently asthma (Black and Sharpe 1997). A suggested mechanism relates increased dietary *n-6*:*n-3* PUFA ratio to increased inflammatory-cell membrane arachidonic acid levels and consequent increased synthesis of prostaglandin (PGE_2) by the action of cyclooxygenase-2. *In vitro*, PGE_2 suppresses Th1 and promotes Th2 differentiation. Although elegant, this proposed mechanism is almost certainly

an oversimplification because the immunological consequences of changing PUFA are very complex. Most research in the field to date, driven by the original 'lipid' hypothesis, has aimed to increase *n-3* PUFA intake; however, a recent detailed review of the available epidemiological evidence concluded that the observational data are more in keeping with reduced levels of *n-6* PUFA being associated with allergy and asthma, and that any intervention should comprise a mixture of long chain *n-3* and *n-6* PUFA (Sala-Vila *et al.* 2008).

13.9.3 Vitamin D hypotheses

Two contradictory hypotheses relate vitamin D to the increase in allergy and asthma. The first proposes the increase in allergy and asthma to be a consequence of widespread early life vitamin D supplementation for rickets prophylaxis in westernised countries (Wjst and Dold 1999), citing immunological studies of high-dose *in vitro* vitamin D supplementation promoting Th2 differentiation. The second hypothesis highlights the widespread vitamin D insufficiency reported in westernised countries, reflecting the increasing tendency to stay indoors, concerns about melanoma and the inability to compensate by dietary-sourced vitamin D. This hypothesis proposes that the increase in allergy and asthma is a consequence of widespread vitamin D insufficiency (Litonjua and Weiss 2007) and cited immunological reports of vitamin D promoting regulatory T-cell function and consequent inhibition of Th2 differentiation.

13.9.4 Maternal antioxidant status during pregnancy and childhood asthma and allergy

The potential for maternal antioxidant intake during pregnancy to modify the risk of childhood asthma has been highlighted by several birth cohort studies. Two such studies have reported wheezing in the first few years of life to be associated with reduced maternal plasma selenium during pregnancy and reduced umbilical cord selenium. Three birth cohort studies in the US, UK and Japan have reported associations between maternal vitamin E status during pregnancy and asthma and allergic outcomes in children (Devereux *et al.* 2006; Litonjua *et al.* 2006; Miyake *et al.* 2010). Two of these studies reported reduced maternal vitamin E intake during pregnancy to be associated with increased neonatal CBMC responses after stimulation with allergens, suggesting that maternal intake of foods containing vitamin E can influence the first interactions between the neonatal immune system and allergens (Devereux *et al.* 2002). All three studies reported childhood wheezing in the first few years of life (up to age 3) to be associated with a reduced maternal dietary vitamin E intake during pregnancy. The UK study further demonstrated reduced first-trimester maternal plasma α-tocopherol to be associated with reduced fetal growth (Turner *et al.* 2010) and at age 5, with reduced lung function and an increased risk of asthma. Furthermore, reduced maternal vitamin E intake during pregnancy was associated with an increased likelihood of wheezing and asthma outcomes in 5-year-old children. None of the studies reported associations between vitamin E and atopic dermatitis. However, the UK study reported that reduced maternal plasma α-tocopherol was associated with increased allergic sensitisation at age 5. Although not considered to be an antioxidant, the US and UK studies reported reduced maternal zinc intake during pregnancy to be associated with an increased likelihood of childhood wheezing, asthma and atopic dermatitis. The Irish Life-ways Cross-Generation Cohort Study reported high maternal fruit and vegetable intake during pregnancy to be associated with a reduced likelihood of asthma in children at age 3. A Menorcan birth cohort study has reported wheeze in children aged 6–7 years to be less frequent if mothers consumed a Mediterranean diet during pregnancy (Chatzi *et al.* 2008). The Menorcan and the UK study quantified the diets of the children, and while maternal and child diets were correlated, there were no associations with children's diets.

The biological mechanisms by which antioxidants could influence the development of childhood asthma are probably independent of their antioxidant properties because the associations appear limited to certain nutrients (with and without antioxidant properties) and not with all antioxidants. The reports from the birth cohort studies are consistent with a mechanism whereby maternal intake of certain nutrients influences fetal lung development, and the first critical interactions between the immune system and allergens. Vitamin E, selenium, zinc and polyphenolic compounds have been reported to influence fetal lung and airway development in animal models (Manthey 2000; Allan *et al.* 2010). They have also been reported to have complex effects on immunological and inflammatory pathways that may be relevant to the development of asthma and allergic disease. It would also appear that the effects of vitamin E on the immune system are age-dependent, becoming less potent as the immune system ages and matures.

13.9.5 Early life polyunsaturated fatty acid status and childhood asthma and allergy

Although many studies have related PUFA status of pregnant women and infants to childhood asthma and allergic disease, the vast majority have been observational, with a handful of intervention trials. Several cross-sectional studies, some with retrospective maternal recall of diet during pregnancy, have reported maternal fish intake during pregnancy to be associated with a reduced likelihood of childhood asthma and allergic sensitisation to inhaled and food allergens. In Japan, high maternal intake of the *n*-3 PUFAs DHA and α-linolenic acid were associated with a reduced likelihood of childhood wheezing at 16–24 months; in addition, higher maternal intakes of the *n*-6 PUFA linoleic acid were associated with an increased risk of childhood atopic dermatitis (Miyake *et al.* 2009). Umbilical cord blood PUFA concentrations have been related to subsequent childhood asthma and allergic disease, and in general, the reported associations have been inconsistent and fail to conform to a consistent pattern. The potential for PUFA to influence the first interactions between the immune system and allergens has been highlighted by a US cohort study reporting that high umbilical cord plasma n-3 and n-6 PUFA concentrations to be associated with reduced neonatal CBMC responses. While these associations are not consistent with the original 'lipid' hypothesis, they are in keeping with the recent suggestion that the most effective form of PUFA intervention will be with a combination of n-3 and n-6 PUFA (Sala-Vila *et al.* 2008).

Several intervention studies have investigated the potential for early life n-3 PUFA supplementation to prevent childhood asthma and allergic disease. A Danish randomised controlled trial investigating pregnancy outcomes supplemented the diets of pregnant women from 30 weeks' gestation with fish oil, olive oil or nothing (no capsules) (Olsen *et al.* 2008). When compared with children of olive oil supplemented mothers, the children of fish oil supplemented women were less likely to develop asthma. However, the study was unable to conclude that fish oil supplementation during pregnancy reduces the risk of childhood asthma because the children of women randomised to 'no capsules' also had a reduced risk of asthma, comparable to fish oil supplementation, possibly because women allocated to 'no capsules' chose to take commercially available fish oil capsules. An Australian randomised controlled trial of fish oil supplementation from 20 weeks' gestation reported that maternal fish oil supplementation was associated with a general reduction in neonatal CBMC cytokine responses. However, only the reduction in IL-10 response after stimulation with cat allergen was statistically significant (Dunstan *et al.* 2003). These two studies suggest that antenatal n-3 PUFA supplementation has the potential to influence neonatal immune responses to allergens, and reduce the likelihood of children developing asthma and allergic disease. However, further work is clearly required. Postnatal infant n-3 PUFA supplementation appears to confer minimal benefit. The Childhood Asthma Prevention Study concluded that while n-3 PUFA-rich fish oil supplementation during infancy reduced the likelihood of early childhood wheeze (at 18 months), it had no effect on the likelihood of asthma, wheeze and allergic disease in later childhood (at 3 and 5 years).

13.9.6 Early life vitamin D status and childhood asthma and allergy

The small number of studies relating early life vitamin D exposure to asthma have reported conflicting results (Devereux *et al.* 2009). Four birth cohort studies have reported low maternal vitamin D intake during pregnancy to be associated with an increased risk of wheeze and asthma outcomes up to the age of 5 years (Nurmatov *et al.* 2011). However, these studies did not assess total vitamin D status as reflected by serum 25-hydroxy vitamin D (25(OH)D). Two cohort studies have reported potentially adverse associations: regular high-dose ($\geq$2000 IU/day) vitamin D supplementation during infancy in a large Northern Finnish study (Hypponen *et al.* 2004) has been associated with an increased likelihood of asthma and allergic outcomes at 31 years, and in a UK birth cohort, elevated maternal blood 25(OH)D in the third trimester was associated with an increased likelihood of childhood asthma at 9 years (Gale *et al.* 2008). However, the study response rate was low (30%) and there was no adjustment for potential confounding. Currently there are at least two intervention studies under way, investigating the effects on childhood asthma and allergic disease from supplementing women during pregnancy (www.vdaart.com; http://clinicaltrials.gov/ct2/show/NCT00856947). The results of these studies will clarify the role of vitamin D in the primary prevention of asthma and allergic disease.

13.9.7 Early life nutrient intake and childhood asthma and allergic disease

The very limited available evidence suggests that maternal nutrient status during pregnancy may influence the development of childhood asthma, and to a lesser extent allergic disease. While this area of active research is scientifically interesting, there is clearly insufficient evidence to advise pregnant women to change or supplement their diet in order to reduce the risk of their children developing asthma and allergic disease.

The observational and very limited intervention data suggest that while there is an association between maternal nutrient intake during pregnancy and childhood asthma and allergic disease, the nature of the association (with PUFA, antioxidants, nutrients, food), the timing (antenatal, infancy, childhood, adulthood) and the therapeutic potential of the association(s) is far from clear. Indeed it remains a distinct possibility that the observed associations are a consequence of confounding by complex social and behavioural factors. The manipulation of maternal diet during pregnancy to reduce the risk of childhood asthma and allergic disease remains a tantalising possibility worthy of further investigation because of the potential benefits for individuals and society. Ultimately, the role of dietary intervention to prevent childhood asthma will only be elucidated by intervention studies. The scientific justification for intervention with single nutrients during pregnancy is severely weakened by the negative results of trials investigating the effects of antioxidant supplementation on cardiovascular disease, cancer and all-cause mortality, despite a wealth of data from observational studies suggesting beneficial associations. The disparity between observational studies and trials has been attributed to a failure to appreciate the complex and important differences between adults with high and low antioxidant intakes. The nature of any intervention needs careful consideration, with dietary-based interventions probably being more acceptable to pregnant women. These have the added advantage of not only including the individual nutrient of interest, but also the nutrients and co-factors that are naturally associated with them.

13.10 Obesity and childhood asthma and allergic disease

The increase in asthma and allergic disease in westernised countries has been paralleled by an increase in the prevalence of obesity in adults and children. The association between obesity, asthma and allergy will be briefly outlined in this section; for a more in-depth discussion of the early life nutritional influences on the development of obesity see Chapter 8.

Numerous cross-sectional and case–control studies have reported significant associations between asthma and body mass index (BMI). Similar associations have also been reported by longitudinal cohort studies with meta-analyses of these studies concluding that being overweight increased the likelihood of incident asthma by 38% (95% CI: 17–62%), with obesity increasing the risk by 92% (95% CI: 43–159%) (Beuther and Sutherland 2007). The association between BMI and allergic disease is less clear. Some studies have reported associations between allergic outcomes and

BMI in one sex, whereas other larger studies fail to report associations with allergic outcomes, despite reporting associations between BMI and asthma.

The mechanisms responsible for the association between BMI and asthma remain unknown. Obesity undoubtedly adversely impacts lung mechanics, with reductions in many parameters of lung function. In addition, obesity can contribute to breathlessness by adversely affecting cardiovascular function and increasing the likelihood of gastro-oesophageal reflux. It is not clear whether asthma and allergic disease are a manifestation of the systematic inflammatory state associated with obesity. Although work in murine models (rats and mice) suggests that obesity modulates airway inflammation, the results of studies in humans are not so clear, with reports that BMI is not associated with inflammatory indices in induced sputum, nor exhaled nitric oxide in subjects with and without asthma. Moreover, while weight loss trials demonstrate that weight loss in obese people with asthma is associated with improved lung function and reduced symptoms, the lack of effect on exhaled nitric oxide levels suggest that any improvement is a consequence of improving lung mechanics rather than reducing airway inflammation.

13.11 Conclusions

There is increasing interest in the early life factors that influence the development of asthma and allergic disease. It seems highly likely that dietary factors can modify the likelihood of asthma and allergic disease by influencing fetal organogenesis and immune development. The main focus of research has undoubtedly been the possible adverse effects of fetal and infant exposure to food allergens. However, the current limited evidence suggests that such exposures may not be as detrimental as originally thought. Indeed, there are ongoing trials attempting to induce oral tolerance by encouraging early life exposure to food allergens. There is now interest in the nutrient content of the maternal diet during pregnancy with the ultimate aim of dietary intervention during pregnancy to reduce the burden of childhood asthma and allergic disease. A very limited evidence base suggests that, while there are associations between components of the maternal diet and childhood asthma, the therapeutic benefit of these is far from clear and further research is required.

13.12 Key points

- Asthma and allergic diseases have increased in prevalence and are now associated with significant morbidity and sizeable use of healthcare resources.
- Asthma and allergic diseases are characterised by an inappropriate immune response biased towards the Th2 phenotype. Tissue-specific deficits probably also critically contribute to the inflammatory process(es).
- It is becoming increasingly apparent that early life influences during fetal development and early childhood critically influence the development of asthma and allergic disease.
- Concerns that maternal ingestion of food allergens during pregnancy and lactation increase the risk of childhood allergic disease have been re-evaluated, and allergen avoidance during pregnancy and lactation is no longer recommended.
- Breastfeeding for 3–4 months reduces the incidence of atopic dermatitis in infants at high risk of allergic disease. While breastfeeding appears to reduce the risk of wheezing and asthma in young children (<6 years), any effects of breastfeeding on these conditions in older children are not so clear.
- Concerns regarding the introduction of potential food allergens into the diets of young children have been reconsidered, and delaying the introduction of potential food allergens beyond 6 months is not widely advocated.
- Although many studies have reported associations between increasing BMI and incident asthma, and that weight loss is associated with improved lung function and reduced asthma symptoms, it is not clear whether the association between obesity and asthma reflects adverse effects on lung mechanics and/or effects on airway inflammation.
- There is increasing interest in the possibility that the nutrient content (e.g. vitamin E, vitamin D, zinc, selenium, PUFA) of the maternal diet during pregnancy can influence the development of childhood asthma and allergic disease.

13.13 Recommendations for future research

- The possible association between early life allergen exposure and subsequent asthma and allergic disease needs to be established by well-conducted pragmatic trials.
- Trials are required to evaluate whether manipulation of maternal nutrient intake during pregnancy can reduce the likelihood of childhood asthma and allergic disease.
- Genetic susceptibilities and interactions with dietary exposures need to be clarified.
- There is still a need to identify novel non-dietary early life influences on asthma and allergic disease and to conduct pragmatic trials to ascertain whether manipulation of these exposures can reduce the prevalence of asthma and allergic disease.

13.14 Key references

Committee on Toxicity of Chemical in Food, Consumer Products and the Environment (2009) *Statement on the review of the 1998 COT recommendations on peanut avoidance.* http://cot.food.gov.uk/pdfs/cotstatement 200807peanut.pdf. (accessed 4 January 2013).

Greer FR, Sicherer SH & Burks AW (2008) Effects of early nutritional interventions on the development of atopic disease in infants and children: the role of maternal dietary restriction, breastfeeding, timing of introduction of complementary foods, and hydrolysed formulas. *Pediatrics*, **121**, 183–91.

Nurmatov U, Devereux G & Sheikh A (2011) Nutrients and foods for the primary prevention of asthma and allergy: systematic review and meta-analysis. *Journal of Allergy and Clinical Immunology*, **127**, 724–33.

Sala-Vila A, Miles EA & Calder PC (2008) Fatty acid composition abnormalities in atopic disease: evidence explored and role in the disease process examined. *Clinical and Experimental Allergy*, **38**, 1432–50.

Sin DD & Sutherland ER (2008) Obesity and the lung: 4. Obesity and asthma. *Thorax*, **63**, 1018–23.

14
Nutrition and Development: Early Nutrition, Mental Development and Mental Ageing

14.1 The importance of mental development and ageing

This chapter focuses on the effects of early nutrition on mental development and ageing. By 'mental' we refer jointly to cognitive function and to mental health; and by 'mental health' we refer essentially to conduct and emotional problems in development, and to emotional problems, such as depression, in ageing. Mental function thus defined has a major impact on life chances, economic productivity, physical morbidity and, ultimately, survival. Cognitive skills in childhood are a strong predictor of educational achievement (Deary *et al.* 2007), which in turn is the principal gateway to adult socioeconomic attainment, especially for contemporary school-leavers. Cognitive skills underlie activities of everyday living, such as learning and retaining new information, multitasking, and reasoning and problem solving. In functional terms, cognitive ability also underpins literacy and numeracy, the significance of which have increased as traditional labour markets in Western countries move towards a more service-based economy, and as people assume more responsibility for self-care in an increasingly complex information age (Richards, Power *et al.* 2009). Childhood cognitive ability also tracks into adulthood (Richards and Sacker 2003), and directly

predicts dementia risk (Whalley *et al.* 2006), a major disease burden in later life.

With regard to mental health, nearly 10% of children aged 5–16 years have a clinically diagnosable mental health problem (Green *et al.* 2005). Childhood behavioural problems have a large negative impact on life chances, particularly socioeconomic attainment and social function (Richards, Abbott *et al.* 2009). Furthermore, most childhood-onset emotional problems persist into adulthood; Rutter *et al.* (2006) estimated that depressed adolescents have 2–7 times the odds of being depressed in adulthood, with 40–70% showing major depressive disorder (MDD) during this phase of the life course. MDD is now the leading cause of disease burden in middle- and high-income countries (World Health Organization (WHO) 2008).

Cognition and mental health are inter-associated at all stages of the life course. They have common early life antecedents; both are regulated by common underlying physiological processes; both track across the life course and influence each other through complex causal chains; depression is also a risk factor for cognitive decline in later life and can coexist with Alzheimer's disease. This chapter focuses on one common early life antecedent – early diet and nutrition. Early diet has been selected as many nutrients that influence brain growth, such as iodine, iron,

Nutrition and Development: Short- and Long-Term Consequences for Health, First Edition. Edited by the British Nutrition Foundation.
© 2013 the British Nutrition Foundation. Published 2013 by Blackwell Publishing Ltd.

folate and essential long-chain polyunsaturated fatty acids (PUFAs), jointly influence cognitive and socio-emotional development (Wachs 2009), with implications for mental ageing.

14.2 Maternal diet during pregnancy

Neural development begins early, soon after conception, and by the time of birth head circumference, an index of brain volume, is far closer to its final size than the rest of the body (see Chapter 2, Section 2.5.2 and Chapter 6, Section 6.2). Thus maternal diet during pregnancy has a fundamental effect on brain development, with implications for mental function across the life course. This is a complex issue; careful analysis showed that a reduction in birthweight after maternal starvation in the Dutch Hunger Winter cohort of the 1940s (see Chapter 1, Section 1.4.1; and Chapter 4, Section 4.4.2) did not have an adverse impact on cognitive development (Stein *et al.* 1975), almost certainly because brain development is protected under such extreme circumstances. More specifically, for example, the fetal requirement for docosahexaenoic acid (DHA), (see Chapter 6, Section 6.4.5) under compromised maternal dietary supply can, to some extent, be met by conservation of essential fatty acids through reduced oxidation; by accessing preformed DHA and eicosapentaenoic acid (EPA) in adipose tissue reserves; and by increased formation from the precursor fatty acid, alpha-linolenic acid (ALA). Nevertheless, intake of this precursor is less effective for DHA deposition in the fetal brain than preformed DHA (Koletzko *et al.* 2007). The extent to which ALA is converted to DHA appears to differ between groups of individuals, with evidence suggesting that the conversion is greater in young women than young men (Burdge *et al.* 2002; Burdge and Wootton 2002). It remains unclear whether the higher ALA conversion observed in women is due to differences in oestrogen exposure or differences in the magnitude and mobilisation of body DHA stores (Burdge and Wootton 2002).

A consensus statement by a panel convened by the European Commission (Koletzko *et al.* 2007) recommends that pregnant and lactating women should aim to achieve a dietary intake of *n*-3 long-chain essential fatty acids to supply a DHA intake of at least 200 mg/day (equivalent to two portions (140 g) of oil-rich fish per week). One effect of this intake is to prolong pregnancy duration, with a beneficial effect on fetal development. In this context, it should be noted that the third trimester of pregnancy is a time of particularly rapid fetal growth, when the brain has a high demand for DHA (Cetin *et al.* 2009). Evidence at the population level tends to support the above European Commission recommendations. In particular, consumption of oil-rich fish during pregnancy in the large UK Avon Longitudinal Study of Parents and Children (ALSPAC) was associated with a range of outcomes including better verbal IQ (at 8 years), fine motor skills at 18 and 42 months (but not at 6 and 30 months), social development at 30 and 42 months (but not at 6 and 18 months) and communication at 6 and 18 months, after controlling for a large number (*n* = 28) of potential confounders (Hibbeln *et al.* 2007). It should be briefly noted that the consumption of oil-rich fish during pregnancy is a controversial topic because of potential exposure to neurotoxins such as mercury; although the European Commission (Koletzko *et al.* 2007) recommendation of two portions of oil-rich fish per week rarely exceeds the tolerable intake of such environmental contaminants.

However, a Cochrane review found no evidence that fatty acid supplementation benefited indicators of early development, such as visual acuity and Bayley scores (Schulzke *et al.* 2011), although this review involved trials conducted in pre-term neonates, rather than drawn from those based on full-term infants.

Finally, pregnancy is associated with a reduction in functional long-chain PUFA status of the mother herself, the so-called maternal depletion syndrome (Hornstra 2000). Since postpartum normalisation is still incomplete after 6 months (Al *et al.* 1995) this may become problematic if the time interval between births is at a minimum.

The emphasis so far has been on long-chain PUFA, but in fact a range of maternal nutrients are important for central nervous system (CNS) development, including the B vitamins. Severe vitamin B_{12} deficiency during pregnancy, caused by untreated malabsorption or certain kinds of extreme vegetarian diet, can lead to a range of neurological deficits in infants, such as delayed myelination, which affects mental development (Dror and Allen 2008). However, these deficits respond well to supplementation (*ibid*). Closely related to homocysteine metabolism is choline, which is necessary for development of the hippocampus, a subcortical structure essential for learning and memory. Animal studies suggest that maternal intake of choline, which is present primarily in liver (note that liver is not advised during pregnancy; see Chapter 3, Table 3.4), eggs and wheat germ, directly influences brain development, and may also reduce behavioural consequences of prenatal stress (Zeisel 2006).

Vitamin D receptors are located in the hippocampus and cerebral cortex, and relevant deficiencies may be found in vegetarians and those who have little exposure to sunlight. However, a recent systematic review of observational studies in adults found no conclusive evidence of an association between intake of this vitamin and cognition (Annweiler *et al.* 2009) and a Cochrane review concluded that there is insufficient evidence to evaluate the effects of supplementation on birth outcomes (Mahomed and Gulmezoglu 2000).

Of greater relevance, several micronutrients such as iodine and iron are critical to mental development; moreover, these are deficient in many regions of the world. More than 200 million children under the age of 5 years in developing countries are not fulfilling their developmental potential (Grantham-McGregor *et al.* 2007) because of some form of malnutrition. The International Child Development Steering Group identified iodine, iron and zinc deficiency as the major sources of nutritional deficiency affecting linear growth (Walker *et al.* 2007).

Iron deficiency anaemia is one of the most prevalent forms of malnutrition in the world (Stoltzfus 2003), and evidence in non-human primates suggests that prenatal iron deprivation leads to behavioural disturbance (Golub *et al.* 2006). The topic of iron deficiency anaemia in children will be returned to in Section 14.4.2. Iodine deficiency can lead to endemic cretinism (whether hypothyroid type, which also occurs in regions deficient in selenium, or neurologic type), and is the most common preventable cause of learning disability (Walker *et al.* 2007); intake of iodine before conception or during pregnancy is important to prevent this (Kretchmer *et al.* 1996), particularly in the first and second trimesters (O'Donnell *et al.* 2002) (see Chapter 15, Section 15.3.3.7). Finally, zinc is important for neurogenesis and establishment of neural cytoarchitecture. Human evidence suggests that low maternal intake of zinc is associated with impaired attention and decreased motor function in infants (Bhatnagar and Taneja 2001), although supplementation trials have

yielded mixed results, possibly because of other micronutrient deficiencies that coexist (Walker *et al.* 2007).

An implicit assumption so far is that the influence of maternal nutrition affecting mental development runs through direct maternal absorption-fetal CNS pathways, and indeed this is the case. However, in the last part of this section we consider other pathways through which this influence is brought to bear; in these cases the topic of behavioural and emotional development is particularly instructive. The first concerns maternal dietary effects on fetal growth, and on the adverse birth outcomes of low birthweight, pre-term birth and intrauterine growth restriction (IUGR). Importantly, birthweight across the full range in the normal population is itself associated with cognitive (e.g. Richards *et al.* 2001; Shenkin *et al.* 2004) and behavioural (Kelly *et al.* 2001) development. This is likely to be related to endocrine systems that regulate physical growth, particularly the growth hormones, hypothalamic–pituitary–adrenal (HPA) and thyroid axes, while targeting brain networks that underpin higher mental function (Berger 2001; Thompson, Syddall *et al.* 2001). In this context the chief nutritional determinant of gestational weight gain is energy (Abu-Saad and Fraser 2010), although effects of protein, essential fatty acids, iron and folate are also reviewed by these authors. The UK Department of Health recommend an additional 0.8 MJ/day (191 kcal/day) during the third trimester only (Department of Health 1991; SACN 2011b) (see Chapter 3, Section 3.4.1.1 and Chapter 15, Section 15.2.1.1).

However, it should be noted that the role of fetal growth as a mediating mechanism between maternal diet and cognitive and behavioural development is far from being fully established.

Wachs (2009) highlights two further mechanisms that extend the influence of maternal diet on mental development beyond direct maternal absorption–fetal CNS pathways. First, maternal nutritional deficits typically concur with other factors that can impair fetal development, such as teratogenic agents at the ecological level, and psychosocial stress. Second, while this might be considered to be a straightforward matter of confounding from an epidemiological perspective, maternal nutrition is capable of influencing the mental health of the mother herself, with indirect effects on the infant via parenting behaviour and infant attachment. For example, synthesis of serotonin, a monoamine neurotransmitter that regulates mood, is influenced by intake of foods containing tryptophan (Christensen 1996). This indirect effect of maternal nutrition through quality of parenting almost certainly influences cognitive development in parallel with behavioural and emotional development.

While fetal life may be thought of as the period of most rapid neural development, dramatic development of this nature also occurs during first 5 years of postnatal life. At this time environmental factors, including nutrients, play a critical role in the 'blooming and pruning' of the cytoarchitecture of the brain (Levitt 2003). Typically the first postnatal nutritional exposure is that of breastfeeding.

14.3 Breastfeeding

Before moving to the specifics of breastfeeding in relation to mental development and ageing, we should note that human breast milk contains numerous macro- and micronutrients that are beneficial to a wide range of health outcomes (see Chapter 3, Section 3.7). These include fatty acids (specific triglycerides e.g. palmitic and oleic acid; lipids e.g. vaccenic acid, and conjugated linoleic acid; and lipase, which breaks down fat for ease of infant absorption and digestion); long-chain PUFAs (see Section 14.3.1); carbohydrates (e.g. lactose bifidus factor, which encourages the growth of lactobacillus bifidus which helps prevent the growth of harmful colonic bacteria); proteins (e.g. casein, alpha-lactalbumin, lysozyme, serum albumin), as well as vitamins and major and trace minerals. Breast milk also provides antibody and lymphocyte defence mechanisms that are individualised to the mother–infant dyad, anti-inflammatory agents and antimicrobial factors (e.g. secretory immunoglobulin A, oligosaccharides and fatty acids). Finally, breast milk provides digestive enzymes (e.g. bile acid stimulated lipase; BASL), and a range of hormones, including nonpeptides (e.g. thyroid hormones, cortisol, progesterone, pregnanediol, oestrogens); peptide and growth factors (e.g. erythropoietin, gonadotropin-releasing hormone, epidermal growth factor insulin, insulin-like growth factor-I, nerve growth factor, transforming growth factor-alpha, gastrointestinal regulatory peptides and thyroid-parathyroid hormones). For further information in this area, and on the relationship between maternal diet and breast milk composition the reader is referred to Chapter 3, Section 3.7.

14.3.1 Breastfeeding and cognitive development

It has been acknowledged since the 1920s that breast-fed infants achieve higher scores on tests of cognitive development than infants fed on formula (Hoefer and Hardy 1929). While there have been many arguments about the possible confounding effects of parental factors, the dominant biomedical model maintains that such cognitive benefit results from the presence of essential long-chain PUFAs in breast milk, particularly arachidonic (AA) and DHA. The latter, which favour the development of the cerebral cortex and retina, accumulate during the last trimester from the placenta and during first year of life (Crawford 1993). These can be synthesised by infants, but only in small amounts. Current evidence indicates that AA (the *n*-6 long-chain PUFA) is more readily synthesised than DHA (Uauy *et al.* 2000; Haggarty 2010).

However, other potential mechanisms, such as the effect of long-chain PUFA control of inflammation, or promotion of the growth hormone pituitary axis, should be considered. Based on these explanations we can understand why this cognitive advantage is observed even when breast milk is delivered via nasal tube rather than during the nurturing contact that typically takes place during mother-infant feeding (Morley *et al.* 1988; Lucas *et al.* 1992). This does not rule out other potentially confounding factors, such as common genetic influences, prenatal maternal diet, which may influence pregnancy duration (see Section 14.2), and parental factors or material home conditions following weaning. Nevertheless, randomised controlled studies in term (Uauy *et al.* 2003) and pre-term (Uauy *et al.* 2000) infants indicate benefits to the CNS, as indicated by improvements in visual function.

A systematic review and meta-analysis of the evidence derived from 16 observational studies in children reported a benefit of 3.16 points (95% CI: 2.35–3.98) in cognitive function during early infancy and adolescence from breastfeeding after adjusting for at least 5 of 15 key covariates (duration of breastfeeding, sex, maternal smoking history, maternal age, maternal cognitive ability, maternal education, maternal training, paternal education, race or ethnicity, socioeconomic status, family size, birth order, birthweight, gestational age and childhood experiences) (Anderson *et al.* 1999). Additional findings of this review were a dose–response effect for duration of breastfeeding, evidence that the cognitive benefit from breastfeeding emerges within the first 2 years of life, and that low-birthweight infants derive more cognitive benefit from breastfeeding than infants within the normal birthweight range.

It should be noted that a subsequent review by Jain *et al.* (2002), which assessed 40 relevant publications according to a range of epidemiological and other quality criteria, concluded that only a minority of these studies provide persuasive evidence that breastfeeding promotes cognitive ability. It could be argued, however, that this conclusion is too conservative, and that some of the criteria used by these authors were either too stringent (e.g. for the 'appropriateness' of the cognitive outcome measure, and size of the effect being sought which needed to demonstrate 'clinical significance'), or potentially misleading (Rutter 1985) (e.g. the role of 'stimulation' of the child, which is likely to correlate with parental socioeconomic status).

Whether the conclusions of Anderson *et al.* (1999) are too optimistic, or those of Jain *et al.* (2002) are too critical, the possibility remains that residual confounding is a serious vulnerability in observational studies, no matter how representative these are of the general population from where they are drawn. Accordingly, there have been several attempts to circumvent this. First, Daniels and Adair (2005) found a 1.6 IQ point advantage at 8.5 years in those breast-fed for 12–18 months compared to those who had been breast-fed for less than 6 months, in a birth cohort in the Philippines, a culture where breastfeeding is inversely associated with socioeconomic status.

Second, Evenhouse and Reilly (2005) studied a range of health outcomes including cognitive function in 2734 sibling pairs drawn from the National Study of Adolescent Health. They reported that the within-family estimate for cognition was robust, suggesting a causal connection between breastfeeding and cognitive development, although this estimate was approximately 25% smaller than that for the between-family comparison. However, these results were not corroborated in the US national longitudinal survey of youth (Der *et al.* 2006), albeit with a smaller number of sibling pairs, and it should be noted that the assumptions of sibling fixed-effect models themselves are not without problems (Strully and Mishra 2009). In the case of breastfeeding, for

example, birth interval effects may operate as an unobserved source of variance.

Third, effects of essential fatty acid supplementation of formula milk have been tested in clinical trials, which aim to remove the influence of confounding through randomisation. A Cochrane systematic review by Simmer *et al.* (2008) concluded that feeding infants with enriched formula milk had no proven benefit to vision, cognition or physical growth. Similar conclusions were reached by these authors in regard to infants born pre-term (Schulzke *et al.* 2011).

Fourth, inconsistencies between studies addressing this issue may partly be explained by evidence that the cognitive benefit of breastfeeding is modified by genetic factors. Specifically, Caspi *et al.* (2007) reported that this benefit was only observed in those with a variant of the *FADS2* gene, which regulates fatty acid metabolism. However, this finding has not been consistently replicated (Steer *et al.* 2010; Martin *et al.* 2011).

14.3.2 Long-term cognitive effects of breastfeeding

While the effects of breastfeeding on cognitive development have been extensively investigated, surprisingly little is known about the long-term effects of this exposure on cognitive ageing. In this context, it should again be noted that cognition tracks (shows a high degree of stability) over the life course. Elwood *et al.* (2005) used retrospective information about birthweight and method of infant feeding from 779 men aged 60–74 years enrolled in the Caerphilly, Wales, cohort study. They found that breastfeeding was associated with higher scores on tests of verbal fluency and crystallised and fluid cognitive abilities, although only in those whose birthweight was below the median.

An apparent beneficial effect of breastfeeding on crystallised ability at age 53 years had also been observed by Richards *et al.* (2002) in the British 1946 birth cohort, although such an effect was not found for verbal memory or speed and concentration. Furthermore, the long-term effect of breastfeeding on crystallised ability was fully mediated by its effect on cognition at age 15 years, suggesting that long-term effects of this exposure are merely tracking across the life course. This qualification is especially relevant in view of the fact that tests of crystallised ability, such as vocabulary and word pronunciation, are particularly stable in ageing, whereas most other types of cognitive function are sensitive to age and morbidity-associated decline.

14.3.3 Breastfeeding and cognitive development: a caveat

While the above studies go some way towards controlling for confounding, few are able to allow for the potentially powerful effect of maternal cognitive ability. In a meta-analysis of nine studies, controlled for this effect, Der *et al.* (2006) found that with full control for covariates there was no statistical effect of breastfeeding on cognition. Following this up with the US national longitudinal survey of youth in the same publication, these authors showed that maternal cognitive ability accounted for most of the effect of breastfeeding on cognitive development, with a residual association fully explained by other covariates including age, education, socioeconomic status and the home environment.

14.3.4 Infant feeding and the central nervous system

While the preceding paragraphs have focused on research using psychometric cognitive abilities as outcomes, far less is known about the effects of infant feeding on CNS systems underlying cognitive function. It is therefore worth noting the study by Isaacs *et al.* (2008), who measured caudate volume by magnetic resonance imaging (MRI) in 76 adolescents who had been born pre-term with similar birth status and neonatal course, but had been fed either standard or nutrient-rich formula milk in infancy.

The caudate nucleus is a component of the basal ganglia, which interconnects with the dorsal frontal cortex to provide a neural system that serves complex higher mental functions, particularly executive control. The enriched formula differed from the standard in terms of energy, protein, calcium, phosphorus, iron, zinc, copper and several other micronutrients, a composition previously shown to benefit cognition (in males) in children born pre-term (Lucas *et al.* 1998). Results indicated that those who had received this enriched formula had significantly larger bilateral caudate volume, although the effect of this intervention on cognitive function fell short of statistical significance in this small sample.

14.3.5 Breastfeeding and behavioural development

Just as essential fatty acids are important for cognitive development, they are also thought to influence the regulation of emotion and conduct in children; in regard to the evidence for continuity between childhood and adult mental health noted above, this has implications for adult mental health. However, the topic of breastfeeding in relation to mental health has received considerably less attention than it has in relation to cognition. One possible reason for this is that maternal stress during the pre- and antenatal phases may confound any observed association by reducing the likelihood of infant exposure to breast milk. This is based on evidence that the oxytocin and prolactin systems are antagonistic to the HPA axis, the principal stress hormone system.

Experimental studies in humans suggest that acute physical and mental stress can impair the milk ejection reflex by reducing the release of oxytocin during a feed (Dewey 2001b). This further suggests that chronic stress may reduce milk production by preventing full emptying of the breast at each feed (*ibid*). Since emotional disorder itself shows intergenerational continuity it is important to determine whether or not apparent effects of breastfeeding on behaviour are independent of this. Of course, this caveat equally applies to breastfeeding in relation to cognitive development; and glucocorticoid overproduction from a poorly regulated stress response can itself impair neural mechanisms underlying cognitive function.

There are, in addition, non-nutritional reasons why breastfeeding may be associated with mental health. Aspects of intimacy such as reciprocity, mutual joy, harmony, concern for other, trust and closeness have all been described as part of successful breastfeeding experiences (Dignam 1995), and it is plausible that a degree of such positive well-being is transferred to the child during rearing. Again, these influences may also directly benefit cognitive development. In addition, the odour of human milk may have a soothing effect on infants; in an experimental study this odour suppressed signs of distress (crying, grimacing and motor activity) during a blood draw (Nishitani *et al.* 2009). To some extent these effects may be determined through epigenetic alteration of gene expression. The best-known demonstration of this in the present context is by Meaney and his colleagues, who showed in rodents that offspring of high-nurturing mothers (in terms of licking or grooming, although these activities may correlate with readiness to feed) tend to have relatively low levels of anxiety. They also show an attenuated HPA axis response to stress, and higher levels of glucocorticoid receptor gene expression in the hippocampus (with parallel implications for cognition), a difference in DNA methylation that persists across the life course (Meaney and Szyf 2005). A detailed consideration of these complex issues is beyond the scope of this report; nevertheless they suggest that the effects of breastfeeding on behavioural development cannot be conceived exclusively at the micronutrient level.

With these cautionary notes in mind, at least three observational studies of childhood mental health in relation to breastfeeding have been conducted in the general population while controlling for maternal mental health factors. The earliest is based on 579 urban and rural high school students in the US (Allen *et al.* 1998); these authors found that breastfeeding was inversely associated with major depression (although not with anxiety, disruptive behaviour or substance abuse), after controlling for maternal emotional health, family cohesion, family conflict and adolescent physical symptoms.

In a more recent, larger study using the Western Australian Pregnancy Cohort Study, Robinson *et al.* (2008) showed that duration of breastfeeding was inversely associated with risk of mental health problems assessed by the Child Behaviour Checklist at age 5 years (although not at age 2 years), after controlling for a wide range of potential confounders: maternal age, education, ethnicity, smoking and stress events during pregnancy and postnatal depressed mood, family income, father living at home, gestational age, gender of the child and number of siblings.

Most recently Waylen *et al.* (2009) studied childhood externalising disorders in relation to dietary essential fatty acid intake in the ALSPAC. These authors found an association between breastfeeding and childhood oppositional defiant disorder or conduct disorder (although not attention deficit hyperactivity disorder); however, this association was explained by a range of confounders including maternal mental health as well as gestational age, birthweight, smoking, and aspects of socioeconomic status.

14.3.6 Optimal duration of breastfeeding

Before leaving the topic of breastfeeding it is worth noting the issue of optimal duration. As discussed in Chapter 3, Section 3.7.3.2) there is a long-standing debate over this duration in middle- and high-income countries – the so-called 'weanling's dilemma' (Fewtrell *et al.* 2007). Briefly, the WHO recommends exclusive breastfeeding for the first 6 months, but there is some concern that this may not fully meet nutritional requirements of the infant, and that complementary feeding may be necessary before this age. For example, a systematic review suggests that, while the mean energy requirement at 6 months is approximately 2.6–2.7 MJ/day (2600–2700 kJ/day), mean metabolised energy intake in exclusively breast-fed infants at this age is lower than this at 2.2–2.4 MJ/day (2200–2400 kJ/day) (Reilly and Wells 2005). In this context, breastfeeding duration has a wide range of determinants (Thulier and Mercer 2009), including demographic factors (e.g. race, age, marital status, education, socioeconomics); biological variables (e.g. insufficient milk supply, infant health problems, maternal obesity, maternal smoking, parity and method of delivery); social variables (including paid work, family support and professional support); and psychological factors such as maternal intention, interest and confidence in breastfeeding. It should also be noted that micronutrients such as iron and zinc require an exogenous source after 6 months (Butte *et al.* 2002; Kramer and Kakuma 2002; Kramer and Kakuma, 2004). This leads to the major topic of post-weaning diet.

14.4 Post-weaning diet

While higher mental function has been extensively studied in relation to pre-weaning diet, we now turn to the effects of infant diet on mental development at the stage of transition to solid foods and beyond. This is an equally important topic because of variation in the composition of infant solid foods (Bolling *et al.* 2007). Looking ahead to childhood, this is a time of gradual transition from parental control of diet-based nutrition to intake based on self-selection and gratification (Rosales *et al.* 2009), where, obviously, healthy intake is equally vulnerable to compromise. The huge topic of childhood dietary choice, including effects of breakfast consumption and snacking, is beyond the scope of this chapter (see, for example, Benton 2008a). However, it is important here to consider nutrition at the macro and micro level in infants and young children while this is still regulated by parental control.

14.4.1 Dietary patterns at the macro level

Little is known about mental development in relation to infant diet at the macro level. However, Gale *et al.* (2009) tested a wide range of cognitive functions in 241 children aged 4 years, drawn from the Southampton Women's Survey, whose diet had been prospectively assessed at ages 6 and 12 months. Patterns of dietary intake at these ages were identified by principal component analysis (PCA), and characterised as 'infant guidelines' (a high frequency of consumption of fruit, vegetables and home-prepared foods, similar to Department of Health guidelines), or 'adult foods' (a high frequency of bread, savoury snacks, biscuits, squash, breakfast cereals and chips). A higher 'infant guidelines' score at 6 and 12 months was associated with higher full scale IQ after controlling for sex, birth order, gestational age, birthweight, maternal age, IQ, social class, education and home conditions. However, no such association was found for attention, sensory-motor ability, memory or language.

In the context of the infant macro diet it is worth briefly referring to the issue of appetitive behaviours, not least because these have potentially serious consequences for obesity (see Chapter 8, Section 8.9), but also because they may themselves be conceptualised as behavioural consequences of dietary intake. These appetitive behaviours refer to low responsiveness to internal satiety signals such as gastric distension and endocrine control mechanisms, high responsiveness to food cues such as taste and smell, the subjective experience of reward during consumption, and over-consumption of energy-dense foods (Carnell and Wardle 2008). The origins of these behaviours are still uncertain, but probably include genetic influence as well as environmental factors such as parental feeding style (*ibid*).

14.4.2 Iron status in childhood

We referred to iron in Section 14.2, but iron uptake into the brain continues throughout life (Kretchmer *et al.* 1996). We should note that iron is potentially neurotoxic, and indeed there is epidemiological evidence that excessive, as well as low concentrations, are associated with poor cognition (Lam *et al.* 2008), although this was observed in older people, suggesting possible effects of accumulation. Nevertheless, iron is essential for the synthesis of major catecholamines, and it is suggested that during shortage it is preferentially directed away from the brain towards manufacture of red blood cells (Benton 2008b). Thus it is of major concern that iron deficiency is highly prevalent, in middle- to high-income as well as developing countries, and can progress to anaemia. The latter is associated with tiredness, low mood and poor concentration (Benton 2008b), variables that themselves impact cognitive function and behaviour (Kretchmer *et al.* 1996). Accordingly, in a systematic review, iron supplementation was found to have a modest but significant benefit to mental and motor development in children, mostly in low-income countries (Sachdev, Gera *et al.* 2005); and as Benton (2008b) comments, it would be surprising if such benefits were not observed in industrialised countries.

14.4.3 Food intolerance and mental development: additives and preservatives

Last but probably not least, we should refer to food intolerance. It should be clarified that this term has been applied to several phenomena, including malabsorption, allergic and other adverse reaction, and psychological avoidance, the latter sometimes following parental input (Benton 2008a). Probably the most widely suspected culprits linked to behaviour problems in children are tartrazine (the yellow food dye), and sodium benzoate (the preservative). These are thought to generate symptoms of hyperactivity (Egger *et al.* 1985), although no responses were observed to these substances alone. It must also be said that research in this area has often involved small selected samples and short duration of monitoring, and with only a tiny fraction of possible additives actually investigated (Benton 2008a). Perhaps the best evidence comes from two large randomised double-blind crossover trials of children drawn from the general population, where food colouring or other additives were associated with an increase in hyperactive symptoms (Bateman *et al.* 2004; McCann *et al.* 2007).

14.5 Conclusions

As Benton (2008b) notes, all nutrients influence brain development, although Georgieff (2007) highlights energy, protein, long-chain PUFAs, iron, zinc, copper, iodine, selenium, vitamin A, choline and folate as particularly important. This chapter has focused on several of these; but perhaps in conclusion it is of interest to step back and address Benton's (2008b) observation that, while received wisdom suggests that intake of key micronutrients is likely to be adequate in a balanced diet in middle- to high-income countries, 'in no instance have psychological or behavioural indices been the measure of adequacy' when deriving relevant nutrient reference values in the UK and US. Yet, as this author notes elsewhere (Benton 1992), psychological symptoms are often the first manifestation of micronutrient deficiencies, and can be improved by supplementation even in well-nourished populations. This should not be surprising, given that the brain is the most complex and metabolically active organ in the body (*ibid*).

14.6 Key points

- Maternal diet during pregnancy is important for brain development, particularly intake of essential long-chain fatty acids, but also B vitamins, iodine, choline, zinc and iron. Intake of essential fatty acids also prolongs pregnancy duration which benefits fetal growth and development (including brain development). A European Commission panel recommends that pregnant and lactating mothers should aim to achieve a dietary intake of long-chain *n*-3 essential fatty acids to supply a DHA intake of at least 200 mg/day (equivalent to two portions (each portion is 140 g) of oil-rich fish per week), although this is not universally agreed.
- During fetal development the brain is protected during periods of poor nutrition, including extreme circumstances such as famine. Maternal starvation in the Dutch Hunger Winter of the 1940s did not have an adverse impact on cognitive development in the offspring.
- Early life nutrition plays an important part in mental health across the life course. Maternal diet during pregnancy has a fundamental effect on brain development, which can track into later life and influence, for example, life chances, economic productivity, physical morbidity and cognitive ageing (e.g. risk of dementia).
- A large body of evidence indicates that breastfeeding benefits cognitive development, with a smaller consensus suggesting benefits to emotional and behavioural development. Again, essential fatty acids are thought to be chiefly responsible. However, in the case of cognitive development there is some evidence that this is explained by maternal IQ. Breastfeeding is also associated with many non-nutritional factors which may be associated with mental health, e.g. aspects of intimacy (such as reciprocity, mutual joy, harmony, concern for others, trust and closeness) and socioeconomic status, maternal smoking history, maternal cognitive ability, maternal education, paternal education, family size and childhood experiences which could potentially confound findings relating to cognitive development in the infant.
- Less is known about the effects of the post-weaning diet on mental development, although high consumption of fruit, vegetables and home-prepared foods at 6 and 12 months has been linked to higher IQ. Relevant micronutrient exposures include essential fatty acids, iron, zinc, iodine, folate and selenium.
- Evidence, including findings from two large randomised controlled trials of infants, indicate an association between some additives and preservatives and hyperactive symptoms, in particular some food colourings or other additives.
- Maternal nutrition may also have an impact on the mental health of the mother herself, as well as influencing the infant via parenting behaviour and infant attachment.

14.7 Recommendations for future research

- The evidence from observational studies conducted in developed countries indicates no objective evidence of a 'weanling's dilemma'. However, there is a need for large randomised trials in both developing and developed countries to rule out potential adverse effects such as not achieving optimal brain and, therefore, mental development, and to confirm the reported health benefits of exclusive breastfeeding for 6 months.

- Research in humans is required to determine the influence of supplementation with nutrients such as iron, zinc, iodine, vitamin D and choline on birth outcomes such as cognitive function. Ideally, randomised controlled trials are required in order to control for potential confounding factors.

14.8 Key references

Anderson JA, Johnstone BM & Remley DT (1999) Breastfeeding and cognitive development: a meta-analysis. *American Journal of Clinical Nutrition*, **70**, 525–35.

Benton D (2008b) Micronutrient status, cognition and behavioural problems in childhood. *European Journal of Nutrition*, **47**, 38–50.

Gale CR, Martyn CN, Marriott LD *et al.* (2009) Southampton Women's Survey Study Group. Dietary patterns in infancy and cognitive and neuropsychological function in childhood. *Journal of Child Psychology and Psychiatry*, **50**, 816–23.

Koletzko B, Cetin I, Brenna JT *et al.* (2007) Dietary fat intakes for pregnant and lactating women. *British Journal of Nutrition*, **98**, 873–7.

Uauy R, Mena P & Rojas C (2000) Essential fatty acids in early life: structural and functional roles. *Proceedings of the Nutrition Society*, **59**, 3–15.

15
Putting the Science into Practice: Public Health Implications

15.1 Introduction

This Task Force has reviewed the effect of nutrition and diet on development in early life and the short- and long-term consequences of these effects for health. The key strands that have emerged are the vulnerability of the fetus in early pregnancy to toxic insults and to inadequate supplies of micronutrients; how the impairment of fetal growth and development in later pregnancy can programme for disease in adult life, especially cardiovascular disease and type 2 diabetes; how maternal over-nutrition may also increase the risk of type 2 diabetes in the offspring; and how infant feeding practices may have lasting effects on long-term mental and physical health. Here we consider how current recommendations may need to be adjusted to take these factors into account.

15.1.1 Critical windows

The fetus is most vulnerable to dietary deficiencies, excesses and toxicity in the first trimester of pregnancy. Once the placenta is fully developed it helps to buffer the fetus from extreme fluctuations. Growth is determined largely by the efficiency of the placenta in delivering nutrients to the fetus. Each organ or tissue has its own phase of rapid growth which, if interrupted, may have long-term consequences if there is no ability to make good any deficit in growth. These

vulnerable periods are termed 'critical windows' in development, during which future health and development can be 'programmed' (see Chapter 4).

Cell division and differentiation occur in phases and the pattern of growth may have long-term consequences, especially if certain phases in the differentiation cycle are arrested. However, besides influencing organ size or cell type, stem cells may be affected by epigenetic changes that programme how those cells derived from them will behave in the future. The extent of the effects of early nutrition varies between organs and is influenced by the stage in pregnancy at which the nutritional insult occurs (see Chapter 2 and Chapter 4).

Concepts such as developmental plasticity or adaptive programming (see Chapter 1, Section 1.3.2 and Chapter 4, Section 4.5) are helpful in explaining how an organism becomes adapted for the environment into which it is born. In other words, the fetus is prepared by environmental cues during the pregnancy to match the predicted postnatal environment. However, a mismatch between the prenatal and postnatal environments may have adverse consequences for health in later life. For example, growth retardation due to an insufficient supply of nutrients, particularly glucose, will prepare an infant for an environment where food supply is limited, but if the infant is born into an environment where the supply is overabundant it may be less able to adapt to exposure to an *ad libitum* food intake, thus resulting in an

Nutrition and Development: Short- and Long-Term Consequences for Health, First Edition. Edited by the British Nutrition Foundation.
© 2013 the British Nutrition Foundation. Published 2013 by Blackwell Publishing Ltd.

increased risk of developing type 2 diabetes in later life (see Chapter 1, Section 1.3.2). These concepts are useful in understanding the changing patterns of disease among communities whose diets are in transition from subsistence on a limited food supply to a situation where food is abundant (see Chapter 6, Section 6.1.4).

The possible mechanisms through which this adaptation may be mediated are discussed in Chapter 4, Section 4.5, and include disruption of normal tissue or organ development and disruption of the endocrine environment, including changes in the hypothalamo–pituitary–adrenal (HPA) axis that regulates response to stress.

Epigenetic modifications are emerging as a likely element involved in this programming activity. These involve changes in DNA and chromatin organisation, which do not alter the DNA sequence but which can affect gene expression patterns by changing the accessibility of specific genes to the transcriptional machinery. Methylation of the DNA bases, cytosine and adenine, alters the gene expression pattern in a stable manner. For example, pancreatic cells programmed to be insulin-producing islets during embryonic development remain islets throughout the life of the offspring. DNA methylation can result in gene repression and, more recently, methylation of RNA has been suggested as an important factor regulating the *FTO* gene that is involved in obesity and type 2 diabetes (Jia *et al.* 2011). Altered nutrient availability has been shown to influence the establishment of DNA methylation in the developing embryo and fetus. Those nutrients and related compounds involved in the methylation cycle (folate, vitamin B_6, vitamin B_{12}, choline and betaine) may have important influences on DNA methylation. Shortening of telomeres that protect the ends of chromosomes (see Chapter 4, Section 4.5.4) is another mechanism by which fetal programming may influence biological ageing (Kirkwood and Mathers 2009). Because several different nutritional insults have common outcomes, the gatekeeper hypothesis (see Chapter 4, Section 4.5.5) proposes that there are a limited number of genes or gene pathways that are altered.

15.1.2 Endocrine system development

The female is the default phenotype, and becoming male (masculinisation) depends on testes formation and the hormones (primarily androgen) they produce.

The masculinisation process occurs around 8–12 weeks' gestation and the vulnerability of this critical window is highlighted by the fact that subtle disorders of masculinisation in males are remarkably common. There is emerging evidence that testicular cancer, which is the leading type of cancer in young men, is related to arrested germ cell line differentiation in fetal life. Other evidence suggests that falling sperm counts in young men may be a consequence of endocrine disruption in early fetal life (Nordkap *et al.* 2012).

The male fetus grows faster than the female and is more vulnerable to growth restriction due to various factors, including maternal diet and lifestyle choices. The masculinisation process exerts effects not only on reproductive organs but throughout the body, and the action of hormones may partly explain the differences between males and females in risk for many chronic diseases, some of which are more common in men (stroke, coronary heart disease) and others such as autoimmune diseases (systemic lupus erythematosus, thyroid disease) and asthma that are more common in women (see Chapter 5, Section 5.4). However, the mechanisms that result in sexual dimorphism are not well understood (see Chapter 5).

15.1.3 Neurological development

The brain is most vulnerable in the first 4 months of pregnancy during the period of rapid neuronal multiplication, as illustrated by the severe effects on fetal brain development in early pregnancy of maternal iodine deficiency (cretinism) or alcoholism resulting in fetal alcohol syndrome (impaired brain development). In later pregnancy, the brain is less vulnerable even though growth is more rapid. The brain growth spurt occurs in the last trimester of pregnancy and extends into the first few years of postnatal life. During this period, accretion of long-chain polyunsaturated fatty acids required for grey matter growth is greatest. Infants born pre-term have a limited capacity to make docosahexaenoic acid (DHA) from linolenic acid and therefore require DHA to be provided preformed to enable the development of normal visual function. In the postnatal period, much of the brain growth is mainly a consequence of myelination (white matter growth). However, there may be subtle effects on brain circuitry and transmitter signalling that may have lifelong consequences (see Chapter 6).

Thus, neurological development in early life may influence cognitive, mental health and behavioural outcomes as well as the risk of disease in later life. For example, the extended central nervous system circuitry which develops during late pregnancy and early neonatal life may be susceptible to nutritionally induced changes in trophic signals such as leptin, which can shape neuronal projections and connectivity between different brain regions in rodents. The potential implications of over-exposure to hormones such as leptin and insulin during gestation, such as in maternal obesity, are now beginning to emerge, especially from studies of laboratory rodent models (see Chapter 8, Section 8.8). Nutritionally acquired epigenetic modification during brain development and exposure to elevated circulating levels of glucocorticoids have both been suggested as possible mechanisms underpinning the influence of early life nutrition on expression of brain transmitters and on aspects of cognitive function or mental health during later life (see Chapter 4, Section 4.5.3 and Chapter 6, Section 6.5.2).

Some nutritional challenges of varying severity may affect brain development and function, including protein/energy malnutrition, global over-nutrition (e.g. maternal obesity, gestational diabetes and over-nutrition prior to weaning), and specific micronutrient and essential fatty acid deficiencies (see Chapter 6, Section 6.4).

15.1.4 Gut flora

Each infant harbours its own unique microbiota determined, to a large degree, by the environment to which the infant is exposed. A healthy gut microbiota plays a vital role in reducing the risk of colonisation of the gut by harmful microorganisms and is also involved in enhancing the bioavailability of some nutrients for the host and stimulating epithelial development and maturation of the immune system (see Chapter 7). The acquisition and development of the infant gut microbiota is affected by a number of factors (genetic, environmental [including infant diet] and health). The addition of probiotics, such as *Bifidobacterium breve* and *Lactobacillus rhamnosus*, to the infant diet may reduce the risk of developing asthma, atopic dermatitis and other common allergies later in childhood. On the other hand, particular bacterial species and microbial profiles have been associated with several severe gastrointestinal disorders in later life (see Chapter 7, Section 7.1).

It is generally accepted that the gut microbiota of breast-fed and formula-fed infants are distinctly different, although recent fortification of infant formulas with prebiotics to simulate breast milk has lessened this distinction. As well as providing all the nutritional requirements of the neonate, human milk delivers a range of other components important to infant health (most notably maternal antibodies and human milk oligosaccharides), which affect the infant gut microbiota (directly or indirectly). In addition, recent research has shown that breast milk contains bacterial DNA and that bacteria (including bifidobacteria and lactic acid bacteria) can be isolated from some breast milk samples. The microbiota is modified by weaning and, between the ages of 12 and 24 months, the profile of microorganisms present converges towards the microbiota present in an adult (see Chapter 7, Section 7.5). However, there is evidence that the oral microbiota, which determines sensitivity to dental caries, may be established in early life and that *Streptococcus mutans*, the main cariogenic species, can be transmitted from mother to infant (Kishi *et al.* 2009).

15.2 Summary of the Task Force's findings for various chronic conditions

This section summarises the evidence from earlier chapters regarding the impact of early life nutrition on the risk of developing a series of chronic conditions in later life and the associated public health recommendations.

15.2.1 Obesity

The prevalence of obesity has been increasing at an alarming rate in recent years in most countries of the world. In the UK, obesity in adults has trebled since the 1980s. With one in four adults currently obese (61% of adults are overweight or obese) (Department of Health 2011b) the UK now has one of the highest prevalence rates in Europe (OECD 2010). However, most obese adults were not obese as children and acquired their increased weight in adult life. More worrying is the high prevalence of obesity among UK children, with 10% of 4- and 5-year-olds and 19% of 10- and 11-year-olds being obese. Moreover, there is a clear social class gradient, with obesity prevalence

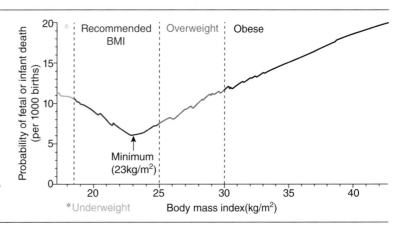

Figure 15.1 Association between maternal body mass index (BMI) and the risk of fetal or infant death. Reproduced from Tennant PW, Rankin J & Bell R (2011) Maternal body mass index and the risk of fetal and infant death: a cohort study from the North of England. *Human Reproduction*, **26**, 1501–11, copyright 2011, with permission from Oxford University Press.

among 4- and 5-year-olds being almost twice as prevalent in the least deprived decile (7%) compared with the most deprived decile (12%) (Health and Social Care Information Centre 2012a). Evidence is now emerging that maternal obesity is fuelling childhood obesity. Tackling the rising rates of obesity is high on the public health agendas both nationally and globally. A recent prediction is that, unless action is taken, the obesity prevalence among UK adults will rise to between 35 and 48% by 2030 (Wang *et al.* 2011).

15.2.1.1 Maternal obesity

Almost half of all women of childbearing age in England are overweight or obese. Epidemiological data comprising three national maternal obesity datasets within the UK have identified a significant increase in maternal obesity in recent years, with a doubling over the last two decades from 7.6% in 1989 to 15.6% in 2007 (Heslehurst 2011), and this number is predicted to rise in the coming years (NHS 2012). There are marked differences in obesity prevalence in women of different socioeconomic status, but not in men. In the UK, prevalence is 28% among women in manual households compared with 19% in non-manual households. The Centre for Maternal and Child Enquiries reported that maternal obesity was more prevalent in the most socially deprived quintile in England: 27.6% of all pregnancies occurred in this quintile, yet this quintile contained 34.6% of those with BMI 35–39.9, 33.8% of those with BMI 40–49.9 and 35.7% of those women with BMI ≥ 50 (Centre

for Maternal and Child Enquiries (CMACE) and Royal College of Obstetricians and Gynaecologists (RCOG) 2010b). Heslehurst *et al.* identified that women with extreme obesity were five times as likely to be living in areas of most deprivation compared with least deprivation according to the index of multiple deprivation (Heslehurst 2011).

Maternal obesity is associated with increased risk of stillbirth, maternal and infant mortality and congenital anomalies that are a major contributor to childhood morbidity (see Fig. 15.1). Obese women are more likely to require a caesarean section and experience serious obstetric complications. The prevalence of gestational diabetes is higher among obese women, which has long-term health implications due to an increased risk of developing type 2 diabetes for these women and their children. There is also a lower breastfeeding rate in this group compared with women with a healthy BMI (CMACE & RCOG 2010b). These statistics need greater recognition by policy makers so that the situation may be improved.

As discussed in Chapter 8, animal studies provide unequivocal evidence for early life origins of obesity and have made a major contribution to understanding the mechanistic basis. In humans, the environmental determinants of obesity may include nutritional status in critical periods in early development. Excessive 'fuel' availability for the fetus, associated with maternal diabetes and obesity, may predispose to enhanced risk of diabetes in later life.

Growth retardation *in utero*, particularly if followed by rapid postnatal growth (sometimes referred to as catch-up growth, see Chapter 8, Section 8.2.2

and Section 15.4.3), may be a determinant of central obesity and type 2 diabetes later in life.

Breastfeeding may protect against later obesity providing the duration of breastfeeding is long enough; the estimated reduction in prevalence being between 7% and 22% but with relatively few women continuing to breastfeed beyond 6 months.

Ideally, women should have a healthy weight prior to conception. However, the current level of evidence (see Chapter 8, Section 8.7) does not support routine provision of public health advice for overweight or obese pregnant women about following energy-restricted diets or following physical activity interventions during pregnancy. A number of randomised trials investigating this aspect, such as UPBEAT (UK Pregnancies: Better Eating and Activity Trial) are in progress, which will enable clearer guidance in the future.

Pre-pregnancy weight and weight gain during pregnancy influence both maternal and infant health outcomes, as well as affecting a healthy weight postpartum. Women who are thin need a greater weight gain to support a good outcome than women who are overweight. At present there are no internationally agreed definitions for the clinical diagnosis of maternal obesity. Although body mass index (BMI) is most commonly used, there are no pregnancy-specific BMI criteria to define maternal obesity. The World Health Organization BMI categories designed for use in the general population are usually used in early pregnancy as a guide for pre-pregnancy weight as there tends to be minimal weight gain in the first trimester (Heslehurst 2011), with the additional category in the UK of BMI ≥ 50 in early pregnancy being described as 'extreme obesity' or 'supermorbid obesity'. In the United States, the Institute of Medicine recently published revised guidelines on gestational weight gain in pregnancy (Institute of Medicine 2009) (see Chapter 3, Section 3.4.1.1), but additional UK-specific evidence is considered necessary before guidance can be implemented in the UK. Current advice in England and Wales (National Institute for Clinical Excellence (NICE) 2010; Riley 2011) is that pregnant women should not be weighed routinely throughout pregnancy as there is insufficient evidence to support the benefits of this intervention. However, this conclusion may need to be reviewed.

Public health policy and practice should have greater focus on interventions and messages to control pre-pregnancy weight so as to reduce the prevalence of obesity in all women of reproductive age, and greater emphasis should be placed on the risk of obesity to mother and child. One vehicle for this could be the UK Department of Health in England's social marketing programme (Change4Life). However, messages need to be embedded throughout policy and practice, and further evaluative research is required to assess the effectiveness of interventions with women before, during and after pregnancy to inform this process.

A recent Scientific Advisory Committee on Nutrition report on energy recommendations for the UK population (SACN 2011b) has concluded that the UK advice related to pregnancy published in 1991 still applies (Department of Health 1991), namely that women do not need to increase their energy intakes during the first two trimesters but, during the last trimester and during lactation, additional energy is required (see below and Chapter 3, Section 3.4.1.2). SACN has set energy requirements for the general adult population at a level that is consistent with a healthy body mass index (BMI 22.5), while recognising that the average BMI is well above this at 27 (SACN 2011b). This approach has been taken to help restore a healthy body weight profile within the UK population. These energy requirements are referred to as 'prescriptive' as they are associated with ideal rather than current BMI levels.

However, for pregnant women, SACN advises that energy requirements should be calculated from actual pre-pregnancy body weights, even if the woman is overweight at the start of the pregnancy, rather than at prescriptive healthy body weights. This is because weight loss during pregnancy is not advisable. The additional requirements during the last trimester should be added to these periconceptual values (i.e. an additional 0.8 MJ/day (800 kJ or 191 kcal/day)). For lactation, an increment of 1.4 MJ/day (1400 kJ or 330 kcal/day) is recommended during the first 6 months, i.e. during the period when exclusive breastfeeding is recommended (SACN 2011b) (see Chapter 3, Section 3.5.1).

Women who weigh over 100 kg (approx. 15 stone 10 lb) may require specific advice from a health professional, although such advice needs to be given sensitively to ensure that women are encouraged not to 'diet' but to control their weight through healthy eating and daily activity and physical activity (NICE 2010). Evidence suggests that many health professionals may be uncomfortable raising and discussing obesity issues with pregnant women, which suggests training is required to help support them in appropriately and effectively addressing weight issues with women (CMACE & RCOG 2010a). There is also a lack of research with women-centred support services to inform sensitive risk communications. The preconception, pregnancy and postnatal periods are important and timely stages in the life course for public health intervention. However, current public health and community service provision lacks structured maternity-related obesity objectives (Smith *et al.* 2011). For example, the transition of care between pregnancy and the postnatal period should be considered, alongside improvements in communication between hospital and public health services, and development of services that will engage pregnant women to recognise and address their obesity problem (Heslehurst, Moore *et al.* 2011).

Maternal obesity and the associated complications are already stretching healthcare budgets and, as the impact of maternal obesity is likely to affect the offspring and their health into adulthood, the healthcare cost will continue to increase for decades.

15.2.1.2 Childhood obesity

Rates of overweight and obesity in UK children have been increasing over recent decades, although in the last few years data suggest a levelling off (Health and Social Care Information Centre 2012b). Higher BMI in childhood or adolescence is associated with increased risk of cardiovascular disease in later life, and cross-sectional data (there are few prospective studies) show associations between BMI and cardiovascular risk factors. A recent prospective study involving over 5200 subjects (Lawlor *et al.* 2010) shows that BMI, waist circumference and total fat mass assessed at age 9–12 years are positively associated with cardiovascular risk factors at age 15–16 years. Lawlor *et al.* report that weight loss in overweight girls between childhood and adolescence normalises their cardiovascular risk profiles, whereas in overweight boys who return to a normal weight in adolescence, risk factor profiles are not fully normalised, being intermediate between those who remain overweight and those who maintain a normal weight. The reason for this difference is not yet understood. These findings highlight the need for interventions that safely and effectively reduce weight and improve cardiovascular risk factors in overweight and obese children.

Evidence suggests that being breast-fed may protect against later obesity in the child (see Chapter 8, Section 8.3). However, the decision to breastfeed is strongly related to education and socioeconomic status, which are inversely related to risk of obesity. Within childhood, no clear age of onset for obesity has been identified, leading some to argue that interventions to prevent childhood obesity should begin in the toddler years or even during infancy. However, this needs to be carefully balanced with the risk of inappropriate energy restriction in normal-weight children, which may lead to stunting of growth. Accelerated weight gain in infancy has been associated with later childhood obesity, which might suggest that infants considered to be at high risk in the first year might be targeted for early intervention. However, poor weight gain in low-birthweight infants is associated with greater risks to health in early life. Differences in responsiveness to external food cues and internal satiety cues are two important aspects of appetite suggested to contribute to a variation in weight gain via the tendency to over-consume or under-consume relative to energy needs.

Appetite at 6 weeks of age was shown to be predictive of weight gain from birth to 12 months in the Gateshead Millennium study, but the association at age 7–8 years was no longer statistically significant although there was an association with height (Parkinson *et al.* 2010). Appetitive traits have been shown to be heritable and satiety responsiveness has been shown to be associated with the common obesity-related gene *FTO* (see Llewellyn *et al.* 2011). Longitudinal analyses of appetitive traits (enjoyment of food, food responsiveness, slowness in eating, satiety responsiveness) in the UK Gemini birth cohort (over 2400 families with twins) at ages 3 and 15 months show that differences in traits, in conjunction with environmental opportunities to overeat, influence weight gain in infancy (Llewellyn *et al.* 2011). Furthermore, associations between traits and subsequent weight were stronger that between weight and subsequent appetitive traits.

Touwslager *et al.* (2011) have estimated the heritability of infant growth and whether any genetic contribution is increased or decreased by birthweight and gestational age. They compared growth (change in weight Z-score) at ages 0–1, 1–6, 6–12 and 12–24 months in a cohort of twins born in East Flanders, and highlight the importance of growth in the first postnatal month as a particular critical window, which is not predicted by genetic factors, unlike growth later in infancy. Variations in growth may lead to lasting epigenetic differences and/or to reprogramming of hormonal axes (see Chapter 5) that regulate food intake and metabolism. Hence intervention to modify growth may be particularly important during this period, particularly in infants born small for gestational age.

Findings from the Gateshead Millennium Study (1029 infants recruited at birth to examine infant feeding behaviour prospectively and relate this to subsequent growth and weight gain) suggest that starting solids and ceasing breastfeeding are a response to rapid early weight gain rather than a cause, and that parents identify and respond to the appetite characteristics of their child (Wright, Cox et al. 2011). The authors concluded that infancy is a period when all children are hungry, reflecting rapid growth, and the hungriest children seem as likely to be growing into tall children as becoming obese. They were not able to identify any behavioural or temperament characteristics that distinguished the two types of growth pattern.

15.2.2 Type 2 diabetes

Both type 1 and type 2 diabetes are increasing in prevalence in the UK and Europe. The increase in childhood diabetes is mainly a consequence of increased type 1 diabetes, which is an autoimmune disease unrelated to obesity but may be related to the more general increase in prevalence of autoimmune disease in young people (see Chapter 9, Section 9.1). However, type 2 diabetes is about twenty times more prevalent than type 1 diabetes in the adult population. Type 2 diabetes is still relatively uncommon in young adults. Most cases of type 2 diabetes arise in middle age and beyond. The risk of type 2 diabetes is enormously increased by unhealthy weight gain, and trailing behind the obesity epidemic is an epidemic of type 2 diabetes. Obesity and physical inactivity cause insulin resistance which causes the pancreas to secrete more insulin. Diabetes results when the pancreas is no longer able to compensate by secreting sufficient insulin. Type 2 diabetes becomes clinically evident when islet beta-cells are no longer able to produce sufficient insulin to maintain glucose homeostasis. The main health risk associated with type 2 diabetes is cardiovascular disease, and the processes that contribute to arterial damage emerge

many years before type 2 diabetes is evident. The longer duration an individual has diabetes (both type 1 and type 2), the greater the risk of developing microvascular disease, which can lead to blindness, kidney failure and limb amputation. Diabetes has major implications for healthcare costs. Diabetes is one of the most common non-communicable diseases globally (World Health Organization 2011). In 2011, an estimated 366 million people worldwide had diabetes and prevalence is expected to rise to 552 million by 2030 (International Diabetes Federation 2011). The prevalence of diabetes in the UK is estimated at approximately 3.8 million people and, by 2035/6, this is expected to increase to 6.25 million; the increase will mainly be in type 2 diabetes (Hex et al. 2012). The direct cost of treating people with diabetes is estimated at £9.8 billion annually and indirect costs of diabetes in terms of increased death, morbidity and loss of work is estimated to be £13.9 billion annually (Hex et al. 2012).

The Health Survey for England in 2004 found that the prevalence of type 2 diabetes was almost three times higher in Pakistani men and increased more than 6-fold among Pakistani women compared with the mainstream population (Mindell and Zaninotto 2006). Furthermore, diabetes tends to develop earlier in minority ethnic groups (in the 4th and 5th decade of life) compared with the White population (typically beyond the 6th decade) (Diabetes UK 2006). Women who develop gestational diabetes have a substantially increased risk of developing diabetes in later life. The prevalence of type 2 diabetes was also higher among Black Caribbean women, being three times higher than in the general female population. Socioeconomic differences in type 2 diabetes prevalence also exist, with women in the highest income quintile having a prevalence of 1.7% compared with 4% for the lowest income quintile (Mindell and Zaninotto 2006).

As discussed in Chapter 9, suboptimal nutrition during early life has a major influence on the risk of developing type 2 diabetes. Compared to the general population, risk of type 2 diabetes in later life appears to be higher among low-birthweight and high-birthweight babies, low-birthweight babies who underwent rapid childhood weight gain and those who experienced poor maternal nutrition. Breastfeeding is associated with lower risk; over the first year of life, breast-fed babies have typically gained less weight than those receiving formula, and are less likely to develop the features of metabolic syndrome (dyslipi-daemia, hypertension, microalbuminuria) that are strongly associated with the development of type 2 diabetes. These associations are supported by evidence from animal studies that suggests that an energy- and/or protein-restricted diet during pregnancy, maternal diabetes, high maternal energy intake and maternal obesity may increase the risk of offspring developing impaired glucose tolerance and type 2 diabetes in later life (see Chapter 9, Section 9.5).

Our understanding at present suggests that earlier onset of type 2 diabetes associated with low birth-weight may be a consequence of decreased beta-cell reserve. Low birthweight followed by accelerated growth rate in infancy may increase the susceptibility to developing insulin resistance in adult life when there is unhealthy weight gain. These changes may be a consequence of changes in the hypothalamus during development. Gestational diabetes also greatly increases the risk of the offspring developing type 2 diabetes but this may be through a different mechanism that involves changes in appetite regulation that predispose to obesity.

15.2.3 Cardiovascular disease

Cardiovascular disease is the leading cause of death worldwide and in the UK it accounts for one in three of all deaths. The major forms of cardiovascular disease are coronary heart disease (CHD) and stroke (cerebrovascular disease). In 2009, CHD caused around one in five deaths in men and one in eight deaths in women in the UK, a total of 82 000 deaths. In the same year, stroke caused more than 49 000 deaths in the UK (Scarborough *et al.* 2010). The estimated cost of cardiovascular disease to the UK economy is around £30 billion per year (Scarborough *et al.* 2010). The incidence of cardiovascular disease has fallen over the past 30 years by as much as 20–30% in many economically developed countries, including the UK. Death rates from CHD have been falling in the UK since the early 1970s and from stroke since the 1950s, but the rates remain relatively high compared to some other Western European countries (Scarborough *et al.* 2010). While cardiovascular mortality from CHD has fallen by 50% in the past decade (Smolina *et al.* 2012), the increased survival rate following myocardial infarction has resulted in a larger number of people living with heart failure, which has

a substantial effect on quality of life. The reasons for the decline are hotly debated but a reduction in cigarette smoking, changes in diet quality and improvements in living conditions are likely to have made a greater contribution than improvements in medical care. Better control of blood pressure through medical intervention has probably contributed to the fall in stroke mortality, and survival following myocardial infarction has been enhanced by thrombolytic therapy and the use of drugs such as aspirin. Further declines are predicted as cholesterol lowering drugs such as statins show their impact.

There are major social, regional and ethnic inequalities in cardiovascular disease morbidity and mortality in the UK, which appear to be widening (Frayn and Stanner 2005).

Men are more likely to die from heart disease than women at any age, with heart disease being uncommon in women below the age of 45. The prevalence then increases, although the risk in women lags 10 years behind that in men. Within the UK, mortality rates from cardiovascular disease have been consistently highest in Scotland and Northern Ireland. Those in the lowest socioeconomic group in the UK have the highest cardiovascular disease, CHD and stroke death rates. These inequalities can be seen clearly in the large metropolitan cities. Much of the variability in risk is also associated with a high prevalence of cigarette smoking. This inequality is even more prominent in women than men, with the CHD death rate in female workers with routine jobs being five times higher than in those with managerial or professional jobs (Langford *et al.* 2009). People from the Indian subcontinent are at particularly high risk of CHD despite a low prevalence of cigarette smoking, and people of African-Caribbean descent in the UK are at greater risk of stroke than the general population but have a lower risk of CHD (Frayn and Stanner 2005). There is a growing body of evidence to suggest that the increased risk in these ethnic minority groups may be a consequence of early life environment but there currently is a lack of evidence to show whether improved pre- and postnatal growth would reduce this risk.

The main modifiable risk factors for cardiovascular disease are dyslipidaemia (raised LDL-cholesterol or low HDL-cholesterol and raised triglycerides), blood pressure, smoking, physical inactivity and elevated body weight. However, an individual's risk of developing cardiovascular disease may also be affected *in utero*. Poor fetal growth, especially when followed by rapid postnatal growth or obesity, increases the risk of cardiovascular disease in adulthood (see Chapter 10, Section 10.3). In particular, the risk of developing the atherogenic lipoprotein phenotype (low HDL-cholesterol, raised fasting triacylglycerol) and micro-albuminuria (an indication of microvascular damage) are all associated positively with low birthweight and with rapid postnatal weight gain followed by over-weight or obesity in adulthood. Both low birthweight and shortness in stature, an integrated measure of childhood growth, are associated with higher blood pressure in adult life. Maternal overweight and obesity increase the risk of intrauterine growth retardation and pre-eclampsia, which may result in higher blood pressure in the offspring, thereby increasing their risk of cardiovascular disease. Maternal smoking habit has a marked effect on fetal growth and risk of intrau-terine growth retardation. It is uncertain whether a high maternal salt intake has an effect on the develop-ment of high blood pressure in the offspring, but low-birthweight infants appear to be more sensitive to the blood pressure lowering effect of salt in adult life. Furthermore, the salt reduction in infant formula that has occurred over the past few decades may have had long-term (beneficial) effects on blood pressure. Fur-thermore, the UK Food Standards Agency's salt reduction programme (undertaken between 2003 and 2010) and similar efforts in other countries have been successful in reducing average population salt intake and increasing consumer awareness of salt (Wyness *et al.* 2011).

Most of the evidence linking programming to car-diovascular disease has focused on poor fetal growth and catch-up growth rather than the other end of the spectrum. It remains unclear whether a birthweight >4 kg, which is often associated with maternal obesity (see Chapter 8), increases the risk of cardiovascular disease in later life, but this will be an important ques-tion to answer, given the rising prevalence of macrosomia.

15.2.4 Cancer

Diet and lifestyle factors can have a major impact on the risk of developing some cancers and it has been estimated that as many as 30% of cancers could be prevented by dietary means in Western countries (World Cancer Research Fund/American Institute for Cancer Research 2007).

Statistics from GLOBOCAN (International Agency for Research on Cancer 2008) indicate that women in the UK are 17% more likely to develop cancer by the age of 75 than the European average. A large proportion of the variation in cancer remains unexplained, especially for the hormonal cancers that afflict women. Obesity is strongly linked to endometrial cancer and weakly to postmenopausal breast cancer, but height is a stronger predictor of risk of breast cancer in pre-menopausal women. This suggests that factors associated with growth in child-hood increase risk. Breast cancer is the most common cancer among women worldwide, accounting for approximately 23% of all cancers in women. With the exception of alcohol intake, few dietary factors have been convincingly linked to risk of breast cancer. Early menarche and a later menopause are associ-ated with increased risk, as is nulliparity or having children later in life. Incidence of breast cancer has been increasing by up to 2% per year over the last decade, which cannot be explained by the implemen-tation of national breast screening programmes in some countries. However, mortality has been falling due to early detection and better treatment.

There is substantial evidence from animal studies that early diet and nutrition might influence later breast cancer risk (see Chapter 11, Section 11.3). The epidemiological evidence from human studies is inconclusive (see Chapter 11, Section 11.3.1).

Evidence from meta-analyses of case–control and cohort studies suggests a lower risk of childhood cancer amongst those who were breast-fed. With breastfeeding rates in the UK substantially lower than in many other European countries (see Chapter 3, Table 3.6); this is an aspect that warrants greater prominence when promoting the benefits of breast-feeding. However, it needs to be recognised that the benefits of breastfeeding regarding risk of breast cancer have never been noted in the UK and are confined to populations where multiple pregnancies are common.

Evidence from some very large studies and meta-analyses indicates a robust relationship between higher birthweight and increased breast cancer risk (see Chapter 11, Section 11.3.4). Postnatal growth and growth during childhood have also been linked to risk of breast cancer (see Chapter 11, Section 11.3.5).

Testicular cancer is the leading cause of cancer in young men; in older men prostate cancer is the most common type (see Chapter 11, Section 11.1). There is very strong evidence that testicular cancer is related to events that occur during fetal growth that may be caused by endocrine disruption (see Section 15.1.2). However, the role of specific dietary components in this process is uncertain, although there is an association between low birthweight and risk of testicular cancer. Prostate cancer mainly affects men over the age of 50 and may share some common features with breast cancer in women that relate to effects of the insulin-like growth factor-I (IGF-I) in promoting the cancer (Key 2011). There is some evidence that IGF-I may be programmed in events in early life and may also be linked to bone growth.

Although less conclusive, evidence from human studies suggests an inverse relationship between birth length and colorectal cancer risk in men but not women. Evidence for a relationship between birth anthropometry and other cancers is either not available or is inconclusive.

Increased body fatness is associated with a higher risk of many types of cancer (see Chapter 11, Section 11.4.3) and possible mechanisms are under investigation. These include peripheral aromatisation of androgens to form oestrogens, as well as the various hormones produced by adipose tissue, such as leptin, that have actions on the hypothalamus. A better understanding of the influence of early nutrition on later adiposity (see Chapter 8) would be particularly useful in determining whether any fetal programming of obesity might influence cancer risk, and whether strategies to tackle obesity in later life can reverse this effect. Various mechanisms linking early diet and nutrition to subsequent cancer risk have been suggested. Besides the effects on endocrine disruption, the most plausible mechanism to date involves epigenetics (see Chapter 11, Section 11.4.2.1). There is now considerable evidence that epigenetic status is heritable and can be modified by environmental and lifestyle factors in humans. A number of imprinted genes are known tumour suppressors or oncogenes involved in cell proliferation. Epigenetic change and loss of imprinting – gain or loss of DNA methylation or the loss of allele-specific gene expression – are common characteristics of tumours. Nutrients that are methyl donors, such as folate and vitamin B_{12}, and the amino acid methionine may have an effect on DNA methylation and, therefore, adequate levels of these nutrients in the maternal diet may be important in reducing risk of cancer in the offspring later in life.

15.2.5 Bone health

Around half of women and one in five men over the age of 50 years are at risk of fracture at the hip, spine or wrist during their remaining lifetime. Bone mass peaks around age 30 years. The amount of bone present in the skeleton in later life is determined by the peak bone mass achieved in early adulthood and its subsequent loss. Peak bone mass is generally lower in women than in men and subsequent bone loss is greater, mainly because of the accelerated loss in the menopausal and postmenopausal periods. Failure to optimise peak bone mass in early adulthood is associated with increased risk of osteoporosis and fractures in later life. Calcium and vitamin D are essential for healthy bones. In the UK, the recommended intake of calcium during pregnancy remains at 700 mg/day, whereas an additional 550 mg/day is recommended for women who breastfeed (Department of Health 1991) (see Chapter 3, Table 3.3). Maternal vitamin D status may be critical for bone development in the offspring and for maintenance of maternal bone mineralisation (see Chapter 12, Section 12.2.1). In the UK, all pregnant women are advised to take a vitamin D supplement of 10 µg/day (40 IU/day). Dark-skinned ethnic minorities or women who conceal most of their skin from sunlight exposure are at particular risk of low vitamin D status and, in the UK, all Asian women and children are advised to take supplementary vitamin D. Exclusively breast-fed babies may also be at increased risk of vitamin D deficiency if the mother has low vitamin D levels. Supplementation of vitamin D for the infant should be considered in this situation. See Chapter 12 and Section 15.3.3.1. To support health professionals, guidance was published by the Department of Health in January 2012 (Department of Health 2012b).

The last trimester of pregnancy is a particularly important period for skeletal growth and the long-term skeletal growth trajectory may be programmed by gene–environment interactions *in utero*. Maternal smoking, excessive physical activity in late pregnancy and limited fat stores all have a detrimental effect on bone mineral accrual by the fetus, leading to reduced bone mass at birth (see Chapter 12, Section 12.1.5). Peak bone mineral density in children and in adults has been positively associated with intake of *n*-3 polyunsaturated fatty acids (PUFAs) (see Chapter 12, Section 12.2.5). Protein is also thought to be of fundamental importance in bone development as bone comprises a protein matrix, but there is little direct evidence.

Regular physical activity seems to be associated with higher bone mineral accrual in children, although it is unclear whether this also results in long-term benefits such as a reduction in fracture risk in later adulthood. Current data suggest that around 30% of boys are meeting the government recommendation of at least 60 minutes of physical activity per day. The corresponding figure among girls is even lower, with for example only 12% of 14-year-old girls achieving the recommended target (Craig *et al.* 2009). As peak bone mass is generally lower in women, and women experience greater bone loss in later life, it is particularly important that girls and young women are encouraged to be physically active.

15.2.6 Allergic disease and asthma

Asthma is currently one of the world's most common chronic diseases with around 300 million sufferers. This figure is estimated to rise to 400 million by 2025. In the UK, there are an estimated 5.2 million people with asthma, 1.1 million of whom are children. The costs to the UK economy are around £2.5 billion per year. Asthma and allergic diseases such as hayfever and eczema (atopic dermatitis) have increased in prevalence in many countries. For example, in Aberdeen, Scotland, the lifetime prevalence of parentally reported asthma in schoolchildren increased from around 4% in 1964 to 26% in 2004, and hayfever increased from about 3% to 19% in the same period. The prevalence of eczema in affluent countries is also common, affecting up to 30% of pre-school children, 15–20% of schoolchildren and 7% of adults. There is some evidence to suggest that prevalence is now plateauing in some countries, particularly in relation to asthma (see Chapter 13, Section 13.3). The same may apply to the IgE sensitisation associated with food allergy, based on follow-up of a series of birth cohorts from the Isle of Wight.

Early life influences, during fetal development and early childhood, may critically influence the development of asthma and allergic disease. Concerns that maternal ingestion of food allergens during pregnancy and lactation increase the risk of childhood allergic disease have been re-evaluated, and allergen avoidance during pregnancy and lactation is no longer recommended (West *et al.* 2011) (see Chapter 13, Section 13.6). Indeed, there is some evidence that fetal and infant exposure to a range of allergens

via the mother and her breast milk is important in the development of normal immune tolerance (see Chapter 2, Section 2.5.12).

Although there are many well-documented benefits of breastfeeding for both mother and child, the effects of breastfeeding on atopic dermatitis, wheezing disease and asthma are less clear (see Chapter 13, Section 13.7). The benefits of exclusive breastfeeding for 3–4 months may be limited to infants with a high risk of allergy. There has been much debate regarding weaning practices and the introduction of potential allergens but there is no convincing evidence that delaying the introduction of allergenic foods during weaning reduces the likelihood of food allergy and allergic disease (Thompson *et al.* 2010) (see Chapter 13, Section 13.8). Several trials are under way that will help inform advice given to parents of young children on the benefits and contraindications associated with allergen avoidance. The advice in the UK for peanut consumption was revised in 2009 (Committee on Toxicity of Chemicals in Food, Consumer Products and the Environment 2009) and now states that if mothers would like to eat peanuts or foods containing peanuts during pregnancy or breastfeeding, then they can choose to do so as part of a healthy balanced diet, irrespective of whether there is a family history of allergies (see Chapter 13, Section 13.6.4).

Although many studies have reported associations between BMI and incident asthma, and that weight loss is associated with improved lung function and reduced asthma symptoms, it is not clear whether the systemic inflammatory state associated with obesity increases the risk of asthma and allergic disease. There is growing interest in the possibility that nutrients such as vitamin E, vitamin D, zinc, selenium and PUFAs in the maternal diet during pregnancy might influence the development of childhood asthma and allergic disease (see Chapter 13, Section 13.9).

There has been considerable change over the past 40 years in the timing of first exposure to solid foods (complementary feeding) (see Misak (2011) for a review). Furthermore, the evidence supporting the benefit of delaying the introduction of allergenic foods (cows' milk, eggs, fish and peanuts) beyond 6 months is contradictory. Current thinking is that tolerance to food allergens appears to be driven by regular, early exposure to potentially allergenic food proteins during a critical window of development (Prescott *et al.* 2008). The EC-funded EuroPreval project has proposed that early complementary food introduction may hasten and/or maintain oral mucosal tolerance rather than increase the risk of food allergy (Grimshaw *et al.* 2009). Current advice from the American Academy of Pediatrics, updated in 2008, is that although solid food should not be introduced before 4–6 months of age, there is currently no convincing evidence that delaying its introduction beyond this age has a significant protective effect in the development of atopic disease (regardless of whether the child is breast-fed or formula-fed). The European Society for Paediatric Gastroenterology, Hepatology and Nutrition (ESPGHAN) has also recently concluded that complementary food may be introduced safely at 4–6 months of age. As evident from Chapter 3 (Section 3.7.3) few UK mothers are compliant with the Department of Health's breastfeeding recommendation. With this in mind, health visitors should provide tailored advice to mothers who choose to introduce complementary foods prior to 6 months, as is common practice in the UK, notwithstanding the recommendation for exclusive breastfeeding.

Early nutrition may have profound implications for long-term health and atopy in later life, and therefore presents an opportunity to prevent or delay the onset of atopic diseases. It is generally agreed that the intestinal microbiota plays an important physiological role in the postnatal development of the immune system. Although pre- and probiotics are theoretically promising candidates for the prevention of atopic diseases, there is currently not enough evidence to support their use in this context (Misak 2011).

15.2.7 Cognitive function/mental health and behaviour

Mental function has a major effect on life chances, economic productivity, physical health and, ultimately, survival. Cognitive skills in childhood are a strong predictor of educational achievement, which in turn is the principal gateway to adult socioeconomic attainment, especially for today's school leavers. Childhood cognitive ability also tracks into adulthood and directly predicts dementia risk, a major disease burden in later life (see Chapter 14, Section 14.1). There are currently 750 000 people living with some form of dementia in the UK and this is expected to increase to over 1 million by 2025. Around one in ten children aged 5–16 years have a clinically diagnosable mental health problem and such problems often persist into adulthood, with

40–70% of depressed adolescents displaying a major depressive disorder during adulthood. The World Health Organization recognises major depressive disorder as the leading cause of disease burden in middle- and high-income countries. Depression is also a risk factor for cognitive decline in later life and can coexist with Alzheimer's disease (see Chapter 14, Section 14.1).

Long-chain PUFAs are known to be particularly important for brain development. A European Commission consensus panel has recommended that pregnant and lactating women consume the fatty acid equivalent of two portions of fish per week to supply at least 200 mg of DHA per day (see Chapter 3, Section 3.4.1.3). In the UK, intake of oil-rich fish is low. Only 28% of women aged 19–64 years consume oil-rich fish and the average weekly consumption of oil-rich fish is currently less than half a portion (56 g), (one portion is typically 140 g) (Bates *et al.* 2012). Only 3% of children in LIDNS (a survey of low-income households) were reported to eat oil-rich fish and dishes containing oil-rich fish (SACN 2011a). Current population-wide advice from the Department of Health in England is consumption of at least two portions of fish per week, of which one should be an oil-rich species. This is subject to the restrictions on consumption of certain fish by pregnant and lactating women – marlin, swordfish, shark and, to a lesser extent, tuna – due to methylmercury contamination (SACN 2004). Fish, especially oil-rich fish, contains long-chain *n*-3 PUFAs and a daily intake of 450 mg/day long-chain *n*-3 PUFAs (chiefly eicosapentaenoic (EPA) and DHA) is recommended in the UK (SACN 2004). The European Food Safety Authority (EFSA) recommends 250 gm/day of EPA plus DHA as an Adequate Intake for the general population, with a further 100–200 mg/day DHA for pregnant and lactating women (EFSA 2010). Pregnancy is associated with a reduction in functional long-chain fatty acid status and, because postpartum normalisation is still incomplete at 6 months, birth spacing is an important factor (see Section 15.3.2.2).

Other nutrients identified as important during pregnancy for neurological and cognitive development in humans are B vitamins (especially B_{12}), iodine, choline, zinc and iron (see Chapter 6 and Chapter 14). Policy on iron varies around the world. In the UK, the view is that physiological adaptations during pregnancy and lactation ensure an adequate supply of iron to the fetus and developing infant, even in the presence of iron deficiency, and so an increment in iron intake is not considered necessary (Department of Health 1991).

Essential fatty acids present in breast milk are thought to be important for cognitive development and perhaps emotional and behavioural development as well, although maternal IQ may also play a role (see Chapter 14, Section 14.3.5). Exclusive breast-feeding beyond 6 months may not fully meet the infant's nutritional requirements; complementary feeding is needed. Some authorities suggest that complementary feeding should begin before 6 months to optimise brain development. However, in the UK for example, the percentage of mothers exclusively breastfeeding at 6 months is negligible, despite recommendations (see Chapter 3, Section 3.7.3.2).

15.3 Diet and lifestyle themes relevant to pregnancy and early life

Excessive exposure to, or insufficiency of, specific nutrients around the time of pregnancy can have a detrimental impact on fetal development. For example, high intakes of vitamin A are associated with teratogenic effects and low maternal folate status is associated with neural tube defects in the fetus. However, it is now understood that fetal growth and development are also affected by more modest variations in nutrition arising from widespread differences in dietary habits and food choice.

Chapter 3 summarises the diet and nutrient recommendations for pre-pregnancy, pregnancy and infancy. In this chapter we focus on a number of themes that have emerged from the Task Force's discussions.

15.3.1 Maternal body weight and energy balance

A recurring theme throughout this report is the importance of maternal weight and energy balance (see, for example, Chapter 3, Section 3.4.1.1 and Chapter 8, Section 8.4.4). The prevalence of obesity among pregnant women and the 2011 SACN recommendations on energy intake during pregnancy are discussed in Section 15.2.1. In summary, the advice is that requirements should be based on pre-pregnancy weight (even if a woman is obese) in order to avoid potential harm to the fetus if energy intakes were to be reduced. Also, no increase in energy intake is needed until the last trimester, when an additional 837 kJ (200 kcal) per day is required. This equates to

a small ham and cheese sandwich, or a banana smoothie, or a medium bowl of porridge with milk, or 30 g of mixed nuts.

Weight gain during pregnancy varies considerably and is often dependent on pre-pregnancy weight, and it influences both maternal and infant health outcomes as well as postpartum weight retention. There are currently no formal, evidence-based guidelines from the UK government or professional bodies on what constitutes appropriate weight gain during pregnancy, but NICE advises that women weighing more than 100 kg may require specific advice from a health professional (NICE 2010) (see Section 15.2.1).

The controversy over the clinical value of monitoring gestational weight gain has been reviewed recently (Amorim *et al.* 2008). While there is a growing body of literature that indicates that weight gain during pregnancy is an inexpensive anthropometric indicator to monitor maternal and fetal nutritional status, predict pregnancy outcomes and identify women at risk, others have argued that the relationship between maternal weight gain and pregnancy outcomes is not strong enough to make it a sensitive or specific screening tool for identifying undesirable outcomes. Much of the contention is related to when weight measurements are taken, and research has suggested that only maternal weight at entry to prenatal care is significantly associated with the infant's birthweight. Possible reasons for weak or non-significant associations between gestational weight gain and maternal and neonatal outcomes are due to the poor quality of obstetric records and selection of the wrong indicators to compute gestational weight gain.

The issue with weight loss after pregnancy is the difference between 'dieting' and sensible eating that results in gradual weight loss. 'Dieting' typically involves a restricted-energy diet and/or avoidance of certain foods or food groups. 'Dieting' is not recommended before, during or immediately after pregnancy. It is particularly important that women who are breastfeeding do not 'diet'. Instead, women should aim to lose weight gradually after childbirth. Gradual weight loss can be achieved through eating a healthy, varied diet and exercising regularly, and is more likely to be maintained long-term if achieved this way. Currently, there are no UK guidelines on the appropriate rate of weight loss postpartum to achieve pre-pregnancy weight. For the general population, gradual weight loss is considered to be no more than 0.5–1 kg per week. A higher rate of weight loss may be experienced by some women postpartum, particularly those who are breastfeeding. In this case, it may be more important to focus on ensuring that the mother's diet is adequate to meet her nutritional requirements (and the additional demand of lactation) rather than the rate of weight loss.

15.3.1.1 Physical activity

Given the high prevalence of obesity in women (almost half of women of childbearing age are either overweight or obese), there is a need for greater recognition of the importance of entering pregnancy with an appropriate body weight (i.e. in the healthy weight range) and the role of physical activity throughout life (including during pregnancy) in maintaining a healthy weight. Only about 30% of women of childbearing age meet the recommendation of 30 minutes or more moderate physical activity on at least 5 days of the week. Guidance on physical activity in pregnancy is available from the Royal College of Obstetricians and Gynaecologists (RCOG 2006). Additional benefits of physical activity during pregnancy include enhanced fitness, and reduced muscle cramps and swelling of legs and feet. Women who have not been habitually active are advised to begin with 15 minutes of continuous aerobic physical activity, three times a week, and to gradually increase this to 30-minute sessions four times a week or more. Physical activity sessions should be accompanied by warm-up and cool-down phases. Contact sports are not advised and hormonal changes cause joints to be more mobile, increasing the risk of injury with weightbearing physical activity. After 16 weeks of pregnancy, physical activities that involve lying on the back are not recommended as the womb is likely to put pressure on major blood vessels. Remaining well hydrated and avoiding hot humid conditions when exercising are also considered important (RCOG 2006). Intervention studies are required to determine effective dietary and physical activity interventions appropriate for overweight and obese pregnant women (see Chapter 8, Section 8.5).

The guidance on physical activity (*Start Active, Stay Active*) published in 2011 by the UK Chief Medical Officers (Chief Medical Officers of England 2011) draws attention to the importance of physical activity for infants and young children, recommending that physical activity should be encouraged from birth, particularly through floor-based play and water-based activities in safe environments. Children of pre-school age who are capable of walking unaided should be physically active daily for at least 180 minutes (3 hours) spread throughout the day. For all under-5s, the amount of time spent being sedentary (being restrained or sitting) for extended periods should be minimised, with the exception of time spent sleeping. As discussed in Chapter 12, Section 12.6, children with habitually greater levels of physical activity have higher bone mineral accrual, although whether this translates into long-term benefits or a reduction in fracture risk, either in childhood or in later adulthood, remains to be established.

15.3.2 Macronutrients

15.3.2.1 Protein

Maternal protein requirements change during pregnancy and lactation (see Chapter 3, Table 3.3). The potential impact of differences in the protein content of breast milk and breast milk substitutes is discussed in Section 15.4.3.

15.3.2.2 Fatty acids

Fatty acids of the *n*-3 and *n*-6 families play major roles during pregnancy, providing precursors for the synthesis of eicosanoids and important constituents of cell membrane phospholipids. An adequate supply of essential fatty acids to the fetus is important for development in general and in particular for cognitive and neural development (see Chapter 6, Section 6.4.5, Chapter 14 and Chapter 15, Sections 15.1.3 and 15.2.7). Two long-chain PUFAs, arachidonic acid (AA; 20:4 *n*-6) and docosahexaenoic acid (DHA; 22:6 *n*-3), are important structural fatty acids in neural tissue. DHA in particular is found in the membranes of neuronal synapses and of photoreceptor outer segments, where it performs an array of membrane-associated functions. There are specific recommendations about intake of long-chain *n*-3 fatty acids (see Chapter 3, Section 3.4.1.3). It has been suggested that birth spacing may be a factor in allowing time for maternal essential fatty acid status to be restored. Research is currently being conducted at the University of Southampton, UK, on the impact of nutritional status on the human reproductive tract and periconceptual interventions to improve fertility outcomes.

15.3.3 Micronutrients

The status of a number of micronutrients is of particular interest during pregnancy and early life, although the specific effects of deficiency are not currently well understood. Table 15.1 summarises the main functions of a selection of nutrients (see also Chapter 3, Section 3.4.1.4). The EC-funded project EURRECA (European Micronutrient Recommendations Aligned) has highlighted the heterogeneity that currently exists in micronutrient recommendations across Europe (as illustrated in Table 15.2), the need for standardised approaches and the importance of establishing recommendations for vulnerable sub-populations of pregnant women, including adolescents and women who have their babies later

Table 15.1 The role and main dietary sources of micronutrients of particular significance during pregnancy

Micronutrient	Functions of particular relevance to pregnancy (1)	UK dietary recommendation during pregnancy (2)	Examples of sources (3)
Folate	Involved in DNA cycle (cell replication); methylation cycle	300 μg/day*	Green leafy vegetables, brown rice, peas, oranges, bananas and fortified breakfast cereals
Vitamin B_{12}	Conversion of homocysteine to methionine as a cofactor of methionine synthase	1.5 μg/day§	Meat, fish, milk, cheese, eggs, fortified yeast extract and fortified breakfast cereals Green plants provide none but it can be synthesised by some algae (although generally not biologically active) and bacteria (but needs to be complexed with intrinsic factor in the stomach for absorption so vitamin B_{12} synthesised in human colon will not be absorbed)
Vitamin A	Growth and differentiation of various cells and tissues	700 μg/day	Retinol: liver, whole milk, cheese, butter, margarine and many reduced fat spreads are dietary sources of retinol. Supplements containing more than 600 μg of retinol should be avoided by pregnant women or women planning a pregnancy. Liver should also be avoided as it contains high levels of retinol Beta-carotene: carrots, dark green leafy vegetables and orange-coloured fruits are dietary sources of beta-carotene In the UK, margarine must be fortified with vitamin A and it is often voluntarily added to reduced fat spreads
Vitamin D	Bone resorption, intestinal calcium transport (calcium and bone homeostasis); modulation of transcription of cell cycle proteins; cell differentiating, anti-inflammatory and immunomodulatory properties	10 μg/day	Dietary sources are relatively insignificant, compared with the synthesis in the skin from exposure to sunlight Vitamin D insufficiency is common in winter months and may be more prevalent in people with darkly melanised skin. Dietary intakes usually only provide 2–3 μg/day Oil-rich fish, eggs, meat, fortified cereals and margarine are the main dietary sources of vitamin D. In the UK, margarine must be fortified with vitamin D and it is often voluntarily added to reduced fat spreads and also to other foods, including some breakfast cereals. Human milk contains low levels of vitamin D, but infant formula is fortified with 0.001–0.0025 mg/100 kcal (418 KJ)

Table 15.1 *(Continued)*

Micronutrient	Functions of particular relevance to pregnancy (1)	UK dietary recommendation during pregnancy (2)	Examples of sources (3)
Iodine	Synthesis of thyroid hormones	140 μg/day§	Sea fish, shellfish and seaweed are rich sources but milk is also a major source (in the UK diet). The amount of iodine in plant foods such as vegetables and cereal grains is determined by the amount of iodine in the growing plant's environment, and the amount in the soil or water can vary dramatically. Iodine is added to salt in iodine deficient areas in many countries
Iron	Haematopoiesis; nucleic acid metabolism; carrier of oxygen to tissues by red blood cell haemoglobin; transport medium for electrons within cells; integral part of important enzyme systems	14.8 mg/day§	Liver, red meat, pulses, nuts, eggs, dried fruits, poultry, fish, whole-grains and dark green leafy vegetables. All wheat flours (other than wholemeal) and many breakfast cereals in the UK are fortified with iron. However, the nature of these foods imposes limitations on the type of iron that can be used as a fortificant and so low bioavailability may be an issue There can also be a significant contribution to iron intake from the use of iron cooking pots and pans
Calcium	Bone formation (fetus) and maintenance (mother)	700 mg/day§	Milk, cheese and other dairy products, some green leafy vegetables, fortified soya products and fish eaten with the bones such as sardines, tinned salmon and whitebait. Bread is an important source in the UK because most bread flour (though not wholemeal) is fortified There is also a contribution from drinking water in hard water areas
Zinc	Structural, regulatory and catalytic functions as cofactor for numerous metalloenzymes	7 mg/day§	Meat, milk, cheese, eggs, shellfish, whole-grain cereals, nuts and pulses (in cereals and pulses bioavailability is limited by phytates)
Selenium	Protection of body systems against oxidative stress; maintenance of defences against infection; modulation of growth and development	60 μg/day§	Brazil nuts, bread, fish, meat and eggs. The selenium content of cereals is directly proportional to the selenium content in the soil. In the UK, selenium intakes have fallen with the decline in import of North American selenium-rich wheat and the increased use of European cereals which are less rich in the mineral

*400 μg/day additionally recommended preconception and for the first 12 weeks of gestation.
§No increment.
Source: (1) information derived from Berti *et al.* (2010); (2) Department of Health (1991); (3) www.nutrition.org.uk.

Table 15.2 An illustration of the variation in current micronutrient recommendations for pregnant women within Europe

	Vitamin A	Vitamin D	Vitamin B$_{12}$	Folate	Iodine	Zinc	Iron
			(µg/day)			(mg/day)	
UK	700	10	1.5§	300**	140§	7§	14.8§¶
Italy	700	10‡	2.2	400‡	175	7	30‡
Nordic countries*	800	10	2.0	500	175	9§§	–†***
Spain¥	800	10	2.2	600††	135	20	18
Germany, Austria, Switzerland	1.1 mg retinol equivalent	5	3.5	600	230 (Switzerland 200)	10	30

Vitamin D: 10 µg/day equates to 400 IU/day.
*Denmark, Finland, Iceland, Norway, Sweden.
**400 µg/day additionally recommended preconception and for the first 12 weeks of gestation.
¥From the second half of pregnancy.
††First and second half of gestation.
‡Dietary supplements or fortified foods may be required.
§No increment.
†The composition of the meal influences the utilisation of dietary iron. The availability increases if the diet contains abundant amounts of vitamin C and meat or fish daily, while it is decreased at simultaneous intake of e.g. polyphenols or phytic acid.
§§Utilisation of zinc is negatively influenced by phytic acid and positively by animal protein. The recommended intakes are valid for a mixed animal/vegetable diet. For a vegetarian cereal-based diets, a 25–30% higher intake is recommended.
¶Insufficient for women with high menstrual losses for whom the most practical approach is to take iron supplements.
***Iron balance during pregnancy requires iron stores of approximately 500 mg at the start of pregnancy. The physiological need of some women for iron cannot be satisfied during the last two-thirds of pregnancy with food alone, and supplemental iron is therefore needed.
Source: Data from Berti *et al.* (2010).

in life (Berti *et al.* 2010) (see Chapter 3, Section 3.2.1). They also highlighted the need for harmonisation because nutrient recommendations form the basis of food policy and food-based dietary guidelines, and are used in nutrition labelling and related legislation (which is harmonised across Europe).

Fetal growth is regulated by the balance between fetal nutrient demand and maternal-placental nutrient supply, the latter being influenced by maternal nutrition and metabolism, utero-placental blood flow, and the size and transfer capabilities of the placenta. Berti and colleagues emphasise the variation in effect depending on when during pregnancy the dietary inadequacy occurs, and also the importance of peri-conceptional nutrition in establishing and developing the pregnancy and the potential for prenatal maternal micronutrient status to condition breast milk composition. The impact of birth spacing is discussed in Chapter 3, Section 3.2.2).

15.3.3.1 Vitamin D

The main source of vitamin D is sunlight (UVB, 290–315 nm) exposure and, in most situations,

approximately 30 minutes of skin exposure during the middle of the day in the summer months can provide 50 000 IU (1.25 mg) of vitamin D for people with white skin (Berti *et al.* 2010). Latitude and season, skin pigmentation, sun avoidance and the use of sunscreen, cloud cover and the extent of clothing cover all influence the capacity of dermal synthesis to fulfil individual vitamin D needs (Lanham-New *et al.* 2011). Those living at a latitude above 52° N (the UK is at a latitude of 50–60° N) may not synthesise enough vitamin D during the winter months (Department of Health 2012b). This affects much of Western Europe (including 90% of the UK), all of Scandinavia and 50% of the North American landmass.

As will be evident from Table 15.2, specific dietary recommendations exist during pregnancy and these vary to some extent from country to country, reflecting the lack of clear evidence upon which recommendations can be based. Typically in Europe (and elsewhere), recommendations are in the range of 5–10 µg/day. Most countries have no official recommendations for ethnic minority groups, in whom risk of deficiency may be greater. Re-emergence of rickets is evident in some sub groups in the UK, predominantly among people of African-Caribbean and South Asian origin (Lanham-New *et al.* 2011). Among the general population, advice to use sunscreen in relation to cancer protection may have contributed to reduced vitamin D status and there is an urgent need for authoritative advice that balances the cancer and vitamin D status aspects. The Department of Health advises that it is wise to stay covered up and use sunscreen (with a high UVB factor) for the majority of time spent outside and to always cover up or protect the skin before it starts to turn red or burn (Department of Health 2012b).

Table 15.3 shows the main contributors to dietary intake of vitamin D in the UK. Dietary sources are few and average intake in women from food is only 2.6 μg/day (Bates *et al.* 2011). Oil-rich fish is the richest source (e.g. in the range 3–8 μg/100 g) but only around 28% of adult women consume oil-rich fish and few achieve the recommendation of one serving per week (see Section 15.2.7). Furthermore, intake of oil-rich fish is very low in adolescent girls and also lower in low-income groups. Eggs provide 3.15 μg/100 g, lamb's liver 0.5 μg/100 g and lean beef 0.7 μg/100 g. Fortified foods also contribute to UK intakes; fortified margarine/spread provides 7.9 μg/100 g and fortified breakfast cereals contain varying amounts usually in the range of 1.5–8.5 μg/100 g.

As illustrated in Fig. 15.2, there is evidence of low vitamin D status (defined as serum 25(OH)D < 25 nmol/L) across the UK population and low vitamin D status is particularly marked in 2-year-old Asian children.

Among pregnant women, low vitamin D status is common. In a study in southern England, 18% of pregnant White women had a serum 25(OH)D < 25 nmol/L and 31% had a level < 50 nmol/L (Javaid *et al.* 2006), and in a study of UK pregnant women from ethnic minorities, >50% had a serum 25(OH)D < 25 nmol/L (Datta *et al.* 2002). Pre-pregnancy BMI is inversely associated with serum vitamin D concentration, causing obese women to be at greater risk of vitamin D deficiency. Neonatal and infant vitamin D status is dependent on maternal vitamin D status, and cord blood vitamin D levels are lower in babies born to obese mothers (Bodnar *et al.*

Table 15.3 Dietary sources of vitamin D in the UK

Source	Contribution to dietary intakes in women (%)
Cereal and cereal products	22
Milk and milk products	3
Egg and egg dishes	9
Fat spreads (included fortified margarine)	15
Meat and meat products	18
Fish and fish dishes	30

Source: Henderson *et al.* (2003).

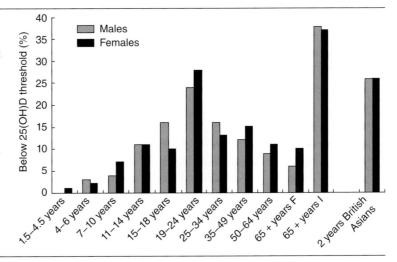

Figure 15.2 Prevalence of vitamin D deficiency defined as serum 25(OH)D < 25 nmol/L in individuals in the UK.
F, free-living; I, institutionalised. British Asians were defined as those of South Asian origin (Pakistani, Indian and Bangladeshi). Reproduced with permission from Lanham-New SA, Buttriss JL, Miles LM *et al.* (2011) Proceedings of the Rank Forum on Vitamin D. *British Journal of Nutrition*, **105**, 144–56, with permission from Cambridge University Press.

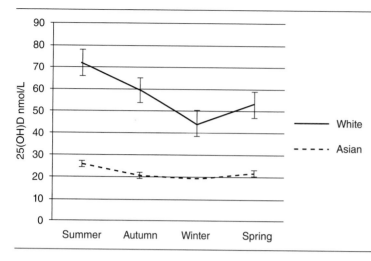

Figure 15.3 Vitamin D status (serum 25(OH)D) by ethnicity and season in a cohort of pre-menopausal women. Reproduced from Osteoporosis International by European Foundation for Osteoporosis; National Osteoporosis Foundation; International Osteoporosis Foundation, with permission from Springer-Verlag London. Darling AL, Hart KH, Macdonald HM *et al.* (2013) Vitamin D deficiency in UK South Asian women of childbearing age: a comparative longitudinal investigation with UK Caucasian women. *Osteoporosis International*, **24**, 477-88.

2007). Current advice in the UK is for pregnant and lactating women, infants, young children (and those over age 65) to supplement their diet with vitamin D. Other risk factors for poor vitamin D status are multiparity, short birth spacing and non-White maternal skin.

The interaction between diet and sunlight exposure on vitamin D status 25(OH)D and functional markers of calcium metabolism and bone health have been studied in Asian and White women living in southern England (who were not taking vitamin D or cod liver oil supplements), in the vitamin D, Food Intake, Nutrition and Exposure to Sunlight in southern England (D-FINES) study. Vitamin D status was consistently higher in pre-menopausal White women compared with pre-menopausal Asian women and showed seasonal variation, being higher in the summer and autumn. There was evidence of poorer status in the winter months (over 60% had 25(OH)D levels below 50 nmol/L). In Asian pre-menopausal women, status was low throughout the year and was below the 25 nmol/L cut-off in the vast majority of women in autumn (79%), winter (81%) and spring (75%) (Darling *et al.* personal communication) (Fig. 15.3).

Similar findings to those illustrated in Fig. 15.2 exist for other European countries, particularly during the winter months, e.g. Denmark, the Netherlands, Germany and Ireland (see Health Council of the Netherlands 2008a). Furthermore, in studies in Denmark, poor vitamin D status was present in over

80% of Pakistani girls and women during the winter months and, in another Danish study of women who wore a veil for religious reasons, 96% had poor status even during the summer (see Health Council of the Netherlands 2008a).

Roles for vitamin D in protection against diabetes, cardiovascular disease and some cancers and in optimising immune function have been proposed recently. This has triggered controversy about the optimal range of serum 25(OH)D (recent estimates have varied between 30 and 80 nmol/L), the threshold concentration below which there are increased risks to health, and also the amount of oral vitamin D required to achieve these various proposals for optimal status (Dawson-Hughes *et al.* 2005; Cashman and Kiely 2011; Lanham-New *et al.* 2011). But the ongoing debate must not be allowed to hinder progress towards the introduction of steps to combat vitamin D deficiency in the context of current guidelines.

Antenatal guidance from the National Institute for Health and Clinical Excellence (NICE 2008) advises on the need to inform pregnant women about the importance of maintaining adequate vitamin D stores during pregnancy and to advise them to take a 10 μg supplement daily; women of South Asian, African, Caribbean or Middle Eastern descent, and those who are housebound, are considered to be at particular risk. Prior to 2008, NICE's position had been that there was insufficient evidence to support routine supplementation and this inconsistency is thought to have led to lack of clarity for health professionals advising the public (SACN 2007). A new Department of Health leaflet on vitamin D deficiency addresses this matter (Department of Health 2012b).

Lack of awareness of the need for vitamin D supplements during pregnancy and lactation is thought to be widespread and there is particular concern about the vitamin D status of teenagers and young women in general, and women in some ethnic minority groups because their darker skin coupled with traditional dress means that skin synthesis is very limited in the British climate. Furthermore, the relatively small amount of vitamin D available from the diet (average intakes from food in adult women in the UK being 2.6 μg/day and in the Netherlands 2.9 μg/day (Health Council of the Netherlands 2008a), means that supplementation (or possibly targeted fortification) is likely to be the most appropriate route. It has also been suggested that those women with darker skins may require a supplement greater than 10 μg/day, especially during pregnancy. Health professionals have been slow to respond to the problem (Pearce and Cheetham 2010).

In the UK, since 2004, 'Healthy Start Vitamins' have been available, free of charge from baby clinics, for pregnant and breastfeeding women and children up to the age of 5 years if the mother is under 18 years of age or on income support, via the Healthy Start scheme (www.healthystart.nhs.uk) (see Chapter 3, Section 3.9.6.4). While there have been reports of problems with the supply chain and lack of awareness among some health professionals (Lanham-New *et al.* 2011), since October 2010, Healthy Start Vitamins have also been available from pharmacists in order to improve availability and uptake. However, it is not only low-income families on benefits who show evidence of low vitamin D status and so there remains a need for enhanced awareness of the problem across the population.

15.3.3.2 *Folate and folic acid*

Since the early 1990s, when research showed that daily consumption of 400 μg of folic acid before conception and during early pregnancy dramatically reduced the occurrence of neural tube defects (NTDs) (Medical Research Council 1991; Czeizel and Dudas 1992), governments and health organisations worldwide have made recommendations for women, before and during early pregnancy, to take folic acid supplements. Adherence to this advice can prevent 50–70% of NTDs, which annually affect more than 300 000 pregnancies worldwide (Centers for Disease Control and Prevention (CDC) 2009; Christianson *et al.* 2006).

In 2000, the UK Department of Health's Committee on Medical Aspects of Food and Nutrition Policy (COMA) concluded that fortification of flour with folic acid would prevent a significant proportion of births affected by NTDs in the UK (COMA 2000). In 2002, the Food Standards Agency (FSA) Board started discussions on the possibility of folic acid fortification in the UK. The Scientific Advisory Committee on Nutrition (SACN), an independent group of scientific experts that succeeded COMA in advising the UK government, also began reviewing the reported risks and the benefits. In 2004, UK Health Ministers requested consideration of the wider impact of folic acid fortification, deciding that at this stage mandatory fortification should not be implemented because of outstanding concerns about vitamin B_{12} deficiency, especially in elderly people. Following its review, in December 2006, SACN recommended that mandatory fortification should be introduced and the FSA launched a consultation on the proposal to fortify flour with folic acid, prior to ministers making a final decision in May 2007 (Medical Research Council (MRC) 2007).

In May 2007, the FSA Board agreed unanimously that mandatory fortification with folic acid of either bread or flour should be implemented, together with recommendations on controls of voluntary fortification for manufacturers and advice for the public on folic acid supplementation. However, mandatory fortification was not introduced at this time because the Chief Medical Officer requested SACN to consider emerging research that suggested folic acid might increase the risk of colorectal cancer. SACN reviewed the evidence and agreed, in October 2009, to support its previous recommendation for the implementation of mandatory fortification with folic acid, with controls on voluntary fortification. In addition, SACN advised that people at higher risk of developing colorectal adenomas or colorectal cancer (i.e. people over 50 and those with a history of colorectal adenomas) should not take folic acid supplements containing more than 200 μg a day without medical advice. At this point there was a change in government and restructuring of the FSA and

Department of Health, and the matter is now in the hands of the Chief Medical Officer. An announcement is expected in 2013.

At the global level, over 70 countries have already introduced mandatory folic acid fortification of flour to prevent NTDs (Table 15.4) (Flour Fortification Initiative (FFI) 2010a), but to date (2012) no countries within the EU have taken this step. Coinciding with the introduction of mandatory folic acid fortification of foods, NTD rates have declined by 27–50% in the US and Canada (see McNulty *et al.* 2011).

The countries that have introduced legislation are at various stages in the flour fortification process and evaluation of the effectiveness of the intervention (Table 15.5).

In the UK, in the absence of fortification, the government continues to advise women of childbearing age to take a daily 400 μg folic acid supplement and to consume foods that provide folate and folic acid. Women who have already experienced an NTD-affected pregnancy are advised to take a 5 mg supplement daily (SACN 2011a). Raised BMI also increases risk of NTD (Rasmussen *et al.* 2008).

There is evidence of ethnic and social disparities relating to use of folic acid supplements. For example, a study of over 400 newly pregnant women in East London found that 42% of Caucasian mothers had taken folic acid supplements prior to neural tube closure compared to only 19% of West Indian and Asian mothers (Brough *et al.* 2009). Similar ethnic disparities have been reported in previous studies conducted in the UK and the US. Pre-conceptional use also appears to be low among teenagers (see Chapter 3, Section 3.3.3).

The main dietary sources of folate in the UK diet are cereals and vegetables (including potatoes), each providing about a third of total intake. A significant amount of that provided by cereals is derived from fortification. Milk and milk products contribute about 8% and fruit 7%. In the National Diet and Nutrition Survey (NDNS) of adults (aged 19–64 years), average intakes of folate among women aged 19–24 and 25–34, respectively, were 248 and 249 μg/day. Among 19- to 24-year-olds, 86% had an intake from all sources below 400 μg/day. In 25- to 34-year-olds and 35- to 49-year-olds, the figures were 92 and 84% respectively (Henderson *et al.* 2003). Among 15- to 18-year-olds, 4% had an intake below the lower reference nutrient intake (LRNI) of 100 μg/day (Smithers *et al.* 2000).

While awareness of the importance of folic acid around the time of conception is high (see Chapter 3, Section 3.3.3), compliance with the recommendation is not reflected in practice among pregnant women. A study in Northern Ireland found that 84% reported taking folic acid supplements in the first trimester but only 19% had started before conception as recom-

Table 15.4 Countries with mandatory fortification of flour with folic acid (as at December 2012)

Central and Eastern Europe	**Asia**	**North America**	**Sub-Saharan Africa**
Kazakhstan, Kosovo, Kyrgyzstan Republic of Moldova, Turkmenistan, Uzbekistan	Indonesia, Nepal	Canada, United States	Benin, Cameroon, Côte d'Ivoire, Ghana, Guinea, Kenya, Mali, Niger, Nigeria, Senegal, Sierra Leone, South Africa, Tanzania, Togo, Uganda
Caribbean	**Middle East/North Africa**	**Latin America**	**Oceania**
Antigua and Barbuda, Bahamas, Barbados, Cuba, Dominica, Dominican Republic, Grenada, Guadeloupe, Guyana, Haiti, Jamaica, Puerto Rico, Saint Kitts and Nevis, Saint Lucia, Saint Vincent and the Grenadines	Bahrain, Egypt, Iran, Iraq, Jordan, Kuwait, Mauritania, Morocco, Oman, Palestine Occupied Territory, Saudi Arabia, Yemen	Argentina, Belize, Bolivia, Brazil, Chile, Colombia, Costa Rica, Ecuador, El Salvador, Guatemala, Honduras, Mexico, Nicaragua, Panama, Paraguay, Peru, Suriname, Uruguay	Australia, Fiji

Note: These countries require fortification of at least one kind of wheat flour. Some countries require fortification of white flours but not wholewheat, for example. Some countries also require fortification of maize flour, but this data has not yet been collected.
Most countries add at least iron and folic acid along with other B vitamins and sometimes zinc.
Wheat Flour Fortification Legislation Status, March 2012, Flour Fortification Initiative, http://www.sph.emory.edu/wheatflour///globalmap.php

Table 15.5 Examples of the impact of global folic acid fortification on neural tube defect (NTD) prevalence

Country	Introduction of mandatory folic acid fortification	Quantity and delivery method	Decrease reported in NTD prevalence since introduction of folic acid fortification
Canada	November 1998	150 µg/100 g wheat flour	46% by 2002[a]
Chile	January 2000	220 µg/100 g wheat flour	40% by 2002[b]
Costa Rica	1999	180 µg/100 g wheat flour	35% by 2000[c]
	2000	180 µg/100 g maize flour	
	2001	40 µg/100 g milk	
South Africa	October 2003	150 µg/100 g wheat flour	31% by 2005[d]
		221 µg/100 g maize meal	
United States	November 1998	140 µg/100 g wheat flour	27% by 2000[e]

[a]De Wals *et al.* (2007),
[b]Hertrampf and Cortes (2004),
[c]Chen and Rivera (2004),
[d]Sayed *et al.* (2008),
[e]Centers for Disease Control and Prevention (CDC) (2004).

mended, despite NTD rates being among the highest in the world (McNulty *et al.* 2011). Furthermore, red cell folate levels in women not complying with recommendations were suboptimal in relation to NTD risk. This indicates the need for a review of current policy as it suggests that in the absence of population-wide food fortification, current recommendations are not being achieved. This is underlined by the findings of a large multicentre study examining 13 million birth records from nine European countries, including the UK, which showed no detectable impact on NTD incidence in any country over the period 1988–98, which included the period when folic acid was actively promoted (Botto *et al.* 2005). There is also a need to understand better and act upon the barriers to supplement use. Higher parity is associated with increased NTD risk and, after their first baby, women appear to be less likely to take folic acid supplementation (McNulty *et al.* 2011).

15.3.3.3 Vitamin B_{12}

Like folate, vitamin B_{12} is important in methylation processes and there is growing awareness of the potential of imbalances in methyl donors to effect changes in disease risk via epigenetic regulation and also (based on animal studies) to influence intergenerational effects. So, vitamin B_{12} may be important during pregnancy and early life (see Chapter 5, Section 5.14, Chapter 11, Section 11.4.2.2 and Chapter 4, Section 4.5.3). A study of pregnant women

in Northern Ireland identified a high prevalence of poor vitamin B_{12} status. This has implications for NTD protection, owing to evidence that vitamin B_{12} status is an independent predictor of NTD risk (Molloy *et al.* 2009), presumably through its involvement in methionine metabolism (see Table 15.1). Almost a third of women had pregnancy vitamin B_{12} levels below 250 ng/L, the level associated (independently of folate status) with an almost three-fold increase in risk of NTD-affected pregnancy compared to a level >400 ng/L (Molloy *et al.* 2009).

15.3.3.4 Calcium

Foods containing calcium should be included in the diet during pregnancy and lactation (see Chapter 3, Section 3.4.1.4). Recommendations are generally being met, but with the exception of some adolescents (see Section 15.5.2). Although higher maternal UVB exposure and 25(OH)D status are associated with greater offspring bone size in later childhood, the relationship with maternal calcium intake or the effects of maternal supplementation are not clear (SACN 2011a).

15.3.3.5 Iron

Iron status during pregnancy and early life is important for a number of reasons, including the risk of iron deficiency impairing neurological/cognitive development, which is rapid during the latter stages of gestation and during infancy (see Chapters 6 and 14), and in relation to diabetes (see Chapter 9). During the third trimester, the fetus accumulates about 2 mg of iron a day and a full-term infant has accumulated 150–250 mg in total, almost 80% of which is in haemoglobin. Fetal haemoglobin has a greater affinity for oxygen than adult haemoglobin, in response to the low availability of oxygen *in utero*. A second difference or adaptation is a higher haemoglobin concentration in the circulation compared to postnatal life (SACN 2010). Following birth, there is a fall in haemoglobin concentration of about 30% in response to the greater abundance of oxygen, and this provides a store of iron (in serum ferritin) of up to 60 mg that can be utilised for lean tissue synthesis during the first 6 months of life. This limits dependence of healthy term infants on dietary iron during this period, particularly if clamping of the umbilical cord is delayed until it has stopped pulsing, which boosts iron levels (SACN 2010). These postnatal changes in haemoglobin synthesis and iron stores occur irrespective of gestational age, which places premature babies at a disadvantage.

In non-pregnant women of childbearing age, intakes are frequently below recommended levels; in women aged 19–64, 23% have intakes below the LRNI for iron and the picture is much worse in girls aged 11–18 in whom the prevalence rate is 46% (Bates *et al.* 2012) (see Section 15.5.2 and Chapter 3, Sections 3.2.1.1 and 3.4.1.4). There is no national data on iron intakes or prevalence of iron deficiency in pregnant women in the UK, but several small British studies suggest that intakes below reference levels are evident. But, there is also little correlation between iron intake and iron status, as measured by haemoglobin. However, there is a strong inverse correlation between parity and ferritin levels that may signify reduced iron stores and potentially the impact of birth spacing. It has been suggested that short inter-pregnancy intervals (<18 months) may provide insufficient time for maternal stores to be replenished and this may compromise the woman's iron status at conception and also her ability to support fetal development, although there are limitations in the quality of the evidence to support this (SACN 2010).

As is apparent in Table 15.2, there is considerable variation in the reference intakes for iron intake during pregnancy, even within Europe (see Chapter 3, Section 3.4.1.4). The opinion of authorities in the UK is that physiological adaptations during preg-

nancy and lactation ensure an adequate supply of iron to the fetus; in particular, changes in structural and compositional characteristics of transferrin favour transfer to the placenta rather than to systemic transferrin receptors (SACN 2010), so reference intakes are the same as for non-pregnant women in the UK, and the same applies in the EU. Nevertheless, severe maternal iron deficiency and anaemia in the early months of pregnancy (and also very high haemoglobin levels) are associated with adverse birth outcomes including low birthweight, pre-term birth and increased perinatal mortality; this association is not necessarily causal (SACN 2010).

In the UK, NICE recommends that iron supplementation should be considered in women with haemoglobin concentrations below 110 g/L in the first trimester and below 105 g/L at 28 weeks (NICE 2008) (and this has been supported by SACN (2011a). In the US, the Centers for Disease Control and Prevention recommend routine iron supplementation (30 mg/ day) for all women during pregnancy (Centers for Disease Control and Prevention 1998) and higher supplementation levels for those identified as having iron deficiency anaemia, whereas the US Preventative Services Task Force, like NICE in the UK, recommends routine screening but not routine supplementation (SACN 2010).

The iron content of breast milk is not influenced by the mother's iron status or by iron supplementation during lactation (SACN 2010). After 6 months of age, when iron reserves have been depleted and growth is rapid, iron requirements rise and the amount provided in breast milk is no longer sufficient, even with upregulation of intestinal absorption. This makes the iron content of the weaning diet of particular importance (see Chapter 3, Section 3.9) as iron deficiency is commonly reported in infants and young children (see Chapter 3, Section 3.9.6.2).

15.3.3.6 Zinc

The importance of zinc in cognitive development is discussed in Chapters 6 and 14, and other relevant functions of zinc are listed in Table 15.1.

15.3.3.7 Iodine

Worldwide, iodine deficiency is widespread and a recent WHO Technical Consultation that focused on the prevention and control of iodine deficiency in pregnant and lactating women and in children under the age of 2 years (Andersson *et al.* 2007) recommended an increase in the WHO reference value for pregnant and lactating women from 200 μg/day to 250 μg/day. No added benefit was associated with intakes over 500 μg/day. For children under the age of 2 years, the recommendation has remained the same at 90 μg/day, and intakes above 180 μg/day are considered to provide no added benefit. Iodised salt is the vehicle recommended by the WHO as the first line of defence in combating conditions caused by iodine deficiency, and supplementation may be required before or during early pregnancy to prevent fetal damage in some countries. In areas of the world where severe iodine deficiency exists, maternal and fetal hypothyroxinaemia can cause cretinism and adversely affect cognitive development in children. Thyroid hormone is required for normal neuronal migration, myelination, and synaptic transmission and plasticity during fetal and early postnatal life. Hypothyroxinaemia at this time leads to irreversible brain damage, mental retardation and neurological abnormalities. Whether mild to moderate maternal deficiency, which is present in parts of Europe, produces more subtle changes in cognitive function in offspring is unclear. This is because the controlled trials of iodine treatment in pregnant women with mild to moderate iodine deficiency have not reported data on infant or child development (Zimmermann 2009).

Few westernised countries have followed the WHO recommendation to provide 20–40 mg iodine per kg table salt although related policies in a number of countries (e.g. Belgium, Germany, France, Switzerland, the Netherlands) permit iodisation of table or bakery salt (and in some countries this is mandatory, e.g. Denmark, Austria) (see Health Council of the Netherlands 2008b for details). There is no such policy in the UK and a pilot study of 227 pregnant women reported that 3.5% had iodine deficiency and 40% had marginal status (Kibirige *et al.* 2004).

In the UK, the reference intake for pregnant and lactating women is currently 140 μg/day, which is the same as for non-pregnant women. Similarly, in the US, the recommended intake in non-pregnant women is 150 μg/day but is increased to 220 μg/day during pregnancy. In the UK, 18% of adolescent girls have an iodine intake below the LRNI, although the picture is of less concern in non-adolescent women (see Section 15.5.2); the implications of this are worthy of investigation. Dietary sources are listed in Table 15.1.

15.3.4 Alcohol

The question of whether moderate alcohol consumption during pregnancy is linked to health risks for the offspring has been widely debated for some years. Despite the lack of evidence of detrimental effects on any outcome at low-to-moderate maternal alcohol consumption (<10 units/week), many professional bodies err on the side of caution. The WHO recommends abstinence from alcohol during pregnancy and similar advice is given in North America (United States and Canada) and Australia. In 2008 the UK's National Institute for Health and Clinical Excellence (NICE) issued revised guidance on alcohol consumption during pregnancy, as part of its clinical guideline on antenatal care, *Antenatal care: routine care for the healthy pregnant woman*, and advised that pregnant women and those planning a pregnancy avoid alcohol in the first 3 months of pregnancy (NICE 2008). This created a number of media headlines (Miles 2008). The new clinical guideline is largely consistent with the Department of Health's advice since 2007, which also advises pregnant women and those trying to conceive to avoid alcohol completely (Department of Health 2007). Before 2007, the Department of Health recommended that pregnant women and those who may become pregnant should drink no more than 1–2 units of alcohol, once or twice a week at any stage of pregnancy, and should avoid binge drinking (Department of Health 1995).

The 2008 NICE advice was not driven by the emergence of new scientific evidence and this is acknowledged by both the Department of Health and NICE. This is perhaps why there is a lack of clarity about the necessity for pregnant women to avoid alcohol completely.

15.3.5 Caffeine

UK government advice on maternal caffeine intake was issued in 2008 following new research that linked levels of caffeine intake above 200 mg/day with an increased risk of giving birth to a baby with low birthweight. Prior to this, the intake guidance figure was no more than 300 mg/day. This benchmark was based on a review conducted in 2001 by the Committee on Toxicity of Chemicals in Food, Consumer

Products and the Environment (COT), which concluded that caffeine intakes above 300 mg/day may be associated with low birthweight and, in some cases, miscarriage. However, COT acknowledged at the time that the evidence was inconclusive. Hence, the FSA funded further research on the effects of caffeine in pregnancy, which supported the new threshold of 200 mg/day as the safe limit to help minimise the risk of fetal growth restriction. This change in advice also caught the attention of the media (Miles and Foxen 2009).

15.4 Diet and lifestyle themes relevant to early feeding and weaning

Recommendations and current practice are summarised in Chapter 3.

15.4.1 Breastfeeding and use of breast milk substitutes

The nature of feeding in infancy influences the rate of growth and the type of tissue deposited and this has the potential to track into adulthood (SACN 2011a). These processes may also be influenced by genetic and ethnic variation, although the extent of this is currently unclear. The pattern of growth exhibited by breast-fed infants is the basis of modern growth charts (see Chapter 2, Section 2.8). The evidence relating infant feeding practices to subsequent cardiovascular disease mortality is inconsistent, but infants who are not breast-fed tend to have a greater risk of type 2 diabetes and are more likely to be obese (SACN 2011a).

15.4.1.1 The impact of the Baby Friendly Initiative

In order to improve breastfeeding rates, training in breastfeeding management is now recommended for health professionals involved in maternity and childcare, using UNICEF's Baby Friendly Initiative (BFI) training as a minimum standard (www.babyfriendly.org.uk) (see NICE 2008). Evaluation of BFI community training in Bristol found improvements in staff breastfeeding attitudes, knowledge and management of problems and a significant increase in breastfeeding rates at 8 weeks: a baby born in 2009 was 1.57 times more likely to be breast-fed than one in 2006 (Ingram *et al.* 2011). However, some women who

cannot breastfeed or those who decide to bottle feed appear to find it difficult to get the information they want from health professionals. Lakshman and colleagues reviewed 23 studies (six qualitative and 17 quantitative) investigating women's experiences of bottle feeding (Lakshman *et al.* 2009). Despite wide differences in study design, context, focus and quality, one of the consistent themes that emerged from the research was that mothers who bottle-fed their babies experienced negative emotions such as guilt, anger, worry, uncertainty and a sense of failure. Some felt that their hospital midwives spent more time with breastfeeding mothers than those choosing to bottle feed and worried about negative opinions from health professionals as a consequence of not breastfeeding. Mothers reported receiving inadequate information on how to bottle feed correctly and consequently did not feel empowered to make decisions about whether to bottle feed, as well as decisions about the frequency of feeding or quantities of formula required. Mistakes in preparation of bottle feeds were therefore common. Related to this, a social marketing intervention to increase breastfeeding rates in a socially deprived area of Leicester, with a cultural tradition of bottle feeding, reported that current policy, which prevents provision of information on use of breast milk substitutes alongside delivery of breastfeeding advice, may have been detrimental in this population group, some of whom had already decided on their method of feeding and were seeking advice and support (Austin and Patterson 2010). The authors argue that, in the absence of readily available, evidence-based information from health professionals, women such as these will draw upon family, friends, magazines and TV programmes where information may be inaccurate or biased. While it is important to promote breastfeeding, it is also necessary to ensure that the needs of bottle-feeding mothers are met. A more open approach to discussions about infant formula alongside the proven benefits of breastfeeding may strengthen the relationship with the midwife and enable her to be more influential with respect to the promotion of breastfeeding.

15.4.2 Weaning onto a family diet

Advice is constrained by the absence of up-to-date information on the diets and nutrient intakes of infants; the most recent survey was conducted in 1995 (Gregory *et al.* 1995). A new survey on the diet and nutrition of infants and young children (aged 4–18 months) is under way. It aims to include provision of quantitative data on the food and nutrient intake, sources of nutrients and nutritional status of 1800 UK infants and young children; quantitative information on breast milk and breast milk substitutes consumed by this age group; and the relationship of anthropometric data with social, dietary and health data.

Meanwhile, the Paediatric Group of the British Dietetic Association, in 2007, proposed a framework for feeding all children from the age of 1 year, based on guidance about the number of servings from each food group in the 'eatwell plate' (Thomas and Bishop 2007) but portion sizes were not provided. To address this, the Infant and Toddler Forum has recently published a factsheet listing appropriate portion size ranges for foods from each of the food groups for children aged 1–3 years (www.infantandtoddlerforum. org). Ranges were thought necessary as the quantities that individual toddlers eat can fluctuate widely from day to day, and the guidance is based on the findings of two large surveys (Avon Longitudinal Study on Parents and Children (ALSPAC) and the NDNS) that were conducted in the early 1990s when obesity levels in toddlers were much lower than today. The guidance is designed to help deliver appropriate amounts of essential nutrients and to limit foods such as confectionery and savoury snacks. In addition to helping to address higher rates of overweight in this age group, the guidance should reassure those parents and carers who are concerned that the children in their care are not eating enough (or are eating too much) and may also help to address problems such as iron deficiency anaemia, dental caries, constipation and diarrhoea (More 2012).

Recommendations and current practice can be found in Chapter 3.

15.4.3 Catch-up growth and accelerated growth

Historically, it has generally been thought that beneficial effects will accrue from optimising neonatal and infant nutrition and preventing growth faltering, particularly in babies who have experienced intrauterine growth restriction. But this approach is now being re-examined as evidence emerges about the potential long-term consequences of growth that is too rapid, including the amplification of later disease risk (see Chapter 2, Section 2.10 and Chapter 8, Section 8.2.2).

In a study of almost 20 000 children, each 100 g increase in weight per month during the first 4 months after birth increased the risk of overweight at age 7 years by around 30% (Stettler *et al.* 2002). More than 25 studies (typically long-term follow-up studies) support the hypothesis that growth acceleration (defined as the upward crossing of weight percentiles) increases the risk of later obesity and this relationship has been demonstrated for obesity in adults and in children, in high- and low-income countries, in breast-fed and formula-fed populations and in a variety of cohorts (Ong and Loos 2006; Singhal *et al.* 2010; Stettler 2007); 20% of the risk of being overweight later in childhood can be attributed to weight gain in the highest quintile in infancy. Follow-up to age 5–8 years of babies in two prospective randomised trials has now demonstrated that a nutrient-enriched diet (micronutrients as well as protein and energy) in infancy, compared to a standard formula, increased fat mass (22–38% greater) later in childhood, supporting a possible causal link between faster early weight gain and later risk of obesity (Singhal *et al.* 2010). These findings are consistent with those of Koletzko and co-workers in a randomised trial (using formulas with different protein contents) that assessed BMI at age 2 years (Koletzko *et al.* 2009) and are also supported by animal studies (Singhal 2010b). Even in breast-fed infants, faster weight gain has been associated with greater adiposity in childhood and shown to programme obesity independently of protein intake and method of infant feeding (see Singhal 2010b). In two prospective randomised trials, Singhal *et al.* (2010) found faster weight gain during the first 3 months to have stronger programming effects on fat mass than on lean mass and on visceral or peritoneal fat (associated with increased cardiovascular disease risk) compared with subcutaneous fat (Singhal 2010b). There appears to be uncertainty about the type of growth; accelerated growth that leads to increased muscle and bone may be different to that which leads to increased fat mass. Under-nutrition followed by over-nutrition results in fat accumulation, and appetite is more likely to be programmed than fat mass.

These findings have important implications for the management of low-birthweight and small-for-gestational-age babies in whom catch-up growth has previously been encouraged, and suggest that primary prevention of obesity could begin in infancy. However, it will be important to also consider outcomes other than adiposity, including neurological development. It is important to note, as mentioned in Chapter 8, Section 8.2.2, that the situation may be different in non-Western populations, where catch-up growth may be important in achieving growth potential.

The slower growth associated with breastfeeding is now reflected in growth charts (see Chapter 2, Section 2.8) and this slower growth in the early postnatal period could explain the long-term advantage regarding obesity and cardiovascular disease for breast-fed compared to formula-fed infants (Singhal and Lucas 2004). The mechanisms linking weight gain with later obesity are poorly understood and there is interest in the effects of infant nutrition on programming of appetite and hormonal systems relevant to appetite and energy metabolism. It has been proposed that specific compositional aspects of breast milk, such as its different (Lonnerdal 2003) and lower protein content compared to conventional infant formula or the presence of endocrine factors, such as IGF-I, leptin, ghrelin and adiponectin, could affect regulation of energy intake and expenditure and growth pattern during infancy.

The effect of protein intake on weight gain has been the focus of a double-blind randomised trial (Koletzko *et al.* 2009). Healthy term infants were randomised to receive either a higher or lower protein cows' milk formula (2.9 vs. 1.8 g protein/100 kcal or 418 kJ; the energy densities were kept constant). A reference group of breast-fed infants was also recruited. Significant differences in weight and weight-for-length in the two formula groups emerged at 6 months of age and remained relatively stable throughout the 24-month study. Compared to the breast-fed group, the higher protein formula group had significantly higher Z-scores of weight, length and weight-for-height at age 2 years. The weight of the lower protein group was closer to the breast-fed group. These findings highlight the growing evidence to support the benefit of lower protein formats for infant formula and follow-on formula in order to deliver growth trajectories more in line with those achieved with breastfeeding.

15.5 Vulnerable groups

15.5.1 Women with poor diets

Women aged 19–24, in particular, have poor dietary variety and have low intakes of some micronutrients.

Consumption of folic acid supplements remains low among women of childbearing age in general and there appears to be a lack of awareness of the recommendation to take vitamin D supplements throughout pregnancy and breastfeeding (SACN 2011a). There is some evidence from national surveys that a woman's educational attainment and income predict her dietary choices and infant feeding behaviour, and the rising prevalence of obesity in girls and young women is a modifiable risk factor for adverse pregnancy outcome and for later health outcomes for both the mother and her baby (SACN 2011a).

To date, information on the proportion of women of childbearing age specifically with micronutrient intakes below the LRNI is not available from the latest NDNS, but the previous NDNS published in 2002 revealed the following for iron: 11–14 years 45%, 15–18 years 50%, 19–24 years 42%, 25–34 years 41%, 35–49 years 27%, compared to 4% in those aged 50–64 years (summarised in SACN 2011a). It also found evidence of relatively poor intakes of vitamin A (19% below the LRNI), riboflavin (15%), calcium (8%), magnesium (22%), zinc (5%), iodine (12%) and potassium (30%) in 19- to 24-year-olds compared with older women (see SACN 2011a). These findings reflect the generally poorer diets of people in their teens and twenties (men and women) compared with older adults and the need to reinforce the principles of healthy eating.

15.5.2 Pregnant adolescents

In the UK, the prevalence of teenage pregnancy is high compared to other parts of Europe (see Chapter 3, Section 3.2.1.1), with as many as 1 in 10 babies being born to a teenage mother. As described in Chapter 3, Section 3.2.1.1, the physiological demands of pregnancy are exacerbated in adolescence. The recent NDNS (Bates *et al.* 2012) has demonstrated the nutrient shortfalls in the diets of girls aged 11–18 years. Related findings are evident for some young women in their late teens and twenties (see Section 15.5.1). Reducing under-18 conceptions is one of the health improvement targets in the *Public Health Outcomes Framework for England 2012–2016* (Department of Health 2011c). Teenage parents are at increased risk of postnatal depression and poor mental health in the three years following birth, are more likely to be living in poverty at age 30 than older mothers, and their children experience

Table 15.6 Percentage of participants with average daily intakes of vitamins and minerals from food sources below the Lower Reference Nutrient Intake (LRNI), by age

	Girls aged 11–18 years (%)	Women aged 19–64 years (%)
Vitamin A	14	6
Thiamin	0	0
Riboflavin	21	12
Niacin equivalent	0	0
Vitamin B$_6$	0	0
Vitamin B$_{12}$	2	2
Folate	7	3
Vitamin C	1	1
Iron	46	23
Calcium	18	8
Magnesium	51	8
Potassium	31	23
Zinc	19	4
Selenium	45	52
Iodine	21	10

Source: Bates *et al.* (2012).

higher rates of infant mortality and low birthweight (Department of Health 2011c).

Table 15.6 compares the prevalence of low intakes of selected vitamins and minerals in adolescents aged 11–18 years and in women aged 19–64 years, illustrating that intakes are typically poorer in the younger age group. For some nutrients, the picture is markedly worse, for example vitamin A, riboflavin, iron, calcium, iodine, zinc, magnesium and potassium. The situation for selenium, which has not been recorded in earlier surveys, is of concern in both adolescents and women. In addition, in girls aged 11–18 years, mean consumption of fruit and vegetables was only 2.8 portions a day (compared to the recommendation of at least 5), the majority did not eat oil-rich fish during the 4-day reporting period and mean consumption was well below the recommended one portion per week (Bates *et al.* 2012) (see also Chapter 3, Section 3.2.1.1 for findings of other studies).

The fat intake of 11- to 18-year-olds now meets recommendations (Bates *et al.* 2012). Although there has been some improvement over time (current NDNS Rolling Programme compared with 1997), saturated fatty acid intakes in 11- to 18-year-olds still exceed recommendations (as in other population groups) at 12.5% of food energy compared with <11% (Bates *et al.* 2012). The biggest contributor is cereal products

(e.g. pasta and rice dishes, pizza, biscuits, cakes and pastries) at 24%, followed by milk and milk products (23%), meat and meat products (21%), fat spreads (8%), confectionery (8%), and vegetables and potatoes cooked with fat (8%) (Bates *et al.* 2011). As in other age groups, fibre intakes are low in 11- to 18-year-olds at 10.8 g non-starch polysaccharides per day (12.8 g in women aged 19–64 years), compared to the recommendation (for adults) of 18 g/day (Bates *et al.* 2012).

Against this background, it will be evident that many adolescent women need guidance on how to eat healthily, even in the absence of pregnancy. Furthermore, pregnant teenagers may be confused and disconcerted by body shape changes associated with pregnancy. Health professionals, particularly midwives, can use this critical period to provide practical advice about the importance of good nutrition, but the approach needs to be carefully targeted and to take account of constraints such as education and work commitments and travel, and to acknowledge that eating habits may be highly variable in this age group (Wrieden and Symon 2003).

As indicated in Table 15.6, 15% of adolescent girls have an inadequate calcium intake, below the LRNI, which will often be associated with low intake of milk and milk products, these being the major source of calcium in the UK diet. A randomised controlled trial (RCT) conducted in the US among adolescent mothers and their babies reported higher intakes of a range of nutrients, higher maternal vitamin D levels (milk is fortified with vitamin D in the US), higher birthweight and increased bone mineralisation in those receiving dairy products (sufficient to provide 1200 mg calcium/day, i.e. four servings a day) compared to controls (usual diet) (Chan *et al.* 2006). This suggests that relatively straightforward dietary changes can have a real impact on the quality of diet.

15.5.3 Ethnic minority groups

Some ethnic minority groups experience an increased risk of cardiovascular disease (see Section 15.2.3). It is currently not clear whether the increased risk in these ethnic minority groups is a consequence of early life environment, and whether improved pre- and postnatal growth would reduce this risk. The limited information available on the diets of ethnic minority groups is discussed in Chapter 3, Section 3.2.3. Non-White ethnicity is associated with an increased risk of poor pregnancy outcome in the UK (Balchin *et al.* 2007); low birthweight is also a characteristic of some groups, e.g. South Asians, and appropriate advice regarding postnatal growth rate is important.

15.5.3.1 Folic acid

Young women from minority ethnic groups and lower socioeconomic backgrounds are least likely to take folic acid supplements pre-conception (Stockley and Lund 2008) (see Section 15.3.3.2).

15.5.3.2 Vitamin D

As is evident from Section 15.3.3.1, there is a need for sustainable strategies that will secure adequate vitamin D status for ethnic minorities and other vulnerable groups as a healthy diet plus sun exposure will not be sufficient. Skin synthesis is reduced for the reasons described earlier and dietary intakes and supplementation are unlikely to increase intakes sufficiently across the whole population, as diets typically provide only 4–7.5 µg/day, depending on the country (Cashman and Kiely 2011), and supplement use is not widespread. An alternative approach would be fortification, perhaps of several widely consumed foods to ensure widespread reach. The Health Council for the Netherlands (2008a) has published some scenario calculations that compare restoration of levels in dairy products, fortification of dairy products and fortification of cooking oils. Consideration of the most effective fortificant is important. Vitamin D_3 is the dominant food-derived form of the vitamin but D_2 is often used as a fortificant and in supplements. More research is needed on differences in physiological responses to the two forms and also on differences with respect to safety, noting that vitamin D_3 supplements are unacceptable to some vegetarians (Cashman and Kiely 2011; O'Connor and Benelam 2011).

15.5.3.3 Iron, zinc and n-3 fatty acids for vegetarians

Additional dietary advice about non-meat sources of these nutrients is important for those who follow a vegetarian diet and on alternate sources of *n*-3 fatty acids for those who exclude oil-rich fish from their diet.

15.5.3.4 Maternal obesity

The Centre for Maternal and Child Enquiries reported a significantly lower proportion of non-White mothers to be obese in pregnancy compared with all maternities in England. However, Heslehurst *et al.* reported that Black women were significantly more likely to be obese in pregnancy (BMI > 30) compared with White women, while some other ethnic groups (e.g. South Asian and Chinese women) were less likely to be obese (Heslehurst *et al.* 2010).

15.5.4 Lower socioeconomic groups

The association between socioeconomic status and health is very strong, and is consistent throughout life (Irwin *et al.* 2007). Low socioeconomic status is associated with many risk factors for poor pregnancy outcome including short stature, low pre-pregnancy body mass index, low weight gain during pregnancy, higher maternal obesity (see Section 15.2.1.1), smoking during pregnancy (NHS Information Centre 2011) and lower uptake of folic acid supplements (see Section 15.3.3.2). Research has shown that mothers from low-income households are nutritionally vulnerable and may go short of food in order to feed their children (Dobson 1994; Dowler and Calvert 1995). Babies born to mothers from lower socioeconomic backgrounds are more likely to be of low birthweight and pre-term and less likely to be breast-fed (see Chapter 3, Section 3.7.3 and Table 3.5). There is also a strong relationship between the duration of breastfeeding and the mother's socioeconomic status, with mothers from higher occupational groups breastfeeding for longer (see Chapter 3, Section 3.8.3 and Table 3.8). Data on physical activity levels in different socioeconomic groups are inconsistent (Weichselbaum and Buttriss 2011). However, action to reduce health disparities needs to start very early in life, and should focus on key issues such as breastfeeding habits and early infant feeding practices, daycare centre attendance and opportunities for physical activity in early childhood and beyond.

15.5.5 Smokers

The adverse consequences of smoking while pregnant are well documented and publicised. These include lowered mean birthweight, and increased risks of pre-term delivery, stillbirth and intrauterine growth restriction (Dietz *et al.* 2010). Nevertheless, despite a decline in all countries in recent years (2005–10), a substantial proportion of pregnant women in the UK smoke. According to the Infant Feeding Survey (NHS Information Centre 2011) a quarter (26%) of mothers in the UK smoked at some point in the year immediately before or during their pregnancy. Of these mothers, just over half (54%) gave up at some point before the birth, while one in eight of all mothers (12%) smoked throughout their pregnancy. The rates are highest among those in manual occupations and the younger age groups (below 24 years). The Tobacco Control Plan aims to reduce the rate of smoking during pregnancy to 11% or less by the end of 2015 (measured at the time of giving birth) (Department of Health 2012b).

Studies have shown that smoking negatively impacts on nutritional intake and status of several micronutrients (Fehily *et al.* 1984; Frisancho *et al.* 1985; Margetts and Jackson 1993; Dallongeville *et al.* 1998; Alberg 2002). However, assessing the effect among pregnant women is difficult due to likely common under-reporting of smoking habits at this time. However, Mathews *et al.* (2000), in their study of 774 women who completed 7-day food diaries at approximately 17 weeks of pregnancy, found significantly lower intakes of vitamin C and carotenoid intakes among smokers compared to non-smokers, which remained significantly lower after adjustment for confounders such as social class and maternal education. A recent study also raised concern about the effect of maternal smoking on folate status in newborns. Oncel *et al.* (2011) assessed neonatal serum folate levels in the newborns of 68 mothers who were non-smokers and 40 smokers. Babies born to smoking mothers had significantly lower serum folate levels compared to those born to non-smoking mothers, both at birth and 1 month after delivery. The authors suggested that folic acid supplementation may be required for expectant smoking mothers throughout pregnancy, rather than just during the first trimester, and that supplementation may also be warranted for infants born to mothers who smoke.

15.5.6 Obese women

Obesity in pregnancy is associated with an increased risk of a number of serious adverse outcomes for both mother and child (see Section 15.2.1.1). There is also a higher caesarean section rate and lower breastfeeding rate in this group of women compared to women with a healthy BMI. It is important that women are aware of these increased risks and advised about the possible strategies to minimise them prior to conception. Women with a raised BMI are at increased risk of neural tube defects. A meta-analysis of 12 observational cohort studies reported an odds ratio of 1.22 (95% CI: 0.99–1.49), 1.70 (95% CI: 1.34–2.15) and 3.11 (95% CI: 1.75–5.46) for women defined as overweight, obese and severely obese, respectively, compared with healthy weight women (Rasmussen *et al.* 2008). Cross-sectional data suggests that, compared to women with a BMI of less than 27, overweight and obese women (BMI > 27) are less likely to use nutritional supplements, and they have a lower folate intake from their diet and lower serum folate levels even after controlling for folate intake (Mojtabai 2004). It has therefore been suggested that obese women should receive higher doses of folic acid supplementation prior to pregnancy and in the first 12 weeks (5 mg/day) in order to minimise the increased risk of fetal neural tube defects. Pre-pregnancy BMI has also been shown to be inversely associated with serum vitamin D concentrations among pregnant women, and obese women are at increased risk of vitamin D deficiency compared to women with a healthy weight (Bodnar *et al.* 2007). Cord serum vitamin D levels in babies of obese women have been found to be lower than in babies born to non-obese women (Bodnar *et al.* 2007). Health professionals, therefore, should take care to check that overweight and obese women in their care are aware of, and following, the advice to take a 10 μg vitamin D supplement daily during pregnancy and while breastfeeding (NICE 2008).

15.6 Diet and lifestyle recommendations

In this section, key messages on specific nutrients and lifestyle factors of importance are summarised in the context of the different stages of early life development (pre-pregnancy, pregnancy, lactation and birth to 2 years) (see Tables 15.7, 15.8, 15.9 and 15.10). Current recommendations and practices can be found in Chapter 3. Dietary sources of the nutrients referred to below can be found in Table 15.1. These recommendations should be considered in the context of a varied diet that follows the principles of

Table 15.7 Pre-pregnancy: diet and lifestyle messages

Diet and lifestyle aspect	Key messages
Body weight	Maintain or attain a healthy body weight (BMI 18.5–25). The importance of this recommendation needs greater emphasis (see Chapter 3, Section 3.3.1)
Folate/folic acid	Take a 400 µg folic acid supplement daily and eat folate-rich foods on a daily basis (see Table 15.1 for food sources). Larger supplements are needed by women who have already had an NTD affected pregnancy and possibly by obese women and smokers (see Chapter 3, Section 3.3.2)
Iron	Build up iron stores prior to conception by eating plenty of iron-rich foods and consuming plant foods containing iron with foods or drinks containing vitamin C, such as fruit or vegetables, or a glass of fruit juice, to assist iron absorption
Vitamin D	Include vitamin D containing foods in the diet and enable skin synthesis while avoiding sunburn (see Section 15.3.3.1). Asian women and those women who conceal most of their skin from sunlight exposure are vulnerable to poor vitamin D status and should consider taking a 10 µg daily supplement (see Section 15.3.3.1)
Zinc	Ensure an adequate dietary supply (see Table 15.1 for food sources)
Iodine	Ensure an adequate dietary supply (see Table 15.1 for food sources)
Vitamin A	Avoid foods with a potentially high vitamin A content, such as liver and liver products (e.g. pâté), supplements containing vitamin A, and fish liver oils that contain high levels of vitamin A
Alcohol	Ideally avoid alcohol while trying to conceive but, if drinking, limit consumption to one or two units of alcohol once or twice a week
Smoking	Do not smoke (see Section 15.5.5)
Physical activity	Ensure regular activity by aiming for at least 150 minutes (2½ hours) of moderate intensity activity per week (one way to approach this is to do 30 minutes on at least 5 days a week) (see Section 15.3.1.1)

Table 15.8 Pregnancy: diet and lifestyle messages

Diet and lifestyle aspect	Key messages
Weight gain	In the UK, at present, there are no formal, evidence-based guidelines from the UK government or professional bodies on what constitutes appropriate weight gain during pregnancy. But avoid poor weight gain and excessive weight gain
	The US Institute of Medicine guidelines state that healthy American women who are of normal weight for their height (BMI 18.5 to 24.9) should gain 11.5–16 kg (25–35 lb) during pregnancy. Overweight women (BMI 25.9 to 29.9) should gain 7–11 kg (15–25 lb) and obese women (BMI > 30.0) should gain only 5–9 kg (11–20 lb) (see Chapter 3, Section 3.4.1.1)
	Never diet when pregnant because this could lead to growth restriction and developmental abnormalities in the baby
Energy	An additional 0.8 MJ/800 kJ (191 kcal)/day is required during the 3rd trimester only. This should be added to energy requirements calculated according to pre-pregnancy body weight (see Section 15.2.1.1)
Protein	Include protein-containing foods such as lean meat, poultry, fish and shellfish, eggs, milk, cheese and other dairy products, beans and soya foods (there is a small increase in protein requirements from 45 to 51 g/day) (see Section 15.3.2.1 and Table 3.3)
Folate/folic acid	Take a 400 µg folic acid supplement daily for the first 12 weeks and eat folate-rich foods on a daily basis (see Table 15.1 for food sources). Larger supplements are needed by women who have already had an NTD affected pregnancy and possibly by obese women
Vitamin D	Take a 10 µg vitamin D supplement daily and include vitamin D containing foods in the diet and enable skin synthesis while avoiding sunburn (see Section 15.3.3.1)
Iron	The Recommended Nutrient Intake (RNI) is 14.8 mg/day, which is the same as pre-pregnancy. Consume plenty of iron-rich foods (see Table 15.1 for sources) preferably with food or drink containing vitamin C for enhancing iron absorption from non-haem sources
Zinc	Maintain an adequate zinc status, RNI is 7 mg/day (see Table 15.1 for food sources)

Table 15.8   *(Continued)*

Diet and lifestyle aspect	Key messages
Iodine	Maintain an adequate iodine status (RNI is 140 µg/day). Women living in iodine-deficient areas, should take iodine supplements to significantly reduce the incidence of iodine-related disorders (see Section 15.3.3.7)
Vitamin A	Avoid foods with potentially high vitamin A content, such as liver and liver products (e.g. paté), supplements containing vitamin A and fish liver oils that contain high levels of vitamin A. The recommended intake for vitamin A is 700 µg/day
Vitamin B$_{12}$	No increment from pre-pregnancy requirement, but if vegan or vegetarian it may be necessary to take a supplement (see Table 15.1 for food sources)
Calcium	There is no increment in calcium requirement during pregnancy but an adequate intake must be maintained as it is important for the development of the baby's bones and teeth, and for preservation of maternal calcium reserves in bone (see Table 15.1 for food sources)
n-3 fatty acids	In the UK, 450 mg/day of DHA and EPA combined is recommended for adults and pregnant women (SACN 2004); this equates to the consumption of two servings of fish a week, one of which is oil-rich. Advice to limit consumption of some types of fish is also relevant (see below) (see Chapter 3, Section 3.4.1.6)
n-6 fatty acids	Seeds and vegetable oils and spreads are rich sources of the *n*-6 essential fatty acid linoleic acid
Foods to avoid	Unpasteurised milk Some types of cheese: mould-ripened cheeses such as Camembert, Brie; some goat cheeses, especially unpasteurised; soft blue cheeses. Paté - all types of paté, including vegetable Raw or partially cooked eggs; raw or undercooked meat; undercooked ready meals; raw shellfish Liver products and supplements containing vitamin A or fish liver oils Some types of fish – shark, swordfish and marlin Intake of tuna should be limited to no more than two tuna steaks a week or four medium-size cans of tuna a week (see Chapter 3, Section 3.4.1.6 and Table 3.4)
Allergens	No specific advice (see Chapter 13, Section 13.8)
Dental health	Attend routine dental check-ups and brush regularly with a fluoride toothpaste. Oral health may require closer attention during pregnancy, e.g. gums bleed more easily. Don't consume high sugar foods and drinks too frequently, to protect against dental caries, or acidic foods and drinks, to prevent dental erosion
Alcohol	Ideally avoid alcohol but if drinking, limit to one or two units of alcohol once or twice a week
Smoking	Do not smoke
Physical activity	Continue to be active in pregnancy via low impact and low-risk activities (e.g. walking and swimming), as it can assist weight control and there appears to be no negative effects on the health of the mother or unborn child (see Section 15.3.1.1)
Pregnant adolescents	Section 15.5.2 summarises areas of particular concern regarding the diets of adolescent girls

the 'eatwell plate', the eight tips for a healthy diet and an active lifestyle (see www.dh.gov.uk/en/Publichealth/Nutrition/index.htm).

15.7 Role of health professionals

Pregnancy is an ideal opportunity for health professionals to encourage positive dietary and lifestyle behaviour change because women are often moti-

vated to adapt their food and lifestyle choices to do the best for their unborn child.

A variety of health professionals will interact with women of childbearing age – general practitioners in the pre-conception stage, midwives and obstetricians during pregnancy, and health visitors after the birth. It is critical that these health professionals provide consistent, evidence-based advice to women about weight management and other aspects of nutrition,

Table 15.9 Lactation: Diet and lifestyle messages for breastfeeding mothers

Diet and lifestyle aspect	Key messages
Body weight	Restore pre-pregnancy weight via healthy eating and regular physical activity. For those women with a pre-pregnancy BMI > 25, plan to reduce BMI by lowering energy intake and increasing physical activity to lose weight gradually once breastfeeding has ceased. If breastfeeding, avoid dieting, especially fad diets that may impair adequate nutrient intake (see Section 15.3.1)
Breastfeeding	Exclusive breastfeeding is recommended for the first 6 months. Maternal requirements during lactation are increased for energy, vitamins A, D, B_2, B_{12}, calcium, magnesium and zinc ((Department of Health 1991). Even a shorter period of breastfeeding is beneficial for a wide range of reasons (see Chapter 3, Section 3.7.1)
Formula feeding	Formula feeding has been associated with a more rapid growth rate – accelerated growth is now considered to have long-term adverse effects (see Chapter 2, Section 2.10) and formulas with a (lower) protein content that is more similar to that of breast milk are now widely available and may be preferable (see Section 15.4.3)
Iron	The RNI remains at 14.8 mg/day. Consume plenty of iron-rich foods (see Table 15.1 for sources) preferably with food or drink containing vitamin C for enhancing iron absorption from non-haem sources
Zinc	Maintain an adequate zinc status, an additional 0.3 mg/day is needed on top of the usual requirement of 7 mg/day (see Table 15.1 for food sources)
Vitamin D	A 10 µg vitamin D supplement daily is recommended
n-3 fatty acids	Ensure an intake of DHA > 200 mg/day (see Chapter 3, Section 3.5.1 and Table 15.8 by including two servings of fish a week, one of which is oil-rich. Do not eat more than one portion of shark, swordfish or marlin a week and no more than two portions a week of oil-rich fish (see Chapter 3, Section 3.4.1.6)
n-6 fatty acids	Seeds and vegetable oils and spreads are rich sources of the n-6 essential fatty acid linoleic acid
Vegan diets	A daily vitamin D supplement is especially important. If women have been taking a vitamin B_{12} supplement, this should be continued during breastfeeding. A varied and balanced diet should be able to provide the other vitamins and minerals required (see Chapter 3, Section 3.4.1.5)
Allergens	No specific advice (see Chapter 13, Section 13.8)
Foods to avoid	Limit certain types of fish (no more than one portion of shark, swordfish or marlin a week and no more than two portions a week of oil-rich fish), alcohol and caffeine intake (see Chapter 3, Section 3.4.1.6 and Table 3.4)
Physical activity	Aim for at least 150 minutes (2½ hours) of moderate intensity activity per week (one way to approach this is to do 30 minutes on at least 5 days a week) (see Section 15.3.1.1)
Weaning (baby-led, introducing solids – when and what)	See Chapter 3, Section 3.9 and Table 15.10

health and lifestyle before, during and after pregnancy. The risks to the mother and unborn baby of the mother being overweight or obese pre-conception and/or gaining excess weight during pregnancy need greater emphasis. These risks should routinely be discussed with all women of childbearing age, particularly those who are overweight or obese. In developing the NICE recommendations on weight management before, during and after pregnancy (NICE 2010), the Public Health Interventions Advisory Committee (PHIAC) noted that

Health professionals recognise the risks but are often unsure what advice to give. In some cases, they lack the training, skills or confidence to discuss weight management. In addition, they may not know how to tailor advice and support for women who are pregnant.

This observation highlights the need for accurate, evidence-based information that health professionals can readily access and communicate to their patients and clients. It also highlights the need for nutrition

Table 15.10 Birth to 2 years: diet and lifestyle messages

Diet and lifestyle aspect	Key messages
Breastfeeding	Exclusive breastfeeding is recommended for the first 6 months. Even a shorter period of breastfeeding is beneficial for a wide range of reasons (see Chapter 3, Section 3.7.1)
Weight gain and catch-up growth	Formula feeding has been associated with a more rapid growth rate – accelerated growth is now considered to have long-term adverse effects (see Chapter 2, Section 2.10) and formulas with a (lower) protein content that is more similar to that of breast milk are now widely available and may be preferable (see Section 15.4.3)
Weaning (baby-led, introducing solids – when and what)	See Chapter 3, Section 3.9
Iron	Ensure an adequate iron intake (see Chapter 3, Section 3.9.6.2)
Zinc	Ensure an adequate zinc intake (see Chapter 3, Section 3.9.6.3)
Vitamin drops (vitamins A, C and D)	Vitamin drops (vitamins A, C and D) should be given from 1 month of age (especially if there is doubt about the mother's vitamin status) and continued until 5 years of age. 'Healthy Start' vitamin supplements are available free to pregnant women, new mothers under 18 years and those on low income (see Chapter 3, Section 3.9.6.4). Babies having >500 mL/day of infant formula do not need to take these supplements as infant formulas have these added
Vitamin D	Children under 5 should take a daily supplement of 7 µg, especially those vulnerable to low status, e.g. Asian and African-Caribbean children. Vitamin drops containing vitamin D together with vitamins A and C may be given in place of a single vitamin D supplement (see above)
n-3 fatty acids	Oil-rich fish is an important provider of n-3 fatty acids. Boys up to the age of 4 should be offered up to four portions of oil-rich fish per week, girls a maximum of two per week (this difference is due to the presence of dioxins and PCBs that can accumulate in body tissues, so girls who may get pregnant in the future have a lower recommended maximum)
n-6 fatty acids	Vegetable oils and spreads are rich sources of the n-6 essential fatty acid linoleic acid
Vegetarian diets	Children weaned onto vegan diets require a variety of protein sources daily, e.g. lentils, tofu, soya, pulses, beans. Advice from a health professional may be required if weaning onto a vegan diet (see Chapter 3, Section 3.9.8 and Section 3.9.9)
Allergens	Current precautionary advice is that foods known to provoke allergies should be avoided before 6 months. After 6 months there is no specific advice unless a food allergy is diagnosed (see Chapter 3, Section 3.10 and Section 15.2.6)
Foods to avoid	See Chapter 3, Table 3.14

and weight management to form part of the training for doctors, midwives and health visitors. The government's NHS Choices website (www.nhs.uk) provides advice on nutrition and pregnancy, including tips on healthy eating, weight management and physical activity. The British Nutrition Foundation's website (www.nutrition.org.uk) is another useful resource for health professionals and the general public, providing evidence-based dietary and lifestyle information and an online resource (www.nutrition4baby.co.uk) designed to deliver practical information for parents, from pre-conception to breastfeeding and weaning. The Foundation is also working with the Royal College of Midwives to improve the nutrition knowledge of UK midwives and to help provide the skills and confidence to discuss weight management issues with women in their care.

The PHIAC also noted that 'women receive a wealth of sometimes conflicting advice on what constitutes a healthy diet and how much physical activity they should do during pregnancy and after childbirth'. Health professionals are often cited as the trusted source of nutrition and weight management advice for these women and, therefore, it is very important that the advice offered is consistent, evidence-based and pitched to enable recipients to counter any conflicting advice they may receive from family, friends and the media.

The importance of improved partnership working was also identified in the 2010 NICE guidelines, which recommend that a range of services is required to address obesity. Heslehurst and colleagues have highlighted the lack of partnership working within maternity, public health, primary care and other community services despite maternal obesity and the health and well-being of mothers and their families being within the role of such organisations. A more 'joined-up' approach is needed, involving a range of agencies to effectively manage diet, physical activity and weight throughout the reproduction cycle, and to achieve long-term benefits of obesity prevention for women and their families (Heslehurst, Bell *et al.* 2011).

The *Public Health Outcomes Framework for England, 2013–2016* (Department of Health 2011c; Department of Health 2012a) published in January 2012, sets out the government's ambitions for a new and reformed public health system. It focuses on two outcomes:

1. Increased healthy life expectancy (taking account of the health quality as well as the length of life).
2. Reduced differences in life expectancy and healthy life expectancy between communities (through greater improvements in more disadvantaged communities).

There are four domains within the framework, the one most relevant to this Task Force Report being Health Improvement. Within this domain there are supporting public health indicators against which annual reports of progress will be made, with involvement of local government, the NHS and Public Health England. Health professionals will have an important role in this process via local authorities. Among these indicators are: low birthweight of term live births, breastfeeding initiation, breastfeeding prevalence at 6–8 weeks after birth, smoking status at the time of delivery, under-18 conception rate, child development at age 2–2.5 years, excess weight at ages 4–5 and 10–11, smoking prevalence in 15-year-olds, comparison of diet against national dietary targets and guidelines, excess weight in adults and physical activity levels in adults.

15.8 Recommendations

It is now clear that growth during early life can be an important determinant of a person's later health and risk of chronic disease. The shape and size of a baby at birth and growth during the first 2 years of postnatal life are predictive of risk of cardiovascular disease, obesity, type 2 diabetes, respiratory disease, osteoporosis, cancer and mental illness. The processes of normal organ growth and development are highly ordered, as discussed in Chapter 2, and hence open to the adverse effects of failure to provide the appropriate mixture of nutrients required at a particular time. Current knowledge about the detailed schedule for nutrient requirements during prenatal and early postnatal growth and development are fragmentary and inadequate to provide the answers needed to secure optimal growth and development. However, the evidence is already sufficiently strong to demand attention because it carries important policy implications (Jackson 2011).

In a recent editorial, Jackson has highlighted fundamental research questions, including: how does nutrition enable linear growth; what are the determinants of individual organ and tissue growth at different ages; how does nutrient availability determine structural and functional development; to what extent is adipose tissue acquisition a reflection of an inability to use energy more effectively for linear growth, lean growth or a functionally beneficial purpose; are there critical ages when these considerations are most sensitive; and does the microbiome play any, or a critically determinant, role in these relationships?

15.8.1 Recommendations to policy makers

The evidence presented in this report that early life nutrition can influence the risk of disease in later life suggests that interventions to improve the diets and lifestyles of women of childbearing age, infants and young children have the potential to improve the health of future generations. Obesity has reached epidemic proportions globally, with a similar rise in prevalence among women in the reproductive age group. This has critical consequences for fetal and maternal health in the pre-pregnancy, pregnancy and postpartum periods as it not only directly influences pregnancy outcome but also impacts on the weight of the child in infancy and beyond. As such, maternal weight may influence the prevalence and severity of obesity in future generations. The wealth of evidence linking maternal obesity with pregnancy outcome also has a direct impact on maternity services' resources. If approached sensitively, pregnancy may be a good time to target health behaviour changes by using the extra motivation women tend to have at this time to maximise the health of their child.

15.8.1.1 Maternal obesity

Despite the numerous challenges, pregnancy and ideally the period when pregnancy is being planned have been identified as key times to target the importance of weight control or a weight loss strategy (either pre-pregnancy or post-lactation). Avoidance of excessive weight gain during pregnancy will help prevent obesity development among women and their children. To date, the policy response to support maternity services in tackling maternal obesity has been weaker than policy initiatives focusing on obesity in childhood. Activity in this area is hampered by the absence of officially accepted guidelines for gestational weight gain, which has been identified by UK health professionals as a barrier to consistent practice (see Section 15.3.1). The lack of evidence supporting the benefit of regular weighing and monitoring after the first antenatal check (and the associated advice from NICE) also serves to underplay the importance of maintaining a healthy body weight. Although health professionals understand their responsibility to explain the potential risks and complications associated with obesity in pregnancy, many report feeling uncomfortable raising and discussing such issues with pregnant women and need greater support and training to deliver effective advice. As differences in the prevalence of maternal obesity reflect broader socio-demographic inequalities, particularly in relation to deprivation, ethnicity and unemployment, a lack of comprehensive policies to tackle this problem will worsen the health inequalities already found in society.

The Task Force supports the calls for clear policy on weight control and avoidance of obesity in pregnancy, including the need for better services for women prior to pregnancy and support for women in achieving and maintaining a healthy body weight after pregnancy.

While the ideal public health solution would be to intervene and support women in achieving a healthy weight prior to pregnancy, women are often hard to reach for targeted interventions before they conceive, and many pregnancies are unplanned. Therefore, broader preventive and public health strategies for young women need to be developed to support this process. Clearly this is a major challenge that can only be met by effective partnership working between maternity and public health services to effectively manage diet, physical activity and weight throughout the 'reproductive cycle' and to provide the necessary training for the professionals involved.

15.8.1.2 Teenage pregnancy

Since the launch of the Teenage Pregnancy Strategy (2010), teenage pregnancy rates have fallen: the under-18 conception rate is now 13.3% lower than in 1998 (Department for Children, Schools and Families and Department of Health 2010) (see Section 15.5.2). While the main policy focus is appropriately on preventing teenage pregnancies, where they do occur, extra support is needed to ensure that young pregnant women are aware of the need for good nutrition, the advice to stop smoking and drinking alcohol, and the recommendations regarding supplementation (folic acid and vitamin D), as well as practical advice regarding breastfeeding and weaning. Family-based programmes, such as the Family Nurse Partnership (FNP) in England (Barnes *et al.* 2008, Department of Health 2011a), and social marketing approaches that provide health professionals with insight and skills to develop targeted interventions that support behaviour change, may be best able to encourage the adoption of a healthier lifestyle in this vulnerable group.

15.8.1.3 Vitamin D

There is evidence of low vitamin D status across the UK population, particularly among young Asian and African-Caribbean children and pregnant women. NICE advises of the need to inform pregnant women about the importance of maintaining adequate vitamin D stores during pregnancy and taking a 10 μg supplement daily. A lack of awareness, particularly among those in vulnerable groups (e.g. ethnic minority groups), is thought to be widespread. Although Healthy Start vitamins are now more widely available, it is not only low-income families who are at risk of poor vitamin D status and there is a need for a public campaign to enhance awareness across the population. A new Department of Health leaflet on vitamin D deficiency, to raise awareness among health professionals, was published at the start of 2012 (Department of Health 2012b) but there is a need for ongoing promotion of the vitamin D message to relevant audiences (e.g. pharmacists, health visitors, midwives and GPs).

15.8.1.4 Folic acid

While awareness of the importance of folic acid seems to be high, compliance with this recommendation is not reflected in practice and many opportunities for health professionals to deliver information on folic acid supplementation are being missed. There is, therefore, a need to understand and act upon common barriers to the uptake of this important health message and to develop a clear public health strategy on supplementation. Campaigns have the potential to exacerbate inequalities in folic acid use between women in lower and higher socioeconomic groups.

Future strategies should include elements that specifically target vulnerable groups such as the less educated and the young, as well as women in general, as many pregnancies are unplanned. To reach the last group, folic acid advice will need to be incorporated into a structure of pre-conception care that reaches high numbers of women of childbearing age. Key barriers relating to training and structural changes would need to be addressed (Stockley 2006). The only other option is likely to be via fortification of foods with folic acid.

15.8.1.5 Breastfeeding

Breastfeeding has a major role to play in promoting health in both the short- and long-term for baby and mother. Evidence-based strategies for promoting the initiation and duration of breastfeeding, particularly in those groups where breastfeeding rates are commonly low, should therefore come high up on the public health agenda. Continued support is required for events, such as National Breastfeeding Week, that offer important opportunities to raise awareness of the health benefits of breastfeeding, increase its social acceptance, and promote support for breastfeeding mothers. However, while promoting the benefits of breastfeeding, health professionals must ensure that mothers who cannot breastfeed or who choose to formula feed are also given the advice and support they need about selecting products, making up feeds, sterilising bottles and storing formula milk. Although the Baby Friendly Hospital Initiative (BFHI) training includes requirements for safe and appropriate formula feeding, it is not easy for midwives to obtain up-to-date information about formula feeding, particularly as the policies of many maternity units preclude manufacturers' representatives from meeting staff to convey information about product composition and innovations.

Consideration needs to be given to ways of ensuring that midwives and health visitors (and also pharmacists) have access to the factual information they require on formula feeding and to prevent them from feeling constrained professionally from supporting all mothers equally in how to feed their babies successfully, regardless of the decision taken by the mother (see Section 15.4.1.1). This is important as the majority of women provide infant formula at some stage during the first year of life (a time when cows' milk is not appropriate as a main drink) and may require advice to ensure that these products are used appropriately and safely.

15.8.1.6 Introduction of solids

Since publication of the COMA report *Weaning and the weaning diet* in 1994, there has not been a thorough risk assessment of the evidence on weaning and the weaning diet in the UK. Advice regarding initiation of weaning onto foods other than milk (breast or infant formula) has changed during this period (from 4–6 months to 6 months). There appears to be confusion among health professionals and mothers alike about current recommendations and also about behavioural aspects of infant feeding such as recommended portion sizes, pace of complementary feeding and the stages at which different textures of food should be offered.

The outcome of the ongoing review of complementary and young child feeding by SACN is, therefore, urgently needed as a stimulus for communicating consistent advice. It will be important that communication of the review's findings includes targeted training to the wide range of health professionals involved in giving advice in this area (including health visitors and other community-based nurses, GPs, pharmacists and nursery and childcare professionals).

15.8.2 Recommendations to health professionals and other educators

All health professionals who are in contact with women prior to, during and immediately after childbirth have an opportunity to discuss diet and lifestyle habits and address individual concerns. This includes midwives, health visitors, dietitians and pharmacists, all of whom need to provide up-to-date, consistent advice tailored to specific needs. Several areas have been identified where more can be done to improve current practice, although consideration must be given to specific training needs to achieve future success, particularly in the context of delivery of the *Public Health Outcomes Framework* and related structural changes (see Section 15.7).

15.8.2.1 *Vitamin D*

It is likely that health professionals could do more to prevent vitamin D deficiency and to improve the uptake of supplements, particularly in vulnerable groups (i.e. those who have limited skin exposure to sunlight or who are of South Asian, African, Caribbean or Middle Eastern descent, and also those who are obese). Studies suggest that training is required to ensure widespread understanding of the current recommendations for supplementation and to improve awareness of the groups most at risk. For example, in a small study of 96 community midwives and health visiting teams, Lockyer *et al.* (2011) reported that less than half had recommended supplements to pregnant women, only 19% correctly identified all the four ethnic groups at increased risk and just over half (52%) were aware of the recommendations for vitamin D supplementation. It is hoped that the new Department of Health leaflet will be a useful resource, but this is unlikely to be sufficient on its own, and ongoing support will be required if progress is to be made.

15.8.2.2 *Folic acid*

Health professionals play an influential role in raising awareness of the importance of folic acid in preventing neural tube defects. As periconceptual supplementation is advised and many pregnancies are unplanned, an opportunistic strategy by all those advising women of childbearing age is required. This includes provision of advice by physicians in obstetrics and gynaecology, internal medicine and family medicine, for example during annual, family planning or infertility visits. Pharmacists also have an important role to play in delivering this message as they may be the first health professional that a

woman sees when she is planning a pregnancy. There is some evidence that pre-conception care can have a positive impact on folic acid uptake, but training and ongoing support is needed to ensure that the messages are being delivered consistently and accurately.

15.8.2.3 *Maternal obesity*

Addressing maternal obesity can be challenging for health professionals, particularly for midwives, who do not want to jeopardise the relationship they have with their patient. However, it is essential that the potential risks and complications associated with maternal obesity are explained to women during early pregnancy. Such communication should be sensitively delivered to encourage continued engagement with antenatal services; midwives are likely to need specific training in this area, as is the case with other public health issues such as smoking cessation. It is important to stress both healthy eating and appropriate activity levels, in order to prevent excess weight gain and gestational diabetes. Women with a BMI > 30 should continue to receive advice on nutrition from appropriately trained professionals, after the birth, to achieve weight reduction. Health professionals should take particular care to check that women with a booking BMI over 30 (i.e. at first antenatal appointment) are following advice to take vitamin D and folic acid supplements.

15.8.2.4 *Catch-up growth*

The rate of weight gain during infancy and childhood might play a role in the development of obesity later in life. Mothers and also some health professionals often perceive early rapid weight gain to be a sign of good feeding practices. This view, however, may encourage faster than optimal growth in early infancy in those who are formula-fed. Health professionals need to be aware of, and communicate to parents and carers, the potential long-term consequences of rapid catch-up growth, particularly in babies who have experienced intrauterine growth restriction (see Section 15.4.3).

15.8.2.5 *Infant feeding and weaning*

Health practitioners, such as midwives, nurses and doctors, have a key role to play in providing support to breastfeeding women, particularly during the first few weeks when discontinuation is greatest. Knowledge of the process of breastfeeding and the ability to adopt a problem-solving approach to the difficulties mothers encounter, in order to give appropriate evidence-based care, are important factors. While all health professionals should continue to promote and support breastfeeding, infant formula is an important source of nutrition for many infants, and parents need education and support in using it appropriately and safely. Being able to give parents advice and help with infant formula feeding requires an up-to-date knowledge of the different formulas available and skills in the safe preparation and storage of formula. Care should be taken in the delivery of advice around choice of infant feeding to prevent the negative emotions described by some women who choose not to breastfeed (see Section 15.4.1.1).

15.8.3 Recommendations to the food industry

The food industry plays a vital role in improving intake of key nutrients such as folic acid and vitamin D to support pregnancy and breastfeeding. As well as providing a range of fortified products and suitable supplements, manufacturers could help to promote their uptake by including information about the importance of these nutrients on relevant pregnancy- and breastfeeding-related products (e.g. pregnancy test kits and breast pumps).

15.8.4 Recommendations to researchers and funders

Research questions relating to the associations between early growth and risk of specific conditions in later life are outlined at the end of the relevant chapters throughout this report and are amalgamated in Chapter 17, Section 17.3. Chapter 15 has also highlighted some general recommendations for researchers and funders.

- There is a need for further evaluative research to assess the effectiveness of interventions to control weight in women before, during and after pregnancy.
- In order to support discussions around vitamin D fortification, more research is needed to clarify differences in physiological responses to vitamin D_3 and vitamin D_2.
- Other research questions that need to be addressed in relation to vitamin D include the extent to which vitamin D insufficiency contributes to geographical health inequalities in the UK, whether there is a causal link between vitamin D status and obesity, and whether individuals are genetically susceptible to vitamin D insufficiency.

15.9 Key points

- There are likely to be periods of fetal and early life development that are particularly sensitive to suboptimal or excessive nutrition. These are 'critical windows' in a child's development during which future health and development can be 'programmed'.
- A fetus is entirely dependent on its mother for its nutrient supply, which is likely to be influenced by a mother's nutritional status prior to conception, and in pregnancy.
- In the UK, teenage pregnancies remain higher than in many other countries in Europe and the diets of adolescents are often poorly balanced with intakes of folate, iron and vitamin D being of particular concern. This has implications for

adolescent girls who become pregnant, especially as many will still be growing themselves.
- The dramatic increase in overweight and obese women in the UK has focused attention on weight management before and during pregnancy. However, efforts in the UK are currently hampered by the lack of formal, evidence-based guidelines. These include gestational weight gain and the need for training for many health professionals to provide the skills and confidence needed for them to appropriately and effectively address sensitive weight issues with pregnant women.
- Only about 30% of women of childbearing age meet current physical activity recommenda-

Continued

tions. This helps maintain an appropriate body weight. Physical activity has many benefits during pregnancy including enhanced fitness, reduced muscles cramps and reduced swelling of the legs and feet.

- Low vitamin D status is common among pregnant women, particularly those of South Asian, African, Caribbean and Middle Eastern descent. Lack of awareness of the recommendation to take vitamin D supplements during pregnancy and lactation is thought to be widespread, particularly in the most vulnerable groups. There is, therefore, a need to enhance awareness of the importance of this health message across the population.

- While awareness of the importance of folic acid around the time of conception is high, compliance with this recommendation is not reflected in practice. One of the key factors associated with lower uptake rates is unplanned pregnancies, which account for around half of all pregnancies in the UK. The only possible way to reach this group of women may be via fortification of foods with folic acid.

- The choice of feeding in infancy influences the rate of growth and the type of tissue deposition, which has the potential to track into adulthood. Infants who are not breast-fed tend to have slightly higher blood pressure and blood cholesterol levels in later life, and are at greater risk of type 2 diabetes and obesity. Promotion and support of breastfeeding therefore offers short- and long-term health benefits. However, it is also necessary for health professionals to ensure that the needs of bottle feeding mothers are met.

- Advice on weaning is constrained by the absence of up-to-date information on the diets and nutrient intakes of infants and a lack of official guidance from the Department of Health on behavioural aspects of infant feeding such as recommended portion sizes, pace of complementary feeding and the stages at which different textures of food should be offered. The ongoing review of complementary and young child feeding by the Scientific Advisory Committee on Nutrition is therefore urgently awaited.

- Evidence is emerging about potential adverse effects of rapid catch-up growth in infancy for risk of later disease. This has important implications for the management of low-birthweight and small-for-gestational-age babies in whom catch-up growth was previously encouraged.

- The slower growth associated with breastfeeding could explain the long-term benefits of breastfeeding in relation to reduced risk of obesity and cardiovascular disease. Some of this may be due to the lower protein content of breast milk, which has led to the recent development of lower protein formulas to deliver growth trajectories more similar to those achieved with breastfeeding.

15.10 Key references

Scientific Advisory Committee on Nutrition (SACN (2011) *The Influence of Maternal, Fetal and Child Nutrition on the Development of Chronic Disease in Later Life.* London, The Stationery Office.

Heslehurst N (2011) Identifying 'at risk' women and the impact of maternal obesity on National Health Service maternity services. *Proceedings of the Nutrition Society,* **70**, 439–49.

Centre for Maternal and Child Enquiries (CMACE) (2010b) *Maternal Obesity in the UK: Findings from a national project.* London, CMACE.

National Institute for Health and Clinical Excellence (NICE) (2010) *NICE Public Health Guidance 27: Dietary interventions and physical activity interventions for weight management before, during and after pregnancy.* London, NICE.

National Institute for Health and Clinical Excellence (NICE) (2008) *NICE Public Health Guidance 11: Improving the nutrition of pregnant and breastfeeding mothers and children in low-income households.* London, NICE.

16
Conclusions of the Task Force

The world's biggest killers include cardiovascular disease, diabetes, chronic lung disease, allergies, some forms of cancer, cognitive decline and osteoporosis. Over the next decade, the World Health Organization (WHO) predicts an increase of 17% in non-communicable diseases such as those mentioned above. The leading causes of death in the UK are circulatory diseases, cancers and respiratory diseases, which, when combined, accounted for 75% of deaths in 2007 (Department of Health 2010). Diseases such as arthritis and type 2 diabetes are expected to rise due to the increasing rates of obesity. Mental health and well-being are also critical dimensions for health. Poor mental health, the prevalence of which has been increasing, is responsible for a high proportion of the overall burden of ill health (Department of Health 2010).

There is now growing evidence that early life nutrition can bring about changes in functional development and, therefore, plays an important role in programming risk of disease in later life. The health of mothers before and during pregnancy, and good parenting, are crucial to getting the best start in life. The number of overweight and obese pregnant women appears to be rising. This poses challenges for our healthcare system as obese women are known to have an increased risk of pregnancy-related complications.

The conditions mentioned above represent a major public health challenge, particularly among vulnerable groups such as women with poor diets, pregnant adolescents, ethnic minorities, lower socioeconomic groups, smokers and obese women. Around four out of ten pregnancies are unplanned (Joshi *et al.* 2001) and an increasing number of women are becoming pregnant in poor health (Confidential Enquiry into Maternal and Child Health (CEMACH) 2007). The Scientific Advisory Committee on Nutrition expressed concern about energy-dense diets with low micronutrient content often consumed by women and girls, and its impact on their offspring (Scientific Advisory Committee on Nutrition (SACN) 2011a). One in five pregnancies during 2009 was in women of Black or minority ethnic groups, and the proportion of pregnant women aged over 35 is increasing (Centre for Maternal and Child Enquiries (CMACE) and Royal College of Obstetricians and Gynaecologists (RCOG) 2010).

From examination of current diets and lifestyles of women of childbearing age, and current practice around early life nutrition, it is clear that there are many aspects requiring improvement. These include the nutritional status of women before and during pregnancy; increased awareness and use of supplements around pregnancy (e.g. folic acid and vitamin D); healthy weight gain and being active during pregnancy; milk feeding and weaning practices. It is vital that these areas are addressed in order to improve the long-term health of the population and to reduce the burden of non-communicable diseases.

Excessive exposure to, or insufficiency of, specific nutrients around the time of pregnancy can have a detrimental impact on fetal development. However, even modest variations in nutrition arising from widespread differences in dietary habits and food choices can influence fetal growth and development.

Research in the area of early life nutrition is still in its infancy, and many gaps in our knowledge need to be addressed by future research (see Chapter 17). However, there is a growing evidence base around the type of adaptive responses, underlying mechanisms, triggers and critical windows in early life development. The challenge is to translate our knowledge and understanding of early life nutrition into effective public health interventions and policies to improve the population's health.

This Task Force Report has reviewed evidence on early life nutrition. First, the Report has described normal growth and development and presented current practice and recommendations relating to diet and lifestyle in pregnancy and in early life. Second, the mechanisms and critical pathways involved in fetal programming and the effect of early life nutrition on specific health consequences in later life have been examined. The conclusions reached by the Task Force are presented below, in chapter order. The recommendations of the Task Force can be found in Chapter 17.

16.1 Chapter 1

- An individual's growth potential is determined by their genome, although adequate nutrient supply is required in early life to realise this growth potential.
- There is strong evidence that some nutrients have clear developmental effects – e.g. vitamin A (excess), iodine and folate insufficiency – but the effects of more modest variations in maternal nutrition are less well understood.
- Fetal programming is defined as a process whereby a stimulus or insult, acting at a critical phase of development, results in long-term changes in the structure or function of the organism.
- Environmental conditions can impact on the genotype, resulting in more than one alternative form of structure, physiological state or behaviour developing. This is referred to as 'developmental plasticity'.
- Epidemiological studies show a link between early experience and adult diseases such as diabetes, cardiovascular disease and cancer.
- Some individuals may be more vulnerable to the effects of stressors in adult life as a result of poor experiences in early life, such as inadequate nutrition.

- Experimental studies provide clear evidence for developmental influences of variations in early nutrition that may be key to the links between early life and adult disease, but our current understanding of how these experimental data inform optimal patterns of maternal and infant nutrition is limited.
- The poor diets of young women observed in the UK are of concern, and may impact on their ability to meet the nutrient needs of future pregnancies.
- Intervention strategies to lower future disease risk will require a very clear understanding of the influence of current variations in diet and nutrition on growth and development in early life and lifelong health.

16.2 Chapter 2

- Development begins with the embryonic period which ends 8 weeks after fertilisation. The fetal period, from week 9 to birth, is characterised by growth and elaboration of structures.
- The first 3 months of pregnancy (the first trimester) is a period of rapid growth. The main external features of the fetus begin to take form by a process of differentiation which produces various cell types (e.g. blood cells, kidney cells and nerve cells). This rapid growth results in the embryo being particularly susceptible to the impact of external factors (e.g. nutrient intake) during this time.
- The developing embryo and then fetus is entirely dependent on the mother and the maternal environment for its nutritional requirements. Therefore, a woman's diet during pregnancy plays a crucial role in determining fetal health and development. There are also particular periods of growth and development of tissues and organs, termed 'critical windows', when susceptibility to damage is elevated.
- The role of the placenta in development is often overlooked, but it plays a central role, as it is the conduit for nutrient and waste transfer between mother and fetus.
- The cardiovascular system is the first major system to function in the embryo. This is because the growing embryo cannot satisfy its nutritional and oxygen requirements by diffusion alone.
- The development of the lungs is a gradual process that can be divided into five stages through embryo

and fetal life. At birth the lungs undergo marked structural changes in order to mature into an adult lung. The lungs continue to develop up to the age of 2 years.

- Infancy (1–24 months) is a period of rapid growth compared to other periods of life. The relative relationships among rates of linear growth, weight gain and brain growth vary greatly during the first few years of life. Although the proportion of energy requirements for body tissue deposition decreases dramatically during infancy, brain energy demands increase markedly during the same period.

- The World Health Organization (WHO) launched new Child Growth Standards in 2006. The UK Department of Health accepted recommendations to replace the UK 1990 reference ('UK90') with the new WHO Growth Standards in 2007. Also in 2007, the Royal College of Paediatricians and Child Health adopted growth charts that combine UK90 and WHO data. These charts represent an international standard of growth for all healthy infants and young children regardless of how they are fed (breast-fed or formula-fed).

- 'Catch-up growth' (the return of the child's growth to its previous normal projectile) may have short-term beneficial health effects, such as lower rates of hospitalisation during infancy and early childhood. However, there is now growing evidence that children who grow rapidly during infancy and childhood are more likely to be obese as adults and are at greater risk of metabolic disturbances such as insulin resistance.

16.3 Chapter 3

- Estimates indicate that around one in five (19%) women of childbearing age in England are obese (BMI $\geq$ 30) and one in 20 women (5%) of women delivering in 2009 had a BMI $\geq$ 35 at any time in pregnancy. It is vital to reverse the trend in obesity in pregnancy to lessen the burden on maternity and health services and to improve the health of mothers and offspring in future generations.

- National surveys show that the majority of women of childbearing age do not reach the recommended intake of 400 µg/day of folic acid from food and supplements. In many countries where supplementation is recommended, data indicate that less than 50% of women have taken folic acid supplement

before becoming pregnant, with some studies finding less than 10% taking supplement.

- Low vitamin D status is common in pregnancy. In the UK, pregnant and lactating women are advised to take vitamin D supplements containing 10 µg/day (400 IU/day). The awareness and compliance of women regarding vitamin D supplementation is low. This is particularly relevant for high-risk groups such as women with darker skin and women who are housebound or who conceal most of their skin.

- The use of supplements during lactation is encouraged in many countries; however, information about how well lactating mothers meet recommendations is even less available than for women during pregnancy. Folate is one of the nutrients commonly found to be low in diets of lactating women, although zinc, calcium, iron, vitamins A, C, D and E and thiamin have also been found to be below the recommended intake.

- Prior to 2001, the WHO global recommendation was that infants should be exclusively breast-fed for 4–6 months before the introduction of complementary foods. Following an Expert Consultation in March 2001 to discuss the scientific evidence on exclusive breastfeeding, the WHO recommended exclusive breastfeeding for 6 months, with introduction of complementary foods and continued breastfeeding thereafter. Like many countries, the UK has adopted this recommendation, but compliance with exclusive breastfeeding for 6 months is low.

- The timing and type of weaning foods introduced is important to help the neuromuscular development of the baby as well as influencing the baby's willingness to experience new tastes and textures. Research indicates that the introduction of solid foods should not be delayed beyond 6 months, with foods with a thicker and lumpier texture being introduced by 9 months to encourage chewing, even before teeth emerge.

16.4 Chapter 4

- Suboptimal nutrition can affect fetal development, both in the short and the long term.
- There are 'critical windows' in development, where the fetus is susceptible to suboptimal nutrition.
- Different organs are most vulnerable to insult during periods of growth and differentiation.

- Many questions remain unanswered in this area of human health and well-being. For example, it is not clear why the placenta, and indeed other homeostatic organs, do not maintain the fetus against the stress of suboptimal nutrition, and further work is needed to prove or disprove the proposed mechanisms of nutritional programming.

16.5 Chapter 5

- Being male or female shapes an individual's risk of certain diseases (cardiovascular disease, autoimmune disease, asthma, depressive illnesses, eating disorders, schizophrenia/autism, gastric ulcers and kidney diseases); the basis for most of these is largely unexplored.
- Masculinsation of the (male) fetus by androgens in fetal and early postnatal life exerts effects throughout the body on non-reproductive organs; this may partly explain male–female differences in disease predisposition.
- Subtle disorders of masculinisation in males are remarkably common, highlighting the inherent vulnerability of this process.
- Maternal body weight, diet and lifestyle choices can impact on growth of the baby before and after birth, and this can exert profound effects on lifelong predisposition to the major 'Western' diseases; these affect males and females differently.
- The male fetus grows faster and is more vulnerable to growth restriction due to various factors, including maternal lifestyle choices.
- Recent discoveries have identified some of the brain mechanisms that interlink the reproductive and metabolic systems of the body; dysfunction of these circuits may underlie disorders such as precocious puberty, eating disorders and susceptibility to obesity.
- Better understanding of the mechanistic bases for male–female differences in disease predisposition and their 'programming' in perinatal life should enable identification of strategies for minimising their impact in later life; modulation of diet is likely to be a factor in this.

16.6 Chapter 6

- The human brain is especially vulnerable to inadequate or inappropriate nutrition during its developmental growth spurt that broadly spans the third trimester of pregnancy and the first two postnatal years. The same period of rapid differentiation takes place in the early postnatal weeks in rodent species that are frequently employed in laboratory studies to mimic early life nutritional challenges.
- Gestational outcome, maternal nutrition and early neonatal diet can affect brain structure and developmental processes such as neurogenesis, synaptogenesis and myelination, as well as more subtle brain circuitry and transmitter signalling.
- Developmental perturbations and beneficial interventions have been studied in human subjects following exposure to adverse conditions during early life, whereas mechanistic studies of the intermediate steps between the nutritional insult and short-term or lifelong functional consequence require examination of appropriate animal models under controlled conditions.
- The extended central nervous system feeding and energy balance circuitry develops during late pregnancy and early neonatal life and is susceptible to nutritionally induced changes in trophic signals such as leptin, which can shape neuronal projections and connectivity between different brain regions. The potential implications of over-exposure to hormones such as leptin and insulin during gestation, such as in maternal obesity, are clear.
- Cognitive, mental health and behavioural outcomes may also be influenced by early life nutrition and pregnancy outcome, processes involving cortical areas and the hippocampus.
- Programming mechanisms linking nutritional or other challenges to functional endpoints may involve epigenetic changes and glucocorticoid exposure.
- A range of nutritional challenges of varying severity affect brain development and function, including protein/energy malnutrition, global over-nutrition (e.g. gestational diabetes, maternal obesity, over-nutrition prior to weaning), and specific micronutrient or essential fatty acid deficiencies.
- Although intervention to counter early life nutritional programming effects will be problematical in humans, more detailed knowledge of underlying mechanisms, and causation, should allow development of an evidence base to be carefully exploited to benefit outcome in compromised pregnancies.

16.7 Chapter 7

- The human gut microbiota comprises more cells than the rest of the human body and plays a role in the health and well-being of the host, including energy harvest (the process by which energy is derived by gut microbiota).
- The acquisition and development of the infant gut microbiota is affected by a number of factors – genetic, environmental (including diet) and health.
- Certain bacterial populations added in the diet in early life as probiotics, such as *Bifidobacterium breve* and *Lactobacillus rhamnosus*, have also been shown to reduce the risk of developing asthma, atopic dermatitis and other common allergies in later life, through infancy, early childhood and into adolescence.
- It is generally accepted that the gut microbiota of breast-fed and formula-fed infants are distinctly different, although fortification of formulas with prebiotics has partially addressed this difference.
- Initial weaning is associated with a transitional phase in the infant gut microbiota succession.
- At between 1 and 2 years of age the infant gut microbiota converges towards the microbiota present in an adult.

16.8 Chapter 8

- The environmental determinants of obesity may include nutritional status in critical periods of early development.
- Growth retardation *in utero*, particularly if followed by rapid postnatal growth, may be a determinant of obesity in later life.
- Breastfeeding may protect against later obesity. The reduction in obesity in later life has been estimated to be between 7% and 22% with breastfeeding of varying degree.
- Excessive 'fuel' availability associated with maternal diabetes and obesity may predispose the developing child to enhanced risk of type 2 diabetes in later life.
- Animal studies provide unequivocal evidence for early life origins of obesity and have made a major contribution to understanding the mechanistic basis.

- The current level of evidence, in the absence of randomised controlled trials, is inadequate to support public health interventions.

16.9 Chapter 9

- Type 1 diabetes arises through the autoimmune destruction of the pancreatic beta-cells (the cells that produce insulin, which is required for the uptake of glucose into muscle and fat cells). Type 1 diabetes accounts for around 10% of all diabetes. It commonly develops in childhood and rarely in individuals aged over 40 years.
- Type 2 diabetes is far more common (accounting for 90% of diabetes). In individuals with type 2 diabetes the body can still produce insulin but not in sufficient quantities (beta-cell dysfunction) and tissues in the body do not respond to insulin appropriately (insulin resistance).
- Obesity is a major risk factor for insulin resistance and consequently type 2 diabetes. Type 2 diabetes was traditionally thought to be a condition of middle age, however, the increasing prevalence of obesity in childhood is resulting in a growing number of cases of type 2 diabetes in children.
- Type 2 diabetes is of great importance to public health and healthcare costs as it is associated with other conditions including cardiovascular disease, stroke, blindness and kidney disease.
- Suboptimal nutrition during early life has a major influence on the risk of an individual developing type 2 diabetes later in life.
- Epidemiological evidence indicates both low and high birthweight is associated with increased risk of type 2 diabetes in later life.
- Over the first year of life breast-fed infants gain less weight than formula-fed infants and are less likely to develop cardiovascular risk factors which are strongly associated with type 2 diabetes.
- A range of different nutrient deficiencies during critical periods of development all lead to increased risk of type 2 diabetes. This is associated with both pancreatic beta-cell dysfunction and insulin resistance.
- Fundamental molecular mechanisms underlying these effects are starting to emerge. These include permanent structural changes and epigenetic programming of gene expression.

- Further understanding of these mechanisms will enable intervention and prevention strategies to be developed.

16.10 Chapter 10

- Poor fetal growth, especially followed by rapid postnatal growth or obesity, increases the risk of cardiovascular disease in adulthood.
- The offspring of mothers with raised blood pressure in pregnancy have increased blood pressure.
- Various animal models can replicate the effects of impaired fetal growth on the development of high blood pressure. Maternal obesity can also result in higher blood pressure in the offspring.
- The mechanism for the increase in blood pressure is uncertain but may be mediated by programming of sympathetic outflow from the central nervous system or impaired renal development making the kidney more sensitive to salt overload.
- The risk of developing the atherogenic lipoprotein phenotype (low HDL-cholesterol, raised fasting triacylglycerol) is greater in infants with low birthweight or those who show rapid postnatal weight gain who become overweight or obese in adult life.

16.11 Chapter 11

- The search for evidence in humans linking early nutrition to later cancer risk has largely been limited by the paucity of large randomised controlled trials of nutrient exposure in early life. While there are a number of plausible mechanisms in humans – and animal models which appear to demonstrate causality – the availability of epidemiological evidence linking early nutrition to later cancer risk in humans is patchy.
- Evidence from meta-analyses of case–control and cohort studies suggest a lower risk of childhood cancer among those who had been breast-fed.
- Evidence indicates a relationship between higher birthweight and increased breast cancer risk. Postnatal growth has also been linked to risk of breast cancer. Rapid growth and falling BMI in childhood through to puberty, early age of peak growth, tall stature and low BMI at age 14 are all strongly related to increased breast cancer risk in later life. On the other hand, greater body fatness during childhood and adolescence are associated with reduced risk of breast cancer.
- There are numerous hypothesised mechanisms through which nutrition can influence the risk of cancer. Likely hypotheses can be categorised into effects on genotype, epigenotype and phenotype.
- It is possible that maternal and paternal periconceptional nutritional status could select for embryos with genotypes that influence cancer risk in later life.
- Diet of the mother before and during pregnancy could plausibly influence later cancer risk via effects on the epigenetic status of particular classes of genes such as the imprinted genes.
- There is some evidence that maternal diet and childhood growth may influence body fatness which has itself been implicated in cancer risk.

16.12 Chapter 12

- Reduced peak bone mass in early adulthood is associated with increased risk of osteoporosis and fractures in later life.
- Maternal smoking, poor fat stores and excessive physical activity in late pregnancy all have a detrimental effect on bone mineral accrual by the fetus, leading to reduced bone mass at birth.
- Maternal vitamin D status may be critical to bone development in the offspring. All pregnant and lactating women are advised to take a vitamin D supplement of 10 µg/day (400 IU/day). Dark-skinned ethnic minorities are at particular risk of low vitamin D and, in the UK, all Asian children and women are advised to take supplementary vitamin D. The Recommended Nutrient Intake (RNI) for calcium among pregnant women, like non-pregnant women, is 700 mg/day, whereas an additional 550 mg/day is recommended for women during lactation.
- Long-term skeletal growth trajectory may be programmed by gene–environment interactions *in utero*. Skeletal growth is particularly important in the last trimester.
- Postnatal modulation of calcium and vitamin D intake may, at least transiently, influence bone mass, but there is a lack of evidence to support any longer-term influence.
- Fatty acid intake also seems to influence bone development; in particular, levels of *n*-3

polyunsaturated fatty acids (PUFAs) have been positively associated with peak bone mineral density (BMD) in adults and children. One study has also suggested a positive link between maternal cord blood levels of long-chain *n*-3 fatty acids and bone mass in offspring.

- Exclusively breast-fed babies may be at increased risk of vitamin D deficiency if the mother is vitamin D deficient and they have minimal effective exposure to sunlight (for example, pigmented skin). Infant supplementation with vitamin D should be considered in these situations.

- As bone is made up of a protein matrix, protein nutrition is likely to be of fundamental importance in bone development. However, there are very few data relating to this directly.

- Several studies have shown beneficial effects of physical activity on bone mass in late childhood. However, the evidence is less clear regarding the influence of physical activity on bone mass in younger children, and in particular, whether bone mineral accrual varies significantly within the normal range of activity for a healthy population. Children with habitually greater levels of physical activity have higher bone mineral accrual; however, whether these observations translate into long-term benefits or a reduction in fracture risk, either in childhood or in later adulthood, remains to be seen.

16.13 Chapter 13

- Asthma and allergic diseases have increased in prevalence and are now associated with significant morbidity and sizeable use of healthcare resources.

- Asthma and allergic diseases are characterised by an inappropriate immune response biased towards the Th2 phenotype. Tissue-specific deficits probably also critically contribute to the inflammatory process(es).

- It is becoming increasingly apparent that early life influences during fetal development and early childhood critically impact on the development of asthma and allergic disease.

- Concerns that maternal ingestion of food allergens during pregnancy and lactation increase the risk of childhood allergic disease have been re-evaluated, and allergen avoidance during pregnancy and lactation is no longer recommended.

- Breastfeeding for 3–4 months reduces the incidence of atopic dermatitis in infants at high risk of allergic disease. While breastfeeding appears to reduce the risk of wheezing and asthma in young children (< 6 years), the effects of breastfeeding on these conditions in older children are not clear.

- Concerns regarding the introduction of potential food allergens into the diets of young children have been reconsidered, and delaying the introduction of potential food allergens beyond 6 months is not widely advocated.

- Although many studies have reported associations between increasing BMI and incident asthma, and that weight loss is associated with improved lung function and reduced asthma symptoms, it is not clear whether the association between obesity and asthma reflects adverse effects on lung mechanics or effects on airway inflammation.

- There is increasing interest in the possibility that the nutrient content (e.g. vitamin E, vitamin D, zinc, selenium, PUFAs) of the maternal diet during pregnancy can influence the development of childhood asthma and allergic disease.

16.14 Chapter 14

- Maternal diet during pregnancy is important for brain development, in particular, intake of essential long-chain fatty acids, but also B vitamins, choline, zinc and iron. Intake of essential fatty acids also prolongs pregnancy duration which benefits fetal growth and development (including brain development). A European Commission panel recommends that pregnant and lactating mothers should aim to achieve a dietary intake of long-chain *n*-3 essential fatty acids to supply a docosahexaenoic acid (DHA) intake of at least 200 mg/day [equivalent to two portions (each portion is 140 g) of oil-rich fish per week), although this is not universally agreed.

- During fetal development the brain is protected during periods of poor nutrition, including extreme circumstances such as famine. Maternal starvation in the Dutch Hunger Winter of the 1940s did not have an adverse impact on cognitive development in the offspring.

- Early life nutrition plays an important part in mental health across the life course. Maternal diet during pregnancy has a fundamental effect on brain development, which can track into later life and influence, for example, life chances, economic productivity, physical morbidity and cognitive ageing (e.g. risk of dementia).

- A large body of evidence indicates that breast-feeding benefits cognitive development, with a smaller consensus suggesting benefits to emotional and behavioural development. Again, essential fatty acids are thought to be chiefly responsible. However, in the case of cognitive development there is some evidence that this is explained by maternal IQ. Breastfeeding is also associated with many non-nutritional factors which may be associated with mental health, e.g. aspects of intimacy (such as reciprocity, mutual joy, harmony, concern for others, trust and closeness) and socioeconomic status, maternal smoking history, maternal cognitive ability, maternal education, paternal education, family size and childhood experiences, which could potentially confound findings relating to cognitive development in the infant.

- Less is known about the effects of the post-weaning diet on mental development, although high consumption of fruit, vegetables and home-prepared foods at 6 and 12 months has been linked to higher IQ. Relevant micronutrient exposures include essential fatty acids, iron, zinc, iodine, folate and selenium.

- Evidence, including findings from two large randomised controlled trials of infants, indicate an association between some additives and preservatives and hyperactive symptoms, in particular some food colourings or other additives.

- Maternal nutrition may also have an impact on the mental health of the mother herself, as well as influencing the infant via parenting behaviour and infant attachment.

16.15 Chapter 15

- There are likely to be periods of fetal and early life development that are particularly sensitive to suboptimal or excessive nutrition. These are 'critical windows' in a child's development during which future health and development can be 'programmed'.

- A fetus is entirely dependent on its mother for its nutrient supply, which is likely to be influenced by a mother's nutritional status prior to conception and during pregnancy.

- In the UK, teenage pregnancy rates remain higher than in many other countries in Europe and the diets of adolescents are often poorly balanced, with low intakes of folate, iron and vitamin D being of particular concern. This has implications for adolescent girls who become pregnant, especially as many will still be growing themselves.

- The dramatic increase in overweight and obese women in the UK has focused attention on weight management before and during pregnancy. However, efforts in the UK are currently hampered by the lack of formal, evidenced-based guidelines. These include gestational weight gain and the need for training for health professionals so that they have the skills and confidence to appropriately and effectively address sensitive weight issues with pregnant women.

- Only about 30% of women of childbearing age meet current recommendations for physical activity. Benefits of physical activity during pregnancy include maintaining an appropriate body weight, enhancing fitness, and reducing muscle cramps and swelling of the legs and feet.

- Low vitamin D status is common among pregnant women, particularly those of South Asian, African, Caribbean and Middle Eastern descent. Lack of awareness of the recommendation to take vitamin D supplements during pregnancy and lactation is thought to be widespread, particularly in the most vulnerable groups. There is, therefore, a need to enhance awareness of the importance of this health message across the population.

- While awareness of the importance of folic acid around the time of conception is high, compliance with this recommendation is not reflected in practice. One of the key factors associated with lower uptake rates is unplanned pregnancies, which account for around half of all pregnancies in the UK. The only possible way to reach this group of women may be via fortification of foods with folic acid.

- The choice of feeding in infancy influences the rate of growth and the type of tissue deposition, which has the potential to track into adulthood. Infants who are not breast-fed tend to have slightly higher blood pressure and blood cholesterol levels in later life, and are at greater risk of type 2 diabetes and obesity. Promotion and support of breastfeeding, therefore, offers short- and long-term health benefits. However, it is also necessary for health professionals to ensure that the needs of bottle-feeding mothers are met.

- Advice on weaning is constrained by the absence of up-to-date information on the diets and nutrient intakes of infants and a lack of official guidance from the Department of Health on behavioural aspects of infant feeding such as recommended portion sizes, pace of complementary feeding and the stages at which different textures of food should be offered. The ongoing review of complementary and young child feeding by the Scientific Advisory Committee on Nutrition is therefore awaited with interest.

- Evidence is emerging about potential adverse effects of rapid 'catch-up' growth in infancy for risk of later disease. This has important implications for the management of low-birthweight and small-for-gestational-age babies in whom 'catch-up' growth was previously encouraged.

- The slower growth associated with breastfeeding could explain the long-term benefits of breastfeeding in relation to reduced risk of obesity and cardiovascular disease. Some of this may be due to the lower protein content of breast milk, which has led to the recent development of lower protein formulas to deliver growth trajectories more similar to those achieved with breastfeeding.

17
Recommendations of the Task Force

This Task Force Report has presented evidence relating to nutrition in early life and its impact on the risk for various chronic diseases in later life. Each chapter has identified specific areas that need to be addressed by further research and these are summarised in this chapter.

17.1 Priorities for future research on current practice in relation to early life development

- There is a need for further evaluative research to assess the effectiveness of interventions to control weight in women before, during and after pregnancy.
- Research is needed to inform UK guidelines on the optimal weight gain during pregnancy for women in different body mass index (BMI) categories.
- In order to support discussions around vitamin D fortification, more research is needed to clarify differences in physiological responses to vitamin D_3 and vitamin D_2.
- Other research questions that need to be addressed in relation to vitamin D include the extent to which vitamin D insufficiency contributes to geographical health inequalities in the UK, whether there is a causal link between vitamin D status and obesity, and whether individuals are genetically susceptible to vitamin D insufficiency.
- The Department of Health advises a gradual transition from spoon-fed puréed foods and baby rice to foods prepared with a coarser texture, finger foods and eventually consumption of family foods by 12 months of age. The baby-led weaning approach proposes that the standard weaning practice of spoon-feeding puréed foods or baby rice is bypassed in favour of introducing foods in their whole form as finger foods, and infants self-feed as opposed to spoon-feeding. Although sparse, research suggests several benefits of baby-led weaning compared to standard weaning practice, but further research is needed in this area.

17.2 Priorities for future research on mechanisms and pathways of early life development

17.2.1 Normal growth and development

- Current research suggests that catch-up growth increases risk of later disease. Further research to determine the reasons for this is needed.
- After birth, all sorts of growth and developmental changes occur. A better understanding is required of the regulation of the timing of development at all stages of life (from fetal life through infancy and early years, and into adolescence, adulthood and older age). Research on what upregulates or downregulates gene expression at any time from conception would be useful.
- Further investigation of how diet and nutrients modulate growth and development is required. For example, what is the influence of phytochemicals on growth and development and could they be used therapeutically?

Nutrition and Development: Short- and Long-Term Consequences for Health, First Edition. Edited by the British Nutrition Foundation.
© 2013 the British Nutrition Foundation. Published 2013 by Blackwell Publishing Ltd.

17.2.2 Mechanisms and pathways of critical windows of development

- Further research is required to confirm or reject the adaptive programming theory as a mechanism for nutritional programming.
- Evidence indicates that the disruption of organ development (organ remodelling) in the kidney can have a direct impact on kidney function. However, research is required to determine whether the remodelling of other organs such as the brain, pancreas and placenta also has a direct impact on their function.
- Further research is required to determine whether a limited number of genes or gene pathways are altered by nutritional insult (the gatekeeper hypothesis).

17.2.3 Perinatal effects of sex hormones in programming of disease susceptibility

- Further research is needed to better understand how modern maternal diet and lifestyle choices may differentially impact male and female offspring, their childhood growth and development and the later impacts on well-being in adulthood.
- Further investigation is required on the fetal mechanisms that underlie male–female differences in disease risk to move them beyond their present descriptive state. In particular, resolution of the role played by hormones (mainly androgens) is needed – this will probably require experimental studies in animal models.

17.2.4 Cognitive and neurological development

- Further research involving human studies and from directed manipulation of appropriate animal models is needed to gain a better understanding of the interaction between early life nutrition and neurological development.
- Further research is required to investigate the hypothesis that over-nutrition during early life is an epigenetic risk factor for obesity and metabolic disorders.
- Current evidence suggests that leptin in breast milk may contribute to the development of energy balance circuitry and to early satiety signalling, although further research is needed to determine whether leptin in breast milk is likely to contribute to the differential growth rates seen in breast-fed and formula-fed infants.
- The potential causality between iron deficiency during development and cognitive or behavioural function in later life requires further investigation.
- Breast milk is a natural source of the *n*-3 polyunsaturated fatty acid DHA, and breastfeeding is generally taken to be associated with better cognitive performance. Consumption of oil-rich fish during pregnancy is also associated with better cognitive performance in children. However, the benefit of supplementing formula milk with DHA is less clear. Further investigation of the potential benefits of DHA on neurological and cognitive development is required.

17.2.5 Establishing gut microbiota and bacterial colonisation of the gut in early life

- Further investigation of the role of the gut microbiota, or specific members thereof, in carbohydrate and fat metabolism is warranted.
- Longitudinal studies and/or prospective studies of cohorts from previous infant studies are needed to understand the impact of the neonatal microbial acquisition and development as a blueprint for gut microbiology, host health and risk of gastrointestinal and/or metabolic disorders later in life.
- Relatively few studies have investigated the impact of weaning (i.e. introduction of solid food to the infant diet) on the infant microbiota. Research investigating this would be very useful.
- In general, findings have shown promising results of using prebiotic-supplemented infant formulas which are now commercially available. However, the longitudinal effects of such prebiotic-supplemented formulas have not been examined. Studies with long-term follow-up are needed to determine whether using such formulas has any implications for health in later life.
- There is increasing interest in the energy-harvesting capacity of human gut microbiota and its potential role in obesity. There is some evidence to suggest that the gut microbiota in lean and obese individuals differ, although further research in this area is needed.

17.3 Priorities for future research: specific diseases

This Task Force Report has highlighted a number of specific areas for future research in relation to early life and various chronic diseases. These are summarised below.

17.3.1 Obesity

- Recent evidence from the European Early Nutritional Programming Project (EARNEST) suggests that lower protein formula feeds may be advantageous in the prevention of childhood obesity. Further cohort studies with longer-term follow-up are required to confirm this.
- Intervention studies are required to determine effective dietary and physical activity interventions appropriate for overweight and obese pregnant women. Some studies designed to improve physical activity or diet in overweight or obese pregnant women are currently under way, and findings are eagerly awaited.

17.3.2 Diabetes

- There is a need to establish biomarkers that could be used to identify individuals who experienced suboptimal nutrition during early life and are therefore at increased disease risk.
- There is a need to assess potential intervention strategies during pregnancy that could prevent suboptimal exposures *in utero*.

17.3.3 Cardiovascular disease

- Further research is needed to ascertain whether the higher risk of stroke in people of African or Caribbean descent and coronary heart disease in South Asian people is a consequence of early life environment and whether improved pre- and postnatal growth will eradicate the differences.
- Further research is needed to understand whether there are critical windows in the differentiation of adipocytes that determine their capacity to produce adipokines.
- Further research is needed to ascertain whether high birthweight associated with maternal obesity increases risk of cardiovascular disease, using disease outcome indicators rather than surrogate risk markers.
- Several lifestyle factors, such as salt intake, have been linked to elevated blood pressure in adult life. Research has mainly focused on developmental influences on blood pressure. However, further research on whether the blood pressure raising effect of salt in adult life is determined by poor growth *in utero* would be useful.

17.3.4 Cancer

- Identification of the mechanism of action and the developmental stage(s) at which early diet and nutrition might influence later cancer risk would be of considerable practical importance.
- The search for evidence in humans linking early nutrition to later cancer risk has largely been limited by the paucity of large randomised controlled trials of nutrient exposure in early life. While few such interventions have been carried out to investigate subsequent cancer risk specifically, there are a number of relatively large historical cohorts where nutritional interventions (e.g. folic acid, fish oils and vitamin D) have been carried out around the time of pregnancy. There are also a number of large historical observational studies where data on nutrient intake or nutrient status in pregnancy are available. Follow-up of the offspring of these studies to assess cancer risk in adult life would be informative. Some of these cohorts have been successfully interrogated to assess links with later disease risk (e.g. Avon Longitudinal Study of Parents and Children [ALSPAC] in the UK) but more could be done to exploit other cohorts if ethical procedures are in place to allow tracing and follow-up.
- In terms of current knowledge, the most plausible mechanism linking early diet to later cancer risk involves the epigenetic status of the imprinted genes. It is important to understand the origin of heterogeneity of imprinted gene epigenetic status in normal tissues and its effects; its heritability, the modulating effect of early influences and later life exposures, and the mechanisms by which this variability might lead to the development of cancer.
- Possible mechanisms linking body fatness to cancer risk are already being studied extensively.

In terms of the early dietary origins of later cancer risk it would be particularly useful to know more about the way in which early nutrition can influence later adiposity and the distribution of body fat, how any programmed pattern of adiposity might impact on cancer risk, and whether this programming can be reversed by strategies to tackle obesity in later life.

- The concept that embryonic stem cells could persist throughout life is particularly important in relation to possible mechanisms linking early diet to later cancer risk. More work is required to establish whether this phenomenon occurs, how widespread it is, and whether these cell types play a role in tumour development.

17.3.5 Bone health

- Investigation of novel public health interventions, such as supplementation of pregnant women with vitamin D, is warranted.
- Many of the trials of calcium intake during pregnancy have focused on preventing pre-eclampsia, with very few studies investigating maternal or neonatal bone mass as an outcome. Research into the effect of maternal calcium intake on the bone mineral density of offspring would be useful.
- It is unclear whether maternal baseline calcium intake is important in the influence of vitamin D supplementation on the fetus. There is also very few data available on the influence of calcium intake on the bone mineral density of offspring.
- There are few dosing studies for calcium intake, particularly in pregnancy and early postnatal life. Gut absorption of calcium is saturable, and the few data that do exist would be consistent with there being a threshold above which further increases yield no additional benefit. However, the optimal levels of 25(OH)D in pregnancy and lactation are currently uncertain.

17.3.6 Allergic disease and asthma

- The possible association between early life allergen exposure and subsequent asthma and allergic disease needs to be established by well-conducted pragmatic trials.
- Trials are required to evaluate whether manipulation of maternal nutrient intake during pregnancy

can reduce the likelihood of childhood asthma and allergic disease.
- Genetic susceptibilities and interactions with dietary exposures need to be clarified.
- There is still a need to identify novel non-dietary early life influences on asthma and allergic disease and to conduct pragmatic trials to ascertain whether manipulation of these exposures can reduce the prevalence of asthma and allergic disease.

17.3.7 Cognitive function

- The evidence from observational studies conducted in developed countries indicate no objective evidence of a 'weanling's dilemma'. However, there is a need for large randomised trials in both developing and developed countries to rule out potential adverse effects such as not achieving optimal brain and, therefore, mental development, and to confirm the reported health benefits of exclusive breastfeeding for 6 months.
- Research in humans is required to determine the influence of supplementation with nutrients such as iron, zinc, iodine, vitamin D and choline on birth outcomes such as cognitive function. Ideally, randomised controlled trials are required in order to control for potential confounding factors.

17.4 Recommendations to key stakeholders

17.4.1 Recommendations to policy makers

The findings of the review of complementary and young child feeding currently being conducted by the Scientific Advisory Committee on Nutrition (SACN) are eagerly awaited. Meanwhile, SACN or other relevant bodies should consider whether dietary recommendations during pregnancy should be modified to take into account the risk of long-term disease in the offspring in relation to pregnancy outcome. The sections below have been identified by the Task Force as key areas for policy makers to consider.

17.4.1.1 Maternal obesity

Despite the numerous challenges, pregnancy and, ideally, the period when pregnancy is being planned have been identified as key times to target the importance of weight control or a weight loss strategy (either pre-pregnancy or post-lactation), and avoidance of excessive weight gain during pregnancy to help prevent the development of obesity in women and their children. To date, the policy response to support maternity services in tackling maternal obesity has been weaker than policy initiatives focusing on obesity in childhood. Activity in this area is hampered by the absence of officially accepted guidelines for gestational weight gain, which has been identified by UK health professionals as a barrier to consistent practice. Although the Institute of Medicine (in the US) published revised guidelines on gestational weight gain in pregnancy, evidence from the UK is required to enable appropriate guidelines to be developed that are relevant for implementing in a UK population. Current advice in England and Wales, from the National Institute for Health and Clinical Excellence (NICE), is that pregnant women should not be weighed routinely throughout pregnancy until such time as an intervention for restriction of weight gain has been shown to safely improve pregnancy outcome.

The lack of evidence supporting the benefit of regular weighing and monitoring after the first antenatal check (and the associated advice from NICE) also serves to underplay the importance of maintaining a healthy body weight. In addition, although health professionals understand their responsibility to explain the potential risks and complications associated with obesity in pregnancy, many report feeling uncomfortable raising and discussing such issues with pregnant women and need greater support and training to deliver effective advice. As differences in the prevalence of maternal obesity reflect broader socio-demographic inequalities, particularly in relation to deprivation, ethnicity and unemployment, a lack of comprehensive policies to tackle this problem will worsen the health inequalities already prevalent in our society.

The Task Force supports the calls for clear policy on weight control and avoidance of obesity in pregnancy, including the need for better services for women prior to pregnancy and support for women in achieving and maintaining a healthy body weight after pregnancy.

While the ideal public health solution would be to intervene and support women in achieving a healthy weight prior to pregnancy, women are often hard to reach for targeted interventions before they conceive,

and many pregnancies are unplanned. Therefore, broader preventive and public health strategies for young women need to be developed to support this process. Clearly this is a major challenge that can only be met by effective partnership working between maternity and public health services to effectively manage diet, physical activity and weight throughout the 'reproductive cycle' and to provide the necessary training for the professionals involved.

17.4.1.2 Teenage pregnancy

While the main policy focus is appropriately on preventing teenage pregnancies, when they occur, extra support is needed to ensure that young pregnant women are aware of the need for good nutrition, the advice to stop smoking and drinking alcohol and the recommendations regarding supplementation (folic acid and vitamin D) in pregnancy, as well as practical advice regarding breastfeeding and weaning.

Family-based programmes, such as the Family Nurse Partnership (FNP) in England, and social marketing approaches that provide health professionals with insight and skills to develop targeted interventions that support behaviour change, may be best able to encourage the adoption of a healthier lifestyle in this vulnerable group.

17.4.1.3 Vitamin D

There is evidence of low vitamin D status across the UK population, particularly among young Asian and African-Caribbean children and pregnant women. NICE advises of the need to inform pregnant women about the importance of maintaining adequate vitamin D stores during pregnancy and taking a 10 µg supplement daily. However, a lack of awareness, particularly among those in vulnerable groups (e.g. ethnic minority groups), is thought to be widespread.

Although Healthy Start vitamins are now more widely available, it is not only low-income families who are at risk of poor vitamin D status and there is a need for a public campaign to enhance awareness across the population. A new Department of Health leaflet on vitamin D deficiency, to raise awareness among health professions, was published at the start of 2012, but there is a need for ongoing promotion of the vitamin D message to relevant audiences.

17.4.1.4 Folic acid

While awareness of the importance of folic acid seems to be high, compliance with this recommendation is not reflected in practice and many opportunities for health professionals to deliver information on folic acid supplementation are being missed. There is, therefore, a need to understand and act upon common barriers to the uptake of this important health message and to develop a clear public health strategy on supplementation. Campaigns have the potential to exacerbate inequalities in folic acid use between women in lower and higher socioeconomic groups. Future strategies should include elements that specifically target vulnerable groups, such as the less educated and the young, as well as women who conceive without planning to. To reach the last group, folic acid advice will need to be incorporated into a structure of preconception care that reaches high numbers of women of childbearing age, although the reality is far from this, and key barriers relating to training and structural changes would need to be addressed. The only other option is likely to be via fortification of foods with folic acid.

17.4.1.5 Breastfeeding and formula feeding

Breastfeeding has a major role to play in promoting health in both the short and long term for baby and mother. Evidence-based strategies for promoting the initiation and duration of breastfeeding, particularly in those groups where breastfeeding rates are commonly low, should therefore come high up on the public health agenda. In addition, continued support is required for events, such as National Breastfeeding Week, that offer important opportunities to raise awareness of the health benefits of breastfeeding, increase its social acceptance, and promote support for breastfeeding mothers. However, while promoting the benefits of breastfeeding, health professionals must ensure that mothers who cannot breastfeed or who choose to formula feed are also given the advice and support they need about selecting products, making up feeds, sterilising bottles and storing formula milk. Although the Baby Friendly Hospital Initiative (BFHI) training includes requirements for safe and appropriate formula feeding, it is not easy for midwives to obtain up-to-date information about formula feeding, particularly as the policies of many maternity units preclude manufacturers' representatives from meeting staff to impart information about product composition and innovations. Consideration needs to be given to ways of ensuring that midwives and health visitors (and also pharmacists) have access to the factual information they require on formula feeding and to prevent them from feeling constrained professionally from supporting all mothers equally in how to feed their babies successfully. This is important as the majority of women provide infant formula at some stage during the first year of life (a time when cows' milk is not appropriate as a drink) and may require advice to ensure that these products are used appropriately and safely.

17.4.1.6 Introduction of solids

Since publication of the COMA report, *Weaning and the weaning diet* in 1994, there has not been a thorough risk assessment of the evidence on weaning and the weaning diet in the UK. Advice regarding initiation of weaning onto foods other than milk (breast or infant formula) has changed during this period (from 4–6 months to 6 months). There appears to be confusion among health professionals and mothers alike about current recommendations and also behavioural aspects of infant feeding such as recommended portion sizes, pace of complementary feeding and the stages at which different textures of food should be offered. The outcome of the ongoing review of complementary and young child feeding by SACN is, therefore, urgently needed as a stimulus for communicating consistent advice. It will be important that communication of the review's findings includes targeted training to the wide range of health professionals involved in giving advice in this area (including health visitors and other community-based nurses, GPs, pharmacists and nursery and childcare professionals).

17.4.2 Recommendations to health professionals and other educators

All health professionals who are in contact with women prior to, during and immediately after childbirth have an opportunity to discuss diet and lifestyle habits and address individual concerns. Among others, this includes midwives, health visitors, dietitians and pharmacists, all of whom need to provide up-to-date, consistent advice tailored to specific needs. Several areas have been identified where more can be done to improve current practice, although consideration must be given to specific training needs to achieve future success, particularly in the context of delivery of the *Public Health Outcomes Framework* and related structural changes.

17.4.2.1 *Vitamin D*

It is likely that health professionals could do more to prevent vitamin D deficiency and to improve the uptake of supplements, particularly in vulnerable groups (i.e. those who have limited skin exposure to sunlight or who are of South Asian, African, Caribbean or Middle Eastern descent, and also those who are obese). Studies suggest that training is required to ensure widespread understanding of the current recommendations for supplementation and to improve awareness of the groups most at risk. It is hoped that the new UK Departments of Health leaflet will be a useful resource, but this is unlikely to be sufficient on its own and ongoing support will be required if progress is to be made.

17.4.2.2 *Folic acid*

Health professionals play an influential role in raising awareness of the importance of folic acid in preventing neural tube defects. As periconceptional supplementation is advised and many pregnancies are unplanned, an opportunistic strategy by all those advising women of childbearing age is required. This includes physicians in obstetrics and gynaecology, internal medicine and family medicine, providing advice, for example during annual visits, family planning visits or infertility visits. Pharmacists also have an important role to play in delivering this message as they may be the first health professional that a woman sees when she is planning a pregnancy. There is some evidence that pre-conception care can have a positive impact on folic acid uptake, but training and ongoing support is needed to ensure that the messages are being delivered consistently and accurately.

17.4.2.3 *Maternal obesity*

Addressing maternal obesity can be challenging for health professionals, particularly for midwives who do not want to jeopardise the relationship they have with their client. However, it is essential that the potential risks and complications associated with maternal obesity are explained to women during early pregnancy. Such communication should be sensitively delivered to encourage continued engagement with antenatal services, and midwives are likely to need specific training in this area, as is the case with other public health issues such as smoking cessation. It is important to stress both healthy eating and appropriate activity levels, in order to prevent excess weight gain and gestational diabetes. Women with a BMI > 30 should continue to receive advice on nutrition from appropriately trained professionals, after the birth, to achieve weight reduction. Health professionals should take particular care to check that women with a booking BMI over 30 are following advice to take vitamin D and folic acid supplements.

17.4.2.4 *Catch-up growth*

The rate of weight accretion during infancy and childhood might play a role in the development of obesity later in life. Mothers and also some health professionals often perceive early rapid weight gain to be a sign of good feeding practices. This view, however, may encourage faster than optimal growth in early infancy in those who are formula-fed. Health professionals need to be aware of, and communicate to parents and carers, the potential long-term consequences of rapid 'catch-up' growth, particularly in babies who have experienced intrauterine growth restriction.

17.4.2.5 *Infant feeding and weaning*

Health practitioners, such as midwives, nurses and doctors, have a key role to play in providing support to breastfeeding women, particularly during the first few weeks when discontinuation is greatest. Health professionals, however, need to have knowledge of the process of breastfeeding and be able to adopt a problem-solving approach to the difficulties mothers encounter, in order to give appropriate evidence-based care. While all health professionals should continue to promote and support breastfeeding, infant formula is an important source of nutrition for many infants, and parents need education and support in using it appropriately and safely. Being able to give parents advice and help with infant formula feeding requires an up-to-date knowledge of the different formulas available and skills in the safe preparation and storage of formula. Care should be taken in the delivery of advice around choice of infant feeding to prevent the negative emotions described by some women who choose not to breastfeed.

17.4.3 Recommendations to the food industry

The food industry plays a vital role in improving intake of key nutrients such as folic acid and vitamin D to support pregnancy and breastfeeding. As well as providing a range of fortified products and suitable supplements, manufacturers could help to promote their uptake by including information about the importance of these nutrients within the packaging of relevant pregnancy- and breastfeeding-related products (e.g. pregnancy test kits and breast pumps).

18
Nutrition and Development: Answers to Common Questions

The purpose of the chapter is to summarise the key points of this report using a question-and-answer format. Many of the questions used are commonly asked by medical journalists. The questions are grouped under headings, and generally follow the same order as the chapters in the report.

18.1 Nutrition and development

Q1: How does nutrition during fetal life influence our long-term health?

Strong evidence from studies in humans and animal models shows that if a baby is exposed to too little or too much nutrition during fetal life he/she is more likely to develop conditions such as type 2 diabetes, heart disease and osteoporosis in later life.

However, it remains to be seen whether altering the mother's nutrient intake during pregnancy can influence her offspring's risk of these conditions.

Q2: At what age does nutrition begin to have an impact on health in later life?

The quality of a mother's diet impacts on her baby's health in early life but there is also evidence that her diet and lifestyle habits (e.g. maternal weight and nutrition), even pre-pregnancy, can impact on her offspring's health in later life. In fact, there are also intergenerational effects: the impact of nutrition on the health of offspring in later life is likely to be influenced by the diet and lifestyle of their grandparents. This is because the nutrition and lifestyle of the grandmother can impact on the development of the offspring's mother, as the egg from which the offspring was formed was created in the offspring's mother while she was developing in the grandmother's womb.

18.2 Developmental programming hypotheses

Q1: What is developmental programming?

The mechanism that underpins the associations between early experience and later disease is described as programming. Developmental programming (also known as fetal programming) is a process whereby a stimulus or insult acting at a critical phase of fetal development or in early postnatal life results in long-term changes in the structure or function of the offspring (see Chapter 1 and Chapter 4).

18.3 Normal growth

Q1: What is an ideal or optimal birthweight?

The ideal birthweight is the weight at birth that is associated with the lowest associated perinatal mortality. The ideal birthweight varies between different populations, as does the average birthweight. The average birthweight of White infants in the UK was

Nutrition and Development: Short- and Long-Term Consequences for Health, First Edition. Edited by the British Nutrition Foundation. © 2013 the British Nutrition Foundation. Published 2013 by Blackwell Publishing Ltd.

reported to be 3.416 kg. Low birthweight is defined by the World Health Organization as a birthweight of less than 2.5 kg at term. High birthweight is defined as a birthweight of more than 4.0 kg at term. There is no ideal birthweight as such, but rather a range of normal birthweights. These are shown on the growth charts used by midwives and health visitors when they assess how a baby is growing. The growth charts and information for parents and carers on what the growth charts mean are available at www.growthcharts.rcpch.ac.uk. Doctors will often make a correction for birthweight which makes allowance for the week of pregnancy at which the baby was born; a baby may therefore be 'small for gestational age' or 'large for gestational age'. This helps more correctly identify those babies that have been adversely influenced by conditions during development (see Chapter 2, Section 2.6).

Q2: Has birthweight been increasing over the last few decades?

There is no clear evidence of an increase in average birthweight over the last decade. However, two factors in recent years are likely to affect such a trend. First, there has been an increase in very premature births due to medical advances that have enabled babies with a very low birthweight to now have a reasonable chance of survival when born as early as 24 weeks' gestation. Second, the proportion of overweight and obese mothers has increased, which impacts directly by increasing the birthweight of their babies. Therefore, the lack of any change in average birthweight over recent decades may have been influenced by changes in birthweight in both directions (see Chapter 2, Section 2.9).

18.4 How development occurs and factors that can affect it

Q1: How much does the environment in which the fetus develops influence the growth of the fetus?

The growth of the fetus is influenced by its genes. However, the environment in which the fetus develops in the womb appears to have a greater effect on the growth achieved than the genetic influence. Evidence suggests that around 62% of the variation in

birthweight is the result of the environment in the womb, 20% the result of maternal genes and 18% is due to fetal genes (see Chapter 1, Section 1.3.1).

Q2: What is the role of the placenta?

The placenta has several important roles (see Chapter 4, Section 4.3). First, the placenta transfers nutrients to the fetus, transports waste away from the fetus, and allows gas exchange between mother and fetus. Second, the placenta releases hormones into the maternal circulation, which affect metabolism in mother and fetus. The placenta plays a key role in the production of the hormones, progesterone and oestrogen, which are essential for a healthy pregnancy. Some placental hormones also help nutrient transfer from mother to fetus and others stimulate blood vessel and placental growth.

Q3: At what stage of pregnancy do the organs begin their development?

Rapid growth of the embryo occurs during the first 3 months of pregnancy. Different types of cell such as blood cells, kidney cells and nerve cells are being formed during this period. Organs begin to take shape around 4 weeks after fertilisation of the egg and develop at different rates throughout pregnancy and during early life. The heart (and cardiovascular system) is the first organ to function in the embryo, with other organs such as the kidney developing later on in pregnancy (see Chapter 4).

Q4: Why are different organs affected differently in terms of growth and development at different stages in pregnancy?

When the embryo becomes a fetus (at around 8 weeks), it signifies that all the major systems have formed. Organs and tissues develop from embryonic cells. These cells follow a distinct pathway. First they develop into different types of cell (e.g. blood cells, kidney cells, heart cells). This stage is known as cell differentiation. Following this, the number of each different type of cell increases. This stage is known as cell proliferation. The timing of the differentiation and proliferation stages is different for each tissue and organ. If the fetus receives poor nutrition during an organ's differentiation stage then it would be expected that the organ would be of normal size, but would have an altered profile of cells. On the other hand, if the fetus receives poor nutrition during an organ's proliferation stage, the organ would have the normal profile of cells, but a reduced total number of cells, which may result in a smaller organ (see Chapter 4, Section 4.5.1).

Q5: How should pregnant women minimise the risk of fetal growth restriction during pregnancy?

There are three important steps that a woman should take when planning a pregnancy, that will minimise the risk of fetal growth restriction during pregnancy. Most important, they should not smoke. It is also important to have a healthy weight and to eat a nutritious, varied diet.

18.5 Influences of perinatal sex hormone exposure on programming of disease susceptibility

Q1: At what stage of fetal development is sex determined?

All fetuses will become female unless testis formation and hormone action (primarily androgen) occurs in fetal life to begin the process of becoming male (masculinisation). Masculinisation of the reproductive tract and genitalia occurs very early in gestation (approx. 8–12 weeks). This time period is known as the *masculinisation programming window*, when the action of male hormones (androgens) in the fetus are critical to the masculinisation process (see Chapter 5, Section 5.2).

Q2: How long does the process of masculinisation take?

The development of the fetus into a male (masculinisation) begins as the result of hormones (primarily androgens) in the fetus, although further androgen-driven development of masculine characteristics occurs immediately after birth ('mini-puberty') and at puberty. Although masculinisation of the reproductive tract and genitalia occurs very early in gestation (approx. 8–12 weeks), masculinisation of different organs and systems does not occur all at the same time. For example, masculinisation of the brain occurs late in gestation (27–35 weeks). It is therefore

possible for the reproductive system and brain to be differentially masculinised if, for example, testosterone production by the fetal testis (which drives masculinisation) was impaired only in early or late pregnancy. Such a differential effect could account for gender dysphoria (when a person feels that they are trapped within a body of the wrong sex) (see Chapter 5, Section 5.2).

Q3: If fetal androgens are so important for the future normality and general well-being of males, is there anything that a pregnant woman can do to ensure maximum androgen exposure; for example, could she take androgens?

To support the masculinisation of her baby, mothers should maintain a healthy, varied diet and healthy lifestyle. Taking androgens should be avoided as these can impair the growth of the fetus (via effects on the mother) and would masculinise a female fetus, if present, resulting in an abnormally masculinised female child. The reproductive organs and genitalia develop at around 8–12 weeks' gestation, so mothers will be unaware of the gender of the baby during early development.

Q4: What role do hormones play in the development of chronic diseases where there are male–female differences in the risk of developing a particular disorder?

We know that hormones play a role in some chronic diseases such as heart disease, as males are more at risk than females, particularly during middle age. In the UK, in 2009 around one in five (20%) deaths in men and one in eight (13%) deaths in women were from heart disease. For male-specific reproductive disorders we know that altered fetal hormones (androgens) are likely to be important, but for kidney, lung and heart disease, we do not know if altered hormones are involved. For cardiovascular disorders, there is more evidence of a relationship as birthweight is related to both adult blood pressure (i.e. lower birthweight is associated with higher adult blood pressure) and to testosterone levels (i.e. lower birthweight is associated with lower testosterone levels), but the interrelationship of the two is still not clear.

Q5: How does the sex of the fetus influence health in later life?

The male fetus grows faster and appears to be more vulnerable to growth restriction due to various factors, including maternal lifestyle choices. Masculinisation of the male fetus by androgens in fetal and early postnatal life exerts effects throughout the body on non-reproductive organs. This may partly explain the fact that being male or female determines an individual's risk of certain diseases, for example, cardiovascular disease, autoimmune disease, asthma, depressive illnesses and kidney disease.

18.6 Cognitive and neurological development

Q1: When does the brain develop?

The time from the third trimester (around 26 weeks) of pregnancy through to birth is one of major and rapid growth of the brain. The brain continues its growth spurt during the first two postnatal years. In children aged 2 years, the human brain is already 80% of the adult weight.

Q2: Can the mother's diet make her offspring more intelligent?

It is extremely difficult to assess whether the mother's diet impacts on her offspring's intelligence, due to the possibility that many other factors may influence intelligence. The mother's diet can affect the brain development and function of the developing fetus in varying severity. Being undernourished, for example not having adequate energy or protein in the diet or not receiving the recommended nutrient intake for specific micronutrients or essential fatty acids, can affect the development and function of the fetal brain. Similarly, being over-nourished, for example having an excessive energy intake, or mothers having gestational diabetes or being overweight or obese during pregnancy, may have a detrimental effect on fetal brain development. Other factors may also affect brain structure and developmental processes and, therefore, influence the intelligence (or IQ) of offspring. These factors include being born small for gestational age, large for gestational age, or premature, as well as the early neonatal diet (milk feeding and early infant diet).

18.7 Influences of gut microbiota on programming of disease susceptibility

Q1: Why is attaining a healthy gut flora (bacteria) important for health?

Having healthy gut bacteria is essential as it reduces opportunity for the gut to be colonised by harmful microorganisms, it enhances the absorption of certain nutrients for the individual and is beneficial for the immune system. Furthermore, certain bacterial species and/or bacterial profiles have been associated with specific disorders (such as autism) and/or gastrointestinal disorders (including colorectal cancer, ulcerative colitis and Crohn's disease), antibiotic-associated diarrhoea and acute diarrhoea. For example, there is good evidence that the probiotic strain called *Lactobacillus rhamnosus* GG (LGG) is effective in decreasing the risk of developing antibiotic-associated diarrhoea and in decreasing the duration of acute diarrhoea in children.

Q2: What are the major changes that occur in the gastrointestinal tract during birth and the first few years of life?

The development of gut bacteria can be described in three stages. The first stage is the birthing process and first hours of life, during which time the infant comes into contact with the maternal microbiota and environmental microorganisms. The second stage of bacterial succession is the period of exclusive milk feeding. The third stage comprises the introduction of solid food into the infant's diet (i.e. weaning). The make-up of the gut bacteria is generally thought to stabilise around 2 years of age.

Q3: Are there differences in gut flora (bacteria) of breast-fed and formula-fed infants?

There are clear differences in the microbiota of breast-fed and formula-fed infants. The bacteria in the gut of breast-fed infants are less diverse than the bacterial profile of formula-fed infants. The main type of bacteria in the gut of breast-fed infants is bifidobacteria, while a wider variety of gut bacteria are found in the gut of formula-fed infants. However, developments in modern milk formulas have led to the addition of prebiotics. These are non-digestible food components that promote the growth and activity of bacteria in the digestive system that are thought to be beneficial to health. These developments in milk formula, together with improved microbiological analysis, may explain why studies published more recently (in the last 20 years) generally demonstrate fewer differences between the gut flora of breast-fed and formula-fed infants (particularly in relation to bifidobacterial levels).

Q4: When do microbes first start to appear in the gastrointestinal tract?

The intestinal tract of unborn infants was thought to be sterile, with microbes starting to appear during or immediately after the birthing process (depending on the mode of delivery). As bacteria have been detected in the placenta and amniotic fluid, scientists now think that the intestinal tract of the fetus may contain microbes.

Q5: What factors influence the numbers and diversity of bacteria present in the gastrointestinal tract of infants?

The major factors affecting early colonisation of the infant intestinal tract include the gestational age, mode of delivery, exposure to bacteria and the genetic make-up of the infant. Babies born pre-term or with very low birthweight tend to have delayed bacterial colonisation of their intestinal tract and less variety of bacteria. This may partially be a result of administration of antibiotics in pre-term infants. The health, nutritional status and gut bacteria of the mother may also be important factors.

18.8 Obesity

Q1: How does what your mother eats during pregnancy influence your risk of obesity as an adult?

When a fetus is faced with inadequate nutrient availability, it can adapt to ensure that these nutrients are channelled to meet the needs of its vital organs such as the brain, heart, adrenal glands and placenta. But this may mean that other organs, such as the bone marrow, muscles, lungs, gastrointestinal tract and kidneys, receive inadequate nutrients. Although this survival strategy is advantageous for the fetus while it is in the womb, it is thought that it can have a longer-term disadvantage when the child experiences ample nutrient availability later in life.

Mothers who are obese in pregnancy are more likely to have high blood sugar levels which increase birthweight. This, in turn, may increase the risk of the child becoming obese as an adult. Animal studies suggest that increased appetite may be programmed *in utero* (in the womb). This may create a vicious cycle of maternal obesity leading to childhood obesity.

Q2: Does breastfeeding reduce the risk of the infant being overweight or obese later in life?

There are many benefits of breastfeeding which appear to include a reduced risk of obesity in later life. But the effect is likely to be more modest than originally thought. It is hard for studies to determine the true effects because of the potential for serious confounding due to the social class differences of women who do and don't choose to breastfeed. The reasons behind the reduced risk of obesity in later life among infants who were breast-fed may be that breast-fed infants gain weight more slowly than formula-fed infants, or that breast-fed infants are likely to take in less milk when dependent on more natural cues to stimulate feeding than bottle-fed infants. Other proposed reasons include factors in breast milk such as leptin (a hormone involved in appetite control and energy expenditure) and insulin levels, or the higher protein content of formula milk (which can lead to accelerated growth – a risk factor for obesity in later life), although innovation in formula development has now resulted in the production of lower protein formulas supporting slower growth in infants.

Q3: Is a child with a higher than average birthweight more likely to be overweight or obese in later life?

There is some indication that babies who are born heavier at term may be more likely to develop obesity in later life. Also, babies who are very small at term also seem to show the same trend. Indeed some researchers suggest that the relationship between birthweight and later obesity follows a J- or U-shaped curve. Pre-term babies that catch up in terms of growth rapidly in early life also seem to have a higher risk for obesity in later life, although some researchers suggest that heavier babies grow into more muscular rather than fatter adults. The more pertinent question is whether a fatter baby, rather than a heavier baby, is more likely to become overweight in later life (in other words, does excessive fat in the baby around the time of birth track into adulthood?). Unfortunately there is currently not enough evidence to be able to answer this question but it is something that should become clearer with further research.

Q4: Are babies of obese mothers more likely to be obese themselves in later life?

Current evidence suggests that babies of obese mothers are more likely to become obese themselves in later life. Obesity increases the risk of complications during early pregnancy, such as pre-eclampsia (where women have high blood pressure, protein in their urine, and may develop other symptoms and problems) that increase the risk of giving birth to a small, growth-retarded baby. If such a baby experiences rapid growth postnatally, it appears to be at greater risk of becoming obese later on. Obese mothers are also more likely to have a baby with an excessive birthweight (a condition known as macrosomia). This is also associated with increased risk of obesity in later life. However, it is very difficult to demonstrate a direct link between the fatness of a mother and the development of obesity in her child because there are so many environmental and lifestyle factors that can influence childhood obesity. Also, many studies investigating the link have used poor measures of body fat in both mothers and children. In obese women, pre-pregnancy body mass index (a measure based on weight and height) is thought to be a more important determinant of pregnancy outcome than weight gain during pregnancy. This is because weight gain during pregnancy is very variable – while many obese mothers gain excessive weight during pregnancy, some can put on less weight than leaner mothers.

Q5: If babies are born with a low birthweight is it beneficial for them to 'catch up' rapidly in weight in the first year?

Infants born small for gestational age who rapidly gain weight ('catch-up' growth) during the first 6–12 months of life are likely to develop an increased body weight or fatness in later life. It is beneficial to

increase weight during infancy at a slower rate consistent with standard growth curves (i.e. to track on the same curve of the growth charts).

18.9 Diabetes

Q1: Why does nutrition during fetal life influence our risk of developing type 2 diabetes?

If tissues, such as the pancreas, are exposed to inadequate levels of nutrients during critical periods of their development, they do not develop properly and, in the case of the pancreas, this can result in a reduced number of the cells that produce insulin.

Insulin is a hormone which helps the body utilise the energy (or glucose) from food. However, in people with diabetes, the body is unable to break down glucose into energy. This may be due to low muscle mass (due to low levels of physical activity) which can reduce the effectiveness of insulin (its ability to remove glucose from blood).

Another reason may be due to insulin resistance which develops in adult life due to unhealthy weight gain and low levels of physical activity. This is a condition in which the body's cells are less responsive (or sensitive) to the action of insulin and, therefore, the pancreas has to secrete more insulin. Eventually, the capacity of the pancreas to secrete insulin fails, blood glucose levels rise and type 2 diabetes results.

Q2: What can I do if I had a low birthweight to stop myself developing diabetes?

Just because you had a low birthweight does not mean that you will definitely develop type 2 diabetes – it just increases your risk, especially if you are overweight and physically inactive. Maintaining a healthy weight, in particular ensuring your waist measurement does not exceed 80 cm for women and 94 cm for men, and doing regular physical activity (equivalent to 30 minutes brisk walking at least five times a week) will reduce your risk.

18.10 Cardiovascular disease

Q1: Is birthweight linked to risk of cardiovascular disease in later life?

Poor fetal growth increases the risk of heart disease and stroke in later life but the risk is much greater in those who become overweight or obese in adult life.

A poor diet and inadequate physical activity will therefore compound the risk.

Q2: If a mother has high blood cholesterol does this affect her offspring's blood cholesterol as an adult?

A mother's cholesterol level during pregnancy should not influence her offspring's cholesterol level. However, if the mother has high blood cholesterol due to her genetic make-up, then her offspring may inherit this from her.

Q3: If a mother has high blood pressure in pregnancy, does this affect the blood pressure of her offspring later in life?

The offspring of mothers with raised blood pressure in pregnancy have increased blood pressure in later life. However, it is a relatively small increase of about 2 mmHg. Other factors, such as maternal obesity and low birthweight, have a greater effect in raising the blood pressure of offspring in adult life.

Q4: Are bottle-fed babies at greater risk of cardiovascular disease than breast-fed babies?

There is no direct evidence to support this. However, babies that put on large amounts of weight in the first 3 months are more at risk of developing metabolic syndrome (a cluster of factors, such as high blood pressure, high cholesterol and obesity, associated with risk of developing type 2 diabetes and heart disease).

Q5: Why are babies who are small at birth and who become overweight as adults more at risk of cardiovascular disease?

The increased risk of heart disease and stroke in babies who were small at birth and overweight as adults is believed to be influenced by increased risk of high blood pressure and developing an abnormal concentration of lipids (fats) in the blood (known as atherogenic lipoprotein phenotype). This is more likely to happen among children who were small at birth but then gained weight rapidly during early childhood (1–5 years). Poor fetal growth may also affect the development of the kidneys, making the

offspring more sensitive to the blood pressure raising effect of salt.

Q6: What effects does maternal obesity have on the offspring's risk of cardiovascular disease?

Although the evidence is not as clear as it is for a link between poor growth in pregnancy and risk of cardiovascular disease in later life, obese mothers are more likely to have high blood pressure in pregnancy and to give birth to large babies which, particularly in the case of female offspring, puts them at increased risk of cardiovascular disease, especially if they become overweight or obese as adults.

Q7: Children are taller nowadays than previous generations; does this affect their risk of cardiovascular disease?

Shortness in height is associated with a 55% greater risk of cardiovascular disease in later life compared with taller adults. Height is largely determined by growth in the first 2 years of life. Increased adult height is also associated with lower blood pressure in adult life.

18.11 Cancer

Q1: Is birthweight linked to risk of cancer in later life?

Most evidence relates to birthweight and risk of breast cancer, where higher birthweight is associated with an increased risk of breast cancer. Evidence on birthweight and risk of other cancers is less clear. Evidence suggests an increased risk of acute lymphocytic leukaemia with higher birthweights. Studies have been conducted to investigate birthweight and risk of colorectal cancer and prostrate cancer, but the findings are inconclusive. Recent research suggests that very tall individuals are at increased risk of cancer.

Q2: How might nutrition lead to increased risk of cancer?

Early nutrition could influence cancer risk by selecting for embryos with particular genes that predispose to cancer. Suboptimal maternal diets can alter the epigenetic code. The epigenetic code is thought to be an extra layer on top of genes (DNA) that can control which genes are switched on or off. Changes to the epigenetic code do not alter the basic structure of DNA; a gene that has had epigenetic changes will still make the same protein, but these changes may affect when the gene is switched on, and the amount of protein the gene makes. Early nutrition could influence cancer risk in later life by affecting body fatness and hormone exposure.

Q3: Does breastfeeding influence the risk of cancer in later life?

This is a difficult question to answer. Rates of breastfeeding tend to be higher among women of higher social class, who are more likely to eat a good diet and have a healthy lifestyle. Cancer rates tend to be lower among those in higher socioeconomic classes. Therefore, it is difficult to determine whether cancer risk is influenced by breastfeeding, or by other socioeconomic factors common to those who breastfeed. Studies in which people who already have cancer are asked about their breastfeeding history can be flawed by 'recall bias'. The more robust data from prospective cohort studies (where people are asked if they were breast-fed and are followed up over time to see if they develop cancer) shows no significant difference.

18.12 Bone health

Q1: What is the recommended dose of vitamin D supplements for pregnant and breastfeeding women?

Recommended doses of vitamin D during pregnancy and before differ between countries. The current UK guidance is to take 400 IU/day (or 10 micrograms/day). The World Health Organization, the United Nations Food and Agricultural Organisation, and the governments of Australia and New Zealand suggest 200 IU/day (or 5 micrograms/day), which is the same amount these organisations and countries suggest for non-pregnant women aged 19–50 years. In the US and Canada 600 IU/day (or 15 micrograms/day) is recommended, assuming minimal exposure to sunlight. Across Europe, recommendations for women vary between 200 IU/day (or 5 micrograms/day) (for example, in Germany, Austria and Switzerland) to 400 IU/day (or 10 micrograms/day) (for example, in

Belgium). A European project called EURRECA (EURopean micronutrient RECommendations Aligned), which aims to establish requirements and recommendations for micronutrients across Europe, suggests 400 IU/day (or 10 micrograms/day) for pregnant and breastfeeding women.

A possible link has been suggested between high levels of vitamin D in pregnant women and increased asthma in their babies, suggesting we must be careful about advising very high dose supplements, and instead aim to achieve adequate (rather than high) levels of the vitamin. In saying this, studies suggest that humans have evolved to cope with as much as 25 000 IU/day (6250 micrograms/day) of vitamin D formed in the skin. Currently, a large randomised controlled trial is under way in Southampton (MAVIDOS; Maternal Vitamin D Osteoporosis Study) which should help to answer this question.

Q2: Should we screen for vitamin D deficiency in pregnancy and/or infancy?

Before implementing a screening programme, there needs to be good evidence that screening for vitamin D would be beneficial to the mother and child. In cases where there is profound vitamin D deficiency with obvious clinical signs, e.g. low calcium levels (hypocalcaemia), bone pain and muscle weakness, treatment is advised for the immediate health of the mother and child. Clinical signs of vitamin D deficiency are likely to be more common in high-risk groups such as dark-skinned ethnic minorities. At the moment, however, where a low level of vitamin D is found incidentally on a blood test in the absence of clinical symptoms, there are very few existing data to inform the correct course of action.

Q3: What aspects of child nutrition and lifestyle might influence their bone health?

There is good evidence to suggest that calcium and vitamin D are necessary for adequate bone development through childhood and adolescence. Evidence suggests that children with greater calcium intake or vitamin D levels have stronger bones (greater bone mineral density). Evidence indicates that physical activity in infants and children has beneficial effects on bone mass in late childhood. Children who do regular physical activity tend to have stronger bones (more bone mineralisation). However, whether these benefits seen in late childhood translate into long-term benefits or a reduction in fracture risk in later adulthood is not yet clear.

Q4: Is there evidence that breast-fed babies are less likely to suffer from osteoporosis than formula-fed babies?

Studies have suggested that bone development may be influenced by different patterns of infant feeding in the short term. However, in the longer-term there is no difference in bone strength among babies who were breast-fed compared to those who were formula-fed. The comparison between breast and bottle feeding may also depend on the calcium content of the formula milk. All infant formulas available in the UK contain levels of calcium set by the European Directive (between 50 and 140 mg calcium per 100 kcal [419 kJ]) (see Infant Formula and Follow-on Formula (England) Regulations, 2007. www.legislation.gov.uk/uksi/2007/3521/contents/made).

18.13 Allergic diseases and asthma

Q1: Why is there an increasing number of people with asthma and allergic disease?

Since the early 1960s there has been a marked increase in the prevalence of asthma and allergic disease throughout the world, particularly in richer, westernised countries. The rapid increase in asthma and allergic disease in recent decades is almost certainly a consequence of the changing environment and lifestyle and there is increasing evidence that exposure to such factors during fetal development and the first few years of life play a particularly important role in modifying the likelihood of asthma and allergic disease in later life.

Q2: Can maternal diet influence the risk of the offspring having an allergy or asthma?

The mother's diet during pregnancy and the offspring's early life nutrition during infancy and early childhood appear to influence the development of asthma and allergic disease. There is increasing interest in the possibility that the nutrient content of the maternal diet during pregnancy, in particular vitamin E, vitamin D, zinc, selenium and polyunsaturated fat, can influence the development of childhood asthma and allergic disease. However, current evidence relating to the effect of nutrients in the maternal diet on the development of asthma and allergic disease in offspring is limited and speculative.

Q3: Should pregnant women avoid eating peanuts?

In 1998, the UK government advised pregnant and breastfeeding women to avoid potential food allergens such as peanuts, as these were thought to increase the risk of childhood allergic disease. However, in 2009, following a review of available evidence, the government revised its advice. Current evidence does not suggest an adverse or a beneficial effect of maternal peanut consumption during pregnancy and lactation in relation to the development of peanut allergy in children. The new advice states that if mothers would like to eat peanuts or foods containing peanuts during pregnancy or breastfeeding, then they can choose to do so as part of a healthy varied diet, irrespective of whether their child has a family history of allergies, unless advised otherwise by their general practitioner.

Q4: Should the introduction of potential food allergens be delayed during weaning?

The commonest allergies are to cows' milk protein, egg, soya, wheat, nuts and shellfish. There is no convincing evidence that delaying the introduction of these potentially allergenic foods will reduce the likelihood of food allergy and allergic disease. In the UK, the advice from the Department of Health is that whole cows' milk is not appropriate as the main drink for infants less than 1 year of age. However, it can be used in foods prepared for babies over 6 months of age. As a baby's immune system is not yet fully developed, they should not be given wheat (including foods such as bread, pasta and breakfast cereals), eggs, fish and shellfish, and soft and unpasteurised cheese before 6 months of age. However, foods containing wheat, cooked eggs, fish (except shark, marlin and swordfish) and soft rind cheeses made with pasteurised milk are OK from 6 months of age. Peanuts or any other nuts or seeds (or foods containing these) should not be fed to a baby until after 6 months of age.

18.14 Mental health and cognitive behaviour

Q1: What is the difference between mental health and cognitive behaviour?

Mental health relates to our emotional well-being and how we behave. It can, therefore, have a major impact on lifestyle behaviours (including food choices), economic productivity, physical morbidity and ultimately life expectancy. Cognitive behaviour relates to the way someone processes information and becomes aware of, perceives or comprehends ideas. It involves all aspects of perception, thinking, reasoning and remembering. Cognitive skills in childhood are a strong predictor of educational achievement, and childhood cognitive ability tracks into adulthood and directly predicts dementia risk in later life.

Q2: How common are mental health problems?

Evidence shows that the prevalence of mental health problems increased between the 1970s and the 1990s. Nearly one in ten children aged 5–16 years has a clinically diagnosable mental health problem. Most childhood-onset emotional problems persist into adulthood. It is estimated that depressed adolescents are 2–7 times more likely to be depressed in adulthood, with 40–70% showing major depressive disorder during this phase of the life course. Major depressive disorder is characterised by a depressed mood, a lack of interest in activities normally enjoyed, changes in weight and sleep, fatigue, feelings of worthlessness and guilt, difficulty concentrating and thoughts of death and suicide. The World Health Organization has identified major depressive disorder as the leading cause of disease burden in middle- and high-income countries (see Chapter 14, Section 14.1). An estimated one in four people globally will experience a mental health condition in their lifetime.

Q3: What should pregnant women be eating to ensure their offspring receive adequate nutrition for their brain development?

All nutrients influence brain development, although nutrients of particular importance are energy, protein, long-chain fatty acids, iron, zinc, copper, iodine, selenium, vitamin A, choline and folate. Rec-ommendations from the European Commission state that pregnant and lactating mothers should consume the fatty acid equivalent of two portions of oil-rich fish per week, although the strength of the evidence is still being debated. One effect of this intake is to prolong pregnancy duration, with a beneficial effect on fetal development. During the third trimester the fetus grows rapidly and the brain has a high demand for DHA (a long-chain omega-3 fatty acid found in oil-rich fish).

Q4: Does being breast-fed improve cognitive function in childhood?

There is good evidence from studies that indicate breastfeeding benefits the baby's cognitive development. Some studies have also suggested breastfeeding benefits the baby's emotional and behavioural development. It is thought that the essential fatty acids found in breast milk are mainly responsible for these benefits. However, a wide range of factors may influence the findings of studies. For example, the benefits observed in some studies may be due to non-nutritional factors such as the mother's socioeconomic status, maternal smoking history, maternal cognitive ability, maternal and paternal education, and family size.

Q5: Does the infant's diet influence mental health in later life?

The effect of the infant's diet on mental development is not well understood. However, evidence suggests that infants aged 6–12 months who are fed a diet high in fruit and vegetables and home-prepared foods are more likely to have a higher IQ. Micronutrients in the infant diet that are thought to be of importance to mental health in later life include the essential fatty acids, iron, zinc, iodine, folate and selenium.

18.15 Dietary and lifestyle advice for early life

Q1: What advice can be followed before becoming pregnant to enhance the health of offspring?

It is important for women to have adequate nutritional stores themselves before becoming pregnant.

This is best achieved by eating a healthy, varied diet. Women of childbearing age should take a daily supplement of 400 micrograms of folic acid. It is also important for women to do regular physical activity as this helps to maintain appropriate body weight. Ideally women should avoid alcohol while trying to conceive but, if drinking, limit consumption to one or two units of alcohol once or twice a week. Most importantly, women should try to be a healthy weight before becoming pregnant.

Q2: What nutrients do pregnant women often have low intakes of?

Low vitamin D status is common in pregnancy. In the UK, pregnant and lactating women are advised to take daily vitamin D supplements containing 10 micrograms (or 400 IU/day). However, awareness of the need for supplements and uptake of the advice by women remains low. This is particularly relevant for women at high risk of low vitamin D status, such as women with darker skin and women who are housebound or who conceal most of their skin. The main dietary sources of vitamin D are oil-rich fish, eggs, meat, fortified cereals and margarine. However, these dietary sources usually only provide 2–3 micrograms in total, and are therefore relatively insignificant compared with the vitamin D synthesised from exposure to sunlight. It is therefore important for pregnant women, especially women with darker skin who are likely to be at more risk of low vitamin D status, to get outside and expose their skin to sunlight on a regular basis, taking care not to burn in the summer months.

Many pregnant women, and women trying for a baby, are aware of the message that increasing folic acid intake in the early stages of pregnancy and before pregnancy is recommended in order to prevent neural tube defects. However, in the UK, a large proportion of pregnancies are unplanned and less than half of women take any folic acid supplements before becoming pregnant. Evidence suggests the use of folic acid supplements in the early stages of pregnancy is particularly low among West Indian and Asian mothers, and teenage mothers in the UK. Women should continue to take a 400 microgram folic acid supplement daily for the first 12 weeks of pregnancy and eat folate-rich foods on a daily basis such as green leafy vegetables, brown rice, peas, oranges, bananas and fortified breakfast cereals.

Adequate omega-3 fatty acids are needed by the baby during pregnancy for healthy development of the brain and nerves. In particular the long-chain omega-3 fatty acids eicosapentaenoic acid (EPA) and docosahexaenoic (DHA) are important to include in the diet of pregnant women. Oil-rich fish, such as herring, mackerel and salmon, are the main dietary source of EPA and DHA. Eggs can also make a significant contribution to intake of DHA. In the UK, 450 mg a day of DHA and EPA is recommended for adults and pregnant women. This can be obtained by eating two servings of fish a week, one of which is oil-rich. Consumption of oil-rich fish should be limited to two portions per week (a portion is around 140 g when cooked) for girls and women of childbearing age. This is because oil-rich fish may contain low levels of pollutants that can build up in the body. Oil-rich fish include anchovies, carp, herring (e.g. kippers), mackerel, pilchards, salmon, sardines, sprats, trout and whitebait.

In the UK, it is thought that the body of pregnant (and lactating) women can adapt to ensure the baby receives an adequate supply of iron, even when the mother is iron deficient. For this reason, extra iron for all pregnant women is not considered necessary. However, pregnant women may develop low iron status, so plenty of iron-rich foods should be eaten and foods containing non-haem iron should be consumed alongside foods or drinks containing vitamin C, such as fruit or vegetables, or a glass of fruit juice, to aid iron absorption. The effect of tea and coffee on iron bioavailability is no longer considered to be of major concern, especially if advice from the Department of Health to limit caffeine intake to 200 mg a day (equivalent to two mugs of coffee/day) while pregnant is followed.

Q3: Is there any specific nutritional advice for particular groups of the population?

Dark-skinned ethnic minorities or women who conceal most of their skin from sunlight exposure are at particular risk of low vitamin D status and, in the UK, all Asian women and children are advised to take supplementary vitamin D. Exclusively breast-fed babies may also be at increased risk of vitamin D deficiency if the mother has low levels. Fewer women from low-income groups take folic acid supplements. Mothers from low-income households are nutritionally vulnerable and may go short of food in order to feed their children. Also, the duration of breastfeeding is shorter among low-income groups. Support and advice from health professionals to women from low-income groups is important in order to lessen inequalities in health. The diets of adolescent girls in the UK are often low in nutrients, in particular folate, iron and vitamin D. This has implications for pregnant adolescents as they may still be growing themselves. Obese women who become pregnant have an increased risk of complications and long-term health implications for their offspring (e.g. increased risk of obesity and diabetes in offspring in later life). Women who weigh over 100 kg (approx. 15 stone 10 lb) may require specific advice from a health professional.

Q4: Should pregnant women 'eat for two'?

No, pregnant women do not need to 'eat for two'. In fact, women do not need any extra energy during the first 6 months of pregnancy. However, during the last trimester (and during lactation) some extra energy is required. An additional 200 calories per day is required during the last trimester of pregnancy. This equates to a small ham and cheese sandwich, or a banana smoothie, or a medium bowl of porridge with milk, or 30 g of mixed nuts.

Q5: How much physical activity should pregnant women do?

Current recommendations suggest women should aim for at least 150 minutes (2½ hours) of moderate intensity activity per week. One way to approach this is to do 30 minutes of physical activity on at least five days a week. Currently, only around 3 in 10 women of childbearing age meet these recommendations. Women should try to keep active during pregnancy, as well as during milk feeding and weaning. Physical activity helps maintain an appropriate body weight and enhances fitness. It also has many benefits during pregnancy such as reducing muscle cramps and swelling of the legs and feet. Women who have not been habitually active should start by doing 15 minutes of continuous aerobic physical activity, three times a week, and gradually increase this to 30-minute sessions four times a week or more. Contact sports are not advised and hormonal changes cause joints to be more mobile, increasing the risk of injury with weightbearing physical activity. However, there are many activities that are suitable during pregnancy, for example, swimming, walking, jogging and taking part in exercise classes. After 16 weeks of pregnancy, physical activities that involve lying on the back are not recommended as the womb is likely to put pressure on major blood vessels. It is also important to keep well hydrated and avoid hot humid conditions when exercising. Women who have any complications or problems that may impact on their ability to be active should seek advice from their GP or midwife.

Q6: Which nutrients are important for women who are breastfeeding?

During the first 6 months of lactation, women require an additional 330 calories per day, if they are exclusively breastfeeding. This is slightly more than the 200 additional calories women need during the last trimester of pregnancy. Breastfeeding women need even more nutrients than when pregnant. When breastfeeding, women require an increased intake of vitamin A, vitamin D, vitamin B_2, vitamin B_{12}, calcium, magnesium and zinc. Adequate levels of these nutrients can be achieved by eating a healthy, varied diet, with the exception of vitamin D. Breastfeeding women should continue to take a daily supplement of 10 micrograms of vitamin D. Folate is one nutrient often found to be low in diets of lactating women. Evidence suggests that the level of folate in breast milk is maintained at the expense of a mother's folate stores. When women do not take a folic acid supplement during pregnancy, their own folate level is likely to be low when breastfeeding.

Q7: How much fluid do pregnant and lactating women need?

'Fluid' includes not only water from the tap or in a bottle, but also other drinks that contain water such as tea, coffee, milk, fruit juices and soft drinks. Pregnant women are advised to consume no more than 200 mg of caffeine a day. This is equivalent to about two mugs of instant coffee or about two and a half mugs of tea. Foods can also provide water – on average food provides about 20% of total fluid intake. The amount of fluid required by adults depends on many things including physical activity levels and the weather, but in general adults should drink about 1.2 litres (6–8 glasses) of fluid per day (on top of the water provided in food). Women need slightly more fluid when pregnant, and significantly more when breast feeding. The estimated additional requirement is 0.3 litres per day (about 2 glasses) during pregnancy and between 0.7 and 1.1 litres per day (about 6 glasses) during lactation.

Q8: When is the best time to wean babies on to solid foods?

The UK's Departments of Health currently recommends that weaning should start at around 6 months. Breastfeeding (and/or breast milk substitutes, if used) should continue beyond the first 6 months, along with appropriate types and amounts of solid foods. Despite this recommendation, virtually all mothers (more than 99%) in the UK report introducing other foods before 6 months, often because they consider their babies to be hungry and not satisfied on breast milk alone. There is a need for clearer advice to mothers and health professionals on weaning. However, this is difficult to provide as there is a lack of up-to-date information about the diets and nutrient intakes of infants. There is also a lack of official guidance from the Department of Health on what appropriate portion sizes are, how long the weaning process should take and when foods with different textures should be offered. The government's advisory body, the Scientific Advisory Committee on Nutrition, is currently reviewing the evidence on complementary and young child feeding, which should help inform future policy and government advice, including the best time to wean.

Q9: What nutrients are most important to include in the weaning and infant diet?

A baby's diet should be varied and balanced as this will help him or her grow up into a healthy child and adult by providing adequate amounts of all of the nutrients an infant needs. Long-chain fatty acids should be included in the weaning diet as these are important for brain development. Rapid brain development occurs during the last trimester of pregnancy and the first year after birth. Oil-rich fish are a great source of long-chain fatty acids. Boys can have up to four portions of oily fish (such as mackerel, salmon and sardines) a week, but girls should have no more than two portions a week. This is because oil-rich fish

may contain low levels of pollutants that can build up in the body and may affect the development of the girl child's future potential offspring already present as eggs in her reproductive system. Vitamin D is also found in oil-rich fish. However, we obtain most of our vitamin D from the action of sunlight on the skin, so playing outdoors should be encouraged. The Department of Health also recommends vitamin drops for infants from 1 month to 5 years of age. In the UK, the 'Healthy Start' vouchers and vitamin supplements are available to pregnant women under 18 years and those on low income (www.healthystart.nhs.uk). The Healthy Start children's vitamin drops contain vitamin A, vitamin C and vitamin D. Children having more than 500 mL (one pint) per day of infant formula do not need to take these vitamins until they are weaned off formula milk.

Other nutrients such as iron and zinc are important for an infant's development. A lack of iron can delay the child's physical and mental development. The iron found in meat and fish is absorbed more easily by the body, compared to the iron found in plant foods. Infants who do not eat meat or fish should be given other sources of iron on a frequent basis (e.g. dark green vegetables, bread, beans, lentils and dhal, and dried fruit such as apricots, figs and prunes). Zinc is important for making new cells and enzymes, healing wounds and helping the body to process carbohydrate, fat and protein in food. Infants are at increased risk of having low iron and zinc intakes if there is a delay in weaning onto foods such as meat.

Q10: How much physical activity should infants and young children do?

Physical activity should be encouraged from birth, particularly through floor-based play and water-based activities in a safe environment. Being active will help the infant develop motor skills, improve cognitive development, support a healthy weight, enhance bone and muscle development and support learning of social skills. Children of pre-school age who are capable of walking unaided should be physically active daily for at least 180 minutes (3 hours) spread throughout the day. For all under-5s, the amount of sedentary time (being restrained or sitting) for extended periods should be minimised, with the exception of time spent sleeping.

18.16 Policies relating to early life nutrition and development

Q1: Are current policies adequately addressing the increasing levels of obesity in pregnancy?

Obese pregnant women are at an increased risk of suffering from complications related to their pregnancy (e.g. stillbirth, maternal and infant mortality and congenital anomalies) and they are more likely to need a caesarean section. The prevalence of gestational diabetes is higher among obese women, which has long-term health implications due to an increased risk among women and their children for developing type 2 diabetes. There is also a lower breastfeeding rate among obese women compared with women with a healthy weight. Policy makers need to place greater focus on interventions and messages to control pre-pregnancy weight, or if approached sensitively, extra support and advice to encourage healthy behaviour changes during and after pregnancy. However, there is currently a lack of officially accepted guidance in the UK for weight gain during pregnancy. To improve the situation, there is a need for a clear policy on weight control and avoidance of obesity in pregnancy, including the need for better services for women before they become pregnant and support for women in achieving and maintaining a healthy body weight after pregnancy.

Q2: Are current policies relating to breastfeeding and bottle feeding adequate?

Breastfeeding has a major role in promoting health in both the short and long term for both the baby and the mother. Therefore, policies that promote breastfeeding should come high up on the public health agenda. This is particularly important among groups where breastfeeding rates are often low (e.g. women from low-income groups, obese mothers and teenage mothers). Activities that raise awareness of the health benefits of breastfeeding, increase its social acceptance and promote support for breastfeeding mothers are essential and should continue. While all health professionals should continue to promote and support breastfeeding, infant formula is an important source of nutrition for many infants. Mothers who cannot breastfeed or who choose to formula feed need education and support in using it appropriately and safely. It is important that health professionals have good, up-to-date knowledge of the different formulas available and are able to provide advice and support to mothers about safely preparing and storing formula.

Glossary

Adaptive programming: See Barker hypothesis.

Adipokine: A type of cytokine produced by adipocytes such as leptin and adiponectin.

Allele: Alternative forms of a gene. A single allele is inherited separately from each parent.

Alpha-linolenic acid (ALA): An *n*-3 polyunsaturated fatty acid (C18:3), the main dietary sources of which include walnuts, rapeseed, soya and blended vegetable oils. Some is also found in green leafy vegetables.

Apoptosis: Programmed cell death ('suicide').

Areal bone mineral density (aBMD): The amount of bone mineral (g) per square centimetre on the projected image derived from a DXA instrument. This measure is used clinically to assess bone density and determine fracture risk for osteoporosis (*cf.* Volumetric bone mineral density).

Atherogenic lipoprotein phenotype (ALP): A form of dyslipidaemia that is characterised by raised fasting triacylglycerol concentrations (>1.7 mmol/L), low HDL-cholesterol concentrations (<1.29 mmol/L in women and <1.03 mmol/L in men) and a predominance of small, dense LDL-cholesterol particles.

Atherosclerosis: A nodular thickening and hardening of large and medium arteries accompanied by the deposition of lipids.

Atopy: Predisposition to immunoglobulin (Ig)E production associated with allergy to several common allergens.

Autocrine: Pertaining to cell messengers that act at, or near, the site where they are produced (*cf.* Endocrine).

Autoimmune diseases: A group of diseases, such as rheumatoid arthritis and systemic lupus erythematosus, in which immune cells turn on the body, attacking various tissues and organs.

Bariatric surgery: Surgery used to promote weight loss.

Barker hypothesis: The hypothesis put forward by Professor David Barker that adverse influences early in development, particularly during intrauterine life, can result in lower birthweight and permanent changes in physiology and metabolism, which result in increased disease risk in adulthood. Also known as fetal programming, and later developed into further hypotheses which are now collectively known as developmental origins of health and disease.

Blood pressure: A measure of the force that the circulating blood exerts on the walls of the main arteries. The pressure wave transmitted along the arteries with each heartbeat is felt as the pulse; the highest (systolic) pressure is created by the heart contracting and the lowest (diastolic) pressure is measured as the heart fills.

Body mass index (BMI): An index used to assess the degree of overweight or obesity; calculated using the equation: weight (kg) divided by height squared (m^2).

Nutrition and Development: Short- and Long-Term Consequences for Health, First Edition. Edited by the British Nutrition Foundation.
© 2013 the British Nutrition Foundation. Published 2013 by Blackwell Publishing Ltd.

Bone mineral content (BMC): The amount of bone mineral within the defined region of interest.

Carcinoma: Malignant cancer that arises from epithelial cells.

Carcinoma in situ: An early cancer that has not broken through the basement membrane of the tissue in which it is growing.

Carnegie stages: In embryology, Carnegie stages are a standardised system of 23 stages used to provide a unified developmental chronology of the vertebrate embryo.

Carunclectomy: The excision of all visible uterine epithelium caruncles (dark spots *in utero*) that will determine the number of cotyledons that will generate the placental mass.

Catch-up growth: Rapid growth following a period of restriction. Ultimately it may redress wholly or partly the accrued deficit in weight or size, though there may be consequences for body composition and metabolic capacity.

Cell proliferation: Reproduction or multiplication of cells.

Centile: Any of the 99 numbered points that divide an ordered set of scores into 100 parts, each of which contains one-hundredth of the total.

Cholesterol ester transfer protein: A protein circulating in blood associated with high-density lipoprotein (HDL) that can catalyse the exchange of triacylglycerol from triacylglycerol-rich lipoproteins to low-density (LDL) and high-density lipoproteins (HDL) in exchange for cholesterol esters.

Choline: A basic constituent of lecithin that is found in many plants and animal organs. It is important as a precursor of acetylcholine, as a methyl donor in various metabolic processes and in lipid metabolism.

Chromosomes: The physically organised form of DNA in a cell nucleus. Chromosomes consist of a double helix of DNA together with associated proteins, such as histone proteins, and other molecules, all of which are responsible for maintaining the chromosome architecture.

Cochrane Review: Systematic reviews of primary research in human health care and health policy.

Coeliac disease: An auto-immune disease, which means that the body's immune system attacks itself. When people with this condition eat gluten, it results in damage to the lining of the small intestine, which stops the intestine properly absorbing nutrients. The symptoms of coeliac disease can range from very mild to severe; for example, diarrhoea and/or constipation, recurrent stomach pain, hair loss, osteoporosis and infertility.

Confounding: A term used in epidemiology to describe factors that travel together that may not be causally related to the disease outcome.

Cognitive function: An intellectual process by which one processes information and becomes aware of, perceives, or comprehends ideas. It involves all aspects of perception, thinking, reasoning and remembering.

Coronary heart disease (CHD): Atherosclerotic disease of the coronary arteries that supply the heart muscle. Also known as ischaemic heart disease or coronary artery disease.

Critical windows of development: Periods during the development of an organ when it is most susceptible to damage.

Cytokines: Small, hormone-like proteins released by leucocytes, endothelial cells and other cells to promote an inflammatory immune response to an injury. Interleukins, interferons and some growth factors are examples of cytokines.

De-methylation: The removal of the methyl group (CH_3) from a compound (*cf.* Methylation and Re-methylation), usually deoxycytosine in DNA.

Dislipidaemia: An abnormal concentration of lipids or lipoproteins in the blood.

Docosahexaenoic acid (DHA): A long-chain *n*-3 (omega-3) fatty acid that is abundant in oil-rich fish (see also Eicosapentaenoic acid). Epidemiological and clinical trial data suggest that these *n*-3 fatty acids may reduce the risk of cardiovascular disease. Possible mechanisms include anti-arrhythmic properties, improved endothelial function, anti-inflammatory action and reductions in blood triacylglycerol concentrations (*cf.* Eicosapentaenoic acid).

Dutch Hunger Winter: The Dutch famine of 1944, which took place in the German-occupied part of the Netherlands, during the winter of 1944–1945, towards the end of the Second World War.

DXA: Dual-energy X-ray absorptiometry. The gold standard clinically used assessment of bone mineral density.

Eicosapentaenoic acid (EPA): A long-chain *n*-3 (omega-3) fatty acid that is abundant in oil-rich fish (*cf.* Docosahexaenoic acid).

Endocrine: Pertaining to hormones and the glands that make and secrete them into the bloodstream, through which they travel to affect distant organs.

Epigenetic: Cellular mechanisms that confer stability of gene expression during development. Epigenetic marking imprints gene expression in somatic tissues and these marks subsequently take form as differential DNA methylation. In general terms, an epigenetic factor is something that changes the phenotype without changing the genotype.

Fetal alcohol spectrum disorders: Describes the range of effects that can occur in an individual whose mother had a high alcohol intake during pregnancy. These effects may include physical, mental, behavioural and/or learning disabilities with possible lifelong implications.

Fetal growth restriction: A fetal weight that is below the 10th percentile for gestational age.

Fetal programming: See Barker hypothesis.

Galactosaemia: A condition in which the body is unable to use (metabolise) the simple sugar, galactose.

Gastrointestinal (GI): Pertaining to the organs of the GI tract, from mouth to anus.

Gatekeeper hypothesis: The suggestion that there are a limited number of genes or gene pathways that are altered by a nutritional insult and that these genes or gene pathways are common to different insults.

Genome: The genetic makeup of a cell, composed of DNA.

Genotype: The genetic makeup of an organism as distinguished from its physical characteristics.

Gestational diabetes: The condition in which glucose intolerance is acquired during pregnancy.

Glial cells: Cells found throughout the nervous system.

Glucocorticoid: A hormone that predominantly affects the metabolism of carbohydrates and, to a lesser extent, fats and proteins (and has other effects). Cortisol is the major natural glucocorticoid in humans.

Glucose tolerance test: A test of the body's ability to metabolise carbohydrate, in which a standard dose of glucose is administered under controlled conditions and the blood and urine are tested for glucose at regular intervals thereafter. The glucose tolerance test is usually used to assist in the diagnosis of diabetes.

Haematopoiesis: The normal formation and development of blood and other tissues in the developing fetus.

Hepatic lipase: An enzyme present in the hepatic sinusoids that can hydrolyse triacylglycerols carried by LDL- and HDL-cholesterol.

High-density lipoproteins (HDL): These are the most dense class of lipoproteins with a density range between 1.063 and 1.21 g/mL. Low levels of HDL-cholesterol are associated with an increased risk of atherosclerosis and coronary heart disease (*cf.* LDL and VLDL).

Hodgkin's lymphoma: Lymphoma is a cancer of the lymphatic system. In Hodgkin's lymphoma, cells in the lymph nodes become cancerous.

Hormone-sensitive lipase: An enzyme located in adipose tissue that hydrolyses triacylglycerols. Its activity is inhibited by insulin and stimulated by noradrenaline.

Hyperglycaemia: A greater than normal concentration of glucose in the blood, most frequently associated with diabetes mellitus.

Hyperinsulinaemia: High blood insulin levels.

Hypertension: Raised blood pressure. A systolic/diastolic blood pressure measured in clinic of 140/90 mmHg or above indicates hypertension.

Hypothalamic–pituitary–adrenal (HPA) axis: The combined system of neuroendocrine units that regulate the adrenal gland's hormonal activities via a negative feedback network.

Immunoglobulin: Any of several types of globulin proteins that function as antibodies.

Impaired glucose tolerance (IGT): A pre-diabetic state of dysglycaemia that is associated with insulin resistance and increased risk of cardiovascular disease. The World Health Organization describes IGT as a fasting blood glucose of less than 7 mmol/L and a blood glucose of 7.8 mmol/L or more but less than 11.1 mmol/L after a 2-hour oral glucose tolerance test.

Insulin: A hormone secreted by the pancreas in response to food intake. It circulates in the blood and assists in the movement of glucose into cells where it is used as a source of energy.

Insulin-like growth factor (IGF): A hormone that promotes growth, whose chemical structure is similar to insulin. While insulin primarily affects the body's metabolic system (energy delivery and use), IGF helps regulate cell growth.

Insulin resistance: A condition in which the body's cells are less responsive (or sensitive) to the action of insulin. This causes more insulin to be released by the pancreas, resulting in an excess amount of insulin circulating in the blood. The metabolic abnormality underlies type 2 diabetes.

Interleukin: One of a large group of proteins produced mainly by T-cells and in some cases by mononuclear phagocytes or other cells. Interleukins participate in communication among leucocytes and are important in the inflammatory response.

Intrauterine: Situated or occurring in the uterus.

Iron-deficient anaemia (IDA): Anaemia due to an inadequate supply of iron for blood cell production. This type of anaemia responds to iron therapy.

Intrauterine growth restriction (IUGR): The faltering of growth *in utero*.

Kisspeptin: A protein involved in the kisspeptin system which translates metabolic signals into hormonal effects within the brain.

Large for gestational age (LGA): LGA babies are above the 90th centile for weight at birth.

Low-density lipoproteins (LDL): A class of lipoproteins with a density of 1.019 to 1.063 g/L. The main protein they carry is apoprotein B100, which is a ligand for the LDL-cholesterol receptor. High levels of LDL-cholesterol cause atherosclerosis and coronary heart disease (*cf.* VLDL and HDL).

Leptin: A hormone produced by the *ob* (obese) gene and secreted by fat tissue that acts on the brain to regulate appetite and has a central role in fat metabolism.

Leukaemia: Cancer of the white blood cells.

Lipolysis: The hydrolysis of triacylglycerols by enzymes called lipases to release fatty acids.

Lipoprotein lipase: An enzyme located on endothelial cells that hydrolyses triacylglycerols carried by lipoproteins. Its activity is enhanced by insulin.

Macrosomia: A term used to describe infants who are large at birth. The cut-off used is typically greater than 4 kg. Macrosomia is usually a result of poorly controlled gestational diabetes.

Major depressive disorder (MDD): A mood disorder characterised by the occurrence of one or more major depressive episodes and the absence of any history of manic, mixed or hypomanic episodes.

Maple syrup urine disease: An inherited metabolic disorder in which an enzyme necessary for the breakdown of the branched chain amino acids valine, leucine and isoleucine is lacking. The disease is usually diagnosed in infancy. It is recog-

nised by the characteristic maple syrup odour of the urine and by hyperreflexia (an exaggeration of reflexes). Stress, fever and infection aggravate the condition. Treatment includes a diet avoiding these amino acids and occasionally dialysis to remove excess protein.

Mast cell: A large cell in connective tissue consisting of granules that release histamine and heparin during allergic reactions.

Mastitis: Inflammation of the breast.

Maternal glycaemia: A measure of the level of glucose in blood during pregnancy. There is evidence that there is a direct relationship between maternal blood glucose levels during pregnancy and fetal growth and size at birth (even when maternal blood glucose levels are within their normal range).

Metabolic syndrome: A cluster of factors associated with risk of developing type 2 diabetes and coronary heart disease. It is defined on the basis of central obesity determined by a waist measurement (≥ 94 cm for Europid men and ≥ 80 cm for Europid women, with ethnicity-specific values for other groups) plus two of the following four factors: raised blood pressure (BP) (systolic BP ≥ 130 or diastolic BP ≥ 85 mmHg); raised fasting plasma glucose > 5.6 mmol/L; raised TAG > 1.7 mmol/L or reduced HDL-cholesterol < 1.03 mmol/L in men and < 1.29 mmol/L in women.

Methylation: The introduction of a methyl group (CH_3) to a compound (*cf.* De-methylation and Re-methylation).

Microbiota: The microorganisms that typically inhabit a bodily organ or part; flora.

Myocardial infarction: More commonly known as a heart attack, the term describes death of heart muscle tissue as a result of being starved of oxygenated blood.

Neonatal: During the first 28 days after birth.

Neural tube defect: Birth defects that occur when the neural tube does not form correctly. Neural tube defects usually occur during the first month of pregnancy, before many women know that they are pregnant.

Neuroblastoma: A cancer that develops from nerve cells called neuroblasts. It affects around 100 children each year in the United Kingdom.

Non-esterified fatty acids (NEFA): Fatty acids released from the hydrolysis of triacylglycerols and derived mainly from adipose tissue. They circulate in the blood, bound to the protein albumin. They are taken up by muscle and liver and can be used as fuel to release energy by beta-oxidation. In the liver they can also be re-esterified into triacylglycerols.

Nucleotide: A building block of DNA or RNA. It includes one base, one phosphate molecule and one sugar molecule (deoxyribose in DNA, ribose in RNA).

***ob/ob* mice:** Mice with mutations on both *ob* genes (*ob/ob* mice) cannot produce leptin so they are unaware of when they have sufficient amounts of fat stored. As a result, these mice overeat and become obese.

Observational studies: A study in which the investigators observe and measure but do not seek to intervene.

Odds ratio (OR): The ratio of the odds of an event occurring in one group to the odds of it occurring in another group.

Oligosaccharides: A carbohydrate molecule composed of between 3 and 20 monosaccharides (simple sugars).

Oncogene: A modified gene, or a set of nucleotides that codes for a protein and is believed to cause cancer.

Osteoporosis: A metabolic bone disease which has two predominant characteristics: low bone mass and micro-architectural deterioration of bone tissue. Both factors lead to enhanced bone fragility and a consequent increase in fracture risk.

Parathyroid hormone (PTH): Hormone secreted by the parathyroid glands to increase the concentration of calcium in the blood.

Paraventricular nuclei: The paraventricular nucleus of the hypothalamus (PVN or PVH) is a neuronal nucleus in the hypothalamus. It contains multiple subpopulations of neurons that are activated by a variety of stressful and/or physiological changes. Many PVN neurons extend directly to the posterior pituitary where they release oxytocin or vasopressin into the general circulation. Other PVN neurons control various anterior pituitary functions, while still others directly regulate appetite and autonomic functions in the brainstem and spinal cord.

Periconceptional: Relating to the period from before conception to early pregnancy.

Perinatal: Relating to the period shortly before and after birth; from the 20th to 29th week of gestation to one to four weeks after birth.

Phenotype: The physical characteristics of an individual that result from the combination of genetic and environmental factors. By contrast, the genotype is solely the genetic constitution (genome) of an individual (*cf.* Genotype).

Phenylketonuria (PKU): A rare genetic condition that is present from birth (congenital). In PKU, the body is unable to break down a chemical called phenylalanine, which then builds up in the blood and in the brain.

Placenta: The organ that allows interchange between the fetus and the mother. Blood from the fetus and the mother do not directly mix, but the placental cell layer allows the fetus to absorb nutrients and oxygen from the mother. Waste products from the fetus can exit through the placenta.

Polycystic ovarian syndrome (PCOS): A hormonal problem of women that causes irregular or no menstrual periods, acne, obesity and excess hair growth. PCOS is a disorder of chronically abnormal ovarian function and hyperandrogenism (abnormally elevated androgen levels).

Ponderal index: An index of fatness, often used as a measure of obesity; the body weight in kilograms divided by the height or length in metres cubed (kg/m^3).

Prebiotics: Nondigestible food components that support overall health by promoting the activity of beneficial bacteria in the large intestine.

Pre-eclampsia: A condition that can occur in pregnant women when there is a problem with the placenta (the organ that links the baby's blood supply to the mother's). As a result, the mother can develop high blood pressure, protein in her urine and fluid retention. In the unborn baby, pre-eclampsia can cause intrauterine growth retardation.

Primordium: The first recognisable stage in the embryonic development and differentiation of a particular organ, tissue, or structure.

Principal component analysis (PCA): A mathematical tool used to derive a small number of linear combinations (principal components) of a set of variables that retain as much of the information in the original variables as possible. This technique is often used when there are large numbers of variables, to reduce to a smaller number of variable combinations by combining similar variables (ones that contain much the same information).

Prolactin: A hormone that helps the breast prepare for milk production during pregnancy.

Proliferation: The reproduction or multiplication of similar forms, especially of cells.

Peripheral quantitative computed tomography (pQCT): A radiation-based imaging modality which allows measurement of true volumetric bone density.

Randomised controlled trial (RCT): In a randomised controlled trial, participants are assigned by chance to receive either an experimental or control treatment. Both groups are followed up for a specified time and the effects of the intervention on a specific outcome (e.g. serum cholesterol level, death rates) are analysed. The idea behind the RCT is that, when it is done properly, the effect of a treatment can be studied in groups of people who are the same at the outset and treated the same way except for the intervention being studied. Any differences then seen in the groups at the end can be attributed to the difference in treatment alone, and not to bias or chance.

Relative risk: An estimate of risk usually derived from comparing the risk in the least exposed group with the most exposed group. However, sometimes comparisons are made with the middle group.

Re-methylation: Methylation that occurs following de-methylation (*cf.* Methylation and De-methylation).

Renin–angiotensin system: A hormone system that regulates sodium balance, fluid volume and blood pressure. In response to reduced kidney perfusion, renin is secreted, which hydrolyses a plasma globulin to release angiotensin I, which is rapidly hydrolysed to angiotensin II, a powerful vasoconstrictor. Angiotension II also stimulates aldosterone secretion, which causes sodium retention, an increase in blood pressure and restoration of renal perfusion, which shuts off the signal for renin release (negative feedback).

Ribonucleic acid (RNA): A nucleic acid, found in both the nucleus and cytoplasm of cells, that plays several roles in the translation of the genetic code and the assembly of proteins. Kinds of RNA include messenger RNA, ribosomal RNA and transfer RNA.

Secular: In the context of epidemiology, changes that occur over time that have no clear causation.

Small for gestational age (SGA): A term used to describe newborns who are below the 10th percentile in height or weight for their estimated gestational age. The gestational age is based upon the date of the mother's last menstrual period.

Stem cells: Parent cells from which other cells are made.

Striatum: Part of the basal ganglia of the brain. The basal ganglia are interconnected masses of grey matter located in the interior regions of the cerebral hemispheres and in the upper part of the brainstem.

Stroke: Rapidly developing clinical signs of focal (at times global) disturbance of cerebral function, lasting more than 24 hours or leading to death, with no apparent cause other than that of vascular origin.

Surrogate risk markers: Factors that are associated with the development of a disease, e.g. blood pressure and serum cholesterol concentrations are surrogate risk markers for coronary heart disease.

T-score: Used in the reporting of bone mineral density derived from DXA scanning, this refers to the number of standard deviations that the individual is away from the sex-matched young healthy adult mean.

Telomeres: Specialised repeated DNA sequences on the ends of chromosomes that protect the chromosomes from degradation.

Teratogenic: Of, relating to, or causing malformations of an embryo or a fetus.

Testosterone: Male hormone produced by the testes and (in small amounts) in the ovaries. Testosterone is responsible for some masculine secondary sex characteristics such as growth of body hair and deepening voice.

Thrifty phenotype hypothesis: See Barker hypothesis, Fetal programming and Adaptive programming.

Thymic: Pertaining to the thymus gland. The thymus gland is a ductless glandular organ at the base of the neck that produces lymphocytes and aids immunity.

Thyroid axis: This is short for the hypothalamic–pituitary–thyroid axis, which is part of the endocrine system responsible for the regulation of metabolism. As its name suggests, it depends upon the hypothalamus, the pituitary gland and the thyroid gland.

Thyroid hormone: A hormone, especially tri-iodothyronine (T3) or thyroxine (T4), produced by the thyroid gland.

Tissue stem cells: Stem cells found in some adult (and fetal) tissue, used to replenish cells in the body, replacing those which naturally wear out. Tissue stem cells have also sometimes been referred to as adult stem cells (*cf.* Stem cells).

Triacylglycerols (TAG): Also referred to as triglycerides. These are stored in adipose tissue and can be obtained from the diet or made in the liver. In the fasting state, the plasma concentration of TAG reflects TAG made in the liver.

Trophic factor: A factor pertaining to a nutritive effect on, or quality of, cellular activity.

Type 1 diabetes: Also known as insulin-dependent diabetes mellitus, this is a disease in which an autoimmune process in the pancreas leads to destruction of the insulin-producing islet cells, producing a form of diabetes characterised by insulin deficiency.

Type 2 diabetes: Previously known as adult-onset diabetes mellitus and non-insulin-dependent diabetes mellitus. This is a disease in which there is both a failure of the body to respond normally to insulin (insulin resistance) and the body does not make enough insulin or is unable to make proper use of it, causing glucose concentrations in the bloodstream to increase.

Vagal nerve: A cranial nerve, i.e. a nerve connected to the brain. The vagus nerve has branches to most of the major organs in the body, including the larynx, throat, windpipe, lungs, heart and most of the digestive system.

Very-low-density lipoprotein (VLDL): A class of lipoprotein with a density of less than 1.006 g/mL. It is secreted from the liver and used to transport triacylglycerols from the liver to other tissues. VLDL particles are eventually converted to low-density lipoproteins (*cf.* LDL and HDL).

Visceral obesity: Excess of body fat around the internal organs of the body, specifically those within the abdomen (e.g. liver or intestines).

Vitamin D receptor (VDR): A structure on the surface of cells that binds the active form of vitamin D 1,25(OH)$_2$D. VDRs receptors are found on cells ubiquitously throughout the body in various tissues.

Volumetric bone mineral density (vBMD): The amount of bone mineral (g) per cubic centimetre of tissue. This cannot be directly measured by DXA and requires a modality such as pQCT (*cf.* Areal bone mineral density).

Weaning: The process of expanding the diet to include foods and drinks other than breast milk or infant formula.

Weanling's dilemma: The choice between the known protective effect of exclusive breastfeeding against infectious morbidity and the (theoretical) insufficiency of breast milk alone to satisfy the infant's energy and micronutrient requirements beyond the age of 4 months.

Z-score: Defined as the difference between an observed value for an individual and the median value of the reference population, divided by the standard deviation value of the reference population. Z-scores are used for height, weight and head circumference. In the reporting of bone mineral density, the term Z-score is used to describe the number of standard deviations an individual is away from the age- and sex-matched healthy mean.

References

Abbott D, Dumesic D & Franks S (2002) Developmental origin of polycystic ovary syndrome – a hypothesis. *Journal of Endocrinology,* **174,** 1–5.

Abel EL & Sokol RJ (1986) Fetal alcohol syndrome is now leading cause of mental retardation. *Lancet,* **2,** 1222.

Abernethy LJ, Cooke RWI & Foulder-Hughes L (2004) Caudate and hippocampal volumes, intelligence, and motor impairment in 7-year-old children who were born preterm. *Pediatric Research,* **55,** 884–93.

Abu-Saad K & Fraser D (2010) Maternal nutrition and birth outcomes. *Epidemiologic Reviews,* **32,** 5–25.

Acerini CL, Miles HL, Dunger DB *et al.* (2009) The descriptive epidemiology of congenital and acquired cryptorchidism in a UK infant cohort. *Archives of Disease in Childhood,* **94,** 868–72.

Aerts L, Sodoyez-Goffaux F, Sodoyez JC *et al.* (1988) The diabetic intrauterine milieu has a long-lasting effect on insulin secretion by B cells and on insulin uptake by target tissues. *American Journal of Obstetrics and Gynecology,* **159,** 1287–92.

Aggarwal BB & Gehlot P (2009) Inflammation and cancer: How friendly is the relationship for cancer patients? *Current Opinion in Pharmacology,* **9,** 351–69.

Aggarwal BB, Vijayalekshmi RV & Sung B (2009) Targeting inflammatory pathways for prevention and therapy of cancer: short-term friend, long-term foe. *Clinical Cancer Research,* **15,** 425–30.

Aguilera G & Catt KJ (1978) Regulation of aldosterone secretion by the renin-angiotensin system during sodium restriction in rats. *Proceedings of the National Academy of Sciences of the USA,* **75,** 4057–61.

Ahima RS, Prabakaran D & Flier JS (1998) Postnatal leptin surge and regulation of circadian rhythm of leptin by feeding: implications for energy homeostasis and neuroendocrine function. *Journal of Clinical Investigation,* **101,** 1020–7.

Ahlgren M, Melbye M, Wohlfahrt J *et al.* (2004) Growth patterns and the risk of breast cancer in women. *New England Journal of Medicine,* **351,** 1619–26.

Ahlgren M, Sorensen T, Wohlfahrt J *et al.* (2003) Birth weight and risk of breast cancer in a cohort of 106, 504 women. *International Journal of Cancer,* **107,** 997–1000.

Ainge H, Thompson C, Ozanne SE *et al.* (2011) A systematic review on animal models of maternal high fat feeding and offspring glycaemic control. *International Journal of Obesity,* **35,** 325–35.

Akobeng AK, Ramanan AV, Buchan I *et al.* (2006) Effect of breast feeding on risk of coeliac disease: a systematic review and meta-analysis of observational studies. *Archives of Disease in Childhood,* **91,** 39–43.

Akre O, Boyd HA, Ahlgren M *et al.* (2008) Maternal and gestational risk factors for hypospadias. *Environmental Health Perspectives,* **116,** 1071–6.

Akre O, Forssell L, Kaijser M *et al.* (2006) Perinatal risk factors for cancer of the esophagus and gastric cardia: a nested case-control study. *Cancer Epidemiology, Biomarkers & Prevention,* **15,** 867–71.

Akyol A, Langley-Evans SC & McMullen S (2009) Obesity induced by cafeteria feeding and pregnancy outcome in the rat. *British Journal of Nutrition,* **102,** 1601–10.

Al MD, van Houwelingen AC, Kester AD *et al.* (1995) Maternal essential fatty acid patterns during normal pregnancy and their relationship to the neonatal essential fatty acid status. *British Journal of Nutrition,* **74,** 55–68.

Ala-Houhala M (1985) 25-Hydroxyvitamin D levels during breast-feeding with or without maternal or infantile supplementation of vitamin D. *Journal of Pediatric Gastroenterology and Nutrition*, **4**, 220–6.

Ala-Houhala M, Koskinen T, Terho A *et al.* (1986) Maternal compared with infant vitamin D supplementation. *Archives of Disease in Childhood*, **61**, 1159–63.

Alberg A (2002) The influence of cigarette smoking on circulating concentrations of antioxidant micronutrients. *Toxicology*, **180**, 121–37.

Alder EM, Williams FL, Anderson AS *et al.* (2004) What influences the timing of the introduction of solid food to infants? *British Journal of Nutrition*, **92**, 527–31.

Alejandro B, Perez R, Pedrana G *et al.* (2002) Low maternal nutrition during pregnancy reduces the number of Sertoli cells in the newborn lamb. *Reproduction, Fertility and Development*, **14**, 333–7.

Alexander BT, Hendon AE, Ferril G *et al.* (2005) Renal denervation abolishes hypertension in low-birth-weight offspring from pregnant rats with reduced uterine perfusion. *Hypertension*, **45**, 754–8.

Allan K, Kelly FJ & Devereux G (2010) Antioxidants and allergic disease: A case of too little or too much? *Clinical and Experimental Allergy*, **40**, 370–80.

Allegrucci C, Thurston A, Lucas E *et al.* (2005) Epigenetics and the germline. *Reproduction*, **129**, 137–49.

Allen NB, Lewinsohn PM & Seeley JR (1998) Prenatal and perinatal influences on risk for psychopathology in childhood and adolescence. *Development and Psychopathology*, **10**, 513–29.

Almeida JR & Mandarim-de-Lacerda CA (2005) Overweight is gender-dependent in prenatal protein-calorie restricted adult rats acting on the blood pressure and the adverse cardiac remodeling. *Life Sciences*, **77**, 1307–18.

AlSaleh A, O'Dell SD, Frost GS *et al.* (2011) Single nucleotide polymorphisms at the ADIPOQ gene locus interact with age and dietary intake of fat to determine serum adiponectin in subjects at risk of the metabolic syndrome. *American Journal of Clinical Nutrition*, **94**, 262–9.

American Academy of Pediatrics (2005) Breastfeeding and the use of human milk. *Pediatrics*, **115**, 496–506.

American Academy of Pediatrics (2000) Hypoallergenic infant formulas. *Pediatrics*, **106**, 346–9.

Amorim AR, Linne Y, Kac G *et al.* (2008) Assessment of weight changes during and after pregnancy: practical approaches. *Maternal and Child Nutrition*, **4**, 1–13.

Anatskaya OV, Sidorenko NV, Beyer TV *et al.* (2010) Neonatal cardiomyocyte ploidy reveals critical windows of heart development. *International Journal of Cardiology*, **141**, 81–91.

Andersen HS, Gambling L, Holtrop G *et al.* (2006) Maternal iron deficiency identifies critical windows for growth and cardiovascular development in the rat postimplantation embryo. *Journal of Nutrition*, **136**, 1171–7.

Anderson JW, Johnstone BM & Remley DT (1999) Breast-feeding and cognitive development: a meta-analysis. *American Journal of Clinical Nutrition*, **70**, 525–35.

Anderson PH & Atkins GJ (2008) The skeleton as an intracrine organ for vitamin D metabolism. *Molecular Aspects of Medicine*, **29**, 397–406.

Andersson M, de Benoist B, Delange F *et al.* (2007) Prevention and control of iodine deficiency in pregnant and lactating women and in children less than 2-years-old: conclusions and recommendations of the Technical Consultation. *Public Health Nutrition*, **10**, 1606–11.

Andersson SW, Bengtsson C, Hallberg L *et al.* (2001) Cancer risk in Swedish women: the relation to size at birth. *British Journal of Cancer*, **84**, 1193–8.

Annweiler C, Allali G, Allain P *et al.* (2009) Vitamin D and cognitive performance in adults: a systematic review. *European Journal of Neurology*, **16**, 1083–9.

Antoniades L, MacGregor AJ, Andrew T *et al.* (2003) Association of birth weight with osteoporosis and osteoarthritis in adult twins. *Rheumatology (Oxford)*, **42**, 791–6.

Ardawi MS, Nasrat HA & BA'Aqueel HS (1997) Calcium-regulating hormones and parathyroid hormone-related peptide in normal human pregnancy and postpartum: a longitudinal study. *European Journal of Endocrinology*, **137**, 402–9.

Arenz S, Ruckerl R, Koletzko B *et al.* (2004) Breast-feeding and childhood obesity: a systematic review. *International Journal of Obesity and Related Metabolic Disorders*, **28**, 1247–56.

Arkkola T, Uusitalo U, Pietikainen M *et al.* (2006) Dietary intake and use of dietary supplements in relation to demographic variables among pregnant Finnish women. *British Journal of Nutrition*, **96**, 913–20.

Armitage JA, Taylor PD & Poston L (2005) Experimental models of developmental programming: consequences of exposure to an energy-rich diet during development. *Journal of Physiology*, **565**, 3–8.

Asher MI, Montefort S, Bjorksten B *et al.* (2006) Worldwide time trends in the prevalence of symptoms of asthma, allergic rhinoconjunctivitis, and eczema in childhood: ISAAC Phases One and Three repeat multicountry cross-sectional surveys. *Lancet*, **368**, 733–43.

Asthma UK (2004) Where do we stand? Asthma in the UK today. www.asthma.org.uk/how-we-help/teachers-and-healthcare-professionals/health-professionals/reports/ (accessed 8 January 2013).

Attig L, Solomon G, Ferezou J *et al.* (2008) Early postnatal leptin blockage leads to a long-term leptin resistance and susceptibility to diet-induced obesity in rats. *International Journal of Obesity*, **32**, 1153–60.

Austin J & Patterson M (2010) *A social marketing intervention to increase breastfeeding rates in Leicester.* www.smahcp.co.uk/professional-know-how/order-literature/literature-order/literature-order-768.aspx (accessed 8 January 2013).

Auyeung B, Baron-Cohen S, Ashwin E *et al.* (2009) Fetal testosterone and autistic traits. *British Journal of Psychology*, **100**, 1–22.

Baade PD, Youlden DR & Krnjacki LJ (2009) International epidemiology of prostate cancer: geographical distribution and secular trends. *Molecular Nutrition and Food Research*, **53**, 171–84.

Bae S, Xiao Y, Li G *et al.* (2003) Effect of maternal chronic hypoxic exposure during gestation on apoptosis in fetal rat heart. *American Journal of Physiology: Heart and Circulatory Physiology*, **285**, H983–90.

Baer HJ, Rich-Edwards JW, Colditz GA *et al.* (2006) Adult height, age at attained height, and incidence of breast cancer in premenopausal women. *International Journal of Cancer*, **119**, 2231–5.

Baird J, Fisher D, Lucas P *et al.* (2005) Being big or growing fast: systematic review of size and growth in infancy and later obesity. *British Medical Journal*, **331**, 929.

Baker PN, Wheeler SJ, Sanders TA *et al.* (2009) A prospective study of micronutrient status in adolescent pregnancy. *American Journal of Clinical Nutrition*, **89**, 1114–24.

Balchin I, Whittaker JC, Patel RR *et al.* (2007) Racial variation in the association between gestational age and perinatal mortality: prospective study. *British Medical Journal*, **334**, 833.

Bansal N, Anderson SG, Vyas A *et al.* (2011) Adiponectin and lipid profiles compared with insulins in relation to early growth of British South Asian and European children: the Manchester children's growth and vascular health study. *Journal of Clinical Endocrinology and Metabolism*, **96**, 2567–74.

Barbour RS, Macleod M, Mires G *et al.* (2011) Uptake of folic acid supplements before and during pregnancy: focus group analysis of women's views and experiences. *Journal of Human Nutrition and Dietetics*, 140–7.

Barker DJ (2002) Fetal programming of coronary heart disease. *Trends in Endocrinology and Metabolism*, **13**, 364–8.

Barker DJ, Forsen T, Uutela A *et al.* (2001) Size at birth and resilience to effects of poor living conditions in adult life: longitudinal study. *British Medical Journal*, **323**, 1273–6.

Barker DJ, Hales CN, Fall CH *et al.* (1993) Type 2 (non-insulin-dependent) diabetes mellitus, hypertension and hyperlipidaemia (syndrome X): relation to reduced fetal growth. *Diabetologia*, **36**, 62–7.

Barker DJ, Meade TW, Fall CH *et al.* (1992) Relation of fetal and infant growth to plasma fibrinogen and factor VII concentrations in adult life. *British Medical Journal*, **304**, 148–52.

Barker DJ & Osmond C (1986) Infant mortality, childhood nutrition, and ischaemic heart disease in England and Wales. *Lancet*, **1**, 1077–81.

Barker DJ, Osmond C, Forsen TJ *et al.* (2005) Trajectories of growth among children who have coronary events as adults. *New England Journal of Medicine*, **353**, 1802–9.

Barker DJ, Osmond C & Law CM (1989) The intrauterine and early postnatal origins of cardiovascular disease and chronic bronchitis. *Journal of Epidemiology and Community Health*, **43**, 237–40.

Barker DJ, Osmond C, Simmonds SJ *et al.* (1993) The relation of small head circumference and thinness at birth to death from cardiovascular disease in adult life. *British Medical Journal*, **306**, 422–6.

Barker DJ, Winter PD, Osmond C *et al.* (1989) Weight in infancy and death from ischaemic heart disease. *Lancet*, **2**, 577–80.

Barnes J, Ball M, Meadows P *et al.* (2008) *Nurse-Family Partnership Programme: Second Year Pilot Sites Implementation in England. The Infancy Period.* www.iscfsi.bbk.ac.uk/projects/files/Second_year.pdf (accessed 8 January 2013).

Bartington S, Griffiths LJ, Tate AR *et al.* (2006) Are breastfeeding rates higher among mothers delivering in Baby Friendly accredited maternity units in the UK? *International Journal of Epidemiology*, **35**, 1178–86.

Basile LA, Taylor SN, Wagner CL *et al.* (2006) The effect of high-dose vitamin D supplementation on serum vitamin D levels and milk calcium concentration in lactating women and their infants. *Breastfeeding Medicine*, **1**, 27–35.

Bass S, Pearce G, Bradney M *et al.* (1998) Exercise before puberty may confer residual benefits in bone density in adulthood: studies in active prepubertal and retired female gymnasts. *Journal of Bone and Mineral Research*, **13**, 500–7.

Bateman B, Warner JO, Hutchinson E *et al.* (2004) The effects of a double blind, placebo controlled, artificial food colourings and benzoate preservative challenge on hyperactivity in a general population sample of preschool children. *Archives of Disease in Childhood*, **89**, 506–11.

Bates B, Lennox A, Bates C *et al.* (2012) *National Diet and Nutrition Survey Headline Results from Years 1, 2 and 3 (combined) of the Rolling Programme (2008/2009–2010/2011). Department of Health.*

Bates B, Lennox A, Bates C *et al.* (2011) *National Diet and Nutrition Survey: Headline results from Years 1 and 2 (combined) of the Rolling Programme (2008/2009–2009/10).* /www.dh.gov.uk/prod_consum_dh/groups/dh_digitalassets/documents/digitalasset/dh_128550.pdf (accessed 9 January 2013).

Bateson P (2007) Developmental plasticity and evolutionary biology. *Journal of Nutrition*, **137**, 1060–2.

Bateson P, Barker D, Clutton-Brock T *et al.* (2004) Developmental plasticity and human health. *Nature*, **430**, 419–21.

Battista M, Calvo E, Chorvatova A *et al.* (2005) Intrauterine growth restriction and the programming of left ventricular remodelling in female rats. *Journal of Physiology*, **565** (Pt 1), 197–205.

Bayol SA, Farrington SJ & Stickland NC (2007) A maternal 'junk food' diet in pregnancy and lactation promotes an exacerbated taste for 'junk food' and a greater propensity for obesity in rat offspring. *British Journal of Nutrition*, **98**, 843–51.

Bayol SA, Simbi BH, Bertrand JA *et al.* (2008) Offspring from mothers fed a 'junk food' diet in pregnancy and lactation exhibit exacerbated adiposity that is more pronounced in females. *Journal of Physiology*, **586**, 3219–30.

Bayol SA, Simbi BH & Stickland NC (2005) A maternal cafeteria diet during gestation and lactation promotes adiposity and impairs skeletal muscle development and metabolism in rat offspring at weaning. *Journal of Physiology*, **567**, 951–61.

Beal VA (1961) Dietary intake of individuals followed through infancy and childhood. *American Journal of Public Health Nations Health*, **51**, 1107–17.

Beauchamp GK & Mennella JA (2009) Early flavor learning and its impact on later feeding behavior. *Journal of Pediatric Gastroenterology and Nutrition*, **48** Suppl 1, S25–30.

Becker GE, Remmington S & Remmington T (2011) Early additional food and fluids for healthy breastfed full-term infants. *Cochrane Database of Systematic Reviews*, **12**, CD006462.

Beckman LM, Beckman TR & Earthman CP (2010) Changes in gastrointestinal hormones and leptin after Roux-en-Y gastric bypass procedure: a review. *Journal of the American Dietetic Association*, **110**, 571–84.

Belkacemi L, Bedard I, Simoneau L *et al.* (2005) Calcium channels, transporters and exchangers in placenta: a review. *Cell Calcium*, **37**, 1–8.

Bellinger L, Lilley C & Langley-Evans SC (2004) Prenatal exposure to a maternal low-protein diet programmes a preference for high-fat foods in the young adult rat. *British Journal of Nutrition*, **92**, 513–20.

Benediktsson R, Lindsay RS, Noble J *et al.* (1993) Glucocorticoid exposure *in utero*: new model for adult hypertension. *Lancet*, **341**, 339–41.

Bennis-Taleb N, Remacle C, Hoet JJ *et al.* (1999) A low-protein isocaloric diet during gestation affects brain development and alters permanently cerebral cortex blood vessels in rat offspring. *Journal of Nutrition*, **129**, 1613–9.

Bentley D, Aubrey S & Bentley M (2004) *Infant Feeding and Nutrition for Primary Care*. Oxford, Radcliffe Publishing Ltd.

Benton D (1992) Vitamin-mineral supplements and intelligence. *Proceedings of the Nutrition Society*, **51**, 295–302.

Benton D (2008a) The influence of children's diet on their cognition and behavior. *European Journal of Nutrition*, **47** Suppl 3, 25–37.

Benton D (2008b) Micronutrient status, cognition and behavioral problems in childhood. *European Journal of Nutrition*, **47** Suppl 3, 38–50.

Berg CM, Lissner L, Aires N *et al.* (2005) Trends in blood lipid levels, blood pressure, alcohol and smoking habits from 1985 to 2002: results from INTERGENE and GOT-MONICA. *European Journal of Cardiovascular Prevention & Rehabilitation*, **12**, 115–25.

Berger A (2001) Insulin-like growth factor and cognitive function. *British Medical Journal*, **322**, 203.

Berger-Achituv S, Shohat T, Romano-Zelekha O *et al.* (2005) Widespread use of soy-based formula without clinical indications. *Journal of Pediatric Gastroenterology and Nutrition*, **41**, 660–6.

Bergvall N, Iliadou A, Tuvemo T *et al.* (2005) Birth characteristics and risk of high systolic blood pressure in early adulthood: socioeconomic factors and familial effects. *Epidemiology*, **16**, 635–40.

Berkowitz GS, Lapinski RH, Godbold JH *et al.* (1995) Maternal and neonatal risk factors for cryptorchidism. *Epidemiology*, **6**, 127–31.

Berti C, Decsi T, Dykes F *et al.* (2010) Critical issues in setting micronutrient recommendations for pregnant women: an insight. *Maternal and Child Nutrition*, **6**, 5–22.

Beuther DA & Sutherland ER (2007) Overweight, obesity, and incident asthma: a meta-analysis of prospective epidemiologic studies. *American Journal of Respiratory and Critical Care Medicine*, **175**, 661–6.

Bhargava SK, Sachdev HS, Fall CH *et al.* (2004) Relation of serial changes in childhood body-mass index to impaired glucose tolerance in young adulthood. *New England Journal of Medicine*, **350**, 865–75.

Bhatia J & Greer F (2008) Use of soy protein-based formulas in infant feeding. *Pediatrics*, **121**, 1062–8.

Bhatnagar S & Taneja S (2001) Zinc and cognitive development. *British Journal of Nutrition*, **85** Suppl 2, S139–45.

Bhutta ZA, Ahmed T, Black RE *et al.* (2008) What works? Interventions for maternal and child undernutrition and survival. *Lancet*, **371**, 417–40.

Birch EE, Carlson SE, Hoffman DR *et al.* (2010) The DIAMOND (DHA Intake and Measurement of Neural Development) Study: a double-masked, randomized controlled clinical trial of the maturation of infant visual acuity as a function of the dietary level of docosahexaenoic acid. *American Journal of Clinical Nutrition*, **91**, 848–59.

Bird A (2007) Perceptions of epigenetics. *Nature*, **447**, 396–8.

Bishop NJ, Dahlenburg SL, Fewtrell MS *et al.* (1996) Early diet of preterm infants and bone mineralization at age five years. *Acta Paediatrica*, **85**, 230–6.

Bishop NJ, King FJ & Lucas A (1993) Increased bone mineral content of preterm infants fed with a nutrient-enriched formula after discharge from hospital. *Archives of Disease in Childhood*, **68**, 573–8.

Bispham J, Gardner DS, Gnanalingham MG *et al.* (2005) Maternal nutritional programming of fetal adipose tissue development: differential effects on messenger ribonucleic acid abundance for uncoupling proteins and peroxisome proliferator-activated and prolactin receptors. *Endocrinology*, **146**, 3943–9.

Bjorksten B, Sepp E, Julge K *et al.* (2001) Allergy development and the intestinal microflora during the first year of life. *Journal of Allergy and Clinical Immunology*, **108**, 516–20.

Black PN & Sharpe S (1997) Dietary fat and asthma: Is there a connection? *European Respiratory Journal*, **10**, 6–12.

Black RE, Williams SM, Jones IE *et al.* (2002) Children who avoid drinking cow milk have low dietary calcium intakes and poor bone health. *American Journal of Clinical Nutrition*, **76**, 675–80.

Blair NJ, Thompson JM, Black PN *et al.* (2007) Risk factors for obesity in 7-year-old European children: the Auckland Birthweight Collaborative Study. *Archives of Disease in Childhood*, **92**, 866–71.

Blanaru JL, Kohut JR, Fitzpatrick-Wong SC *et al.* (2004) Dose response of bone mass to dietary arachidonic acid in piglets fed cow milk-based formula. *American Journal of Clinical Nutrition*, **79**, 139–47.

Bloom L & Escuro A (2008) Adolescent pregnancy: where do we start? *Handbook of Nutrition and Pregnancy*. Ed. Lammi-Keefe CJ, Couch SC & Philipson EH. Towtowa, New Jersey, Humana Press.

Blouin K, Veilleux A, Luu-The V *et al.* (2009) Androgen metabolism in adipose tissue: recent advances. *Molecular and Cellular Endocrinology*, **301**, 97–103.

Bodnar LM, Catov JM, Roberts JM *et al.* (2007) Prepregnancy obesity predicts poor vitamin D status in mothers and their neonates. *Journal of Nutrition*, **137**, 2437–42.

Bodnar LM, Himes KP, Venkataramanan R *et al.* (2010) Maternal serum folate species in early pregnancy and risk of preterm birth. *American Journal of Clinical Nutrition*, **92**, 864–71.

Bogdarina I, Welham S, King PJ *et al.* (2007) Epigenetic modification of the renin-angiotensin system in the fetal programming of hypertension. *Circulation Research*, **100**, 520–6.

Bolling K, Grant C, Hamlyn B *et al.* (2007) *Infant Feeding Survey 2005*. London, The NHS Information Centre.

Boney CM, Verma A, Tucker R *et al.* (2005) Metabolic syndrome in childhood: association with birth weight, maternal obesity, and gestational diabetes mellitus. *Pediatrics*, **115**, e290–6.

Bonjour JP, Carrie AL, Ferrari S *et al.* (1997) Calcium-enriched foods and bone mass growth in prepubertal girls: a randomized, double-blind, placebo-controlled trial. *Journal of Clinical Investigation*, **99**, 1287–94.

Bonjour JP, Chevalley T, Ammann P *et al.* (2001) Gain in bone mineral mass in prepubertal girls 3.5 years after discontinuation of calcium supplementation: a follow-up study. *Lancet*, **358**, 1208–12.

Bonsch D, Lenz B, Kornhuber J *et al.* (2005) DNA hypermethylation of the alpha synuclein promoter in patients with alcoholism. *Neuroreport*, **16**, 167–70.

Bonsch D, Lenz B, Reulbach U *et al.* (2004) Homocysteine associated genomic DNA hypermethylation in patients with chronic alcoholism. *Journal of Neural Transmission*, **111**, 1611–16.

Botto LD, Lisi A, Robert-Gnansia E *et al.* (2005) International retrospective cohort study of neural tube defects in relation to folic acid recommendations: Are the recommendations working? *British Medical Journal*, **330**, 571.

Bouret SG (2010a) Neurodevelopmental actions of leptin. *Brain Research*, **1350**, 2–9.

Bouret SG (2010b) Development of hypothalamic neural networks controlling appetite. *Forum of Nutrition*, **63**, 84–93.

Bouret SG, Draper SJ & Simerly RB (2004) Trophic action of leptin on hypothalamic neurons that regulate feeding. *Science*, **304**, 108–10.

Bouret SG & Simerly RB (2007) Development of leptin-sensitive circuits. *Journal of Neuroendocrinology*, **19**, 575–82.

Bourguignon J-P, Rasier G, Lebrethon M-C *et al.* (2010) Neuroendocrine disruption of pubertal timing and interactions between homeostasis of reproduction and energy balance. *Molecular and Cellular Endocrinology*, **324**, 110–20.

Bradney M, Pearce G, Naughton G *et al.* (1998) Moderate exercise during growth in prepubertal boys: changes in bone mass, size, volumetric density, and bone strength: a controlled prospective study. *Journal of Bone and Mineral Research*, **13**, 1814–21.

Brameld JM, Buttery PJ, Dawson JM *et al.* (1998) Nutritional and hormonal control of skeletal-muscle cell growth and differentiation. *Proceedings of the Nutrition Society*, **57**, 207–17.

Bray F, McCarron P & Parkin DM (2004) The changing global patterns of female breast cancer incidence and mortality. *Breast Cancer Research*, **6**, 229–39.

Brekke HK, Ludvigsson JF, van Odijk J *et al.* (2005) Breastfeeding and introduction of solid foods in Swedish infants: the All Babies in Southeast Sweden study. *British Journal of Nutrition*, **94**, 377–82.

Brenna JT, Varamini B, Jensen RG *et al.* (2007) Docosa-hexaenoic and arachidonic acid concentrations in human breast milk worldwide. *American Journal of Clinical Nutrition*, **85**, 1457–64.

Brion MJ, Lawlor DA, Matijasevich A *et al.* (2011) What are the causal effects of breastfeeding on IQ, obesity and blood pressure? Evidence from comparing high-income with middle-income cohorts. *International Journal of Epidemiology*, **40**, 670–80.

British Medical Association (2009) *Early life nutrition and long life health.* London. http://www.derbyshirelmc.org.uk/Guidance/Early%20Life%20Nutrition%20and%20 Lifelong%20Health.pdf (accessed 9 January 2013).

Broekman BF, Chan YH, Chong YS *et al.* (2009) The influence of birth size on intelligence in healthy children. *Pediatrics*, **123**, e1011–16.

Brooke OG, Brown IR, Bone CD *et al.* (1980) Vitamin D supplements in pregnant Asian women: effects on calcium status and fetal growth. *British Medical Journal*, **280**, 751–4.

Brooke OG, Brown IR, Cleeve HJ *et al.* (1981) Observations on the vitamin D state of pregnant Asian women in London. *British Journal of Obstetrics and Gynaecology*, **88**, 18–26.

Brooks AA, Johnson MR, Steer PJ *et al.* (1995) Birth weight: Nature or nurture? *Early Human Development*, **42**, 29–35.

Brough L, Rees GA, Crawford MA *et al.* (2009) Social and ethnic differences in folic acid use preconception and during early pregnancy in the UK: effect on maternal folate status. *Journal of Human Nutrition and Dietetics*, **22**, 100–7.

Brown A & Lee M (2011) An exploration of experiences of mothers following a baby-led weaning style: developmental readiness for complementary foods. *Maternal and Child Nutrition*, Nov 28. doi: 10.1111/j.1740-8709.2011.00360.x.

Brown JD & Vannucci RC (1978) Cerebral oxidative metabolism during intrauterine growth retardation. *Biology of the Neonate*, **34**, 170–3.

Buckley AJ, Keseru B, Briody J *et al.* (2005) Altered body composition and metabolism in the male offspring of high fat-fed rats. *Metabolism*, **54**, 500–7.

Burdette HL, Whitaker RC, Hall WC *et al.* (2006) Maternal infant-feeding style and children's adiposity at 5 years of age. *Archives of Pediatric and Adolescent Medicine*, **160**, 513–20.

Burdge GC, Jones AE & Wootton SA (2002) Eicosapentaenoic and docosapentaenoic acids are the principal products of alpha-linolenic acid metabolism in young men. *British Journal of Nutrition*, **88**, 355–63.

Burdge GC & Lillycrop KA (2010) Nutrition, epigenetics, and developmental plasticity: implications for understanding human disease. *Annual Review of Nutrition*, **30**, 315–39.

Burdge GC, Slater-Jefferies J, Torrens C *et al.* (2007) Dietary protein restriction of pregnant rats in the F0 generation induces altered methylation of hepatic gene promoters in the adult male offspring in the F1 and F2 generations. *British Journal of Nutrition*, **97**, 435–9.

Burdge GC & Wootton SA (2002) Conversion of alpha-linolenic acid to eicosapentaenoic, docosapentaenoic and docosahexaenoic acids in young women. *British Journal of Nutrition*, **88**, 411–20.

Burns S, Desai M, Cohen R *et al.* (1997) Gluconeogenesis, glucose handling, and structural changes in livers of the adult offspring of rats partially deprived of protein during pregnancy and lactation. *Journal of Clinical Investigation*, **100**, 1768–74.

Burri P (1997) Structural aspects of prenatal and postnatal development and growth of the lung. In: *Lung Growth and Development.* Ed. McDonald, JA. New York, Marcel Dekker, Inc.

Buschman NA, Foster G & Vickers P (2001) Adolescent girls and their babies: achieving optimal birthweight. Gestational weight gain and pregnancy outcome in terms of gestation at delivery and infant birth weight: a comparison between adolescents under 16 and adult women1. *Child: Care, Health and Development*, **27**, 163–71.

Butler TG, Schwartz J & McMillen IC (2002) Differential effects of the early and late intrauterine environment on corticotrophic cell development. *Journal of Clinical Investigation*, **110**, 783–91.

Butte N, Lopez-Alarcon G & Garza C (2002) *Nutrient adequacy of exclusive breastfeeding for the term infant during the first six months of life.* Geneva, World Health Organization.

Buttriss J (2002) *Adverse Reactions to Food: The Report of the British Nutrition Foundation Task Force.* Oxford, Wiley-Blackwell Publishing Ltd.

Caire-Juvera G, Ortega MI, Casanueve E *et al.* (2007) Food components and dietary patterns of the two different groups of Mexican lactating women. *Journal of the American College of Nutrition*, **26**, 88–9.

Calle EE & Kaaks R (2004) Overweight, obesity and cancer: epidemiological evidence and proposed mechanisms. *Nature Reviews Cancer*, **4**, 579–91.

Calvert JW, Lefer DJ, Gundewar S *et al.* (2009) Developmental programming resulting from maternal obesity in mice: effects on myocardial ischaemia-reperfusion injury. *Experimental Physiology*, **94**, 805–14.

Calvi LM & Schipani E (2000) The PTH/PTHrP receptor in Jansen's metaphyseal chondrodysplasia. *Journal of Endocrinological Investigation*, **23**, 545–54.

Calvi LM, Sims NA, Hunzelman JL *et al.* (2001) Activated parathyroid hormone/parathyroid hormone-related protein receptor in osteoblastic cells differentially affects cortical and trabecular bone. *Journal of Clinical Investigation*, **107**, 277–86.

Cancer Research UK (2010a) Breast Cancer. http://info. cancerresearchuk.org/cancerstats/types/breast/index. htm?script=true.

Cancer Research UK (2010b) UK incidence Statistics. http://info.cancerresearchuk.org/cancerstats/types/ bowel/incidence/index.htm.

Cancer Research UK (2010c) UK incidence statistics. http://info.cancerresearchuk.org/cancerstats/types/ stomach/incidence/ 21st

Cancer Research UK (2010d) Oesophageal cancer survival statistics. http://info.cancerresearchuk.org/cancerstats/ types/oesophagus/survival/index.htm.

Cancer Research UK (2010e) Incidence. http://info. cancerresearchuk.org/cancerstats/childhoodcancer/ incidence/index.htm.

Cancer Research UK (2012) Testicular cancer statistics – UK. http://info.cancerresearchuk.org/cancerstats/types/ testis/.

Care AD, Caple IW, Abbas SK *et al.* (1986) The effect of fetal thyroparathyroidectomy on the transport of calcium across the ovine placenta to the fetus. *Placenta*, **7**, 417–24.

Carey MA, Card JW, Voltz JW *et al.* (2007) It's all about sex: gender, lung development and lung disease. *Trends in Endocrinology and Metabolism*, **18**, 308–13.

Carlson SE (2009) Docosahexaenoic acid supplementation in pregnancy and lactation. *American Journal of Clinical Nutrition*, **89**, 678S-84S.

Carnell S & Wardle J (2008) Appetitive traits and child obesity: measurement, origins and implications for intervention. *Proceedings of the Nutrition Society*, **67**, 343–55.

Carruth BR & Skinner JD (2002) Feeding behaviors and other motor development in healthy children (2–24 months). *Journal of the American College of Nutrition*, **21**, 88–96.

Casas JP, Bautista LE, Smeeth L *et al.* (2005) Homocysteine and stroke: evidence on a causal link from mendelian randomisation. *Lancet*, **365**, 224–32.

Cashman KD & Kiely M (2011) Towards prevention of vitamin D deficiency and beyond: knowledge gaps and research needs in vitamin D nutrition and public health. *British Journal of Nutrition*, **106**, 1617–27.

Caspi A, Williams B, Kim-Cohen J *et al.* (2007) Moderation of breastfeeding effects on the IQ by genetic variation in fatty acid metabolism. *Proceedings of the National Academy of Sciences of the USA*, **104**, 18860–5.

Castellano JM, Roa J, Luque RM *et al.* (2009) KiSS-1/ kisspeptins and the metabolic control of reproduction: physiologic roles and putative physiopathological implications. *Peptides*, **30**, 139–45.

Catalano PM, Drago NM & Amini SB (1995) Maternal carbohydrate metabolism and its relationship to fetal growth and body composition. *American Journal of Obstetrics and Gynaecology*, **172**, 1464–70.

Catalano PM & Ehrenberg HM (2006) The short- and long-term implications of maternal obesity on the mother and her offspring. *An International Journal of Obstetrics and Gynaecology*, **113**, 1126–33.

Catalano PM, Farrell K, Thomas A *et al.* (2009) Perinatal risk factors for childhood obesity and metabolic dysregulation. *American Journal of Clinical Nutrition*, **90**, 1303–13.

Catalano PM, Presley L, Minium J *et al.* (2009) Fetuses of obese mothers develop insulin resistance *in utero*. *Diabetes Care*, **32**, 1076–80.

Catta-Preta M, Oliveira DA, Mandarim-de-Lacerda CA *et al.* (2006) Adult cardiorenal benefits from postnatal fish oil supplement in rat offspring of low-protein pregnancies. *Life Sciences*, **80**, 219–29.

Cawthorn RM, Smith KR, O'Brien E *et al.* (2003) Association between telomere length in blood and mortality in people aged 60 years or older. Lancet, **361**, 393–5.

Centers for Disease Control and Prevention (CDC) (2004) Spina bifida and anencephaly before and after folic acid mandate : United States, 1995–1996 and 1999–2000. www.cdc.gov/mmwr/preview/mmwrhtml/mm5317a3. htm (accessed 8 January 2013).

Centers for Disease Control and Prevention (CDC) (2009) Facts about folic acid. www.cdc.gov/ncbddd/folicacid/ about.html (accessed 8 January 2013).

Centers for Disease Control and Prevention (2010) Vital signs: state-specific obesity prevalence among adults. United States, 2009. *Morbidity and Mortality Weekly Report*, **59**, 951–5.

Centers for Disease Control and Prevention (1998) Recommendations to prevent and control iron deficiency in the United States. *Morbidity and Mortality Weekly Report*, **47**.

Centre for Maternal and Child Enquiries (CMACE) & Royal College of Obstetricians and Gynaecologists (RCOG) (2010a) *Management of Women with Obesity in Pregnancy*. London.

Centre for Maternal and Child Enquiries (CMACE) & Royal College of Obstetricians and Gynaecologists (RCOG) (2010b) *Maternal obesity in the UK: Findings from a national project*. London.

Ceravolo GS, Franco MC, Carneiro-Ramos MS *et al.* (2007) Enalapril and losartan restored blood pressure and vascular reactivity in intrauterine undernourished rats. *Life Sciences*, **80**, 782–7.

Cetin I & Alvino G (2008) Intrauterine growth restriction: implications for placental metabolism and transport. A review. *Placenta*, **30**, 77–82.

Cetin I, Alvino G & Cardellicchio M (2009) Long chain fatty acids and dietary fats in fetal nutrition. *Journal of Physiology*, **587**, 3441–51.

Chamberlain G & Steer PJ (2001) *Turnbull's Obstetrics*. London, Churchill Livingstone.

Chan GM, McElligott K, McNaught T *et al.* (2006) Effects of dietary calcium intervention on adolescent mothers and newborns: a randomized controlled trial. *Obstetrics and Gynecology*, **108**, 565–71.

Chan LL, Sebert SP, Hyatt MA *et al.* (2009) Effect of maternal nutrient restriction from early to midgestation on cardiac function and metabolism after adolescent-onset obesity. *American Journal of Physiology – Regulatory, Integrative and Comparative Physiology*, **296**, R1455–63.

Chapman KE & Seckl JR (2008) 11beta-HSD1, inflammation, metabolic disease and age-related cognitive (dys) function. *Neurochemical Research*, **33**, 624–36.

Chatzi L, Torrent M, Romieu I *et al.* (2008) Mediterranean diet in pregnancy is protective for wheeze and atopy in childhood. *Thorax*, **63**, 507–13.

Cheema KK, Dent MR, Saini HK *et al.* (2005) Prenatal exposure to maternal undernutrition induces adult cardiac dysfunction. *British Journal of Nutrition*, **93**, 471–7.

Chen H, Simar D, Lambert K *et al.* (2008) Maternal and postnatal overnutrition differentially impact appetite regulators and fuel metabolism. *Endocrinology*, **149**, 5348–56.

Chen LT & Rivera MA (2004) The Costa Rican experience: reduction of neural tube defects following food fortification programs. *Nutrition Reviews*, **62**, S40–3.

Chen ZP & Hetzel BS (2010) Cretinism revisited. *Best Practice and Research: Clinical Endocrinology & Metabolism*, **24**, 39–50.

Cheng S, Tylavsky F, Kroger H *et al.* (2003) Association of low 25-hydroxyvitamin D concentrations with elevated parathyroid hormone concentrations and low cortical bone density in early pubertal and prepubertal Finnish girls. *American Journal of Clinical Nutrition*, **78**, 485–92.

Chief Medical Officers of England, Scotland, Wales, and Northern Ireland (2011) *Start Active, Stay Active: A Report on physical activity from the four home countries' Chief Medical Officers*. www.dh.gov.uk/en/Publicationsandstatistics/Publications/PublicationsPolicyAndGuidance/DH_128209 (accessed 8 January 2013).

Cho NH, Silverman BL, Rizzo TA *et al.* (2000) Correlations between the intrauterine metabolic environment and blood pressure in adolescent offspring of diabetic mothers. *Journal of Pediatrics*, **136**, 587–92.

Christensen L (1996) *Diet Behavior Relationships: Focus on Depression*. Washington, DC, American Psychological Association.

Christianson A, Howson CP & Modell B (2006) *March of Dimes Global Report on Birth Defects: The hidden toll of dying and disabled children*. New York March of Dimes Birth Defects Foundation. www.marchofdimes.com/downloads/BirthDefects/ExecutiveSummary.pdf (accessed 8 January 2013).

Cianfarani S, Germani D & Branca F (1999) Low birthweight and adult insulin resistance: the 'catch-up growth'

hypothesis. *Archives of Disease in Childhood, Fetal and Neonatal Edition*, **81**, F71–3.

Cifkova R, Skodova Z, Bruthans J *et al.* (2010) Longitudinal trends in major cardiovascular risk factors in the Czech population between 1985 and 2007/8. Czech MONICA and Czech post-MONICA. *Atherosclerosis*, **211**, 676–81.

Cinti S (2009) Reversible physiological transdifferentiation in the adipose organ. *Proceedings of the Nutrition Society*, **68**, 340–9.

Clausen TD, Mathiesen ER, Hansen T *et al.* (2008) High prevalence of type 2 diabetes and pre-diabetes in adult offspring of women with gestational diabetes mellitus or type 1 diabetes: the role of intrauterine hyperglycemia. *Diabetes Care*, **31**, 340–6.

Clayton PE & Gill MS (2001) Normal growth and its endocrine control. In *Clinical Paediatric Endocrinology*. Ed. Brook C & Hindmarsh PC. Oxford, Blackwell Publishing Ltd.

Cockburn F, Belton NR, Purvis RJ *et al.* (1980) Maternal vitamin D intake and mineral metabolism in mothers and their newborn infants. *British Medical Journal*, **281**, 11–14.

Cockell KA, Miller DC & Lowell H (2009) Application of the Dietary Reference Intakes in developing a recommendation for pregnancy iron supplements in Canada. *American Journal of Clinical Nutrition*, **90**, 1023–8.

Codex Alimentarius (2007) Standard for infant forumla and formulas for special medical purposes intended for infants. Vol. CODEX STAN 72–1981.

Cole TJ (2000) Secular trends in growth. *Proceedings of the Nutrition Society*, **59**, 317–24.

Cole TJ (2003) The secular trend in human physical growth: a biological view. *Economics & Human Biology*, **1**, 161–8.

Coll O, Pisa S, Palacio M *et al.* (2004) Awareness of the use of folic acid to prevent neural tube defects in a Mediterranean area. *European Journal of Obstetrics & Gynecology and Reproductive Biology*, **115**, 173–7.

Commission of the European Communities (1983) *First Report of the Scientific Committee for Food on the Essential Requirements of Infant Formulae and Follow-up Milks Based on Cow's Milk Protein*. Luxembourg. Commission of the European Communities.

Commission of the European Communities (1989) *The Minimum Requirements for Soya-Based Infant Formulas and Follow-up Milks*. Luxembourg, European Commission.

Committee on Medical Aspects of Food and Nutrition Policy (COMA) (2000) *Folic Acid and the Prevention of Disease: Report of the Committee on Medical Aspects of Food and Nutrition Policy*. http://www.dh.gov.uk/en/Publicationsandstatistics/Publications/PublicationsPolicyAndGuidance/DH_4005805 (accessed 8 January 2013).

Committee on Medical Aspects of Food Policy (COMA) (1980) *Artificial Feeds for the Young Infant*. London, Her Majesties Stationery Office.

Committee on Medical Aspects of Food Policy (COMA) (1996) *Guirdelines on the Nutritonal Assessment of Infant Formulas: Report of the Working Group on Nutritional Assessment of Infant Formulas*. London, The Stationery Office.

Committee on Toxicity of Chemicals in Food Consumer Products and the Environment (1998) *Peanut Allergy*. London, Department of Health.

Committee on Toxicity of Chemicals in Food Consumer Products and the Environment (2008) Statement on the Reproductive Effects of Caffeine. http://cot.food.gov.uk/cotstatements/cotstatementsyrs/cotstatements2008/cot200804.

Committee on Toxicity of Chemicals in Food Consumer Products and the Environment (2009) Statement on the review of the 1998 COT recommendations on peanut avoidance. http://cot.food.gov.uk/pdfs/cotstatement200807peanut.pdf (accessed 4 January 2013).

Confidential Enquiry into Maternal and Child Health (CEMACH) (2007) *Saving Mothers' Lives: Reviewing Maternal Deaths to Make Motherhood Safer 2003–2005. The Seventh Report on Confidential Enquiries into Maternal Deaths in the United Kingdom*. London. CEMACH.

Confidential Enquiry into Maternal and Child Health (CEMACH) (2009) *Perinatal Mortality 2007: United Kingdom*. London. CEMACH.

Congdon P, Horsman A, Kirby PA *et al.*(1983) Mineral content of the forearms of babies born to Asian and white mothers. *British Medical Journal (Clinical Research ed.)*, **286**, 1233–5.

Constancia M, Angiolini E, Sandovici I *et al.* (2005) Adaptation of nutrient supply to fetal demand in the mouse involves interaction between the Igf2 gene and placental transporter systems. *Proceedings of the National Academy of Sciences of the USA*, **102**, 19219–24.

Conway P (1997) Development of intestinal microbiota *Gastrointestinal Microbiology*. Ed. Mackie RI, White BA & Isaacson RE. New York, Chapman & Hall: 3–38.

Cooper C, Eriksson JG, Forsen T *et al.* (2001) Maternal height, childhood growth and risk of hip fracture in later life: a longitudinal study. *Osteoporosis International*, **12**, 623–9.

Cottrell EC, Mercer JG & Ozanne SE (2010) Postnatal development of hypothalamic leptin receptors. In *Vitamins & Hormones*. Ed. Gerald L. London, Academic Press: 201–17.

Cottrell EC & Ozanne SE (2007) Developmental programming of energy balance and the metabolic syndrome. *Proceedings of the Nutrition Society*, **66**, 198–206.

Cottrell EC & Seckl JR (2009) Prenatal stress, glucocorticoids and the programming of adult disease. *Frontiers in Behavioral Neuroscience*, **3**, 19.

Coulthard H, Harris G & Emmett P (2009) Delayed introduction of lumpy foods to children during the complementary feeding period affects child's food acceptance and feeding at 7 years of age. *Maternal and Child Nutrition*, **5**, 75–85.

Craig R, Mindell J & Hirani V (2009) *Health Survey for England 2008: Physical Activity and Fitness*. London. The NHS Information Centre.

Crawford MA (1993) The role of essential fatty acids in neural development: implications for perinatal nutrition. *American Journal of Clinical Nutrition*, **57**, 703S–9S; discussion 9S–10S.

Crawley H & Westland S (2011) *Infant milks in the UK*. Herts, Caroline Walker Trust. www.cwt.org.uk/pdfs/infantsmilk_web.pdf (accessed 8 January 2013).

Crespi EJ, Steckler TL, Mohankumar PS *et al.* (2006) Prenatal exposure to excess testosterone modifies the developmental trajectory of the insulin-like growth factor system in female sheep. *Journal of Physiology*, **572**, 119–30.

Crew KD & Neugut AI (2006) Epidemiology of gastric cancer. *World Journal of Gastroenterology*, **12**, 354–62.

Cripps RL, Martin-Gronert MS, Archer ZA *et al.* (2009) Programming of hypothalamic neuropeptide gene expression in rats by maternal dietary protein content during pregnancy and lactation. *Clinical Science*, **117**, 85–93.

Crowe C, Dandekar P, Fox M *et al.* (1995) The effects of anaemia on heart, placenta and body weight, and blood pressure in fetal and neonatal rats. *Journal of Physiology*, **488**, 515–19.

Crowther NJ, Cameron N, Trusler J *et al.* (1998) Association between poor glucose tolerance and rapid postnatal weight gain in seven-year-old children. *Diabetologia*, **41**, 1163–7.

Crozier SR, Inskip HM, Godfrey KM *et al.* (2010) Weight gain in pregnancy and childhood body composition: findings from the Southampton Women's Survey. *American Journal of Clinical Nutrition*, **91**, 1745–51.

Crozier SR, Robinson SM, Borland SE *et al.* (2009) Do women change their health behaviours in pregnancy? Findings from the Southampton Women's Survey. *Paediatric and Perinatal Epidemiology*, **23**, 446–53.

Cryer A & Jones HM (1980) The development of white adipose tissue: effect of litter size on the lipoprotein lipase activity of four adipose-tissue depots, serum immunoreactive insulin and tissue cellularity during the first year of life in male and female rats. *Biochemical Journal*, **186**, 805–15.

Curhan GC, Chertow GM, Willett WC *et al.* (1996) Birth weight and adult hypertension and obesity in women. *Circulation*, **94**, 1310–15.

Czeizel AE & Dudas I (1992) Prevention of the first occurrence of neural-tube defects by periconceptional vitamin supplementation. *New England Journal of Medicine*, **327**, 1832–5.

Dabelea D, Hanson RL, Lindsay RS *et al.* (2000) Intrauterine exposure to diabetes conveys risks for type 2 diabetes and obesity: a study of discordant sibships. *Diabetes*, **49**, 2208–11.

Dabelea D, Knowler WC & Pettitt DJ (2000) Effect of diabetes in pregnancy on offspring: follow-up research in the Pima Indians. *Journal of Maternal and Fetal Medicine*, **9**, 83–8.

Dallongeville J, Marecaux N, Fruchart JC *et al.* (1998) Cigarette smoking is associated with unhealthy patterns of nutrient intake: a meta-analysis. *Journal of Nutrition*, **128**, 1450–7.

Daly LE, Kirke PN, Molloy A *et al.* (1995) Folate levels and neural tube defects: implications for prevention. *The Journal of the American Medical Association*, **274**, 1698–702.

Dampney RA, Horiuchi J, Killinger S *et al.* (2005) Long-term regulation of arterial blood pressure by hypothalamic nuclei: some critical questions. *Clinical and Experimental Pharmacology and Physiology*, **32**, 419–25.

Daniels MC & Adair LS (2005) Breast-feeding influences cognitive development in Filipino children. *Journal of Nutrition*, **135**, 2589–95.

Darling AL, Hart KH, Macdonald HM *et al.* (2013) Vitamin D deficiency in UK South Asian women of childbearing age: a comparative longitudinal investigation with UK Caucasian women. *Osteoporosis International*, **24**, 477–88.

Datta S, Alfaham M, Davies DP *et al.* (2002) Vitamin D deficiency in pregnant women from a non-European ethnic minority population: an interventional study. *British Journal of Obstetrics and Gynaecology*, **109**, 905–8.

Davidowa H, Li Y & Plagemann A (2003) Altered responses to orexigenic (AGRP, MCH) and anorexigenic (alpha-MSH, CART) neuropeptides of paraventricular hypothalamic neurons in early postnatally overfed rats. *European Journal of Neuroscience*, **18**, 613–21.

Davidowa H & Plagemann A (2001) Inhibition by insulin of hypothalamic VMN neurons in rats overweight due to postnatal overfeeding. *Neuroreport*, **12**, 3201–4.

Davis L, Roullet JB, Thornburg KL *et al.* (2003) Augmentation of coronary conductance in adult sheep made anaemic during fetal life. *Journal of Physiology*, **547**, 53–9.

Dawson-Hughes B, Heaney RP, Holick MF *et al.* (2005) Estimates of optimal vitamin D status. *Osteoporosis International*, **16**, 713–6.

de Boer MP, Ijzerman RG, de Jongh RT *et al.* (2008) Birth weight relates to salt sensitivity of blood pressure in healthy adults. *Hypertension*, **51**, 928–32.

de Escobar GM, Obregón MJ & del Rey FE (2007) Iodine deficiency and brain development in the first half of pregnancy. *Public Health Nutrition*, **10**, 1554–70.

de Lange T (2005) Shelterin: the protein complex that shapes and safeguards human telomeres. *Genes & Development*, **19**, 2100–10.

de Onis M, Villar J & Gulmezoglu M (1998) Nutritional interventions to prevent intrauterine growth retardation: evidence from randomized controlled trials. *European Journal of Clinical Nutrition*, **52** Suppl 1, S83–93.

de Rooij SR, Painter RC, Phillips DI *et al.* (2006) Impaired insulin secretion after prenatal exposure to the Dutch famine. *Diabetes Care*, **29**, 1897–901.

De Stavola BL, dos Santos Silva I & Wadsworth MJ (2005) Birth weight and breast cancer. *New England Journal of Medicine*, **352**, 304–6.

De Wals P, Tairou F, Van Allen MI *et al.* (2007) Reduction in neural-tube defects after folic acid fortification in Canada. *New England Journal of Medicine*, **357**, 135–42.

de Zegher F & Ibanez L (2009) Early Origins of polycystic ovary syndrome: hypotheses may change without notice. *Journal of Clinical Endocrinology and Metabolism*, **94**, 3682–5.

Deary IJ, Strand S, Smith P *et al.* (2007) Intelligence and educational achievement. *Intelligence*, **35**, 13–21.

Delvin EE, Salle BL, Glorieux FH *et al.* (1986) Vitamin D supplementation during pregnancy: effect on neonatal calcium homeostasis. *Journal of Pediatrics*, **109**, 328–34.

Demerath EW, Cameron N, Gillman MW *et al.* (2004) Telomeres and telomerase in the fetal origins of cardiovascular disease: a review. *Human Biology*, **76**, 127–46.

Demmelmair H, von Rosen J & Koletzko B (2006) Long-term consequences of early nutrition. *Early Human Development*, **82**, 567–74.

Dennison EM, Aihie-Sayer A, Syddall H *et al.* (2003) Birth-weight is associated with bone mass in the seventh decade: the Hertfordshire 31–39 Study. *Pediatric Research*, **53**, S525A.

Department for Children Schools and Families & Department of Health (2010) *Teenage Pregnancy Strategy: Beyond 2010.* www.education.gov.uk/publications/standard/publicationDetail/Page1/DCSF-00224-2010 (accessed 8 January 2013).

Department of Health (1980) *Present Day Practice in Infant Feeding: 1980.* London, Her Majesties Stationery Office.

Department of Health (1989) *Present Day Practice in Infant feeding: Third Report.* London: Her Majesties Stationery Office.

Department of Health (1991) *Dietary Reference Values for Food Energy and Nutrients for the United Kingdom. Report of the panel on dietary reference values of the*

Committee on Medical Aspects of Food Policy. London, Her Majesties Stationery Office.

Department of Health (1994) *Weaning and the Weaning Diet*. London, Her Majesties Stationery Office.

Department of Health (1995) *Sensible Drinking. The Report of an Inter-departmental Working Group*. London, Her Majesties Stationery Office.

Department of Health (2007) *Updated alcohol advice for pregnant women*. http://webarchive.nationalarchives.gov. uk/+/www.direct.gov.uk/en/Nl1/Newsroom/DG_068143.

Department of Health (2009a) *The Pregnancy Book*. London, The Stationery Office.

Department of Health (2009b) *Birth to Five*. London, Department of Health.

Department of Health (2010) *Healthy Lives, Healthy People: Our Strategy for Public Health in England*. London, The Stationery Office.

Department of Health (2011a) The Family Nurse Partnership Programme. www.dh.gov.uk/en/Publicationsand statistics/Publications/PublicationsPolicyAndGuidance/ DH_118530 (accessed 8 January 2013).

Department of Health (2011b) *Healthy Lives, Healthy People: A call to action on obesity in England*. The Central Office of Information. www.dh.gov.uk/en/Publication sandstatistics/Publications/PublicationsPolicyAndGuid ance/DH_130401 (accessed 8 January 2013).

Department of Health (2011c) *The NHS Outcomes Framework 2012/2013*. www.dh.gov.uk/prod_consum_dh/ groups/dh_digitalassets/@dh/@en/@ps/documents/ digitalasset/dh_123138.pdf (accessed 8 January 2013).

Department of Health (2012a) *Healthy Lives, Healthy People: Improving outcomes and supporting transparency. Part 1: A public health outcomes framework for England, 2013–2013*. www.dh.gov.uk/prod_consum_dh/groups/ dh_digitalassets/@dh/@en/documents/digitalasset/ dh_132559.pdf (accessed 8 January 2013).

Department of Health (2012b) Vitamin D: an essential nutrient for all . . . but who is at risk of vitamin D deficiency? Important information for healthcare professionals (leaflet).

Der G, Batty GD & Deary IJ (2006) Effect of breast feeding on intelligence in children: prospective study, sibling pairs analysis, and meta-analysis. *British Medical Journal*, **333**, 945.

De-Regil LM, Fernandez-Gaxiola AC, Dowswell T *et al.* (2010) Effects and safety of periconceptional folate supplementation for preventing birth defects. *Cochrane Database of Systematic Reviews*, CD007950.

Desai M, Byrne CD, Meeran K *et al.* (1997) Regulation of hepatic enzymes and insulin levels in offspring of rat dams fed a reduced-protein diet. *American Journal of Physiology*, **273**, G899–904.

Desoye G, Gauster M & Wadsack C (2011) Placental transport in pregnancy pathologies. *American Journal of Clinical Nutrition*, **94**, 1896S–902S.

Devenny A, Wassall H, Ninan T *et al.* (2004) Respiratory symptoms and atopy in children in Aberdeen: questionnaire studies of a defined school population repeated over 35 years. *British Medical Journal*, **329**, 489–90.

Devereux G, Barker RN & Seaton A (2002) Antenatal determinants of neonatal immune responses to allergens. *Clinical and Experimental Allergy*, **32**, 43–50.

Devereux G, Macdonald H & Hawrylowicz C (2009) Vitamin D and asthma: time for intervention? *American Journal of Respiratory and Critical Care Medicine*, **179**, 739–40.

Devereux G, Seaton A & Barker RN (2001) *in utero* priming of allergen-specific helper T cells. *Clinical and Experimental Allergy*, **31**, 1686–95.

Devereux G, Turner SW, Craig LC *et al.* (2006) Low maternal vitamin E intake during pregnancy is associated with asthma in 5-year-old children. *American Journal of Respiratory and Critical Care Medicine*, **174**, 499–507.

Dewey KG (2001a) Nutrition, growth, and complementary feeding of the breastfed infant. *Pediatric Clinics of North America*, **48**, 87–104.

Dewey KG (2001b) Maternal and fetal stress are associated with impaired lactogenesis in humans. *Journal of Nutrition*, **131**, 3012S–5S.

Dewey KG & Cohen RJ (2007) Does birth spacing affect maternal or child nutritional status? A systematic literature review. *Maternal & Child Nutrition*, **3**, 151–73.

Diabetes UK (2006) *Causes and risk factors*. www.diabetes. org.uk/Guide-to-diabetes/Introduction-to-diabetes/ Causes_and_Risk_Factors/ (accessed 8 January 2013).

Diabetes UK (2010) *Diabetes in the UK 2012: Key Statistics on Diabetes*. www.diabetes.org.uk/Documents/Reports/ Diabetes_in_the_UK_2010.pdf (accessed 8 January 2013).

Diabetes UK (2012) Diabetes in the UK 2012: Key Statistics on Diabetes. www.diabetes.org.uk/Documents/Reports/ Diabetes-in-the-UK-2012.pdf (accessed 11 January 2013).

Dicksved J, Floistrup H, Bergstrom A *et al.* (2007) Molecular fingerprinting of the fecal microbiota of children raised according to different lifestyles. *Applied and Environmental Microbiology*, **73**, 2284–9.

Dietz PM, England LJ, Shapiro-Mendoza CK *et al.* (2010) Infant morbidity and mortality attributable to prenatal smoking in the U.S. *American Journal of Preventive Medicine*, **39**, 45–52.

Dignam DM (1995) Understanding intimacy as experienced by breastfeeding women. *Health Care Women International*, **16**, 477–85.

Dobbing J (1971) Vulnerable periods of brain development. In: lipids, malnutrition & the developing brain. *Ciba Foundation Symposium*, 9–29.

Dobson B (1994) *Diet, Choice and Poverty: Social, Cultural and Nutritional Aspects of Food Consumption among Low-income Families (Family & Parenthood: Policy and Practice)*. Family Policy Studies Centre.

Dockerty JD, Herbison P, Skegg DC *et al.* (2007) Vitamin and mineral supplements in pregnancy and the risk of childhood acute lymphoblastic leukaemia: a case-control study. *BioMed Central Public Health,* **7,** 136.

Dodic M, Abouantoun T, O'Connor A *et al.* (2002) Programming effects of short prenatal exposure to dexamethasone in sheep. *Hypertension,* **40,** 729–34.

Dodic M, May CN, Wintour EM *et al.* (1998) An early prenatal exposure to excess glucocorticoid leads to hypertensive offspring in sheep. *Clinical Science,* **94,** 149–55.

Dolinoy DC, Weidman JR & Jirtle RL (2007) Epigenetic gene regulation: linking early developmental environment to adult disease. *Reproductive Toxicology,* **23,** 297–307.

Dolinoy DC, Weidman JR, Waterland RA (2006) Maternal genistein alters coat color and protects Avy mouse offspring from obesity by modifying the fetal epigenome. *Environmental Health Perspectives,* **114,** 567–72.

Doran L & Evers S (1997) Energy and nutrient inadequacies in the diets of low-income women who breast-feed. *Journal of the American Dietetic Association,* **97,** 1283–7.

dos Santos Silva I, De Stavola BL, Hardy RJ *et al.* (2004) Is the association of birth weight with premenopausal breast cancer risk mediated through childhood growth? *British Journal of Cancer,* **91,** 519–24.

Douglas JW (1950) The extent of breast feeding in Great Britain in 1946, with special reference to the health and survival of children. *Journal of Obstetrics and Gynaecology of the British Empire,* **57,** 335–61.

Dowler E & Calvert C (1995) *Nutrition and Diet in Lone Parent Families in London (Family & Parenthood: Policy & Practice).* Family Policy Studies Centre.

Dror DK & Allen LH (2008) Effect of vitamin B_{12} deficiency on neurodevelopment in infants: current knowledge and possible mechanisms. *Nutrition Reviews,* **66,** 250–5.

Drover JR, Hoffman DR, Castaneda YS *et al.* (2011) Cognitive function in 18-month-old term infants of the DIAMOND study: a randomized, controlled clinical trial with multiple dietary levels of docosahexaenoic acid. *Early Human Development,* **87,** 223–30.

Druet C & Ong KK (2008) Early childhood predictors of adult body composition. *Best Practice & Research: Clinical Endocrinology & Metabolism,* **22,** 489–502.

Du Toit G, Katz Y, Sasieni P *et al.* (2008) Early consumption of peanuts in infancy is associated with a low prevalence of peanut allergy. *Journal of Allergy and Clinical Immunology,* **122,** 984–91.

Dubos R (1987) *Mirage of Health: Utopias, Progress, and Biological Change.* New Brunswick, New Jersey, Rutgers University Press.

Dumortier O, Blondeau B, Duvillie B *et al.* (2007) Different mechanisms operating during different critical time-windows reduce rat fetal beta cell mass due to a maternal low-protein or low-energy diet. *Diabetologia,* **50,** 2495–503.

Dunger DB, Ong KK, Huxtable SJ *et al.* (1998) Association of the INS VNTR with size at birth. ALSPAC Study Team. Avon Longitudinal Study of Pregnancy and Childhood. *Nature Genetics,* **19,** 98–100.

Dunlop AL, Kramer MR, Hogue CJ *et al.* (2011) Racial disparities in preterm birth: an overview of the potential role of nutrient deficiencies. *Acta Obstetricia Gynecologica Scandinavica,* **90,** 1332–41.

Dunn GA & Bale TL (2009) Maternal high-fat diet promotes body length increases and insulin insensitivity in second-generation mice. *Endocrinology,* **150,** 4999–5009.

Dunstan JA, Mori TA, Barden A *et al.* (2003) Fish oil supplementation in pregnancy modifies neonatal allergen-specific immune responses and clinical outcomes in infants at high risk of atopy: a randomized, controlled trial. *Journal of Allergy and Clinical Immunology,* **112,** 1178–84.

Durnin JV (1991) Energy requirements of pregnancy. *Acta Paediatrica Scandinavica. Supplement,* **373,** 33–42.

Dwyer CM & Stickland NC (1992) The effects of maternal undernutrition on maternal and fetal serum insulin-like growth factors, thyroid hormones and cortisol in the guinea pig. *Journal of Developmental Physiology,* **18,** 303–13.

Dyer AR, Elliott P, Marmot M *et al.* (1996) Commentary: strength and importance of the relation of dietary salt to blood pressure. Intersalt Steering and Editorial Committee. *British Medical Journal,* **312,** 1661–4.

Edelbauer M, Loibichler C, Nentwich I *et al.* (2004) Maternally delivered nutritive allergens in cord blood and in placental tissue of term and preterm neonates. *Clinical and Experimental Allergy,* **34,** 189–93.

Edwards CR, Benediktsson R, Lindsay RS *et al.* (1996) 11 beta-Hydroxysteroid dehydrogenases: key enzymes in determining tissue-specific glucocorticoid effects. *Steroids,* **61,** 263–9.

Edwards LJ & McMillen IC (2001) Maternal undernutrition increases arterial blood pressure in the sheep fetus during late gestation. *Journal of Physiology,* **533,** 561–70.

Egger J, Carter CM, Graham PJ *et al.* (1985) Controlled trial of oligoantigenic treatment in the hyperkinetic syndrome. *Lancet,* **1,** 540–5.

Ekbom A (1998) Growing evidence that several human cancers may originate *in utero*. *Seminars in Cancer Biology,* **8,** 237–44.

Ekbom A, Hsieh CC, Lipworth L *et al.* (1997) Intrauterine environment and breast cancer risk in women: a population-based study. *Journal of the National Cancer Institute,* **89,** 71–6.

Ekbom A, Wuu J, Adami HO *et al.* (2000) Duration of gestation and prostate cancer risk in offspring. *Cancer Epidemiology, Biomarkers & Prevention,* **9,** 221–3.

El-Hajj Fuleihan G, Nabulsi M, Tamim H *et al.* (2006) Effect of vitamin D replacement on musculoskeletal parameters in school children: a randomized controlled trial. *Journal of Clinical Endocrinology and Metabolism,* **91**, 405–12.

Elliott P, Stamler J, Nichols R *et al.* (1996) Intersalt revisited: further analyses of 24 hour sodium excretion and blood pressure within and across populations. Intersalt Cooperative Research Group. *British Medical Journal,* **312**, 1249–53.

Ellis-Hutchings RG, Cherr GN, Hanna LA *et al.* (2009) The effects of marginal maternal vitamin A status on penta-brominated diphenyl ether mixture-induced alterations in maternal and conceptal vitamin A and fetal development in the Sprague-Dawley rat. *Birth Defects Research Part B–Developmental and Reproductive Toxicology,* **86**, 48–57.

Elmes MJ, Gardner DS & Langley-Evans SC (2007) Fetal exposure to a maternal low-protein diet is associated with altered left ventricular pressure response to ischaemia-reperfusion injury. *British Journal of Nutrition,* **98**, 93–100.

Elmes MJ, McMullen S, Gardner DS *et al.* (2008) Prenatal diet determines susceptibility to cardiac ischaemia-reperfusion injury following treatment with diethylmaleic acid and N-acetylcysteine. *Life Sciences,* **82**, 149–55.

Elwood PC, Pickering J, Gallacher JE *et al.* (2005) Long-term effect of breast feeding: cognitive function in the Caerphilly cohort. *Journal of Epidemiology and Community Health,* **59**, 130–3.

Emery JL, Scholey S & Taylor EM (1990) Decline in breast feeding. *Archives of Disease in Childhood,* **65**, 369–72.

Emmett P, North K & Noble S (2000) Types of drinks consumed by infants at 4 and 8 months of age: a descriptive study. The ALSPAC Study Team. *Public Health Nutrition,* **3**, 211–17.

Eriksson J (2001) Commentary: 'Early catch-up' growth is good for later health. *International Journal of Epidemiology,* **30**, 1330–1.

Eriksson J, Forsen T, Tuomilehto J *et al.* (2000) Fetal and childhood growth and hypertension in adult life. *Hypertension,* **36**, 790–4.

Eriksson JG, Forsen T, Tuomilehto J *et al.* (1999) Catch-up growth in childhood and death from coronary heart disease: longitudinal study. *British Medical Journal,* **318**, 427–31.

Eriksson S, Mellstrom D & Strandvik B (2009) Fatty acid pattern in serum is associated with bone mineralisation in healthy 8-year-old children. *British Journal of Nutrition,* **102**, 407–12.

Esmaillzadeh A & Azadbakht L (2006) Whole-grain intake, metabolic syndrome, and mortality in older adults. *American Journal of Clinical Nutrition,* **83**, 1439–40; author reply 1441–2.

European Food Safety Authority (EFSA) (2010) Scientific Opinion on Dietary Reference Values for fats, including saturated fatty acids, polyunsaturated fatty acids, monounsaturated fatty acids, trans fatty acids, and cholesterol. *EFSA Journal,* **8**, 1461.

EURO-PERISTAT (2008) *European Perinatal Health Report by the EURO-PERISTAT project in collaboration with SCPE, EUROCAT and EURONEOSTAT* http://www.sante.public.lu/publications/sante-fil-vie/petite-enfance/european-perinatal-health-report/european-perinatal-health-report.pdf (accessed 7 March 2013).

Evenhouse E & Reilly S (2005) Improved estimates of the benefits of breastfeeding using sibling comparisons to reduce selection bias. *Health Services Research,* **40**, 1781–802.

Fall C (2005) Fetal and Maternal Nutrition. In *Cardiovascular Disease: Diet, Nutrition and Emerging Risk Factors.* Ed. Stanner S. Oxford, Blackwell Publishing Ltd.: 177–95.

Fall CH, Borja JB, Osmond C *et al.* (2011) Infant-feeding patterns and cardiovascular risk factors in young adulthood: data from five cohorts in low- and middle-income countries. *International Journal of Epidemiology,* **40**, 47–62.

Fall CH, Osmond C, Barker DJ *et al.* (1995) Fetal and infant growth and cardiovascular risk factors in women. *British Medical Journal,* **310**, 428–32.

Fanaro S, Chierici R, Guerrini P *et al.* (2003) Intestinal microflora in early infancy: composition and development. *Acta Paediatrica Supplement,* **91**, 48–55.

Favier CF, Vaughan EE, De Vos WM *et al.* (2002) Molecular monitoring of succession of bacterial communities in human neonates. *Applied and Environmental Microbiology,* **68**, 219–26.

Fehily AM, Phillips KM & Yarnell JW (1984) Diet, smoking, social class, and body mass index in the Caerphilly Heart Disease Study. *American Journal of Clinical Nutrition,* **40**, 827–33.

Feigelman S (2007) The second year. In *Nelson Textbook of Pediatrics.* Ed. Kliegman, Behrman, Jenson & Stanton. Philadelphia, Saunders, Elsevier.

Feinberg AP, Ohlsson R & Henikoff S (2006) The epigenetic progenitor origin of human cancer. *Nature Reviews Genetics,* **7**, 21–33.

Ferezou-Viala J, Roy AF, Serougne C *et al.* (2007) Long-term consequences of maternal high-fat feeding on hypothalamic leptin sensitivity and diet-induced obesity in the offspring. *American Journal of Physiology – Regulatory, Integrative and Comparative Physiology,* **293**, R1056–62.

Ferlay J, Bray F, Pisani P *et al.* (2004) *Cancer Incidence, Mortality and Prevalence Worldwide.* Lyon, France, IARC CancerBase.

Fernandez-Twinn DS, Ekizoglou S, Wayman A *et al.* (2006) Maternal low protein diet programs cardiac beta-adrenergic response and signalling in 3 month old male offspring. *American Journal of Physiology – Regulatory, Integrative and Comparative Physiology*, **291**, R429–36.

Fewtrell M, Wilson DC, Booth I *et al.* (2011) When to wean? How good is the evidence for six months' exclusive breastfeeding? *British Medical Journal*, **342**, 209–12.

Fewtrell MS, Morgan JB, Duggan C *et al.* (2007) Optimal duration of exclusive breastfeeding: What is the evidence to support current recommendations? *American Journal of Clinical Nutrition*, **85**, 635S–8S.

Fewtrell MS, Prentice A, Jones SC *et al.* (1999) Bone mineralization and turnover in preterm infants at 8–12 years of age: the effect of early diet. *Journal of Bone and Mineral Research*, **14**, 810–20.

Fildes V (1982) The age of weaning in Britain 1500–1800. *Journal of Biosocial Science*, **14**, 223–40.

Fish EN (2008) The X-files in immunity: sex-based differences predispose immune responses. *Nature Reviews. Immunology*, **8**, 737–44.

Fisher D, Baird J, Payne L *et al.* (2006) Are infant size and growth related to burden of disease in adulthood? A systematic review of literature. *International Journal of Epidemiology*, **35**, 1196–210.

Fisk CM, Crozier SR, Inskip HM *et al.* (2011) Influences on the quality of young children's diets: the importance of maternal food choices. *British Journal of Nutrition*, **105**, 287–96.

Flour Fortification Initiative (FFI) (2010a) Effectiveness, Safety and Economics of Fortifying Flour with Folic Acid. www.FFInetwork.org (accessed 18 January 2013).

Flour Fortification Initiative (FFI) (2010b) Fortification Status – June 2010 www.sph.emory.edu/wheatflour/globalmap.php (accessed 18 January 2013).

Fomon S (2001) Infant feeding in the 20th century: formula and beikost. *Journal of Nutrition*, **131**, 409S-20S.

Foo LL, Quek SJ, Ng SA *et al.* (2005) Breastfeeding prevalence and practices among Singaporean Chinese, Malay and Indian mothers. *Health Promotion International*, **20**, 229–37.

Food and Agriculture Organization of the United Nations, World Health Organization & United Nations University (2004) *Human Energy Requirements. Report of a Joint FAO/WHO/UNU Expert Consultation: Rome, October (2001)*. www.fao.org/docrep/007/y5686e/y5686e00.htm#Contents (accessed 18 January 2013).

Food and Agriculture Organization of the United Nations & World Health Organization (2011) *Report of the joint FAO/WHO Expert consultation on the risks and benefits of fish consumption*. Rome, Food and Agriculture Organization of the United Nations; Geneva, World Health Organization.

Food and Drug Administration (1996) Food additives permitted for direct addition to food for human consumption; folic acid (Folacin), Final Rule. *Federal Register*, **61**, 8797–807.

Food Standards Agency (FSA) (2003) Intense sweeteners survey: your questions answered. www.food.gov.uk/multimedia/faq/intense_sweeteners/ (accessed 18 January 2013).

Ford L, Graham V, Wall A *et al.* (2006) Vitamin D concentrations in an UK inner-city multicultural outpatient population. *Annals of Clinical Biochemistry*, **43**, 468–73.

Ford MA, Bass MA, Turner LW *et al.* (2004) Past and recent physical activity and bone mineral density in college-aged women. *Journal of Strength and Conditioning Research*, **18**, 405–9.

Forman MR, Cantwell MM, Ronckers C *et al.* (2005) Through the looking glass at early-life exposures and breast cancer risk. *Cancer Investigation*, **23**, 609–24.

Forsdahl A (1977) Are poor living conditions in childhood and adolescence an important risk factor for arteriosclerotic heart disease? *British Journal of Preventative and Social Medicine*, **31**, 91–5.

Forsen T, Eriksson J, Tuomilehto J *et al.* (2000) The fetal and childhood growth of persons who develop type 2 diabetes. *Annals of Internal Medicine*, **133**, 176–82.

Forsen T, Eriksson JG, Tuomilehto J *et al.* (1999) Growth *in utero* and during childhood among women who develop coronary heart disease: longitudinal study. *British Medical Journal*, **319**, 1403–7.

Forsen T, Eriksson JG, Tuomilehto J *et al.* (1997) Mother's weight in pregnancy and coronary heart disease in a cohort of Finnish men: follow up study. *British Medical Journal*, **315**, 837–40.

Forsyth JS, Willatts P, Agostoni C *et al.* (2003) Long chain polyunsaturated fatty acid supplementation in infant formula and blood pressure in later childhood: follow up of a randomised controlled trial. *British Medical Journal*, **326**, 953.

Fraga MF, Ballestar E, Villar-Garea A *et al.* (2005) Loss of acetylation at Lys16 and trimethylation at Lys20 of histone H4 is a common hallmark of human cancer. *Nature Genetics*, **37**, 391–400.

Franco MC, Akamine EH, Di Marco GS *et al.* (2003) NADPH oxidase and enhanced superoxide generation in intrauterine undernourished rats: involvement of the renin-angiotensin system. *Cardiovascular Research*, **59**, 767–75.

Franco MC, Arruda RM, Dantas AP *et al.* (2002) Intrauterine undernutrition: expression and activity of the endothelial nitric oxide synthase in male and female adult offspring. *Cardiovascular Research*, **56**, 145–53.

Frank NY, Schatton T & Frank MH (2010) The therapeutic promise of the cancer stem cell concept. *Journal of Clinical Investigation*, **120**, 41–50.

Frankel S, Elwood P, Sweetnam P *et al.* (1996) Birthweight, adult risk factors and incident coronary heart disease: the Caerphilly Study. *Public Health*, **110**, 139–43.

Franks PW, Hanson RL, Knowler WC *et al.* (2010) Childhood obesity, other cardiovascular risk factors, and premature death. *New England Journal of Medicine*, **362**, 485–93.

Franks PW, Looker HC, Kobes S *et al.* (2006) Gestational glucose tolerance and risk of type 2 diabetes in young Pima Indian offspring. *Diabetes*, **55**, 460–5.

Franzek EJ, Sprangers N, Janssens AC, *et al.* (2008) Prenatal exposure to the 1944–45 Dutch 'hunger winter' and addiction later in life. *Addiction*, **103**, 433–8.

Fraser A, Tilling K, Macdonald-Wallis C *et al.* (2010) Association of maternal weight gain in pregnancy with offspring obesity and metabolic and vascular traits in childhood. *Circulation*, **121**, 2557–64.

Frayling TM, Timpson NJ, Weedon MN *et al.* (2007) A common variant in the FTO gene is associated with body mass index and predisposes to childhood and adult obesity. *Science*, **316**, 889–94.

Frayn K & Stanner S (2005) The aetiology and epidemiology of cardiovascular disease. In *Cardiovascular Disease: Diet, Nutrition and Emerging Risk Factors*. Ed. Stanner S. Oxford, Blackwell Publishing Ltd.

Freeman V, van't Hof M & Haschke F (2000) Patterns of milk and food intake in infants from birth to age 36 months: the Euro-growth study. *Journal of Pediatric Gastroenterology and Nutrition*, **31** Suppl 1, S76–85.

Frisancho AR, Matos J, Leonard WR *et al.* (1985) Developmental and nutritional determinants of pregnancy outcome among teenagers. *American Journal of Physical Anthropology*, **66**, 247–61.

Friso S, Choi SW, Girelli D *et al.* (2002) A common mutation in the 5,10-methylenetetrahydrofolate reductase gene affects genomic DNA methylation through an interaction with folate status. *Proceedings of the National Academy of Sciences of the USA*, **99**, 5606–11.

Gabory A, Attig L & Junien C (2009) Sexual dimorphism in environmental epigenetic programming. *Molecular and Cellular Endocrinology*, **304**, 8–18.

Gale CR, Javaid MK, Robinson SM *et al.* (2007) Maternal size in pregnancy and body composition in children. *Journal of Clinical Endocrinology and Metabolism*, **92**, 3904–11.

Gale CR, Martyn CN, Kellingray S *et al.* (2001) Intrauterine programming of adult body composition. *Journal of Clinical Endocrinology and Metabolism*, **86**, 267–72.

Gale CR, Martyn CN, Marriott LD *et al.* (2009) Dietary patterns in infancy and cognitive and neuropsychological function in childhood. *Journal of Child Psychology and Psychiatry*, **50**, 816–23.

Gale CR, Robinson SM, Harvey NC *et al.* (2008) Maternal vitamin D status during pregnancy and child outcomes. *European Journal of Clinical Nutrition*, **62**, 68–77.

Galler JR & Tonkiss J (1991) Prenatal protein malnutrition and maternal behavior in Sprague-Dawley rats. *Journal of Nutrition*, **121**, 762–9.

Gambling L, Charania Z, Hannah L *et al.* (2002) Effect of iron deficiency on placental cytokine expression and fetal growth in the pregnant rat. *Biology of Reproduction*, **66**, 516–23.

Gambling L, Czopek A, Andersen HS *et al.* (2009) Fetal iron status regulates maternal iron metabolism during pregnancy in the rat. *American Journal of Physiology*, **296**, R1063–R70.

Gambling L, Danzeisen R, Gair S *et al.* (2001) Effect of iron deficiency on placental transfer of iron and expression of iron transport proteins in vivo and in vitro. *Biochemical Journal*, **356**, 883–9.

Gambling L, Dunford S, Wallace DI *et al.* (2003) Iron deficiency during pregnancy affects postnatal blood pressure in the rat. *Journal of Physiology*, **552**, 603–10.

Gambling L & McArdle HJ (2004) Iron, copper and fetal development. *Proceedings of the Nutrition Society*, **63**, 553–62.

Gamborg M, Byberg L, Rasmussen F *et al.* (2007) Birth weight and systolic blood pressure in adolescence and adulthood: meta-regression analysis of sex- and age-specific results from 20 Nordic studies. *American Journal of Epidemiology*, **166**, 634–45.

Gardner DS, Tingey K, Van Bon BW *et al.* (2005) Programming of glucose-insulin metabolism in adult sheep after maternal undernutrition. *American Journal of Physiology – Regulatory, Integrative and Comparative Physiology*, **289**, R947–54.

Garofalo C & Surmacz E (2006) Leptin and cancer. *Journal of Cellular Physiology*, **207**, 12–22.

Garofano A, Czernichow P & Breant B (1999) Effect of ageing on beta-cell mass and function in rats malnourished during the perinatal period. *Diabetologia*, **42**, 711–18.

Gauguier D, Bihoreau MT, Picon L *et al.* (1991) Insulin secretion in adult rats after intrauterine exposure to mild hyperglycemia during late gestation. *Diabetes*, **40** Suppl 2, 109–14.

Geary MP, Pringle PJ, Rodeck CH *et al.* (2003) Sexual dimorphism in the growth hormone and insulin-like growth factor axis at birth. *Journal of Clinical Endocrinology and Metabolism*, **88**, 3708–14.

Geary N (2004) Is the control of fat ingestion sexually differentiated? *Physiology and Behavior*, **83**, 659–71.

Georgieff MK (2007) Nutrition and the developing brain: nutrient priorities and measurement. *American Journal of Clinical Nutrition*, **85**, 614S–20S.

Giammarioli S, Sanzini E, Ambruzzi AM *et al.* (2002) Nutrient intake of Italian women during lactation. *International Journal for Vitamin and Nutrition Research*, **72**, 329–35.

Gilbert JS, Lang AL, Grant AR *et al.* (2005) Maternal nutrient restriction in sheep: hypertension and decreased nephron number in offspring at 9 months of age. *Journal of Physiology*, **565**, 137–47.

Gilbert JS & Nijland MJ (2008) Sex differences in the developmental origins of hypertension and cardiorenal disease. *American Journal of Physiology – Regulatory, Integrative and Comparative Physiology*, **295**, R1941–52.

Gilchrist JM, Moore MB, Andres A (2010) *et al.* Ultrasonographic patterns of reproductive organs in infants fed soy formula: comparisons to infants fed breast milk and milk formula. *Journal of Pediatrics*, **156**, 215–20.

Gillman MW, Oakey H, Baghurst PA *et al.* (2010) Effect of treatment of gestational diabetes mellitus on obesity in the next generation. *Diabetes Care*, **33**, 964–8.

Gillman MW, Rifas-Shiman S, Berkey CS *et al.* (2003) Maternal gestational diabetes, birth weight, and adolescent obesity. *Pediatrics*, **111**, e221–6.

Gilsanz V & Nelson DA (2003) Childhood and adolescence. In *Primer on the Metabolic Bone Diseases and Disorders of Mineral Metabolism*. Ed. Favus MJ. Washington, American Society for Bone and Mineral Research.

Ginde AA, Liu MC & Camargo CA, Jr. (2009) Demographic differences and trends of vitamin D insufficiency in the US population, 1988–2004. *Archives of Internal Medicine*, **169**, 626–32.

Giraud GD, Louey S, Jonker S *et al.* (2006) Cortisol stimulates cell cycle activity in the cardiomyocyte of the sheep fetus. *Endocrinology*, **147**, 3643–9.

Glazier JD, Atkinson DE, Thornburg KL *et al.* (1992) Gestational changes in Ca2+ transport across rat placenta and mRNA for calbindin9K and Ca(2+)-ATPase. *American Journal of Physiology*, **263**, R930–5.

Glazier M (1933) Advantages of strained solids in the early months of infancy. *Journal of Paediatrics*, **3**, 883–90.

Glinoer D, De Nayer P, Delange F *et al.* (1995) A randomised trial for the treatment of mild iodine deficiency during pregnancy: maternal and neonatal effects. *Journal of Clinical Endocrinology and Metabolism*, **80**, 258–69.

GLOBOCAN (2002) *Cancer Incidence, Mortality and Prevalence Worldwide*. Lyon, France, CancerBase.

Gluckman PD, Cutfield W, Hofman P *et al.* (2005) The fetal, neonatal, and infant environments: the long-term consequences for disease risk. *Early Human Development*, **81**, 51–9.

Gluckman PD, Hanson MA, Cooper C *et al.* (2008) Effect of *in utero* and early-life conditions on adult health and disease. *New England Journal of Medicine*, **359**, 61–73.

Godfrey K, Walker-Bone K, Robinson S *et al.* (2001) Neonatal bone mass: influence of parental birthweight, maternal smoking, body composition, and activity during pregnancy. *Journal of Bone and Mineral Research*, **16**, 1694–703.

Godfrey KM, Barker DJ & Osmond C (1994) Disproportionate fetal growth and raised IgE concentration in adult life. *Clinical and Experimental Allergy*, **24**, 641–8.

Goh YI, Bollano E, Einarson TR *et al.* (2006) Prenatal multivitamin supplementation and rates of congenital anomalies: a meta-analysis. *Journal of Obstetrics and Gynaecology*, **28**, 680–9.

Golub MS, Hogrefe CE, Germann SL *et al.* (2006) Behavioral consequences of developmental iron deficiency in infant rhesus monkeys. *Neurotoxicology and Teratology*, **28**, 3–17.

Goodenday LS & Gordon GS (1971) No risk from vitamin D in pregnancy. *Annals of Internal Medicine*, **75**, 807–8.

Graafmans WC, Richardus JH, Borsboom GJ *et al.* (2002) Birth weight and perinatal mortality: a comparison of 'optimal' birth weight in seven Western European countries. *Epidemiology*, **13**, 569–74.

Grantham-McGregor S, Cheung YB, Cueto S *et al.* (2007) Developmental potential in the first 5 years for children in developing countries. *Lancet*, **369**, 60–70.

Grayson BE, Allen SE, Billes SK *et al.* (2006) Prenatal development of hypothalamic neuropeptide systems in the nonhuman primate. *Neuroscience*, **143**, 975–86.

Grayson BE, Kievit P, Smith MS *et al.* (2010) Critical determinants of hypothalamic appetitive neuropeptide development and expression: species considerations. *Frontiers in Neuroendocrinology*, **31**, 16–31.

Grayson BE, Levasseur PR, Williams SM *et al.* (2010) Changes in melanocortin expression and inflammatory pathways in fetal offspring of nonhuman primates fed a high-fat diet. *Endocrinology*, **151**, 1622–32.

Green H, McGinnity A, Meltzer H *et al.* (2005) *Mental Health of Children and Young People in Great Britain, 2004*. Basingstoke, Palgrave Macmillan.

Greer FR (2008) 25-Hydroxyvitamin D: functional outcomes in infants and young children. *American Journal of Clinical Nutrition*, **88**, 529S–33S.

Greer FR, Hollis BW & Napoli JL (1984) High concentrations of vitamin D2 in human milk associated with pharmacologic doses of vitamin D2. *Journal of Pediatrics*, **105**, 61–4.

Greer FR & Marshall S (1989) Bone mineral content, serum vitamin D metabolite concentrations, and ultraviolet B light exposure in infants fed human milk with and without vitamin D2 supplements. *Journal of Pediatrics*, **114**, 204–12.

Greer FR, Searcy JE, Levin RS *et al.* (1982) Bone mineral content and serum 25-hydroxyvitamin D concentrations in breast-fed infants with and without supplemental vitamin D: one-year follow-up. *Journal of Pediatrics*, **100**, 919–22.

Greer FR, Sicherer SH & Burks AW (2008) Effects of early nutritional interventions on the development of atopic disease in infants and children: the role of maternal dietary restriction, breastfeeding, timing of introduction of complementary foods, and hydrolyzed formulas. *Pediatrics*, **121**, 183–91.

Gregory J, Lowe S, Bates CJ *et al.* (2000) *National Diet and Nutrition Survey: Young People Aged 4–18 Years. Vol. 1. Report of the Diet and Nutrition Survey*. London, The Stationery Office.

Gregory JR, Collins DL, Davies PSW *et al.* (1995) *National Diet and Nutrition Survey: children aged 1.5–4.5 years. Volume I: report of the diet and nutrition survey*. London, HMSO.

Griffiths LJ, Tate AR & Dezateux C (2005) The contribution of parental and community ethnicity to breastfeeding practices: evidence from the Millennium Cohort Study. *International Journal of Epidemiology*, **34**, 1378–86.

Griffiths LJ, Tate AR & Dezateux C (2007) Do early infant feeding practices vary by maternal ethnic group? *Public Health Nutrition*, **10**, 957–64.

Grigore D, Ojeda NB & Alexander BT (2008) Sex differences in the fetal programming of hypertension. *Gender Medicine*, **5** Suppl A, S121–32.

Grigore D, Ojeda NB, Robertson EB *et al.* (2007) Placental insufficiency results in temporal alterations in the renin angiotensin system in male hypertensive growth restricted offspring. *American Journal of Physiology – Regulatory, Integrative and Comparative Physiology*, **293**, R804–11.

Grimshaw KE, Allen K, Edwards CA *et al.* (2009) Infant feeding and allergy prevention: a review of current knowledge and recommendations. A EuroPrevall state of the art paper. *Allergy*, **64**, 1407–16.

Grote V, von Kries R, Closa-Monasterolo R, *et al.* (2010) Protein intake and growth in the first 24 months of life. European Childhood Obesity Trial Study Group. *Journal of Pediatric Gastroenterology and Nutrition*, **51**(Supp 3), S117–18.

Grove KL, Grayson BE, Glavas MM *et al.* (2005) Development of metabolic systems. *Physiology and Behaviour*, **86**, 646–60.

Grummer-Strawn LM (1996) The effect of changes in population characteristics on breastfeeding trends in fifteen developing countries. *International Journal of Epidemiology*, **25**, 94–102.

Grummer-Strawn LM, Scanlon KS & Fein SB (2008) Infant feeding and feeding transitions during the first year of life. *Pediatrics*, **122** Suppl 2, S36–42.

Grundy J, Matthews S, Bateman B *et al.* (2002) Rising prevalence of allergy to peanut in children: Data from 2 sequential cohorts. *Journal of Allergy and Clinical Immunology*, **110**, 784–9.

Guelinckx I, Devlieger R, Beckers K *et al.* (2008) Maternal obesity: pregnancy complications, gestational weight gain and nutrition. *Obesity Review*, **9**, 140–50.

Gunnell D, Okasha M, Smith GD *et al.* (2001) Height, leg length, and cancer risk: a systematic review. *Epidemiologic Reviews*, **23**, 313–42.

Gunnell DJ, Davey Smith G, Frankel S *et al.* (1998) Childhood leg length and adult mortality: follow up of the Carnegie (Boyd Orr) Survey of Diet and Health in Pre-war Britain. *Journal of Epidemiology and Community Health*, **52**, 142–52.

Gupta A, Srinivasan M, Thamadilok S *et al.* (2009) Hypothalamic alterations in fetuses of high fat diet-fed obese female rats. *Journal of Endocrinology*, **200**, 293–300.

Gupta R, Sheikh A, Strachan DP *et al.* (2004) Burden of allergic disease in the UK: secondary analyses of national databases. *Clinical and Experimental Allergy*, **34**, 520–6.

Haddad JG Jr., Boisseau V & Avioli LV (1971) Placental transfer of vitamin D3 and 25-hydroxycholecalciferol in the rat. *Journal of Laboratory and Clinical Medicine*, **77**, 908–15.

Haggarty P (2004) Effect of placental function on fatty acid requirements during pregnancy. *European Journal of Clinical Nutrition*, **58**, 1559–70.

Haggarty P (2007) B-vitamins, genotype and disease causality. *Proceedings of the Nutrition Society*, **66**, 539–47.

Haggarty P (2010) Fatty acid supply to the human fetus. *Annual Review of Nutrition*, **30**, 237–55.

Haggarty P, Campbell DM, Duthie S *et al.* (2008) Folic acid use in pregnancy and embryo selection. *British Journal of Obstetrics and Gynaecology*, **115**, 851–6.

Haggarty P, Campbell DM, Duthie S *et al.* (2009) Diet and deprivation in pregnancy. *British Journal of Nutrition*, **102**, 1487–97.

Haider BA & Bhutta ZA (2006) Multiple-micronutrient supplementation for women during pregnancy. *Cochrane Database of Systematic Reviews*, CD004905.

Haland G, Carlsen KC, Sandvik L *et al.* (2006) Reduced lung function at birth and the risk of asthma at 10 years of age. *New England Journal of Medicine*, **355**, 1682–9.

Hales CN & Barker DJ (1992) Type 2 (non-insulin-dependent) diabetes mellitus: the thrifty phenotype hypothesis. *Diabetologia*, **35**, 595–601.

Hales CN, Barker DJ, Clark PM *et al.* (1991) Fetal and infant growth and impaired glucose tolerance at age 64. *British Medical Journal*, **303**, 1019–22.

Hall JE, Brands MW & Henegar JR (1999) Angiotensin II and long-term arterial pressure regulation: the overriding dominance of the kidney. *Journal of the American Society of Nephrology*, **10** Suppl 12, S258–65.

Hamilton JK, Odrobina E, Yin J *et al.* (2010) Maternal insulin sensitivity during pregnancy predicts infant weight gain and adiposity at 1 year of age. *Obesity*, **18**, 340–6.

Hamlyn B, Brooker S, Oleinikova K *et al.* (2002) *Infant Feeding Survey 2000*. London, The Stationery Office.

Han HC, Austin KJ, Nathanielsz PW *et al.* (2004) Maternal nutrient restriction alters gene expression in the ovine fetal heart. *Journal of Physiology*, **558**, 111–21.

Hannah ML (2000) *Prescriber Update No. 20:22–26. Peanut Allergy.* www.medsafe.govt.nz/profs/PUarticles/peanut.htm (accessed 8 January 2013).

HAPO Study Cooperative Research Group (2009) Hyperglycemia and Adverse Pregnancy Outcome (HAPO) Study: associations with neonatal anthropometrics. *Diabetes*, **58**, 453–9.

Harder T, Plagemann A, Rohde W *et al.* (1998) Syndrome X-like alterations in adult female rats due to neonatal insulin treatment. *Metabolism*, **47**, 855–62.

Harding JE (2001) The nutritional basis of the fetal origins of adult disease. *International Journal of Epidemiology*, **30**, 15–23.

Harding R & Bocking A (2001) *Fetal Growth and Development.* Cambridge, Cambridge University Press.

Harmsen HJ, Wildeboer-Veloo AC, Raangs GC *et al.* (2000) Analysis of intestinal flora development in breast-fed and formula-fed infants by using molecular identification and detection methods. *Journal of Pediatric Gastroenterology and Nutrition*, **30**, 61–7.

Harris WS, Connor WE & Lindsey S (1984) Will dietary omega-3 fatty acids change the composition of human milk? *American Journal of Clinical Nutrition*, **40**, 780–5.

Harvey N & Cooper C (2004a) Disease prevention: osteoporosis and hip fracture. In *Public Health Nutrition.* Ed. Gibney M, Margetts B, Kearney J & Arab L. Oxford, Blackwell Publishing Ltd.: 357–69.

Harvey N & Cooper C (2004b) The developmental origins of osteoporotic fracture. *Journal of the British Menopause Society*, **10**, 14–29.

Harvey NC, Cole ZA, Crozier SR *et al.* (2012) Physical activity, calcium intake and childhood bone mineral: a population-based cross-sectional study. *Osteoporosis International*, **23**, 121–30.

Harvey NC, Javaid MK, Bishop N *et al.* (2012) MAVIDOS Maternal Vitamin D Osteoporosis Study: study protocol for a randomized controlled trial. *Trials*, **13**, 13.

Harvey NC, Javaid MK, Arden NK *et al.* (2010) Maternal predictors of neonatal bone size and geometry: the Southampton Women's Survey. *Journal of Developmental Origins of Health and Disease*, **1**, 35–41.

Harvey NC, Javaid MK, Poole JR *et al.* (2008) Paternal skeletal size predicts intrauterine bone mineral accrual. *Journal of Clinical Endocrinology and Metabolism*, **93**, 1676–81.

Hattersley AT, Beards F, Ballantyne E *et al.* (1998) Mutations in the glucokinase gene of the fetus result in reduced birth weight. *Nature Genetics*, **19**, 268–70.

Hauger MS, Gibbons L, Vik T *et al.* (2008) Prepregnancy weight status and the risk of adverse pregnancy outcome. *Acta Obstetricia Gynecologica Scandinavica*, **87**, 953–9.

Hawkesworth S, Prentice AM, Fulford AJ *et al.* (2009) Maternal protein-energy supplementation does not affect adolescent blood pressure in the Gambia. *International Journal of Epidemiology*, **38**, 119–27.

Hawkesworth S, Walker CG, Sawo Y *et al.* (2011) Nutritional supplementation during pregnancy and offspring cardiovascular disease risk in the Gambia. *American Journal of Clinical Nutrition*, **94**, 1853–60S.

Hawkins P, Steyn C, McGarrigle HH *et al.* (1999) Effect of maternal nutrient restriction in early gestation on development of the hypothalamic-pituitary-adrenal axis in fetal sheep at 0.8–0.9 of gestation. *Journal of Endocrinology*, **163**, 553–61.

Hawkins P, Steyn C, Ozaki T *et al.* (2000) Effect of maternal undernutrition in early gestation on ovine fetal blood pressure and cardiovascular reflexes. *American Journal of Physiology – Regulatory, Integrative and Comparative Physiology*, **279**, R340–8.

Haydon O (1919) The Midwife. *British Journal of Nursing*, **230**.

Hayes RB, Ziegler RG, Gridley G *et al.* (1999) Dietary factors and risks for prostate cancer among blacks and whites in the United States. *Cancer Epidemiology, Biomarkers & Prevention*, **8**, 25–34.

Health Council of the Netherlands (2008a) *Towards an adequate intake of vitamin D.* The Hague, Health Council of the Netherlands.

Health Council of the Netherlands (2008b) *Towards maintaining an optimum iodine intake.* The Hague, Health Council of the Netherlands.

Health Council of the Netherlands (2012) Evaluation of dietary reference values for vitamin D. The Hague: Health Council of the Netherlands, Publication no. 2012/15E.

Health & Social Care Information Centre (2012a) National Child Measurement Programme: England 2011/12 school year. www.ic.nhs.uk/ncmp (accessed 16 January 2013).

Health & Social Care Information Centre (2012b) Health Survey for England – 2011, Health, Social Care and Lifestyles. www.ic.nhs.uk/catalogue/PUB09300 (accessed 16 January 2013).

Heaney RP (2004) Functional indices of vitamin D status and ramifications of vitamin D deficiency. *American Journal of Clinical Nutrition*, **80**, 1706S–9S.

Heaney RP (2006) Normal/abnormal vitamin D physiology. In *Contemporary Diagnosis and Treatment of Vitamin D-Related Disorders.* American Society for Bone and Mineral Research,. Virginia, USA.

Heaney RP, Dowell MS, Hale CA & Bendich A (2003) Calcium absorption varies within the reference range for serum 25-hydroxyvitamin D. *Journal of the American College of Nutrition*, **22**, 142–6.

Heddleston JM, Li Z, Lathia JD *et al.* (2010) Hypoxia inducible factors in cancer stem cells. *British Journal of Cancer*, **102**, 789–95.

Heijmans BT, Tobi EW, Stein AD *et al.* (2008) Persistent epigenetic differences associated with prenatal exposure to famine in humans. *Proceedings of the National Academy of Sciences of the USA*, **105**, 17046–9.

Heinig MJ, Follett JR, Ishii KD *et al.* (2006) Barriers to compliance with infant-feeding recommendations among low-income women. *Journal of Human Lactation*, **22**, 27–38.

Hemachandra AH, Howards PP, Furth SL *et al.* (2007) Birth weight, postnatal growth, and risk for high blood pressure at 7 years of age: results from the Collaborative Perinatal Project. *Pediatrics*, **119**, e1264–e70.

Hemachandra AH & Klebanoff MA (2006) Use of serial ultrasound to identify periods of fetal growth restriction in relation to neonatal anthropometry. *American Journal of Human Biology*, **18**, 791–7.

Henderson L, Irving K, Gregory J *et al.* (2003) *The National Diet & Nutrition Survey: adults aged 19 to 64 years. Vitamin and mineral intake and urinary analytes.* London, The Stationery Office. www.food.gov.uk/multimedia/pdfs/ndnsv3.pdf (accessed 18 January 2013).

Hernandez CJ, Beaupre GS & Carter DR (2003) A theoretical analysis of the relative influences of peak BMD, age-related bone loss and menopause on the development of osteoporosis. *Osteoporosis International*, **14**, 843–7.

Hernell O (2011) Human milk vs. cow's milk and the evolution of infant formulas. *Nestlé Nutrition workshop series. Paediatric programme*, **67**, 17–28.

Hertrampf E & Cortes F (2004) Folic acid fortification of wheat flour: Chile. *Nutrition Reviews*, **62**, S44–8; discussion S49.

Heslehurst N (2011) Identifying 'at risk' women and the impact of maternal obesity on National Health Service maternity services. *Proceedings of the Nutrition Society*, **70**, 439–49.

Heslehurst N, Bell R & Rankin J (2011) Tackling maternal obesity: the challenge for public health. *Perspectives in Public Health*, **131**, 161–2.

Heslehurst N, Moore H, Rankin J *et al.* (2011) How can maternity services be developed to effectively address maternal obesity? A qualitative study. *Midwifery*, **27**, e170–7.

Heslehurst N, Rankin J, Wilkinson JR *et al.* (2010) A nationally representative study of maternal obesity in England, UK: trends in incidence and demographic inequalities in 619 323 births, 1989–2007. *International Journal of Obesity*, **34**, 420–8.

Hess SY, Zimmermann MB, Brogli S *et al.* (2001) A national survey of iron and folate status in pregnant women in Switzerland. *International Journal for Vitamin and Nutrition Research*, **71**, 268–73.

Hetzel BS (2000) Iodine and neuropsychological development. *Journal of Nutrition*, **130**, 493–5S.

Hex N, Bartlett C, Wright D *et al.* (2012) Estimating the current and future costs of Type 1 and Type 2 diabetes in the UK, including direct health costs and indrect societal and productivity costs. *Diabetic Medicine*, **29**, 855–62.

Hibbeln JR, Davis JM, Steer C *et al.* (2007) Maternal seafood consumption in pregnancy and neurodevelopmental outcomes in childhood (ALSPAC study): an observational cohort study. *Lancet*, **369**, 578–85.

Hikino S, Nakayama H, Yamamoto J *et al.* (2001) Food allergy and atopic dermatitis in low birthweight infants during early childhood. *Acta Paediatrica*, **90**, 850–5.

Hilakivi-Clarke L & de Assis S (2006) Fetal origins of breast cancer. *Trends in Endocrinology and Metabolism*, **17**, 340–8.

Hillier TA, Pedula KL, Schmidt MM (2007) *et al.* Childhood obesity and metabolic imprinting: the ongoing effects of maternal hyperglycemia. *Diabetes Care*, **30**, 2287–92.

Hirschman C & Hendershot GE (1979) Trends in breast feeding among American mothers. *Vital Health Statistics, series 23*, **23**, 1–39.

Hjalgrim LL, Rostgaard K, Hjalgrim H *et al.* (2004) Birth weight and risk for childhood leukemia in Denmark, Sweden, Norway, and Iceland. *Journal of the National Cancer Institute*, **96**, 1549–56.

Hjalgrim LL, Westergaard T, Rostgaard K *et al.* (2003) Birth weight as a risk factor for childhood leukemia: a meta-analysis of 18 epidemiologic studies. *American Journal of Epidemiology*, **158**, 724–35.

Hochner H, Friedlander Y, Calderon-Margalit R (2012) Associations of maternal prepregnancy body mass index and gestational weight gain with adult offspring cardiometabolic risk factors, the Jerusalem Perinatal Family Follow-up study. *Circulation*, **25**, 1381–9.

Hoefer C & Hardy MC (1929) Later development of breast fed and artificially fed infants. *JAMA*, **92**, 615–9.

Hoek HW, Susser E, Buck KA *et al.* (1996) Schizoid personality disorder after prenatal exposure to famine. *American Journal of Psychiatry*, **153**, 1637–9.

Hofmeyr GJ, Duley L & Atallah A (2007) Dietary calcium supplementation for prevention of pre-eclampsia and related problems: a systematic review and commentary. *British Journal of Obstetrics and Gynaecology*, **114**, 933–43.

Hogstrom M, Nordstrom P & Nordstrom A (2007) n-3 fatty acids are positively associated with peak bone mineral density and bone accrual in healthy men: the NO2 Study. *American Journal of Clinical Nutrition*, **85**, 803–7.

Holden C (2005) Sex and the suffering brain. *Science*, **308**, 1574.

Holemans K, Caluwaerts S, Poston L *et al.* (2004) Diet-induced obesity in the rat: a model for gestational diabetes mellitus. *American Journal of Obstetrics and Gynaecology*, **190**, 858–65.

Holemans K, Gerber R, Meurrens K, *et al.* (1999) Maternal food restriction in the second half of pregnancy affects vascular function but not blood pressure of rat female offspring. *British Journal of Nutrition*, **81**, 73–9.

Holgate ST, Church MK & Lichtenstein LM (2006) *Allergy*. Philadelphia, USA, Mosby Elseview.

Holgate ST, Davies DE, Lackie PM *et al.* (2000) Epithelial-mesenchymal interactions in the pathogenesis of asthma. *Journal of Allergy and Clinical Immunology*, **105**, 193–204.

Hollis BW & Wagner CL (2004) Vitamin D requirements during lactation: high-dose maternal supplementation as therapy to prevent hypovitaminosis D for both the mother and the nursing infant. *American Journal of Clinical Nutrition*, **80**, 1752–8S.

Holt RI (2002) Fetal programming of the growth hormone-insulin-like growth factor axis. *Trends in Endocrinology and Metabolism*, **13**, 392–7.

Hoppe CC, Evans RG, Bertram JF *et al.* (2007) Effects of dietary protein restriction on nephron number in the mouse. *American Journal of Physiology – Regulatory, Integrative and Comparative Physiology*, **292**, R1768–74.

Hornstra G (2000) Essential fatty acids in mothers and their neonates. *American Journal of Clinical Nutrition*, **71**, 1262–9S.

Horta BL, Bahl R, Martines JC *et al.* (2007) *Evidence on the Long-Term Effects of Breastfeeding: Systematic Reviews and Meta-Analyses*. Geneva, World Health Organization.

Horvath TL & Bruning JC (2006) Developmental programming of the hypothalamus: a matter of fat. *Nature Medicine*, **12**, 52–3; discussion 53.

Houdijk EC, Engelbregt MJ, Popp-Snijders C *et al.* (2000) Endocrine regulation and extended follow up of longitudinal growth in intrauterine growth-retarded rats. *Journal of Endocrinology*, **166**, 599–608.

Howie PW & McNeilly AS (1980) The initiation of lactation. *Midwife Health Visit Community Nurse*, **16**, 142–7.

Howlader N, Noone AM, Krapcho M *et al.* (2012) SEER Cancer Statistics Review. 1975–2009 (Vintage 2009 Populations), Bethesda, MD, National Cancer Institute. http://seer.cancer.gov/csr/1975_2009_pops09/ (accessed 21 January 2013).

Hoyme HE, May PA, Kalberg WO *et al.* (2005) A practical clinical approach to diagnosis of fetal alcohol spectrum disorders: clarification of the 1996 Institute of Medicine criteria. *Pediatrics*, **115**, 39–47.

Huang Y, Yan X, Zhao JX *et al.* (2010) Maternal obesity induces fibrosis in fetal myocardium of sheep. *American Journal of Physiology – Endocrinology and Metabolism*, **299**, E968–75.

Huxley R, Neil A & Collins R (2002) Unravelling the fetal origins hypothesis: is there really an inverse association between birthweight and subsequent blood pressure? *Lancet*, **360**, 659–65.

Huxley R, Owen CG, Whincup PH *et al.* (2007) Is birth weight a risk factor for ischemic heart disease in later life? *American Journal of Clinical Nutrition*, **85**, 1244–50.

Huxley RR, Shiell AW & Law CM (2000) The role of size at birth and postnatal catch-up growth in determining systolic blood pressure: a systematic review of the literature. *Journal of Hypertension*, **18**, 815–31.

Hypponen E & Power C (2007) Hypovitaminosis D in British adults at age 45y: nationwide cohort study of dietary and lifestyle predictors. *American Journal of Clinical Nutrition*, **85**, 860–8.

Hypponen E, Sovio U, Wjst M *et al.* (2004) Infant vitamin D supplementation and allergic conditions in adulthood: northern Finland birth cohort 1966. *Annals of the New York Academy of Sciences*, **1037**, 84–95.

Hytten FE (1974) Weight gain in pregnancy. In *Clinical Physiology in Obstetrics*. Ed. Hytten FE & Chamberlain JG. Oxford, Blackwell Scientific Publications: 129–233.

Ibanez L, Ong K, Dunger DB *et al.* (2006) Early development of adiposity and insulin resistance after catch-up weight gain in small-for-gestational-age children. *Journal of Clinical Endocrinology and Metabolism*, **91**, 2153–8.

Igosheva N, Taylor PD, Poston L *et al.* (2007) Prenatal stress in the rat results in increased blood pressure responsiveness to stress and enhanced arterial reactivity to neuropeptide Y in adulthood. *Journal of Physiology*, **582**, 665–74.

Illingworth RS & Lister J (1964) The critical or sensitive period, with special reference to certain feeding problems in infants and children. *Journal of Paediatrics*, **65**, 839–48.

Imamura M, Tucker J, Hannaford P *et al.* (2007) Factors associated with teenage pregnancy in the European Union countries: a systematic review. *European Journal of Public Health*, **17**, 630–6.

Ingram J, Johnson D & Condon L (2011) The effects of Baby Friendly Initiative training on breastfeeding rates and the breastfeeding attitudes, knowledge and self-efficacy of community health-care staff. *Primary Health Care Research & Development*, **12**, 266–75.

Inskip HM, Crozier SR, Godfrey KM *et al.* (2009) Women's compliance with nutrition and lifestyle recommendations before pregnancy: general population cohort study. *British Medical Journal*, **338**, b481.

Institute of Medicine (2005) *Dietary Reference Intakes for energy, carbohydrate, fibre, fat, fatty acids, cholesterol, protein, and amino acids (macronutrients)*. Washington, DC, National Academies Press.

Institute of Medicine (2009) *Weight Gain During Pregnancy: Reexamining the Guidelines.* Washington, DC, National Academies Press.

Institute of Medicine (2011) Dietary Reference Intakes for Calcium and Vitamin D. Washington, DC: The National Academies Press.

International Agency for Research on Cancer (2008) GLOBOCAN 2008 Cancer Incidence, Mortality and Prevalence Worldwide in 2008. http://globocan.iarc.fr/.

International Diabetes Federation (IDF) (2011) The Global Burden. www.idf.org/diabetesatlas/5e/the-global-burden (accessed 18 January 2013).

Irwin L, Siddiqi A & Hertzman C (2007) *Early Child Development: A Powerful Equalizer.* http://whqlibdoc.who.int/hq/2007/a91213.pdf (accessed 18 January 2013).

Isaacs EB, Gadian DG, Sabatini S *et al.* (2008) The effect of early human diet on caudate volumes and IQ. *Pediatric Research*, **63**, 308–14.

Iwamoto M, Jikko A, Murakami H *et al.* (1994) Changes in parathyroid hormone receptors during chondrocyte cytodifferentiation. *Journal of Biological Chemistry*, **269**, 17245–51.

Jackson AA (1996) Perinatal nutrition: the impact on postnatal growth and development. In *Pediatrics and Perinatology: The Scientific Basis.* Ed. Gluckman & Heymann M. London, Hodder Arnold.

Jackson AA (2011) Nutrient requirements to optimize neonatal growth. *American Journal of Clinical Nutrition*, **94**, 1394–5.

Jackson AA & Robinson SM (2001) Dietary guidelines for pregnancy: a review of current evidence. *Public Health Nutrition*, **4**, 625–30.

Jackson K, Yu MC, Arakawa K *et al.* (2004) DNA hypomethylation is prevalent even in low-grade breast cancers. *Cancer Biology & Therapy*, **3**, 1225–31.

Jacob RA, Gretz DM, Taylor PC *et al.* (1998) Moderate folate depletion increases plasma homocysteine and decreases lymphocyte DNA methylation in postmenopausal women. *Journal of Nutrition*, **128**, 1204–12.

Jaffe CA, Ocampo-Lim B, Guo W *et al.* (1998) Regulatory mechanisms of growth hormone secretion are sexually dimorphic. *Journal of Clinical Investigation*, **102**, 153–64.

Jain A, Concato J & Leventhal JM (2002) How good is the evidence linking breastfeeding and intelligence? *Pediatrics*, **109**, 1044–53.

Janakiraman V, Ettinger A, Mercado-Garcia A *et al.* (2003) Calcium supplements and bone resorption in pregnancy: a randomized crossover trial. *American Journal of Preventative Medicine*, **24**, 260–4.

Janz KF, Burns TL, Levy SM *et al.* (2004) Everyday activity predicts bone geometry in children: the Iowa bone development study. *Medicine and Science in Sports and Exercise*, **36**, 1124–31.

Janz KF, Burns TL, Torner JC *et al.* (2001) Physical activity and bone measures in young children: the Iowa bone development study. *Pediatrics*, **107**, 1387–93.

Javaid MK, Crozier SR, Harvey NC *et al.* (2006) Maternal vitamin D status during pregnancy and childhood bone mass at age 9 years: a longitudinal study. *Lancet*, **367**, 36–43.

Jenner N, Campbell J & Marks R (2004) Morbidity and cost of atopic eczema in Australia. *Australasian Journal of Dermatology*, **45**, 16–22.

Jensen RB, Vielwerth S, Larsen T *et al.* (2007) Pituitary-gonadal function in adolescent males born appropriate or small for gestational age with or without intrauterine growth restriction. *Journal of Clinical Endocrinology and Metabolism*, **92**, 1353–7.

Jensen TK, Jacobsen R, Christensen K *et al.* (2009) Good semen quality and life expectancy: a cohort study of 43,277 men. *American Journal of Epidemiology*, **170**, 559–65.

Jia G, Fu Y, Zhao X *et al.* (2011) N6-methyladenosine in nuclear RNA is a major substrate of the obesity-associated FTO. *Nature Chemical Biology*, **7**, 885–7.

Jimenez E, Fernandez L, Marin ML *et al.* (2005) Isolation of commensal bacteria from umbilical cord blood of healthy neonates born by cesarean section. *Current Microbiology*, **51**, 270–4.

Jirtle RL & Skinner MK (2007) Environmental epigenomics and disease susceptibility. *Nature Reviews Genetics*, **8**, 253–62.

Jones AP & Friedman MI (1982) Obesity and adipocyte abnormalities in offspring of rats undernourished during pregnancy. *Science*, **215**, 1518–19.

Jones CT, Gu W, Harding JE, *et al.* (1988) Studies on the growth of the fetal sheep. Effects of surgical reduction in placental size, or experimental manipulation of uterine blood flow on plasma sulphation promoting activity and on the concentration of insulin-like growth factors I and II. *Journal of Developmental Physiology*, **10**, 179–89.

Jones G, Riley M & Dwyer T (1999) Maternal smoking during pregnancy, growth, and bone mass in prepubertal children. *Journal of Bone and Mineral Research*, **14**, 146–51.

Jones HN, Ashworth CJ, Page KR *et al.* (2006a) Cortisol stimulates System A amino acid transport and SNAT2 expression in a human placental cell line (BeWo). *American Journal of Physiology (Endocrinology)*, **291**, E596–603.

Jones HN, Ashworth CJ, Page KR *et al.* (2006b) Expression and adaptive regulation of amino acid transport system A in a placental cell line under amino acid restriction. *Reproduction*, **131**, 591–60.

Jones HN, Powell TL & Jansson T (2007) Regulation of placental nutrient transport: a review. *Placenta*, **28**, 763–74.

Jones IE, Williams SM & Goulding A (2004) Associations of birth weight and length, childhood size, and smoking with bone fractures during growth: evidence from a birth cohort study. *American Journal of Epidemiology*, **159**, 343–50.

Jones RJ (2009) Cancer stem cells: clinical relevance. *Journal of Molecular Medicine*, **87**, 1105–10.

Jonker SS, Faber JJ, Anderson DF *et al.* (2007) Sequential growth of fetal sheep cardiac myocytes in response to simultaneous arterial and venous hypertension. *American Journal of Physiology – Regulatory, Integrative and Comparative Physiology*, **292**, R913–9.

Joost HG & Thorens B (2001) The extended GLUT-family of sugar/polyol transport facilitators: nomenclature, sequence characteristics, and potential function of its novel members (review). *Molecular Membrane Biology*, **18**, 247–56.

Joshi H, Hawkes D & Ward K (2001) *Unequal entry to motherhood and unequal starts in life: evidence from the first survey of the UK Millennium Cohort*. London, Centre for Longitudinal Research, Institute of Education, University of London.

Judex S, Wohl GR, Wolff RB *et al.* (2000) Dietary fish oil supplementation adversely affects cortical bone morphology and biomechanics in growing rabbits. *Calcified Tissue International*, **66**, 443–8.

Kaaks R & Lukanova A (2001) Energy balance and cancer: the role of insulin and insulin-like growth factor-I. *Proceedings of the Nutrition Society*, **60**, 91–106.

Kaijser M, Akre O, Cnattingius S *et al.* (2005) Preterm birth, low birth weight, and risk for esophageal adenocarcinoma. *Gastroenterology*, **128**, 607–9.

Kaijser M, Lichtenstein P, Granath F *et al.* (2001) *In utero* exposures and breast cancer: a study of opposite-sexed twins. *Journal of the National Cancer Institute*, **93**, 60–2.

Kamangar F, Dores GM & Anderson WF (2006) Patterns of cancer incidence, mortality, and prevalence across five continents: defining priorities to reduce cancer disparities in different geographic regions of the world. *Journal of Clinical Oncology*, **24**, 2137–50.

Kaminsky ZA, Tang T, Wang SC *et al.* (2009) DNA methylation profiles in monozygotic and dizygotic twins. *Nature Genetics*, **41**, 240–5.

Kannus P, Haapasalo H, Sankelo M *et al.* (1995) Effect of starting age of physical activity on bone mass in the dominant arm of tennis and squash players. *Annals of Internal Medicine*, **123**, 27–31.

Kappei D & Londono-Vallejo JA (2008) Telomere length inheritance and aging. *Mechanisms of Ageing and Development*, **129**, 17–26.

Karaplis AC, Luz A, Glowacki J *et al.* (1994) Lethal skeletal dysplasia from targeted disruption of the parathyroid hormone-related peptide gene. *Genes & Development*, **8**, 277–89.

Karlberg J, Jalil F, Lam B *et al.* (1994) Linear growth retardation in relation to the three phases of growth. *European Journal of Clinical Nutrition*, **48** Suppl 1, S25–43; discussion S44.

Karlsson MK, Johnell O & Obrant KJ (1995) Is bone mineral density advantage maintained long-term in previous weight lifters? *Calcified Tissue International*, **57**, 325–8.

Kato Y, Shimazu A, Nakashima K *et al.* (1990) Effects of parathyroid hormone and calcitonin on alkaline phosphatase activity and matrix calcification in rabbit growth-plate chondrocyte cultures. *Endocrinology*, **127**, 114–8.

Katz KA, Pocock SJ & Strachan DP (2003) Neonatal head circumference, neonatal weight, and risk of hayfever, asthma and eczema in a large cohort of adolescents from Sheffield, England. *Clinical & Experimental Allergy*, **33**, 737–45.

Kautzky-Willer A & Handisurya A (2009) Metabolic diseases and associated complications: sex and gender matter! *European Journal of Clinical Investigation*, **39**, 631–48.

Keller G, Zimmer G, Mall G *et al.* (2003) Nephron number in patients with primary hypertension. *New England Journal of Medicine*, **348**, 101–8.

Kelly T, Yang W, Chen C-S *et al.* (2008) Global burden of obesity in 2005 and projections to 2030. *International Journal of Obesity*, **32**, 1431–7.

Kelly Y, Panico L, Bartley M *et al.* (2009) Why does birthweight vary among ethnic groups in the UK? Findings from the Millennium Cohort Study. *Journal of Public Health*, **31**, 131–7.

Kelly YJ, Nazroo JY, McMunn A *et al.* (2001) Birthweight and behavioural problems in children: A modifiable effect? *International Journal of Epidemiology*, **30**, 88–94.

Kelsey G (2011) Epigenetics and the brain: transcriptome sequencing reveals new depths to genomic imprinting. *Bioessays*, **33**, 362–7.

Kennedy K, Ross S, Isaacs EB *et al.* (2010) The 10-year follow-up of a randomised trial of long-chain polyunsaturated fatty acid supplementation in preterm infants: effects on growth and blood pressure. *Archives of Disease in Childhood*, **95**, 588–95.

Kensara OA, Wootton SA, Phillips DI *et al.* (2005) Fetal programming of body composition: relation between birth weight and body composition measured with dual-energy X-ray absorptiometry and anthropometric methods in older Englishmen. *American Journal of Clinical Nutrition*, **82**, 980–7.

Key TJ (2011) Diet, insulin-like growth factor-1 and cancer risk. *Proceedings of the Nutrition Society*, 1–4.

Khan IY, Dekou V, Douglas G *et al.* (2005) A high-fat diet during rat pregnancy or suckling induces cardiovascular dysfunction in adult offspring. *American Journal of Physiology – Regulatory, Integrative and Comparative Physiology*, **288**, R127–33.

Khan IY, Dekou V, Hanson M *et al.* (2004) Predictive adaptive responses to maternal high fat diet prevent endothelial dysfunction but not hypertension in adult rat offspring. *Circulation*, **110**, 1097–102.

Khan IY, Taylor PD, Dekou V *et al.* (2003) Gender-linked hypertension in offspring of lard-fed pregnant rats. *Hypertension*, **41**, 168–75.

Kibirige MS, Hutchison S, Owen CJ *et al.* (2004) Prevalence of maternal dietary iodine insufficiency in the north east of England: implications for the fetus. *Archives of Disease in Childhood, Fetal and Neonatal Edition*, **89**, F436–9.

Kim SY, Dietz PM, England L *et al.* (2007) Trends in prepregnancy obesity in nine states, 1993–2003. *Obesity* **15**, 986–93.

King AJ, Olivier NB, Mohankumar PS *et al.* (2007) Hypertension caused by prenatal testosterone excess in female sheep. *American Journal of Physiology – Endocrinology and Metabolism*, **292**, E1837–41.

Kip SN & Strehler EE (2004) Vitamin D3 upregulates plasma membrane Ca2+-ATPase expression and potentiates apico-basal Ca2+ flux in MDCK cells. *American Journal of Physiology – Regulatory, Integrative and Comparative Physiology*.

Kirk SL, Samuelsson AM, Argenton M *et al.* (2009) Maternal obesity induced by diet in rats permanently influences central processes regulating food intake in offspring. *PLoS One*, **4**, e5870.

Kirkwood TBL & Mathers JC (2009) The basic biology of ageing. In *Healthy Ageing: The Role of Nutrition and Lifestyle*. Ed. Stanner S, Thompson R & Buttriss J. Oxford, Blackwell Publishing Ltd.: 29.

Kishi M, Abe A, Kishi K *et al.* (2009) Relationship of quantitative salivary levels of Streptococcus mutans and S. sobrinus in mothers to caries status and colonization of mutans streptococci in plaque in their 2.5-year-old children. *Community dentistry and oral epidemiology*, **37**, 241–9.

Kleiser C, Schaffrath Rosario A, Mensink GB *et al.* (2009) Potential determinants of obesity among children and adolescents in Germany: results from the cross-sectional KiGGS Study. *BioMed Central Public Health*, **9**, 46.

Klerk M, Verhoef P, Clarke R *et al.* (2002) MTHFR 677C- ->T polymorphism and risk of coronary heart disease: a meta-analysis. *Journal of the American Medical Association*, **288**, 2023–31.

Knudsen VK, Orozova-Bekkevold I, Rasmussen LB *et al.* (2004) Low compliance with recommendations on folic acid use in relation to pregnancy: is there a need for fortification? *Public Health Nutrition*, **7**, 843–50.

Koletzko B, Cetin I & Brenna JT (2007) Dietary fat intakes for pregnant and lactating women. *British Journal of Nutrition*, **98**, 873–7.

Koletzko B, Lien E, Agostoni C *et al.* (2008) The roles of long-chain polyunsaturated fatty acids in pregnancy, lactation and infancy: review of current knowledge and consensus recommendations. *Journal of Perinatal Medicine*, **36**, 5–14.

Koletzko B & Shamir R (2006) Standards for infant formula milk. *British Medical Journal*, **332**, 621–2.

Koletzko B, von Kries R, Closa R *et al.* (2009) Lower protein in infant formula is associated with lower weight up to age 2y: a randomized clinical trial. *American Journal of Clinical Nutrition*, **89**, 1836–45.

Kollarova H, Machova L, Horakova D *et al.* (2007) Epidemiology of esophageal cancer: an overview article. *Biomedical Papers of the Medical Faculty of the University Palacky, Olomouc, Czechoslovakia*, **151**, 17–20.

Korotkova M, Ohlsson C, Hanson LA *et al.* (2004) Dietary n-6:n-3 fatty acid ratio in the perinatal period affects bone parameters in adult female rats. *British Journal of Nutrition*, **92**, 643–8.

Koupil I & Toivanen P (2008) Social and early-life determinants of overweight and obesity in 18-year-old Swedish men. *International Journal of Obesity*, **32**, 73–81.

Kovacs C (2003) Skeletal physiology: fetus and neonate. In *Primer on the metabolic bone diseases and disorders of mineral metabolism*. Ed. Favus M. Washington, American Society for Bone and Mineral Research: 65–71.

Kovacs CS, Chafe LL, Fudge NJ *et al.* (2001) PTH regulates fetal blood calcium and skeletal mineralization independently of PTHrP. *Endocrinology*, **142**, 4983–93.

Kovacs CS, Lanske B, Hunzelman JL *et al.* (1996) Parathyroid hormone-related peptide (PTHrP) regulates fetal-placental calcium transport through a receptor distinct from the PTH/PTHrP receptor. *Proceedings of the National Academy of Sciences of the USA*, **93**, 15233–8.

Kovacs CS, Manley NR, Moseley JM *et al.* (2001) Fetal parathyroids are not required to maintain placental calcium transport. *Journal of Clinical Investigation*, **107**, 1007–15.

Koyama Y & Kotake K (1997) Overview of colorectal cancer in Japan: report from the Registry of the Japanese Society for Cancer of the Colon and Rectum. *Diseases of the Colon and Rectum*, **40**, S2–9.

Kramer MS & Kakuma R (2002) Optimal duration of exclusive breastfeeding. *Cochrane Database of Systematic Reviews*, (1) CD003517.

Kramer MS & Kakuma R (2004) The optimal duration of exclusive breastfeeding: a systematic review. *Advances in Experimental Medicine and Biology*, **554**, 63–77.

Kramer MS, Chalmers B, Hodnett ED *et al.* (2001) Promotion of Breastfeeding Intervention Trial (PROBIT): a randomized trial in the Republic of Belarus. *Journal of the American Medical Association*, **285**, 413–20.

Kramer MS, Chalmers B, Hodnett ED *et al.* (2000) Promotion of breastfeeding intervention trial (PROBIT): a cluster-randomized trial in the Republic of Belarus.

Design, follow-up, and data validation. *Advances in Experimental Medicine and Biology*, **478**, 327–45.

Kramer MS & Kakuma R (2002) Optimal duration of exclusive breastfeeding. *Cochrane Database of Systematic Reviews*, CD003517.

Kretchmer N, Beard JL & Carlson S (1996) The role of nutrition in the development of normal cognition. *American Journal of Clinical Nutrition*, **63**, 997–1001S.

Kris-Etherton PM, Innis S, American Dietetic Association & Dietitians of Canada (2007) Position of the American Dietetic Association and Dietitians of Canada: dietary fatty acids. *Journal of the American Dietetic Association*, **107**, 1599–611.

Krtolica A (2005) Stem cell: balancing aging and cancer. *International Journal of Biochemistry & Cell Biology*, **37**, 935–41.

Kupelian V, Hayes FJ, Link CL *et al.* (2008) Inverse association of testosterone and the metabolic syndrome in men is consistent across race and ethnic groups. *Journal of Clinical Endocrinology and Metabolism*, **93**, 3403–10.

Kwon TH, Nielsen J, Kim YH *et al.* (2003) Regulation of sodium transporters in the thick ascending limb of rat kidney: response to angiotensin II. *American Journal of Physiology - Renal Physiology*, **285**, F152–65.

Lack G, Fox D, Northstone K *et al.* (2003) Factors associated with the development of peanut allergy in childhood. *New England Journal of Medicine*, **348**, 977–85.

Laitinen J, Power C & Jarvelin MR (2001) Family social class, maternal body mass index, childhood body mass index, and age at menarche as predictors of adult obesity. *American Journal of Clinical Nutrition*, **74**, 287–94.

Lakshman R, Ogilvie D & Ong KK (2009) Mothers' experiences of bottle-feeding: a systematic review of qualitative and quantitative studies. *Archives of Disease in Childhood*, **94**, 596–601.

Lam PK, Kritz-Silverstein D, Barrett Connor E *et al.* (2008) Plasma trace elements and cognitive function in older men and women: the Rancho Bernardo study. *Journal of Nutrition, Health and Aging*, **12**, 22–7.

Lamberg-Allardt CJ & Viljakainen HT (2008) 25-Hydroxyvitamin D and functional outcomes in adolescents. *American Journal of Clinical Nutrition*, **88**, 534S–6S.

Landon MB, Spong CY, Thom E *et al.* (2009) A multicenter, randomized trial of treatment for mild gestational diabetes. *New England Journal of Medicine*, **361**, 1339–48.

Lane IR (2011) Preventing neural tube defects with folic acid: nearly 20 years on, the majority of women remain unprotected. *Journal of Obstetrics and Gynaecology*, **31**, 581–5.

Langford A, Johnson B & Al-Hamad A (2009) Social inequalities in female mortality by region and by selected causes of death, England and Wales, 2001–03. *Health Statistics Quarterly*, **Winter**, 7–26.

Langley SC & Jackson AA (1994) Increased systolic blood pressure in adult rats induced by fetal exposure to maternal low protein diets. *Clinical Science*, **86**, 217–22; discussion 121.

Langley-Evans SC (1997) Maternal carbenoxolone treatment lowers birthweight and induces hypertension in the offspring of rats fed a protein-replete diet. *Clinical Science*, **93**, 423–9.

Langley-Evans SC (2006) Developmental programming of health and disease. *Proceedings of the Nutrition Society*, **65**, 97–105.

Langley-Evans SC (2009) Nutritional programming of disease: unravelling the mechanism. *Journal of Anatomy*, **215**, 36–51.

Langley-Evans SC & Jackson AA (1996) Rats with hypertension induced by *in utero* exposure to maternal low-protein diets fail to increase blood pressure in response to a high salt intake. *Annals of Nutrition and Metabolism*, **40**, 1–9.

Langley-Evans SC, Phillips GJ, Benediktsson R *et al.* (1996) Protein intake in pregnancy, placental glucocorticoid metabolism and the programming of hypertension in the rat. *Placenta*, **17**, 169–72.

Langley-Evans SC, Phillips GJ & Jackson AA (1994) *In utero* exposure to maternal low protein diets induces hypertension in weanling rats, independently of maternal blood pressure changes. *Clinical Nutrition*, **13**, 319–24.

Langley-Evans SC, Sherman RC, Welham SJ *et al.* (1999) Intrauterine programming of hypertension: the role of the renin- angiotensin system. *Biochemical Society Transactions*, **27**, 88–93.

Langley-Evans SC, Welham SJ & Jackson AA (1999) Fetal exposure to a maternal low protein diet impairs nephrogenesis and promotes hypertension in the rat. *Life Sciences*, **64**, 965–74.

Langley-Evans SC, Welham SJ, Sherman RC *et al.* (1996) Weanling rats exposed to maternal low-protein diets during discrete periods of gestation exhibit differing severity of hypertension. *Clinical Science*, **91**, 607–15.

Lanham-New SA, Buttriss JL, Miles LM *et al.* (2011) Proceedings of the Rank Forum on Vitamin D. *British Journal of Nutrition*, **105**, 144–56.

Lanigan JA, Bishop J, Kimber AC *et al.* (2001) Systematic review concerning the age of introduction of complementary foods to the healthy full-term infant. *European Journal of Clinical Nutrition*, **55**, 309–20.

Lanske B, Amling M, Neff L *et al.* (1999) Ablation of the PTHrP gene or the PTH/PTHrP receptor gene leads to distinct abnormalities in bone development. *Journal of Clinical Investigation*, **104**, 399–407.

Lanske B, Karaplis AC, Lee K *et al.* (1996) PTH/PTHrP receptor in early development and Indian hedgehog-regulated bone growth. *Science*, **273**, 663–6.

Laughlin GA, Barrett-Connor E & Bergstrom J (2008) Low serum testosterone and mortality in older men. *Journal of Clinical Endocrinology and Metabolism*, **93**, 68–75.

Law CM, Barker DJ, Osmond C *et al.* (1992) Early growth and abdominal fatness in adult life. *Journal of Epidemiology and Community Health*, **46**, 184–6.

Lawlor DA, Benfield L, Logue J *et al.* (2010) Association between general and central adiposity in childhood, and change in these, with cardiovascular risk factors in adolescence: prospective cohort study. *British Medical Journal*, **341**, c6224.

Lawlor DA, Fraser A, Lindsay RS *et al.* (2010) Association of existing diabetes, gestational diabetes and glycosuria in pregnancy with macrosomia and offspring body mass index, waist and fat mass in later childhood: findings from a prospective pregnancy cohort. *Diabetologia*, **53**, 89–97.

Lawlor DA, Leon DA & Davey Smith G (2005) The association of ambient outdoor temperature throughout pregnancy and offspring birthweight: findings from the Aberdeen Children of the 1950s cohort. *British Journal of Obstetrics and Gynaecology*, **112**, 647–57.

Lawlor DA, Macdonald-Wallis C, Fraser A *et al.* (2012) Cardiovascular biomarkers and vascular function during childhood in the offspring of mothers with hypertensive disorders of pregnancy: findings from the Avon Longitudinal Study of Parents and Children. *European Heart Journal*, **33**, 335–45.

Lawlor DA, Najman JM, Sterne J *et al.* (2004) Associations of parental, birth, and early life characteristics with systolic blood pressure at 5 years of age: findings from the Mater-University study of pregnancy and its outcomes. *Circulation*, **110**, 2417–23.

Lawlor DA, Ronalds G, Clark H *et al.* (2005) Birth weight is inversely associated with incident coronary heart disease and stroke among individuals born in the 1950s: findings from the Aberdeen Children of the 1950s prospective cohort study. *Circulation*, **112**, 1414–18.

Lawlor DA, Smith GD, O'Callaghan M *et al.* (2007) Epidemiologic evidence for the fetal overnutrition hypothesis: findings from the mater-university study of pregnancy and its outcomes. *American Journal of Epidemiology*, **165**, 418–24.

Lawlor DA, Timpson NJ, Harbord RM *et al.* (2008) Exploring the developmental overnutrition hypothesis using parental-offspring associations and FTO as an instrumental variable. *PLoS Medicine*, **5**, e33.

Leahy JL (2005) Pathogenesis of type 2 diabetes mellitus. *Archives of Medical Research*, **36**, 197–209.

Lee CF, Qiao M, Schroder K *et al.* (2010) Nox4 is a novel inducible source of reactive oxygen species in monocytes and macrophages and mediates oxidized low density lipoprotein-induced macrophage death. *Circulation Research*, **106**, 1489–97.

Lee CM, Barzi F, Woodward M *et al.* (2009) Adult height and the risks of cardiovascular disease and major causes of death in the Asia-Pacific region: 21,000 deaths in 510,000 men and women. *International Journal of Epidemiology*, **38**, 1060–71.

Leon DA, Lithell HO, Vagero D *et al.* (1998) Reduced fetal growth rate and increased risk of death from ischaemic heart disease: cohort study of 15000 Swedish men and women born 1915–29. *British Medical Journal*, **317**, 241–5.

Leon DA & Moser (2012) KA Low birth weight persists in South Asian babies born in England and Wales regardless of maternal country of birth. Slow pace of acculturation, physiological constraint or both? Analysis of routine data. *Journal of Epidemiology and Community Health*, **66** 544–51.

Lester GE (1986) Cholecalciferol and placental calcium transport. *Federation Proceedings*, **45**, 2524–7.

Leunissen RW, Kerkhof GF, Stijnen T *et al.* (2009) Timing and tempo of first-year rapid growth in relation to cardiovascular and metabolic risk profile in early adulthood. *Journal of the American Medical Association*, **301**, 2234–42.

Levitt NS, Lindsay RS, Holmes MC *et al.* (1996) Dexamethasone in the last week of pregnancy attenuates hippocampal glucocorticoid receptor gene expression and elevates blood pressure in the adult offspring in the rat. *Neuroendocrinology*, **64**, 412–8.

Levitt P (2003) Structural and functional maturation of the developing primate brain. *Journal of Pediatrics*, **143**, S35–45.

Lewington S, Clarke R, Qizilbash N *et al.* (2002) Age-specific relevance of usual blood pressure to vascular mortality: a meta-analysis of individual data for one million adults in 61 prospective studies. *Lancet*, **360**, 1903–13.

Lewis DS, Bertrand HA, McMahan CA *et al.* (1986) Preweaning food intake influences the adiposity of young adult baboons. *Journal of Clinical Investigation*, **78**, 899–905.

Lewis RM, Doherty CB, James LA *et al.* (2001) Effects of maternal iron restriction on placental vascularization in the rat. *Placenta*, **22**, 534–9.

Lewis RM, Petry CJ, Ozanne SE *et al.* (2001) Effects of maternal iron restriction in the rat on blood pressure, glucose tolerance, and serum lipids in the 3-month-old offspring. *Metabolism*, **50**, 562–7.

Li C, Goran MI, Kaur H *et al.* (2007) Developmental trajectories of overweight during childhood: role of early life factors. *Obesity*, **15**, 760–71.

Li C, Kaur H, Choi WS *et al.* (2005b) Additive interactions of maternal prepregnancy BMI and breast-feeding on childhood overweight. *Obesity Research*, **13**, 362–71.

Li F, Wang X, Capasso JM *et al.* (1996) Rapid transition of cardiac myocytes from hyperplasia to hypertrophy during postnatal development. *Journal of Molecular and Cellular Cardiology*, **28**, 1737–46.

Li H, Stein AD, Barnhart HX *et al.* (2003a) Associations between prenatal and postnatal growth and adult body size and composition. *American Journal of Clinical Nutrition*, **77**, 1498–505.

Li L, Fink GD, Watts SW *et al.* (2003b) Endothelin-1 increases vascular superoxide via endothelin(A)-NADPH oxidase pathway in low-renin hypertension. *Circulation*, **107**, 1053–8.

Li R, Darling N, Maurice E *et al.* (2005a) Breastfeeding rates in the United States by characteristics of the child, mother, or family: the 2002 National Immunization Survey. *Pediatrics*, **115**, e31–7.

Liem JJ, Kozyrskyj AL, Huq SI *et al.* (2007) The risk of developing food allergy in premature or low-birth-weight children. *Journal of Allergy and Clinical Immunology*, **119**, 1203–9.

Lillycrop KA, Phillips ES, Jackson AA *et al.* (2005) Dietary protein restriction of pregnant rats induces and folic acid supplementation prevents epigenetic modification of hepatic gene expression in the offspring. *Journal of Nutrition*, **135**, 1382–6.

Lillycrop KA, Phillips ES, Torrens C *et al.* (2008) Feeding pregnant rats a protein-restricted diet persistently alters the methylation of specific cytosines in the hepatic PPAR alpha promoter of the offspring. *British Journal of Nutrition*, **100**, 278–82.

Lillycrop KA, Slater-Jefferies JL, Hanson MA *et al.* (2007) Induction of altered epigenetic regulation of the hepatic glucocorticoid receptor in the offspring of rats fed a protein-restricted diet during pregnancy suggests that reduced DNA methyltransferase-1 expression is involved in impaired DNA methylation and changes in histone modifications. *British Journal of Nutrition*, **97**, 1064–73.

Lindzon G & O'Connor DL (2007) Folate during reproduction: the Canadian experience with folic acid fortification. *Nutrition Research and Practice*, **1**, 163–74.

Lisle SJ, Lewis RM, Petry CJ *et al.* (2003) Effect of maternal iron restriction during pregnancy on renal morphology in the adult rat offspring. *British Journal of Nutrition*, **90**, 33–9.

Litonjua AA, Rifas-Shiman SL, Ly NP *et al.* (2006) Maternal antioxidant intake in pregnancy and wheezing illnesses in children at 2 y of age. *American Journal of Clinical Nutrition*, **84**, 903–11.

Litonjua AA & Weiss ST (2007) Is vitamin D deficiency to blame for the asthma epidemic? *Journal of Allergy and Clinical Immunology*, **120**, 1031–5.

Liu L, Li A & Matthews SG (2001) Maternal glucocorticoid treatment programs HPA regulation in adult offspring: sex-specific effects. *American Journal of Physiology – Endocrinology and Metabolism*, **280**, E729–39.

Liu PY, Death AK & Handelsman DJ (2003) Androgens and cardiovascular disease. *Endocrine Reviews*, **24**, 313–40.

Llewellyn CH, van Jaarsveld CH, Johnson L *et al.* (2011) Development and factor structure of the Baby Eating Behaviour Questionnaire in the Gemini birth cohort. *Appetite*, **57**, 388–96.

Locker J, Reddy TV & Lombardi B (1986) DNA methylation and hepatocarcinogenesis in rats fed a choline-devoid diet. *Carcinogenesis*, **7**, 1309–12.

Locyer V, Porcellato L & Gee I (2011) Vitamin D deficiency and supplementation: are we failing to prevent the preventable? *Community Practitioner*, **84**, 23–6.

Longstreth GF (1995) Epidemiology of hospitalization for acute upper gastrointestinal hemorrhage: a population-based study. *American Journal of Gastroenterology*, **90**, 206–10.

Lonnerdal B (2003) Nutritional and physiologic significance of human milk proteins. *American Journal of Clinical Nutrition*, **77**, 1537S–43S.

Lopuhaa CE, Roseboom TJ, Osmond C *et al.* (2000) Atopy, lung function, and obstructive airways disease after prenatal exposure to famine. *Thorax*, **55**, 555–61.

Louey S, Jonker SS, Giraud GD *et al.* (2007) Placental insufficiency decreases cell cycle activity and terminal maturation in fetal sheep cardiomyocytes. *Journal of Physiology*, **580**, 639–48.

Lucas A (1991) Programming by early nutrition in man. *Ciba Foundation Symposium*, **156**, 38–50; discussion 50–5.

Lucas A, Morley R & Cole TJ (1998) Randomised trial of early diet in preterm babies and later intelligence quotient. *British Medical Journal*, **317**, 1481–7.

Lucas A, Morley R, Cole TJ *et al.* (1992) Breast milk and subsequent intelligence quotient in children born preterm. *Lancet*, **339**, 261–4.

Lucock M & Yates Z (2005) Folic acid: Vitamin and panacea or genetic time bomb? *Nature Reviews Genetics*, **6**, 235–40.

Luke B, Hediger M, Min SJ *et al.* (2005) Gender mix in twins and fetal growth, length of gestation and adult cancer risk. *Paediatric and Perinatal Epidemiology*, **19** Suppl 1, 41–7.

Lumey LH, Stein AD, Kahn HS *et al.* (2007) Cohort profile: the Dutch Hunger Winter families study. *International Journal of Epidemiology*, **36**, 1196–204.

Luo J, Yin X, Ma T *et al.* (2010) Stem cells in normal mammary gland and breast cancer. *American Journal of the Medical Sciences*, **339**, 366–70.

Lussana F, Painter RC, Ocke MC *et al.* (2008) Prenatal exposure to the Dutch famine is associated with a preference for fatty foods and a more atherogenic lipid profile. *American Journal of Clinical Nutrition*, **88**, 1648–52.

Luther JS, Redmer DA, Reynolds LP *et al.* (2005) Nutritional paradigms of ovine fetal growth restriction:

implications for human pregnancy. *Human Fertility*, **8**, 179–87.

Macintyre K, Stewart S, Chalmers J *et al.* (2001) Relation between socioeconomic deprivation and death from a first myocardial infarction in Scotland: population based analysis. *British Medical Journal*, **322**, 1152–3.

Mackay H (1957) Infant feeding: 1936–1957. Progress and changes in two decades. *Nutrition*, **11**, 158–64.

Mackey AD & Picciano MF (1999) Maternal folate status during extended lactation and the effect of supplemental folic acid. *American Journal of Clinical Nutrition*, **69**, 285–92.

Mackey AD, Picciano MF, Mitchell DC *et al.* (1998) Self-selected diets of lactating women often fail to meet dietary recommendations. *Journal of the American Dietetic Association*, **98**, 297–302.

Macleod DJ, Sharpe RM, Welsh M *et al.* (2010) Androgen action in the masculinization programming window and development of male reproductive organs. *International Journal of Andrology*, **33**, 279–87.

Mahomed K, Bhutta Z & Middleton P (2007) Zinc supplementation for improving pregnancy and infant outcome. *Cochrane Database of Systematic Reviews*, CD000230.

Mahomed K & Gulmezoglu AM (2000) Vitamin D supplementation in pregnancy. *Cochrane Database of Systematic Reviews*, CD000228.

Malcolm JC, Lawson ML, Gaboury I *et al.* (2006) Glucose tolerance of offspring of mother with gestational diabetes mellitus in a low-risk population. *Diabetic Medicine*, **23**, 565–70.

Mallet E, Gugi B, Brunelle P *et al.* (1986) Vitamin D supplementation in pregnancy: a controlled trial of two methods. *Obstetrics and Gynecology*, **68**, 300–4.

Mamun AA, O'Callaghan M, Callaway L *et al.* (2009) Associations of gestational weight gain with offspring body mass index and blood pressure at 21 years of age: evidence from a birth cohort study. *Circulation*, **119**, 1720–7.

Manikkam M, Crespi EJ, Doop DD *et al.* (2004) Fetal programming: prenatal testosterone excess leads to fetal growth retardation and postnatal catch-up growth in sheep. *Endocrinology*, **145**, 790–8.

Manthey JA (2000) Biological properties of flavonoids pertaining to inflammation. *Microcirculation*, **7**, S29–34.

Margetts BM & Jackson AA (1993) Interactions between people's diet and their smoking habits: the dietary and nutritional survey of British adults. *British Medical Journal*, **307**, 1381–4.

Maric C (2007) Mechanisms of fetal programming of adult hypertension: role of sex hormones. *Hypertension*, **50**, 605–6.

Marmot M & Wilkinson RG (2001) Psychosocial and material pathways in the relation between income and health: a response to Lynch *et al. British Medical Journal*, **322**, 1233–6.

Marmot MG & McDowall ME (1986) Mortality decline and widening social inequalities. *Lancet*, **2**, 274–6.

Martin JT (2000) Sexual dimorphism in immune function: the role of prenatal exposure to androgens and estrogens. *European Journal of Pharmacology*, **405**, 251–61.

Martin NW, Benyamin B, Hansell NK *et al.* (2011) Cognitive function in adolescence: testing for interactions between breast-feeding and FADS2 polymorphisms. *Journal of the American Academy of Child and Adolescent Psychiatry*, **50**, 55–62 e4.

Martin R, Harvey NC, Crozier SR *et al.* (2007) Placental calcium transporter (PMCA3) gene expression predicts intrauterine bone mineral accrual. *Bone*, **40**, 1203–8.

Martin RM, Ben-Shlomo Y, Gunnell D *et al.* (2005) Breast feeding and cardiovascular disease risk factors, incidence, and mortality: the Caerphilly study. *Journal of Epidemiology and Community Health*, **59**, 121–9.

Martin RM, Davey SG, Mangtani P *et al.* (2004) Breast-feeding and cardiovascular mortality: the Boyd Orr cohort and a systematic review with meta-analysis. *European Heart Journal*, **25**, 778–86.

Martin RM, Gunnell D, Owen CG *et al.* (2005) Breast-feeding and childhood cancer: A systematic review with metaanalysis. *International Journal of Cancer*, **117**, 1020–31.

Martín R, Langa S, Reviriego C *et al.* (2004) The commensal microflora of human milk: new perspectives for food bacteriotherapy and probiotics. *Trends in Food Science & Technology*, **15**, 121–7.

Martins EB & Carvalho MS (2006) Birth weight and over-weight in childhood: a systematic review. *Cadernos Saúde Pública*, **22**, 2281–300.

Marya RK, Rathee S, Dua V *et al.* (1988) Effect of vitamin D supplementation during pregnancy on foetal growth. *Indian Journal of Medical Research*, **88**, 488–92.

Marya RK, Rathee S, Lata V *et al.* (1981) Effects of vitamin D supplementation in pregnancy. *Gynecologic and Obstetric Investigation*, **12**, 155–61.

Masoli M, Fabian D, Holt S *et al.* (2004) The global burden of asthma: executive summary of the GINA Dissemination Committee report. *Allergy*, **59**, 469–78.

Massot C & Vanderplas J (2003) A survey of iron deficinecy anaemia during pregnancy in Belgium: ananlysis of routine hosptial laboratory data in Mons. *Acta Clinica Belgica*, **58**, 169–77.

Mathers JC & McKay JA (2009) Epigenetics: potential contribution to fetal programming. *Advances in Experimental Medicine and Biology*, **646**, 119–23.

Mathews F, Yudkin P, Smith RF *et al.* (2000) Nutrient intakes during pregnancy: the influence of smoking status and age. *Journal of Epidemiology and Community Health*, **54**, 17–23.

Matthews S, Owen D, Banjanin S *et al.* (2002) Glucocorticoids, hypothatlamo-pituitary-adrenal (HPA) development and life after birth. *Endocrine Research*, **28**, 709–18.

McAndrew F, Thompson J, Fellows L *et al.* (2012) Infant Feeding Survey 2010. NHS The Information Centre. http://data.gov.uk/dataset/infant-feeding-survey-2010.

McArdle HJ, Andersen HS, Jones H *et al.* (2006) Fetal programming: causes and consequences as revealed by studies of dietary manipulation in rats. A review. *Placenta*, **27** Supplement A, S56–60.

McArdle HJ, Andersen HS, Jones H *et al.* (2008) Copper and iron transport across the placenta: regulation and interactions. *Journal of Neuroendocrinology*, **20**, 427–31.

McCance DR, Pettitt DJ, Hanson RL *et al.* (1994) Birth weight and non-insulin dependent diabetes: thrifty genotype, thrifty phenotype, or surviving small baby genotype? *British Medical Journal*, **308**, 942–5.

McCance RA (1962) Food, growth, and time. *Lancet*, **2**, 671–6.

McCann D, Barrett A, Cooper A *et al.* (2007) Food additives and hyperactive behaviour in 3-year-old and 8/9-year-old children in the community: a randomised, double-blinded, placebo-controlled trial. *Lancet*, **370**, 1560–7.

McCann JC & Ames BN (2005) Is docosahexaenoic acid, an n-3 long-chain polyunsaturated fatty acid, required for development of normal brain function? An overview of evidence from cognitive and behavioral tests in humans and animals. *American Journal of Clinical Nutrition*, **82**, 281–95.

McCann JC & Ames BN (2007) An overview of evidence for a causal relation between iron deficiency during development and deficits in cognitive or behavioral function. *American Journal of Clinical Nutrition*, **85**, 931–45.

McCormack VA, dos Santos Silva I, Koupil I *et al.* (2005) Birth characteristics and adult cancer incidence: Swedish cohort of over 11,000 men and women. *International Journal of Cancer*, **115**, 611–17.

McCormick MC (1985) The contribution of low birth weight to infant mortality and childhood morbidity. *New England Journal of Medicine*, **312**, 82–90.

McCurdy CE, Bishop JM, Williams SM *et al.* (2009) Maternal high-fat diet triggers lipotoxicity in the fetal livers of nonhuman primates. *Journal of Clinical Investigation*, **119**, 323–35.

McFadyen IR, Campbell-Brown M, Abraham R *et al.* (1984) Factors affecting birthweights in Hindus, Moslems and Europeans. *British Journal of Obsetrics and Gynaecology*, **91**, 968–72.

McGowan PO, Meaney MJ & Szyf M (2008) Diet and the epigenetic (re)programming of phenotypic differences in behavior. *Brain Research*, **1237**, 12–24.

McIntosh N, Helms PJ, Smyth RL *et al.* (2008) *Forfar and Arneil's Textbook of Pediatrics* 7th Edition. London, Churchill Livingstone.

McMillen IC & Robinson JS (2005) Developmental origins of the metabolic syndrome: prediction, plasticity, and programming. *Physiological Reviews*, **85**, 571–633.

McMullen S, Langley-Evans SC, Gambling L *et al.* (2012) A common cause for a common phenotype: the gatekeeper hypothesis in fetal programming. *Medical Hypotheses*, **78**, 88–94.

McMullen S & Mostyn A (2009) Animal models for the study of the developmental origins of health and disease. *Proceedings of the Nutrition Society*, **68**, 306–20.

McNeill G, Tagiyeva N, Aucott L *et al.* (2009) Changes in the prevalence of asthma, eczema and hay fever in prepubertal children: a 40-year perspective. *Paediatric and Perinatal Epidemiology*, **23**, 506–12.

McNulty B, Pentieva K, Marshall B *et al.* (2011) Women's compliance with current folic acid recommendations and achievement of optimal vitamin status for preventing neural tube defects. *Human Reproduction*, **26**, 1530–6.

Meade TW, Ruddock V, Stirling Y *et al.* (1993) Fibrinolytic activity, clotting factors, and long-term incidence of ischaemic heart disease in the Northwick Park Heart Study. *Lancet*, **342**, 1076–9.

Meaney MJ & Szyf M (2005) Environmental programming of stress responses through DNA methylation: life at the interface between a dynamic environment and a fixed genome. *Dialogues in Clinical Neuroscience*, **7**, 103–23.

Medical Research Council (MRC) (2007) Folic acid. www.mrc.ac.uk/Achievementsimpact/Storiesofimpact/Folicacid/index.htm (accessed 13 January 2013).

Medical Research Council (1991) Prevention of neural tube defects: results of the Medical Research Council Vitamin Study. MRC Vitamin Study Research Group. *Lancet*, **338**, 131–7.

Mendez MA, Anthony MS & Arab L (2002) Soy-based formulae and infant growth and development: a review. *Journal of Nutrition*, **132**, 2127–30.

Mennella JA, Jagnow CP & Beauchamp GK (2001) Prenatal and postnatal flavor learning by human infants. *Pediatrics*, **107**, E88.

Mensink RP, Zock PL, Kester AD *et al.* (2003) Effects of dietary fatty acids and carbohydrates on the ratio of serum total to HDL cholesterol and on serum lipids and apolipoproteins: a meta-analysis of 60 controlled trials. *American Journal of Clinical Nutrition*, **77**, 1146–55.

Mercer JG & Archer ZA (2008) Putting the diet back into diet-induced obesity: diet-induced hypothalamic gene expression. *European Journal of Pharmacology*, **585**, 31–7.

Merezak S, Reusens B, Renard A *et al.* (2004) Effect of maternal low-protein diet and taurine on the vulnerability of adult Wistar rat islets to cytokines. *Diabetologia*, **47**, 669–75.

Mess A & Carter AM (2007) Evolution of the placenta during the early radiation of placental mammals. *Comparative Biochemistry and Physiology Part B: Biochemistry and Molecular Biology*, **148A**, 769–79.

Metzger BE, Lowe LP, Dyer AR *et al.* (2008) Hyperglycemia and adverse pregnancy outcomes. *New England Journal of Medicine*, **358**, 1991–2002.

Michail S & Sherman PM (2009) *Probiotics in Pediatric Medicine*. Totowa, New Jersey, Humana Press.

Miles EA, Warner JA, Jones AC *et al.* (1996) Peripheral blood mononuclear cell proliferative responses in the first year of life in babies born to allergic parents. *Clinical & Experimental Allergy*, **26**, 780–8.

Miles HL, Gidlof S, Nordenstrom A *et al.* (2010) The role of androgens in fetal growth: observational study in two genetic models of disordered androgen signalling. *Archives of Disease in Childhood, Fetal and Neonatal Edition*, **95**, F435–8.

Miles L (2008) Alcohol in pregnancy: Is there a safe amount? *Nutrition Bulletin*, **33**, 224–6.

Miles L & Foxen R (2009) New guidelines on caffeine in pregnancy. *Nutrition Bulletin*, **34**, 203–6.

Miller GJ (1975) Plasma-high-density-lipoprotein concentration and development of ischaemic heart-disease. *Lancet*, **1** 16–9

Miller GJ (1982) Serum lipoproteins and susceptibility of men of Indian descent to coronary heart disease. The St James Survey, Trinidad. *Lancet*, **1**, 16–9.

Miller RK, Hendrickx AG, Mills JL *et al.* (1998) Periconceptional vitamin A use: How much is teratogenic? *Reproductive Toxicology*, **12**, 75–88.

Mills A & Tyler H (1992) *Food and nutrient intakes of British infants aged 6–12 months*. London, Her Majesties Stationery Office.

Milne E, Royle JA, Miller M *et al.* (2010) Maternal folate and other vitamin supplementation during pregnancy and risk of acute lymphoblastic leukemia in the offspring. *International Journal of Cancer.* **126**, 2690–9.

Mindell J & Zaninotto P (2006) Cardiovascular disease and diabetes. In *Health Survey for England 2004: The health of minority ethnic groups*. Ed. Sproston K & Mindell J. The NHS Information Centre, London.

Mingrone G, Manco M, Mora ME *et al.* (2008) Influence of maternal obesity on insulin sensitivity and secretion in offspring. *Diabetes Care*, **31**, 1872–6.

Ministry of Agriculture Fisheries and Food (1995) *The infant formula and follow-on regulations 1995*. London, MAFF.

Miralles O, Sanchez J, Palou A *et al.* (2006) A physiological role of breast milk leptin in body weight control in developing infants. *Obesity*, **14**, 1371–7.

Misak Z (2011) Infant nutrition and allergy. *Proceedings of the Nutrition Society*, **70**, 465–71.

Misra A & Khurana L (2008) Obesity and the metabolic syndrome in developing countries. *Journal of Clinical Endocrinology and Metabolism*, **93**, S9–30.

Miyake Y, Sasaki S, Tanaka K *et al.* (2010) Consumption of vegetables, fruit, and antioxidants during pregnancy and wheeze and eczema in infants. *Allergy*, **65**, 758–65.

Miyake Y, Sasaki S, Tanaka K *et al.* (2009) Maternal fat consumption during pregnancy and risk of wheeze and eczema in Japanese infants aged 16–24 months: the Osaka Maternal and Child Health Study. *Thorax*, **64**, 815–21.

Mocarelli P, Gerthoux PM, Patterson DG, Jr. *et al.* (2008) Dioxin exposure, from infancy through puberty, produces endocrine disruption and affects human semen quality. *Environmental Health Perspectives*, **116**, 70–7.

Moinuddin MM, Jameson KA, Syddall HE *et al.* (2008) Cigarette smoking, birthweight and osteoporosis in adulthood: results from the hertfordshire cohort study. *Open Rheumatology Journal*, **2**, 33–7.

Mojtabai R (2004) Body mass index and serum folate in childbearing age women. *European Journal of Epidemiology*, **19**, 1029–36.

Moller H (1993) Clues to the aetiology of testicular germ cell tumours from descriptive epidemiology. *European Urology*, **23**, 8–13; discussion 14–15.

Molloy AM, Kirke PN, Troendle JF *et al.* (2009) Maternal vitamin B12 status and risk of neural tube defects in a population with high neural tube defect prevalence and no folic Acid fortification. *Pediatrics*, **123**, 917–23.

Monasta L, Batty GD, Cattaneo A *et al.* (2010) Early-life determinants of overweight and obesity: a review of systematic reviews. *Obesity Review*, **11**, 695–708.

Monteiro PO & Victora CG (2005) Rapid growth in infancy and childhood and obesity in later life: a systematic review. *Obesity Review*, **6**, 143–54.

Moore K & Persaud T (1998) *The developing human*. Philadelphia, W.B. Saunders.

Moorman JE, Rudd RA, Johnson CA *et al.* (2007) National surveillance for asthma: United States, 1980–2004. *Morbidity and Mortality Weekly Report Surveillance Summaries*, **56**, 1–54.

Moran VH (2006) Nutrition during adolescent pregnancy *Maternal and Infant Nutrition and Nurture: Controversies and Challenges*. Ed. Moran VH & Dykes. London, Quay Books.

Moran VH (2007a) A systematic review of dietary assessments of pregnant adolescents in industrialised countries. *British Journal of Nutrition*, **97**, 411–25.

Moran VH (2007b) Nutritional status in pregnant adolescents: a systematic review of biochemical markers. *Maternal & Child Nutrition*, **3**, 74–93.

More J (2012) Evidence-based portion sizes for toddlers (aged 1–3 years). *Nutrition Bulletin*, **37**, 64–6.

Moreira P, Padez C, Mourao-Carvalhal I *et al.* (2007) Maternal weight gain during pregnancy and overweight in Portuguese children. *International Journal of Obesity*, **31**, 608–14.

Morgan HD, Santos F, Green K *et al.* (2005) Epigenetic reprogramming in mammals. *Human Molecular Genetics*, **14**, R47–58.

Moritz KM, Johnson K, Douglas-Denton R *et al.* (2002) Maternal glucocorticoid treatment programs alterations in the renin-angiotensin system of the ovine fetal kidney. *Endocrinology*, **143**, 4455–63.

Morleo M, Woolfall K, Dedman D *et al.* (2011) Under-reporting of foetal alcohol spectrum disorders: an analysis of hospital episode statistics. *BioMed Central Pediatrics*, **11**, 14.

Morley R, Cole TJ, Powell R *et al.* (1988) Mother's choice to provide breast milk and developmental outcome. *Archives of Disease in Childhood*, **63**, 1382–5.

Morris FL, Naughton GA, Gibbs JL *et al.* (1997) Prospective ten-month exercise intervention in premenarcheal girls: positive effects on bone and lean mass. *Journal of Bone and Mineral Research*, **12**, 1453–62.

Morris MJ (2009) Early life influences on obesity risk: maternal overnutrition and programming of obesity. *Expert Review of Endocrinology and Metabolism*, **4**, 625–37.

Morris MJ & Chen H (2009) Established maternal obesity in the rat reprograms hypothalamic appetite regulators and leptin signaling at birth. *International Journal of Obesity*, **33**, 115–22.

Mortaz M, Fewtrell MS, Cole TJ *et al.* (2001) Birth weight, subsequent growth, and cholesterol metabolism in children 8–12 years old born preterm. *Archives of Disease in Childhood*, **84**, 212–7.

Mortensen LH, Diderichsen F, Davey SG *et al.* (2009) Time is on whose side? Time trends in the association between maternal social disadvantage and offspring fetal growth. A study of 1 409 339 births in Denmark, 1981–2004. *Journal of Epidemiology and Community Health*, **63**, 281–5.

Mostyn A & Symonds ME (2009) Early programming of adipose tissue function: a large-animal perspective. *Proceedings of the Nutrition Society*, **68**, 393–400.

Mountzouris KC, McCartney AL & Gibson GR (2002) Intestinal microflora of human infants and current trends for its nutritional modulation. *British Journal of Nutrition*, **87**, 405–20.

Mouritsen A, Aksglaede L, Sorensen K *et al.* (2010) Hypothesis: exposure to endocrine-disrupting chemicals may interfere with timing of puberty. *International Journal of Andrology*, **33**, 346–59.

Muhlhausler B & Smith SR (2009) Early-life origins of metabolic dysfunction: role of the adipocyte. *Trends in Endocrinology and Metabolism*, **20**, 51–7.

Muhlhausler BS, Adam CL & McMillen IC (2008) Maternal nutrition and the programming of obesity: the brain. *Organogenesis*, **4**, 144–52.

Munoz-Moran E, Dieguez-Lucena JL, Fernandez-Arcas N *et al.* (1998) Genetic selection and folate intake during pregnancy. *Lancet*, **352**, 1120–1.

Murphy MJ, Metcalf BS, Jeffery AN *et al.* (2006) Does lean rather than fat mass provide the link between birth weight, BMI, and metabolic risk? EarlyBird 23. *Pediatric Diabetes*, **7**, 211–14.

Mustalahti K, Catassi C, Reunanen A *et al.* (2010) The prevalence of celiac disease in Europe: results of a centralized, international mass screening project. *Annals of Medicine*, **42**, 587–95.

Naef L, Srivastava L, Gratton A *et al.* (2008) Maternal high fat diet during the perinatal period alters mesocorticolimbic dopamine in the adult rat offspring: reduction in the behavioral responses to repeated amphetamine administration. *Psychopharmacology*, **197**, 83–94.

Naja RP, Dardenne O, Arabian A *et al.* (2009) Chondrocyte-specific modulation of Cyp27b1 expression supports a role for local synthesis of 1,25-dihydroxyvitamin D3 in growth plate development. *Endocrinology*, **150**, 4024–32.

Nakahara K, Nakagawa M, Baba Y *et al.* (2006) Maternal ghrelin plays an important role in rat fetal development during pregnancy. *Endocrinology*, **147**, 1333–42.

Nathanielsz PW, Poston L & Taylor PD (2007) *In utero* exposure to maternal obesity and diabetes: animal models that identify and characterize implications for future health. *Clinics in Perinatology*, **34**, 515–26.

National Health Service Information Centre and IFF Research (NHS IC & IFF Research) (2011) *Infant Feeding Survey 2010: Early results*. London.

National Institute for Health and Clinical Excellence (NICE) (2008) *Antenatal Care, Routine Care for the Healthy Pregnant Woman*. London, NICE.

National Institute for Health and Clinical Excellence (NICE) (2008) *NICE Public Health Guidance 11: Improving the nutrition of pregnant and breastfeeding mothers and children in low-income households*. London, NICE.

National Institute for Health and Clinical Excellence (NICE) (2010) *NICE Public Health Guidance 27: Dietary interventions and physical activity interventions for weight management before, during and after pregnancy*. www.nice.org.uk/guidance/PH27 (accessed 18 January 2013).

National Obesity Observatory (2010) National Child Measurement Programme. www.noo.org.uk/NCMP (accessed 18 January 2013).

Nawapun K & Phupong V (2007) Awareness of the benefits of folic acid and prevalence of the use of folic acid supplements to prevent neural tube defects among Thai women. *Archives of Gynecology and Obstetrics*, **276**, 53–7.

Nelson M, Erens B, Bates B *et al.* (2007) *Low Income Diet and Nutrition Survey Volume 2: Food consumption nutrient intake*. London, The Stationery Office.

Nelson SM, Matthews P & Poston L (2010) Maternal metabolism and obesity: modifiable determinants of pregnancy outcome. *Human Reproduction Update*, **16**, 255–75.

Neugebauer R, Hoek HW & Susser E (1999) Prenatal exposure to wartime famine and development of antisocial personality disorder in early adulthood. *Journal of the American Medical Association*, **282**, 455–62.

Newsome CA, Shiell AW, Fall CHD *et al.* (2003) Is birth weight related to later glucose and insulin metabolism? A systematic review. *Diabetic Medicine*, **20**, 339–48.

NHS (2012) The NHS Information Centre: for health and social care. www.ic.nhs.uk/ (accessed 18 January 2013).

NHS Choices (2011) Birth to Five. Healthy Diet: Weaning and Beyond. www.nhs.uk/Planners/birthtofive/Pages/Healthydietweaninghub.aspx (accessed 18 January 2013).

NHS Choices (2012) Your Pregnancy and Baby Guide. www.nhs.uk/conditions/pregnancy-and-baby/pages/pregnancy-and-baby-care.aspx (accessed 17 January 2013).

NHS Information Centre (2011) *Infant Feeding Survey 2010: Early Results*. www.ic.nhs.uk/pubs/infantfeeding10 (accessed 18 January 2013).

NHS Information Centre (2011) *Health Survey for England 2010: Trend tables*. www.ic.nhs.uk (accessed 18 January 2013).

NHS Information Centre (2008) *Statistics on Obesity, Physical Activity and Diet: England, January 2008*. www.ic.nhs.uk (accessed 18 January 2013).

Niculescu MD, Craciunescu CN & Zeisel SH (2006) Dietary choline deficiency alters global and gene-specific DNA methylation in the developing hippocampus of mouse fetal brains. *FASEB Journal*, **20**, 43–9.

Nilsen TI, Romundstad PR, Troisi R *et al.* (2005) Birth size and colorectal cancer risk: a prospective population based study. *Gut*, **54**, 1728–32.

Nishitani S, Miyamura T, Tagawa M *et al.* (2009) The calming effect of a maternal breast milk odor on the human newborn infant. *Neuroscience Research*, **63**, 66–71.

Nivoit P, Morens C, Van Assche FA *et al.* (2009) Established diet-induced obesity in female rats leads to off-spring hyperphagia, adiposity and insulin resistance. *Diabetologia*, **52**, 1133–42.

Noble S & Emmett P (2001) Food and nutrient intake in a cohort of 8-month-old infants in the south-west of England in 1993. *European Journal of Clinical Nutrition*, **55**, 698–707.

Noble S & Emmett P (2006) Differences in weaning practice, food and nutrient intake between breast- and formula-fed 4-month-old infants in England. *Journal of Human Nutrition and Dietetics* **19**, 303–13.

Nohr EA, Vaeth M, Baker JL *et al.* (2008) Combined associations of prepregnancy body mass index and gestational weight gain with the outcome of pregnancy. *American Journal of Clinical Nutrition*, **87**, 1750–9.

Nordkap L, Joensen UN, Blomberg Jensen M *et al.* (2012) Regional differences and temporal trends in male reproductive health disorders: semen quality may be a sensitive marker of environmental exposures. *Molecular and Cellular Endocrinology*, **355**, 221–30.

Norgan NG (1998) Body composition. In *The Cambridge Encyclopaedia of Human Growth and Development*. Ed. Ulijaszek SJ, Johnston FE & Preece MA. Cambridge, Cambridge University Press.

Norris FJ, Larkin MS, Williams CM *et al.* (2002) Factors affecting the introduction of complementary foods in the preterm infant. *European Journal of Clinical Nutrition*, **56**, 448–54.

Northstone K, Emmett P & Nethersole F (2001) The effect of age of introduction to lumpy solids on foods eaten and reported feeding difficulties at 6 and 15 months. *Journal of Human Nutrition and Dietetics*, **14**, 43–54.

Norval MA (1947) Some factors which influence the duration of breast feeding. *Journal of Pediatrics*, **31**, 415–9.

Nurmatov U, Devereux G & Sheikh A (2011) Nutrients and foods for the primary prevention of asthma and allergy: systematic review and meta-analysis. *Journal of Allergy and Clinical Immunology*, **127**, 724–33 e1–30.

Oakley AE, Clifton DK & Steiner RA (2009) Kisspeptin signaling in the brain. *Endocrine Reviews*, **30**, 713–43.

O'Connor A & Benelam B (2011) An update on UK vitamin D intakes and status, and issues for food fortification and supplementation. *Nutrition Bulletin*, **36**, 389–95.

O'Donnell KJ, Rakeman MA, Zhi-Hong D *et al.* (2002) Effects of iodine supplementation during pregnancy on child growth and development at school age. *Developmental Medicine and Child Neurology*, **44**, 76–81.

Organisation for Economic Co-operation and Development (OECD) (2010) *Health at a Glance: Europe 2010*. Paris, OECD. www.oecd.org/dataoecd/21/44/46464231.pdf (accessed 18 January 2013).

Office for National Statistics (ONS) (2000) *Birth Statistics: Review of the Register General on births and patterns of family building in England and Wales*. London, Office for National Statistics.

Office for National Statistics (ONS) (2005) *Focus on Ethnicity and Identity*. Newport, Office for National Statistics.

Office for National Statistics (ONS) (2011) *Births and Deaths in England and Wales, 2010*. Newport, Office for National Statistics.

Ojeda NB, Grigore D & Alexander BT (2008) Developmental programming of hypertension: insight from animal models of nutritional manipulation. *Hypertension*, **52**, 44–50.

Ojeda NB, Grigore D, Robertson EB *et al.* (2007) Estrogen protects against increased blood pressure in postpubertal female growth restricted offspring. *Hypertension*, **50**, 679–85.

Okasha M, McCarron P, Gunnell D *et al.* (2003) Exposures in childhood, adolescence and early adulthood and breast cancer risk: a systematic review of the literature. *Breast cancer research and treatment*, **78**, 223–76.

Oken E, Levitan EB & Gillman MW (2008) Maternal smoking during pregnancy and child overweight: systematic review and meta-analysis. *International Journal of Obesity*, **32**, 201–10.

Oken E, Rifas-Shiman SL, Field AE *et al.* (2008) Maternal gestational weight gain and offspring weight in adolescence. *Obstetrics and Gynecology*, **112**, 999–1006.

Oken E, Taveras EM, Kleinman KP *et al.* (2007) Gestational weight gain and child adiposity at age 3 years. *American Journal of Obstetrics and Gynaecology*, **196**, 322 e1–8.

Olsen SF, Halldorsson TI, Willett WC *et al.* (2007) Milk consumption during pregnancy is associated with increased infant size at birth: prospective cohort study. *American Journal of Clinical Nutrition*, **86**, 1104–10.

Olsen SF, Osterdal ML, Salvig JD *et al.* (2008) Fish oil intake compared with olive oil intake in late pregnancy and asthma in the offspring: 16 y of registry-based follow-up from a randomized controlled trial. *American Journal of Clinical Nutrition*, **88**, 167–75.

Olshansky SJ, Passaro DJ, Hershow RC *et al.* (2005) A potential decline in life expectancy in the United States in the 21st century. *New England Journal of Medicine*, **352**, 1138–45.

Oncel MY, Ozdemir R, Erdeve O *et al.* (2011) Influence of maternal cigarette smoking during pregnancy on neonatal serum folate levels. *European Journal of Nutrition*, **51**, 385–7.

Ong KK, Ahmed ML, Emmett PM *et al.* (2000) Association between postnatal catch-up growth and obesity in childhood: prospective cohort study. *British Medical Journal*, **320**, 967–71.

Ong KK & Loos RJ (2006) Rapid infancy weight gain and subsequent obesity: systematic reviews and hopeful suggestions. *Acta Paediatrica Scandinavica*, **95**, 904–8.

Ong KK, Preece MA, Emmett PM *et al.* (2002) Size at birth and early childhood growth in relation to maternal smoking, parity and infant breast-feeding: longitudinal birth cohort study and analysis. *Pediatric Research*, **52**, 863–7.

Ong ZY & Muhlhausler BS (2011) Maternal 'junk-food' feeding of rat dams alters food choices and development of the mesolimbic reward pathway in the offspring. *FASEB Journal*, **25**, 2167–79.

O'Rahilly R & Müller F (1999) Minireview: summary of the initial development of the human nervous system. *Teratology*, **60**, 39–41.

O'Rahilly R & Müller F (2000) Prenatal ages and stages: measures and errors. *Teratology*, **61**, 382–4.

O'Regan D, Kenyon CJ, Seckl JR *et al.* (2008) Prenatal dexamethasone 'programmes' hypotension, but stress-induced hypertension in adult offspring. *Journal of Endocrinology*, **196**, 343–52.

Ormond G, Nieuwenhuijsen MJ, Nelson P *et al.* (2009) Endocrine disruptors in the workplace, hair spray, folate supplementation, and risk of hypospadias: case–control study. *Environmental Health Perspectectives*, **117**, 303–7.

Osmond C, Barker DJ, Winter PD *et al.* (1993) Early growth and death from cardiovascular disease in women. *British Medical Journal*, **307**, 1519–24.

Owen CG, Martin RM, Whincup PH *et al.* (2005) Effect of infant feeding on the risk of obesity across the life course: a quantitative review of published evidence. *Pediatrics*, **115**, 1367–77.

Owen CG, Whincup PH, Kaye SJ *et al.* (2008) Does initial breastfeeding lead to lower blood cholesterol in adult life? A quantitative review of the evidence. *American Journal of Clinical Nutrition*, **88**, 305–14.

Owen CG, Whincup PH, Orfei L *et al.* (2009) Is body mass index before middle age related to coronary heart disease risk in later life? Evidence from observational studies. *International Journal of Obesity*, **33**, 866–77.

Owen D (2006) Profile of Black and Minority ethnic groups in the UK. Background paper. In *ESRC Seminar Series 'Understanding and tackling ethnic inequalities in health'*.

Ozaki T, Hawkins P, Nishina H *et al.* (2000) Effects of undernutrition in early pregnancy on systemic small artery function in late-gestation fetal sheep. *American Journal of Obstetrics and Gynaecology*, **183**, 1301–7.

Ozaki T, Nishina H, Hanson MA *et al.* (2001) Dietary restriction in pregnant rats causes gender-related hypertension and vascular dysfunction in offspring. *Journal of Physiology*, **530**, 141–52.

Ozanne SE, Fernandez-Twinn D & Hales CN (2004) Fetal growth and adult diseases. *Seminars in Perinatology*, **28**, 81–7.

Ozanne SE, Jensen CB, Tingey KJ *et al.* (2005) Low birthweight is associated with specific changes in muscle insulin-signalling protein expression. *Diabetologia*, **48**, 547–52.

Ozanne SE, Lewis R, Jennings BJ *et al.* (2004) Early programming of weight gain in mice prevents the induction of obesity by a highly palatable diet. *Clinical Science*, **106**, 141–5.

Ozanne SE, Nave BT, Wang CL *et al.* (1997) Poor fetal nutrition causes long-term changes in expression of insulin signaling components in adipocytes. *American Journal of Physiology*, **273**, E46–51.

Ozanne SE, Olsen GS, Hansen LL *et al.* (2003) Early growth restriction leads to down regulation of protein kinase C zeta and insulin resistance in skeletal muscle. *Journal of Endocrinology*, **177**, 235–41.

Ozanne SE, Wang CL, Coleman N *et al.* (1996) Altered muscle insulin sensitivity in the male offspring of protein-malnourished rats. *American Journal of Physiology*, **271**, E1128–34.

Paajanen TA, Oksala NK, Kuukasjarvi P *et al.* (2010) Short stature is associated with coronary heart disease: a systematic review of the literature and a meta-analysis. *European Heart Journal*, **31**, 1802–9.

Page K (1993) *The Physiology of the Human Placenta*. London, Taylor & Francis.

Painter RC, de Rooij SR, Bossuyt PM *et al.* (2006a) Early onset of coronary artery disease after prenatal exposure to the Dutch famine. *American Journal of Clinical Nutrition*, **84**, 322–7; quiz 466–7. Ch1

Painter RC, de Rooij SR, Bossuyt PM *et al.* (2006b) Blood pressure response to psychological stressors in adults after prenatal exposure to the Dutch famine. *Journal of Hypertension*, **24**, 1771–8.

Painter RC, De Rooij SR, Bossuyt PM *et al.* (2006c) A possible link between prenatal exposure to famine and breast cancer: a preliminary study. *American Journal of Human Biology*, **18**, 853–6.

Painter RC, Roseboom TJ & Bleker OP (2005) Prenatal exposure to the Dutch famine and disease in later life: an overview. *Reproductive Toxicology*, **20**, 345–52.

Pal BR & Shaw NJ (2001) Rickets resurgence in the United Kingdom: improving antenatal management in Asians. *Journal of Pediatrics*, **139**, 337–8.

Palmer C, Bik EM, DiGiulio DB *et al.* (2007) Development of the human infant intestinal microbiota. *PLoS Biology*, **5**, e177.

Paltiel O, Harlap S, Deutsch L *et al.* (2004) Birth weight and other risk factors for acute leukemia in the Jerusalem Perinatal Study cohort. *Cancer Epidemiology, Biomarkers & Prevention*, **13**, 1057–64.

Pan American Health Organisation/ World Health Organization (PAHO/WHO) (2003) *Guiding Principles for Complementary Feeding of the Breastfed Child*. Washington, DC.

Parente LB, Aguila MB & Mandarim-de-Lacerda CA (2008) Deleterious effects of high-fat diet on perinatal and postweaning periods in adult rat offspring. *Clinical Nutrition*, **27**, 623–34.

Park JH, Stoffers DA, Nicholls RD *et al.* (2008) Development of type 2 diabetes following intrauterine growth retardation in rats is associated with progressive epigenetic silencing of Pdx1. *Journal of Clinical Investigation*, **118**, 2316–24.

Park SK, Kang D, McGlynn KA *et al.* (2008) Intrauterine environments and breast cancer risk: meta-analysis and systematic review. *Breast Cancer Research*, **10**, R8.

Parkinson KN, Drewett RF, Le Couteur AS *et al.* (2010) Do maternal ratings of appetite in infants predict later Child Eating Behaviour Questionnaire scores and body mass index? *Appetite*, **54**, 186–90.

Parsons TJ, Power C & Manor O (2001) Fetal and early life growth and body mass index from birth to early adulthood in 1958 British cohort: longitudinal study. *British Medical Journal*, **323**, 1331–5.

Paulozzi LJ (1999) International trends in rates of hypospadias and cryptorchidism. *Environmental Health Perspectives*, **107**, 297–302.

Paunier L, Lacourt G, Pilloud P *et al.* (1978) 25-hydroxyvitamin D and calcium levels in maternal, cord and infant serum in relation to maternal vitamin D intake. *Helvetica Paediatrica Acta*, **33**, 95–103.

Pearce SH & Cheetham TD (2010) Diagnosis and management of vitamin D deficiency. *British Medical Journal*, **340**, b5664.

Pehlivan I, Hatun S, Aydogan M *et al.* (2003) Maternal vitamin D deficiency and vitamin D supplementation in healthy infants. *Turkish Journal Pediatrics*, **45**, 315–20.

Penrose LS (1954) Some recent trends in human genetics. *Carylogia*, **6**, 521–30.

Pepe A, Ferlin A, Gianesello L *et al.* (2009) INSL3 plays a role in the balance between bone formation and resorption. *Annals of the New York Academy of Sciences*, **1160**, 219–20.

Perala MM, Moltchanova E, Kaartinen NE *et al.* (2011) The association between salt intake and adult systolic blood pressure is modified by birth weight. *American Journal of Clinical Nutrition*, **93**, 422–6.

Petry CJ, Dorling MW, Pawlak DB *et al.* (2001) Diabetes in old male offspring of rat dams fed a reduced protein diet. *International Journal of Experimental Diabetes Research*, **2**, 139–43.

Petry CJ, Dorling MW, Wang CL *et al.* (2000) Catecholamine levels and receptor expression in low protein rat offspring. *Diabetic Medicine*, **17**, 848–53.

Pettitt DJ, Baird HR, Aleck KA *et al.* (1983) Excessive obesity in offspring of Pima Indian women with diabetes during pregnancy. *New England Journal of Medicine*, **308**, 242–5.

Pettitt DJ, Bennett PH, Saad MF *et al.* (1991) Abnormal glucose tolerance during pregnancy in Pima Indian women. Long-term effects on offspring. *Diabetes*, **40** Suppl 2, 126–30.

Pettitt DJ, Knowler WC, Bennett PH *et al.* (1987) Obesity in offspring of diabetic Pima Indian women despite normal birth weight. *Diabetes Care*, **10**, 76–80.

Pettitt DJ, McKenna S, McLaughlin C *et al.* (2010) Maternal glucose at 28 weeks of gestation is not associated with obesity in 2-year-old offspring: the Belfast Hyperglyc-emia and Adverse Pregnancy Outcome (HAPO) family study. *Diabetes Care*, **33**, 1219–23.

Pettitt DJ, Nelson RG, Saad MF *et al.* (1993) Diabetes and obesity in the offspring of Pima Indian women with dia-betes during pregnancy. *Diabetes Care*, **16**, 310–14.

Phillips DI, Walker BR, Reynolds RM *et al.* (2000) Low birth weight predicts elevated plasma cortisol concentra-tions in adults from 3 populations. *Hypertension*, **35**, 1301–6.

Phillips K & Matheny AP, Jr. (1990) Quantitative genetic analysis of longitudinal trends in height: preliminary results from the Louisville Twin Study. *Acta Geneticae Medicae et Gemellologiae*, **39**, 143–63.

Picciano MF (2003) Pregnancy and lactation: physiological adjustments, nutritional requirements and the role of dietary supplements. *Journal of Nutrition*, **133**, 1997S–2002S.

Picciano MF & McGuire MK (2009) Use of dietary sup-plements by pregnant and lactating women in North America. *American Journal of Clinical Nutrition*, **89**, 663–7S.

Pinney SE & Simmons RA (2010) Epigenetic mechanisms in the development of type 2 diabetes. *Trends in Endo-crinology and Metabolism*, **21**, 223–9.

Pischon T, Nothlings U & Boeing H (2008) Obesity and cancer. *Proceedings of the Nutrition Society*, **67**, 128–45.

Pladys P, Lahaie I, Cambonie G *et al.* (2004) Role of brain and peripheral angiotensin II in hypertension and altered arterial baroreflex programmed during fetal life in rat. *Pediatric Research*, **55**, 1042–9.

Plagemann A (2005) Perinatal programming and func-tional teratogenesis: impact on body weight regulation and obesity. *Physiology and Behaviour*, **86**, 661–8.

Plagemann A (2006) Perinatal nutrition and hormone-dependent programming of food intake. *Hormone Research*, **65** Suppl 3, 83–9.

Plagemann A, Harder T, Brunn M *et al.* (2009) Hypotha-lamic proopiomelanocortin promoter methylation becomes altered by early overfeeding: an epigenetic model of obesity and the metabolic syndrome. *Journal of Physiology*, **587**, 4963–76.

Plagemann A, Harder T, Janert U *et al.* (1999c) Malforma-tions of hypothalamic nuclei in hyperinsulinemic off-spring of rats with gestational diabetes. *Developmental Neuroscience*, **21**, 58–67.

Plagemann A, Harder T, Kohlhoff R *et al.* (1997) Over-weight and obesity in infants of mothers with long-term insulin-dependent diabetes or gestational diabetes. *Inter-national Journal of Obesity and Related Metabolic Disor-ders*, **21**, 451–6.

Plagemann A, Harder T, Melchior K *et al.* (1999b) Eleva-tion of hypothalamic neuropeptide Y-neurons in adult offspring of diabetic mother rats. *Neuroreport*, **10**, 3211–16.

Plagemann A, Harder T, Rake A *et al.* (1999a) Morpho-logical alterations of hypothalamic nuclei due to intrahy-pothalamic hyperinsulinism in newborn rats. *International Journal of Developmental Neuroscience*, **17**, 37–44. Ch6

Plagemann A, Harder T, Rake A *et al.* (1998) Hypotha-lamic insulin and neuropeptide Y in the offspring of gestational diabetic mother rats. *Neuroreport*, **9**, 4069–73.

Plagemann A, Heidrich I, Gotz F *et al.* (1992) Obesity and enhanced diabetes and cardiovascular risk in adult rats due to early postnatal overfeeding. *Experimental and Clinical Endocrinology & Diabetes*, **99**, 154–8.

Platz EA, Giovannucci E, Rimm EB *et al.* (1998) Retro-spective analysis of birth weight and prostate cancer in the Health Professionals Follow-up Study. *American Journal of Epidemiology*, **147**, 1140–4.

Poore KR & Fowden AL (2004) The effects of birth weight and postnatal growth patterns on fat depth and plasma leptin concentrations in juvenile and adult pigs. *Journal of Physiology*, **558**, 295–304.

Porrello ER, Bell JR, Schertzer JD *et al.* (2009) Heritable pathologic cardiac hypertrophy in adulthood is preceded by neonatal cardiac growth restriction. *American Journal of Physiology – Regulatory, Integrative and Comparative Physiology*, **296**, R672–80.

Poston L (2010) Developmental programming and diabe-tes: the human experience and insight from animal models. *Best Practice & Research: Clinical Endocrinology & Metabolism*, **24**, 541–52.

Poulsen P, Vaag AA, Kyvik KO *et al.* (1997) Low birth weight is associated with NIDDM in discordant monozy-gotic and dizygotic twin pairs. *Diabetologia*, **40**, 439–46.

Powell SE & Aberle ED (1980) Effects of birth weight on growth and carcass composition of swine. *Journal of Animal Science*, **50**, 860–8.

Prader A, Tanner JM & von HG (1963) Catch-up growth following illness or starvation. An example of develop-mental canalization in man. *Journal of Pediatrics*, **62**, 646–59.

Prasad M, Lumia M, Erkkola M *et al.* (2010) Diet com-position of pregnant Finnish women: changes over time and across seasons. *Public Health Nutrition*, **13**, 939–46.

Preece MA (1996) The genetic contribution to stature. *Hormone Research*, **45** Suppl 2, 56–8.

Prescott SL, Smith P, Tang M *et al.* (2008) The importance of early complementary feeding in the development of oral tolerance: concerns and controversies. *Pediatric Allergy and Immunology*, **19**, 375–80.

Prescott SL & Tang ML (2005) The Australasian Society of Clinical Immunology and Allergy position statement:

Summary of allergy prevention in children. *Medical Journal of Australia*, **182**, 464–7.

Pritchard E (1920) The feeding of young children during and after weaning. *Maternity and Child Welfare*, **1v**, 39–42.

Pritchard E (1928) A few reflections on the present position of infant feeding in England. *American Medicine*, **23**, 881–3.

Purvis RJ, Barrie WJ, MacKay GS *et al.* (1973) Enamel hypoplasia of the teeth associated with neonatal tetany: a manifestation of maternal vitamin-D deficiency. *Lancet*, **2**, 811–14.

Rahmouni K, Correia ML, Haynes WG *et al.* (2005) Obesity-associated hypertension: new insights into mechanisms. *Hypertension*, **45**, 9–14.

Raman L, Rajalakshmi K, Krishnamachari KA *et al.* (1978) Effect of calcium supplementation to undernourished mothers during pregnancy on the bone density of the bone density of the neonates. *American Journal of Clinical Nutrition*, **31**, 466–9.

Ramlau-Hansen CH, Nohr EA, Thulstrup AM *et al.* (2007) Is maternal obesity related to semen quality in the male offspring? A pilot study. *Human Reproduction*, **22**, 2758–62.

Ramsay JE, Ferrell WR, Crawford L *et al.* (2002) Maternal obesity is associated with dysregulation of metabolic, vascular, and inflammatory pathways. *Journal of Clinical Endocrinology and Metabolism*, **87**, 4231–7.

Rapley G & Murkett T (2008) *Baby-Led Weaning: Helping your baby to love good food.* London, Vermillion.

Rasmussen KM & Yaktine AL (2009) *Committee to Reexamine IOM Pregnancy Weight Guidelines.* Washington, DC, National Academies Press.

Rasmussen SA, Chu SY, Kim SY *et al.* (2008) Maternal obesity and risk of neural tube defects: a metaanalysis. *American Journal of Obstetrics and Gynaecology*, **198**, 611–19.

Ratajczak MZ, Shin DM & Kucia M (2009) Very small embryonic/epiblast-like stem cells: a missing link to support the germ line hypothesis of cancer development? *American Journal of Pathology*, **174**, 1985–92.

Ratajczak MZ, Shin DM, Liu R *et al.* (2010) Epiblast/germ line hypothesis of cancer development revisited: lesson from the presence of Oct-4+ cells in adult tissues. *Stem Cell Reviews*, **6**, 307–16.

Rautava S & Walker WA (2009) Academy of Breastfeeding Medicine founder's lecture 2008: breastfeeding – an extrauterine link between mother and child. *Breastfeeding Medicine*, **4**, 3–10.

Ravelli AC, van der Meulen JH, Michels RP *et al.* (1998) Glucose tolerance in adults after prenatal exposure to famine. *Lancet*, **351**, 173–7.

Ravelli AC, van der Meulen JH, Osmond C *et al.* (1999) Obesity at the age of 50 y in men and women exposed to

famine prenatally. *American Journal of Clinical Nutrition*, **70**, 811–16.

Ravelli GP, Stein ZA & Susser MW (1976) Obesity in young men after famine exposure *in utero* and early infancy. *New England Journal of Medicine*, **295**, 349–53.

Reaven GM (1988) Banting lecture 1988. Role of insulin resistance in human disease. *Diabetes*, **37**, 1595–607.

Rebhan B, Kohlhuber M, Schwegler U *et al.* (2009) Infant feeding practices and associated factors through the first 9 months of life in Bavaria, Germany. *Journal of Pediatric Gastroenterology and Nutrition*, **49**, 467–73.

Reckelhoff JF (2001) Gender differences in the regulation of blood pressure. *Hypertension*, **37**, 1199–208.

Reddy S, Sanders TA & Obeid O (1994) The influence of maternal vegetarian diet on essential fatty acid status of the newborn. *European Journal of Clinical Nutrition*, **48**, 358–68.

Reece EA, Leguizamon G & Homko C (1998) Pregnancy performance and outcomes associated with diabetic nephropathy. *American Journal of Perinatology*, **15**, 413–21.

Rees S, Mallard C, Breen S *et al.* (1998) Fetal brain injury following prolonged hypoxemia and placental insufficiency: a review. *Comparative Biochemistry and Physiology Part A: Molecular & Integrative Physiology*, **119**, 653–60.

Reeves GK, Pirie K, Beral V *et al.* (2007) Cancer incidence and mortality in relation to body mass index in the Million Women Study: cohort study. *British Medical Journal*, **335**, 1134.

Regitz-Zagrosek V, Lehmkuhl E & Weickert MO (2006) Gender differences in the metabolic syndrome and their role for cardiovascular disease. *Clinical Research in Cardiology*, **95**, 136–47.

Regnault TRH, Limesand SW & Hay WW (2006) Aspects of fetoplacental nutrition in intrauterine growth restriction and macrosomia. In *Neonatal Nutrition and Metabolism*. Ed. Thureen PJ & Hay WW. Cambridge, Cambridge University Press.

Reif S, Katzir Y, Eisenberg Z *et al.* (1988) Serum 25-hydroxyvitamin D levels in congenital craniotabes. *Acta Paediatrica Scandinavica*, **77**, 167–8.

Reik W & Walter J (2001) Genomic imprinting: parental influence on the genome. *Nature Reviews Genetics*, **2**, 21–32.

Reilly JJ, Armstrong J, Dorosty AR *et al.* (2005) Early life risk factors for obesity in childhood: cohort study. *British Medical Journal*, **330**, 1357.

Reilly JJ, Methven E, McDowell ZC *et al.* (2003) Health consequences of obesity. *Archives of Disease in Childhood*, **88**, 748–52.

Reilly JJ & Wells JC (2005) Duration of exclusive breastfeeding: introduction of complementary feeding may be necessary before 6 months of age. *British Journal of Nutrition*, **94**, 869–72.

Reilly MP & Rader DJ (2003) The metabolic syndrome: More than the sum of its parts? *Circulation*, **108**, 1546–51.

Reinhardt C, Reigstad CS & Backhed F (2009) Intestinal microbiota during infancy and its implications for obesity. *Journal of Pediatric Gastroenteroogy and Nutrition*, **48**, 249–56.

Renehan AG, Tyson M, Egger M *et al.* (2008) Body-mass index and incidence of cancer: a systematic review and meta-analysis of prospective observational studies. *Lancet*, **371**, 569–78.

Rewers M (2005) Epidemiology of celiac disease: What are the prevalence, incidence, and progression of celiac disease? *Gastroenterology*, **128**, S47–51.

Reyes-Engel A, Munoz E, Gaitan MJ *et al.* (2002) Implications on human fertility of the 677C-->T and 1298A-->C polymorphisms of the MTHFR gene: consequences of a possible genetic selection. *Molecular Human Reproduction*, **8**, 952–7.

Richards M, Abbott R, Collis G *et al.* (2009) Childhood mental health and life chances in post-war Britain. www. scmh.org.uk/pdfs/life_chances_report.pdf (accessed 18 January 2013).

Richards M, Hardy R, Kuh D *et al.* (2001) Birth weight and cognitive function in the British 1946 birth cohort: longitudinal population-based study. *British Medical Journal*, **322**, 199–203.

Richards M, Hardy R & Wadsworth ME (2002) Long-term effects of breast-feeding in a national birth cohort: educational attainment and midlife cognitive function. *Public Health Nutrition*, **5**, 631–5.

Richards M, Power C & Sacker A (2009) Paths to literacy and numeracy problems: evidence from two British birth cohorts. *Journal of Epidemiology and Community Health*, **63**, 239–44.

Richards M & Sacker A (2003) Lifetime antecedents of cognitive reserve. *Journal of Clinical and Experimental Neuropsychology*, **25**, 614–24.

Rich-Edwards JW, Kleinman K, Michels KB *et al.* (2005) Longitudinal study of birth weight and adult body mass index in predicting risk of coronary heart disease and stroke in women. *British Medical Journal*, **330**, 1115.

Rich-Edwards JW, Stampfer MJ, Manson JE *et al.* (1997) Birth weight and risk of cardiovascular disease in a cohort of women followed up since 1976. *British Medical Journal*, **315**, 396–400.

Rifas-Shiman SL, Rich-Edwards JW, Kleinman KP *et al.* (2009) Dietary quality during pregnancy varies by maternal characteristics in Project Viva: a US cohort. *Journal of the American Dietetic Association*, **109**, 1004–11.

Riggs AD, Martienssen RA & Russo VE (1996) Introduction. In *Epigenetic Mechanisms of Gene Regulation*. Ed.

Russo VE, Martienssen RA & Riggs AD. Plainview, NY, Cold Spring Harbor Laboratory Press: 1–4.

Riley H (2011) Weight management before, during and after pregnancy: What are the 'rules'? *Nutrition Bulletin*, **36**, 212–5.

Rinaudo P & Wang E (2012) Fetal programming and metabolic syndrome. *Annual Review of Physiology*, **74**, 107–30.

Robertson KD (2005) DNA methylation and human disease. *Nature Reviews Genetics*, **6**, 597–610.

Robertson A, Lobstein T & Knai C (2007) *Obesity and Socio-Economic Groups in Europe: Evidence review and implications for action*. http://ec.europa.eu/health/ph_determinants/life_style/nutrition/documents/ev20081028_rep_en.pdf (accessed 18 January 2013).

Robinson M, Oddy WH, Li J *et al.* (2008) Pre- and postnatal influences on preschool mental health: a large-scale cohort study. *Journal of Child Psychology and Psychiatry*, **49**, 1118–28.

Robinson PD, Hogler W, Craig ME *et al.* (2006) The re-emerging burden of rickets: a decade of experience from Sydney. *Archives of Disease in Childhood*, **91**, 564–8.

Robinson S, Marriott L, Poole J *et al.* (2007) Dietary patterns in infancy: the importance of maternal and family influences on feeding practice. *British Journal of Nutrition*, **98**, 1029–37.

Robinson SM, Batelaan SF, Syddall HE *et al.* (2006) Combined effects of dietary fat and birth weight on serum cholesterol concentrations: the Hertfordshire Cohort Study. *American Journal of Clinical Nutrition*, **84**, 237–44.

Roger LC, Costabile A, Holland DT *et al.* (2010) Examination of faecal Bifidobacterium populations in breast- and formula-fed infants during the first 18 months of life. *Microbiology*, **156**, 3329–41.

Roger LC & McCartney AL (2010) Longitudinal investigation of the faecal microbiota of healthy full-term infants using fluorescence in situ hybridization and denaturing gradient gel electrophoresis. *Microbiology*, **156**, 3317–28.

Rogers I (2003) The influence of birthweight and intrauterine environment on adiposity and fat distribution in later life. *International Journal of Obesity and Related Metabolic Disorders*, **27**, 755–77.

Rogers IS, Ness AR, Steer CD *et al.* (2006) Associations of size at birth and dual-energy X-ray absorptiometry measures of lean and fat mass at 9 to 10 y of age. *American Journal of Clinical Nutrition*, **84**, 739–47.

Roigas J, Roigas C, Heydeck D *et al.* (1996) Prenatal hypoxia alters the postnatal development of beta-adrenoceptors in the rat myocardium. *Biology of the Neonate*, **69**, 383–8.

Ronnberg A & Nilsson K (2010) Interventions during pregnancy to reduce excessive gestational weight gain: a systematic review assessing current clinical evidence using the Grading of Recommendations, Assessment, Development and Evaluation (GRADE) system. *British Journal of Obstetrics and Gynaecology*, **117**, 1327–34.

Rosales FJ, Reznick JS & Zeisel SH (2009) Understanding the role of nutrition in the brain and behavioral development of toddlers and preschool children: identifying and addressing methodological barriers. *Nutritional Neuroscience*, **12**, 190–202.

Rose DP, Komninou D & Stephenson GD (2004) Obesity, adipocytokines, and insulin resistance in breast cancer. *Obesity Reviews*, **5**, 153–65.

Roseboom T, de Rooij S & Painter R (2006) The Dutch famine and its long-term consequences for adult health. *Early Human Development*, **82**, 485–91.

Roseboom TJ, van der Meulen JH, Osmond C *et al.* (2000c) Coronary heart disease after prenatal exposure to the Dutch famine, 1944–45. *Heart*, **84**, 595–8.

Roseboom TJ, van der Meulen JH, Ravelli AC *et al.* (2000b) Plasma fibrinogen and factor VII concentrations in adults after prenatal exposure to famine. *British Journal of Haematology*, **111**, 112–17.

Roseboom TJ, van der Meulen JHP, Osmond C *et al.* (2000a) Plasma lipid profile in adults after prenatal exposure to the Dutch famine. *American Journal of Clinical Nutrition*, **72**, 1101–6.

Roseboom TJ, van der Meulen JH, Ravelli AC *et al.* (1999) Blood pressure in adults after prenatal exposure to famine. *Journal of Hypertension*, **17**, 325–30.

Rosengren A, Eriksson H, Larsson B *et al.* (2000) Secular changes in cardiovascular risk factors over 30 years in Swedish men aged 50: the study of men born in 1913, 1923, 1933 and 1943. *Journal of Internal Medicine*, **247**, 111–18.

Ross R (1999) Atherosclerosis: -an inflammatory disease. *New England Journal of Medicine*, **340**, 115–26.

Rothman KJ, Moore LL, Singer MR *et al.* (1995) Teratogenicity of high vitamin A intake. *New England Journal of Medicine*, **333**, 1369–73.

Rowe J, Kusel M, Holt BJ *et al.* (2007) Prenatal versus postnatal sensitization to environmental allergens in a high-risk birth cohort. *Journal of Allergy and Clinical Immunology*, **119**, 1164–73.

Roy DK, Berry JL, Pye SR *et al.* (2007) Vitamin D status and bone mass in UK South Asian women. *Bone*, **40**, 200–4.

Royal College of Obstetricians and Gynaecologists (RCOG) (2006) *Statement No.4: Exercise in Pregnancy.* www.rcog.org.uk/womens-health/clinical-guidance/exercise-pregnancy (accessed 18 January 2013).

Royal College of Paediatricians and Child Health (2009) UK-WHO growth charts: early years. www.rcpch.ac.uk/child-health/research-projects/uk-who-growth-charts-early-years/uk-who-growth-charts-early-years (accessed 18 January 2013).

Rump P, Zeegers MP & van Essen AJ (2005) Tumor risk in Beckwith-Wiedemann syndrome: a review and meta-analysis. *American Journal of Medical Genetics, Part A*, **136**, 95–104.

Russo VEA, Martienssen RA & Riggs AD (1996) *Epigenetic Mechanisms of Gene Regulation*. Plainview, New York, Cold Spring Harbor Laboratory Press.

Rutter M (1985) Family and school influences on cognitive development. *Journal of Child Psychology and Psychiatry, and Allied Disciplines*, **26**, 683–704.

Rutter M, Kim-Cohen J & Maughan B (2006) Continuities and discontinuities in psychopathology between childhood and adult life. *Journal of Child Psychology and Psychiatry*, **47**, 276–95.

Ryan AS, Wenjun Z & Acosta A (2002) Breastfeeding continues to increase into the new millennium. *Pediatrics*, **110**, 1103–9.

Saadi HF, Dawodu A, Afandi BO *et al.* (2007) Efficacy of daily and monthly high-dose calciferol in vitamin D-deficient nulliparous and lactating women. *American Journal of Clinical Nutrition*, **85**, 1565–71.

Saarinen UM & Kajosaari M (1995) Breastfeeding as prophylaxis against atopic disease: prospective follow-up study until 17 years old. *Lancet*, **346**, 1065–9.

Sachdev H, Gera T & Nestel P (2005) Effect of iron supplementation on mental and motor development in children: systematic review of randomised controlled trials. *Public Health Nutrition*, **8**, 117–32.

Sachdev HS, Fall CH, Osmond C *et al.* (2005) Anthropometric indicators of body composition in young adults: relation to size at birth and serial measurements of body mass index in childhood in the New Delhi birth cohort. *American Journal of Clinical Nutrition*, **82**, 456–66.

Sahota O, Mundey MK, San P *et al.* (2006) Vitamin D insufficiency and the blunted PTH response in established osteoporosis: the role of magnesium deficiency. *Osteoporosis International*, **17**, 1013–21.

Sajjad Y, Quenby S, Nickson P *et al.* (2007) Androgen receptors are expressed in a variety of human fetal extragenital tissues: an immunohistochemical study. *Asian Journal of Andrology*, **9**, 751–9.

Sala-Vila A, Miles EA & Calder PC (2008) Fatty acid composition abnormalities in atopic disease: evidence explored and role in the disease process examined. *Clinical & Experimental Allergy*, **38**, 1432–50.

Salsberry PJ & Reagan PB (2005) Dynamics of early childhood overweight. *Pediatrics*, **116**, 1329–38.

Samuelsson AM, Matthews PA, Argenton M *et al.* (2008) Diet-induced obesity in female mice leads to offspring hyperphagia, adiposity, hypertension, and insulin resistance: a novel murine model of developmental programming. *Hypertension*, **51**, 383–92.

Samuelsson AM, Morris A, Igosheva N *et al.* (2010) Evidence for sympathetic origins of hypertension in juvenile offspring of obese rats. *Hypertension*, **55**, 76–82.

Sanders M, Fazzi G, Janssen G *et al.* (2004a) Prenatal stress changes rat arterial adrenergic reactivity in a regionally selective manner. *European Journal of Pharmacology*, **488**, 147–55.

Sanders MW, Fazzi GE, Janssen GM, *et al.* (2004b) Reduced uteroplacental blood flow alters renal arterial reactivity and glomerular properties in the rat offspring. *Hypertension*, **43**, 1283–9.

Sandhu MS, Dunger DB & Giovannucci EL (2002) Insulin, insulin-like growth factor-I (IGF-I), IGF binding proteins, their biologic interactions, and colorectal cancer. *Journal of the National Cancer Institute*, **94**, 972–80.

Sandhu MS, Luben R, Day NE *et al.* (2002) Self-reported birth weight and subsequent risk of colorectal cancer. *Cancer Epidemiology, Biomarkers & Prevention*, **11**, 935–8.

Sandstrom O, Lonnerdal B, Graverholt G *et al.* (2008) Effects of alpha-lactalbumin-enriched formula containing different concentrations of glycomacropeptide on infant nutrition. *American Journal of Clinical Nutrition*, **87**, 921–8.

Sasaki H & Matsui Y (2008) Epigenetic events in mammalian germ-cell development: reprogramming and beyond. *Nature Reviews Genetics*, **9**, 129–40.

Savage S-AH, Reilly JJ, Edwards CA *et al.* (1998) Weaning practice in the Glasgow longitudinal infant growth study. *Archives of Disease in Childhood*, **79**, 153–6.

Sayed AR, Bourne D, Pattinson R *et al.* (2008) Decline in the prevalence of neural tube defects following folic acid fortification and its cost-benefit in South Africa. *Birth Defects Research. Part A, Clinical and Molecular Teratology*, **82**, 211–16.

Sayer AA, Syddall HE, Dennison EM *et al.* (2004) Birth weight, weight at 1 y of age, and body composition in older men: findings from the Hertfordshire Cohort Study. *American Journal of Clinical Nutrition*, **80**, 199–203.

Scarborough P, Bhatnagar P, Wickramasinghe K *et al.* (2010) *Coronary Heart Disease Statistics*. www.bhf.org.uk/publications/view-publication.aspx?ps=1001546 (accessed 18 January 2013).

Schaefer-Graf UM, Pawliczak J, Passow D *et al.* (2005) Birth weight and parental BMI predict overweight in children from mothers with gestational diabetes. *Diabetes Care*, **28**, 1745–50.

Schaub B, Liu J, Schleich I *et al.* (2008) Impairment of T helper and T regulatory cell responses at birth. *Allergy*, **63**, 1438–47.

Schlotz W & Phillips DI (2009) Fetal origins of mental health: evidence and mechanisms. *Brain Behavior and Immunity*, **23**, 905–16.

Scholl TO (1998) Teenage pregnancy. In *The Cambridge Encyclopaedia of Human Growth and Development*. Ed.

Ulijaszek SJ, Johnston FE & Preece MA. Cambridge, Cambridge University Press.

Schulzke SM, Patole SK & Simmer K (2011) Longchain polyunsaturated fatty acid supplementation in preterm infants. *Cochrane Database of Systematic Reviews*, CD000375.

Scientific Advisory Committee on Nutrition (SACN) (2004) *Advice on Fish Consumption: Benefits and Risks*. London, The Stationery Office.

Scientific Advisory Committee on Nutrition (SACN) (2007) *Update on Vitamin D*. London, The Stationery Office. www.sacn.gov.uk/pdfs/sacn_position_vitamin_d_2007_05_07.pdf (accessed 18 January 2013).

Scientific Advisory Committee on Nutrition (SACN) (2008) *The Nutritional Wellbeing of the British Population: An analysis of British dietary surveys*. London, The Stationery Office.

Scientific Advisory Committee on Nutrition (SACN) (2010) *Iron and Health*. London, The Stationery Office.

Scientific Advisory Committee on Nutrition (SACN) (2011a) *The Influence of Maternal, Fetal and Child Nutrition on the Development of Chronic Disease in Later Life*. London, The Stationery Office. www.sacn.gov.uk/pdfs/sacn_early_nutrition_final_report_20_6_11.pdf (accessed 18 January 2013).

Scientific Advisory Committee on Nutrition (SACN) (2011b) *Dietary Recommendations for Energy*. Uncorrected proofs. www.sacn.gov.uk (accessed 18 January 2013).

Scientific Advisory Committee on Nutrition (SACN) & Committee on Toxicology (COT) (2011) *Timing of Introduction of Gluten into the Infant Diet*. www.sacn.gov.uk/reports_position_statements/position_statements/index.html (accessed 18 January 2013).

Scientific Advisory Committee on Nutrition (SACN) & Royal College of Paediatrics and Child Health (2007) *Application of WHO Growth Standards in the UK*. London, The Stationery Office.

Scott HM, Hutchison GR, Mahood IK *et al.* (2007) Role of androgens in fetal testis development and dysgenesis. *Endocrinology*, **148**, 2027–36.

Scott WR (2011) Roux-en-Y gastric bypass and laparoscopic sleeve gastrectomy: understanding weight loss and improvements in type 2 diabetes after bariatric surgery. *American Journal of Physiology – Regulatory, Integrative and Comparative Physiology*, **301**, R15–27.

Seaton A, Godden DJ & Brown K (1994) Increase in asthma: A more toxic environment or a more susceptible population? *Thorax*, **49**, 171–4.

Seckl JR (2001) Glucocorticoid programming of the fetus; adult phenotypes and molecular mechanisms. *Molecular and Cellular Endocrinology*, **185**, 61–71.

Sekiya N, Anai T, Matsubara M *et al.* (2007) Maternal weight gain rate in the second trimester are associated with birth weight and length of gestation. *Gynecologic and Obstetric Investigation*, **63**, 45–8.

Sergeant G, Vankelecom H, Gremeaux L *et al.* (2009) Role of cancer stem cells in pancreatic ductal adenocarcinoma. *Nature Reviews Clinical Oncology*, **6**, 580–6.

Sewell MF, Huston-Presley L, Super DM *et al.* (2006) Increased neonatal fat mass, not lean body mass, is associated with maternal obesity. *American Journal of Obstetrics and Gynaecology*, **195**, 1100–3.

Shah PS & Shah V (2009) Influence of the maternal birth status on offspring: a systematic review and meta-analysis. *Acta Obstetricia Gynecologica Scandinavica*, **88**, 1307–18.

Shams M, Kilby MD, Somerset DA *et al.* (1998) 11Beta-hydroxysteroid dehydrogenase type 2 in human pregnancy and reduced expression in intrauterine growth restriction. *Human Reproduction*, **13**, 799–804.

Shankar K, Harrell A, Liu X *et al.* (2008) Maternal obesity at conception programs obesity in the offspring. *American Journal of Physiology – Regulatory, Integrative and Comparative Physiology*, **294**, R528–38.

Sharkey D, Gardner DS, Fainberg HP *et al.* (2009) Maternal nutrient restriction during pregnancy differentially alters the unfolded protein response in adipose and renal tissue of obese juvenile offspring. *FASEB Journal*, **23**, 1314–24.

Sharpe RM (2010) Environmental/lifestyle effects on spermatogenesis. *Philosophical transactions of the Royal Society of London. Series B, Biological Sciences*, **365**, 1697–712.

Sharpe RM, Martin B, Morris K *et al.* (2002) Infant feeding with soy formula milk: effects on the testis and on blood testosterone levels in marmoset monkeys during the period of neonatal testicular activity. *Human Reproduction*, **17**, 1692–703.

Sharpe RM, McKinnell C, Kivlin C *et al.* (2003) Proliferation and functional maturation of Sertoli cells, and their relevance to disorders of testis function in adulthood. *Reproduction*, **125**, 769–84.

Shehadeh N, Khaesh-Goldberg E, Shamir R *et al.* (2003) Insulin in human milk: postpartum changes and effect of gestational age. *Archives of Disease in Childhood, Fetal and Neonatal Edition*, **88**, F214–16.

Shelley P, Martin-Gronert MS, Rowlerson A *et al.* (2009) Altered skeletal muscle insulin signaling and mitochondrial complex II-III linked activity in adult offspring of obese mice. *American Journal of Physiology – Regulatory, Integrative and Comparative Physiology*, **297**, R675–81.

Shenkin SD, Starr JM & Deary IJ (2004) Birth weight and cognitive ability in childhood: a systematic review. *Psychological Bulletin*, **130**, 989–1013.

Sherman RC & Langley-Evans SC (1998) Early administration of angiotensin-converting enzyme inhibitor captopril, prevents the development of hypertension programmed by intrauterine exposure to a maternal low-protein diet in the rat. *Clinical Science*, **94**, 373–81.

Sherman RC & Langley-Evans SC (2000) Antihypertensive treatment in early postnatal life modulates prenatal dietary influences upon blood pressure in the rat. *Clinical Science*, **98**, 269–75.

Sherwood KL, Houghton LA, Tarasuk V *et al.* (2006) One-third of pregnant and lactating women may not be meeting their folate requirements from diet alone based on mandated levels of folic acid fortification. *Journal of Nutrition*, **136**, 2820–6.

Shi H, Seeley RJ & Clegg DJ (2009) Sexual differences in the control of energy homeostasis. *Frontiers in Neuroendocrinology*, **30**, 396–404.

Sidnell A & Greenstreet E (2009) Infant nutrition: protein and its influence on growth rate. *Nutrition Bulletin*, **34**, 395–400.

Sidnell A & Greenstreet E (2011) Infant nutrition: review of lipid innovation in infant formula. *Nutrition Bulletin*, **36**, 373–80.

Silano M, Agostoni C & Guandalini S (2010) Effect of the timing of gluten introduction on the development of celiac disease. *World Journal of Gastroenterology*, **16**, 1939–42.

Silva Idos S, De Stavola B & McCormack V (2008) Birth size and breast cancer risk: re-analysis of individual participant data from 32 studies. *PLoS Medicine*, **5**, e193.

Silventoinen K, Kaprio J, Lahelma E *et al.* (2000) Relative effect of genetic and environmental factors on body height: differences across birth cohorts among Finnish men and women. *American Journal of Public Health*, **90**, 627–30.

Silverman BL, Rizzo TA, Cho NH *et al.* (1998) Long-term effects of the intrauterine environment: The Northwestern University Diabetes in Pregnancy Center. *Diabetes Care*, **21** Suppl 2, B142–9.

Simmer K, Schulzke S & Patole S (2008) Longchain polyunsaturated fatty acid supplementation in infants born at term. *Cochrane Database of Systematic Reviews*, CD000375.

Sin DD & Sutherland ER (2008) Obesity and the lung: 4. Obesity and asthma. *Thorax*, **63**, 1018–23.

Sinclair KD, Allegrucci C, Singh R *et al.* (2007) DNA methylation, insulin resistance, and blood pressure in offspring determined by maternal periconceptional B vitamin and methionine status. *Proceedings of the National Academy of Sciences of the USA*, **104**, 19351–6.

Singhal A (2010a) Does early growth affect long-term risk factors for cardiovascular disease? *Nestlé Nutrition workshop series. Paediatric programme*, **65**, 55–64; discussion 65–9.

Singhal A (2010b) Does weight gain in infancy influence the later risk of obesity? *Journal of Pediatric Gastroenterology and Nutrition*, **51** Suppl 3, S119–20.

Singhal A, Cole TJ, Fewtrell M *et al.* (2004) Breastmilk feeding and lipoprotein profile in adolescents born preterm: follow-up of a prospective randomised study. *Lancet*, **363**, 1571–8.

Singhal A, Fewtrell M, Cole TJ *et al.* (2003) Low nutrient intake and early growth for later insulin resistance in adolescents born preterm. *Lancet*, **361**, 1089–97.

Singhal A, Kennedy K, Lanigan J *et al.* (2010) Nutrition in infancy and long-term risk of obesity: evidence from 2 randomized controlled trials. *American Journal of Clinical Nutrition*, **92**, 1133–44.

Singhal A & Lucas A (2004) Early origins of cardiovascular disease: Is there a unifying hypothesis? *Lancet*, **363**, 1642–5.

Singhal A, Wells J, Cole TJ *et al.* (2003) Programming of lean body mass: A link between birth weight, obesity, and cardiovascular disease? *American Journal of Clinical Nutrition*, **77**, 726–30.

Siri-Tarino PW, Williams PT, Fernstrom HS *et al.* (2009) Reversal of small, dense LDL subclass phenotype by normalization of adiposity. *Obesity*, **17**, 1768–75.

Smith GC & Pell JP (2001) Teenage pregnancy and risk of adverse perinatal outcomes associated with first and second births: population based retrospective cohort study. *British Medical Journal*, **323**, 476.

Smith J, Cianflone K, Biron S *et al.* (2009) Effects of maternal surgical weight loss in mothers on intergenerational transmission of obesity. *Journal of Clinical Endocrinology and Metabolism*, **94**, 4275–83.

Smith SA, Heslehurst N, Ells LJ *et al.* (2011) Community-based service provision for the prevention and management of maternal obesity in the North East of England: a qualitative study. *Public Health*, **125**, 518–24.

Smithers G, Gregory JR, Bates CJ *et al.* (2000) The National Diet and Nutrition Survey: young people aged 4–18 years. *Nutrition Bulletin*, **25**, 105–11.

Smolina K, Wright FL, Rayner M *et al.* (2012) Determinants of the decline in mortality from acute myocardial infarction in England between 2002 and 2010: linked national database study. *British Medical Journal*, **344**, d8059.

Snell C, Krypuy M, Wong EM *et al.* (2008) BRCA1 promoter methylation in peripheral blood DNA of mutation negative familial breast cancer patients with a BRCA1 tumour phenotype. *Breast Cancer Research*, **10**, R12.

Snoeck A, Remacle C, Reusens B *et al.* (1990) Effect of a low protein diet during pregnancy on the fetal rat endocrine pancreas. *Biology of the Neonate*, **57**, 107–18.

Soonpaa MH & Field LJ (1998) Survey of studies examining mammalian cardiomyocyte DNA synthesis. *Circulation Research*, **83**, 15–26.

Spalding KL, Arner E, Westermark PO *et al.* (2008) Dynamics of fat cell turnover in humans. *Nature*, **453**, 783–7.

Sparks J & Cetin I (2006) Determinants of intrauterine growth. In *Neonatal Nutrition and Metabolism*. Ed. Thureen, P & Hay, W. Cambridge, Cambridge University Press: 23–32.

Specker B (2004) Nutrition influences bone development from infancy through toddler years. *Journal of Nutrition*, **134**, 691S-5S.

Specker BL, Beck A, Kalkwarf H *et al.* (1997) Randomized trial of varying mineral intake on total body bone mineral accretion during the first year of life. *Pediatrics*, **99**, E12.

Specker BL, Ho ML, Oestreich A *et al.* (1992) Prospective study of vitamin D supplementation and rickets in China. *Journal of Pediatrics*, **120**, 733–9.

Specker BL, Mulligan L & Ho M (1999) Longitudinal study of calcium intake, physical activity, and bone mineral content in infants 6–18 months of age. *Journal of Bone and Mineral Research*, **14**, 569–76.

Srinivasan M, Katewa SD, Palaniyappan A *et al.* (2006) Maternal high-fat diet consumption results in fetal malprogramming predisposing to the onset of metabolic syndrome-like phenotype in adulthood. *American Journal of Physiology – Endocrinology and Metabolism*, **291**, E792–9.

Stanner S, Thompson R & Buttriss J (2009) *Healthy Ageing: The Role of Nutrition and Lifestyle: The Report of the British Nutrition Foundation*. Oxford, Blackwell Publishing Ltd.

Stanner S & Yudkin JS (2001) Fetal programming and the Leningrad Siege study. *Twin Research*, **4**, 287–92.

Stanner SA, Bulmer K, Andrès C *et al.* (1997) Does malnutrition *in utero* determine diabetes and coronary heart disease in adulthood? Results from the Leningrad siege study, a cross sectional study. *British Journal of Nutrition*, **315**, 1342–5.

Stanner SA & Yudkin JS (2001) Fetal programming and the Leningrad Siege study. *Twin Research*, **4**, 287–92.

Stauffer TP, Hilfiker H, Carafoli E *et al.* (1993) Quantitative analysis of alternative splicing options of human plasma membrane calcium pump genes. *Journal of Biological Chemistry*, **268**, 25993–6003.

Stavola BL, Hardy R, Kuh D *et al.* (2000) Birthweight, childhood growth and risk of breast cancer in a British cohort. *British Journal of Cancer*, **83**, 964–8.

Steegers-Theunissen RP, Obermann-Borst SA, Kremer D *et al.* (2009) Periconceptional maternal folic acid use of 400 microg per day is related to increased methylation of the IGF2 gene in the very young child. *PLoS One*, **4**, e7845.

Steer CD, Davey Smith G, Emmett PM *et al.* (2010) FADS2 polymorphisms modify the effect of breastfeeding on child IQ. *PLoS One*, **5**, e11570.

Stein AD, Melgar P, Hoddinott J *et al.* (2008) Cohort Profile: the Institute of Nutrition of Central America and Panama (INCAP) Nutrition Trial Cohort Study. *International Journal of Epidemiology*, **37**, 716–20.

Stein AD, Wang M, Ramirez-Zea M *et al.* (2006) Exposure to a nutrition supplementation intervention in early childhood and risk factors for cardiovascular disease in adulthood: evidence from Guatemala. *American Journal of Epidemiology*, **164**, 1160–70.

Stein AD, Zybert PA, van de Bor M *et al.* (2004) Intrauterine famine exposure and body proportions at birth: the Dutch Hunger Winter. *International Journal of Epidemiology*, **33**, 831–6.

Stein AD, Zybert PA, van der Pal-de Bruin K *et al.* (2006) Exposure to famine during gestation, size at birth, and blood pressure at age 59 y: evidence from the Dutch Famine. *European Journal of Epidemiology*, **21**, 759–65.

Stein CE, Fall CH, Kumaran K *et al.* (1996) Fetal growth and coronary heart disease in south India. *Lancet*, **348**, 1269–73.

Stein Z, Susser M, Saenger G *et al.* (1975) *Famine and Human Development: The Dutch Hunger Winter of 1944/45.* New York, Oxford University Press.

Stephen A, Alles M, de Graaf C *et al.* (2012) The role and requirements of digestible dietary carbohydrates in infants and toddlers. *European Journal of Clinical Nutrition*, **66**, 765–79.

Stern LL, Mason JB, Selhub J *et al.* (2000) Genomic DNA hypomethylation, a characteristic of most cancers, is present in peripheral leukocytes of individuals who are homozygous for the C677T polymorphism in the methylenetetrahydrofolate reductase gene. *Cancer Epidemiology, Biomarkers & Prevention*, **9**, 849–53.

Stettler N (2007) Nature and strength of epidemiological evidence for origins of childhood and adulthood obesity in the first year of life. *International Journal of Obesity*, **31**, 1035–43.

Stettler N, Stallings VA, Troxel AB *et al.* (2005) Weight gain in the first week of life and overweight in adulthood: a cohort study of European American subjects fed infant formula. *Circulation*, **111**, 1897–903.

Stettler N, Zemel BS, Kumanyika S *et al.* (2002) Infant weight gain and childhood overweight status in a multicenter, cohort study. *Pediatrics*, **109**, 194–9.

Stevenson RD & Allaire JH (1991) The development of normal feeding and swallowing. *Pediatric Clinics of North America*, **38**, 1439–53.

Stevenson SS (1949) Comparison of breast and artificial feeding. *Journal of the American Dietetic Association*, **25**, 752–6.

Stewart A & Westropp C (1953) Breast-feeding in the Oxford Child Health Survey. *British Medical Journal*, **2**, 305–8.

Stewart BW & Kleihues P (2003) *World Cancer Report.* Lyon, France, International Agency for Research on Cancer.

Stewart RJ, Sheppard H, Preece R *et al.* (1980) The effect of rehabilitation at different stages of development of rats marginally malnourished for ten to twelve generations. *British Journal of Nutrition*, **43**, 403–12.

Stewart T, Jung FF, Manning J *et al.* (2005) Kidney immune cell infiltration and oxidative stress contribute to prenatally programmed hypertension. *Kidney International*, **68**, 2180–8.

Stites DP & Pavia CS (1979) Ontogeny of human T cells. *Pediatrics*, **64**, 795–802.

Stockley L (2006) *Folic acid: influencing low-income groups.* www.food.gov.uk/multimedia/pdfs/influencinglowin comers.pdf (accessed 18 January 2013).

Stockley L & Lund V (2008) Use of folic acid supplements, particularly by low-income and young women: a series of systematic reviews to inform public health policy in the UK. *Public Health Nutrition*, **11**, 807–21.

Stoltzfus RJ (2003) Iron deficiency: global prevalence and consequences. *Food and Nutrition Bulletin*, **24**, S99–103.

Story & Alton (1995) Nutrition issues and adolescent pregnancy *Nutrition Today*, **30**, 142–51.

Strachan T & Read AP (2004) *Human Molecular Genetics.* New York, Garland Science.

Strom BL, Schinnar R, Ziegler EE *et al.* (2001) Exposure to soy-based formula in infancy and endocrinological and reproductive outcomes in young adulthood. *Journal of the American Medical Association*, **286**, 807–14.

Strully K & Mishra G (2009) Theoretical underpinning for the use of sibling studies in life course epidemiology. In *Family Matters: Designing, analysing and understanding family-based studies in life course epidemiology.* Ed. Lawlor D & Mishra G. Oxford, Oxford University Press.

Stultz EE, Stokes JL, Shaffer ML *et al.* (2007) Extent of medication use in breastfeeding women. *Breastfeeding Medicine*, **2**, 145–51.

Sullivan EL, Grayson B, Takahashi D *et al.* (2010) Chronic consumption of a high-fat diet during pregnancy causes perturbations in the serotonergic system and increased anxiety-like behavior in nonhuman primate offspring. *Journal of Neuroscience*, **30**, 3826–30.

Sweeney L, J. (1998) *Basic Concepts in Embryology: A Student's Survival Guide.* New York, McGraw Hill.

Symonds ME, Pearce S, Bispham J *et al.* (2004) Timing of nutrient restriction and programming of fetal adipose tissue development. *Proceedings of the Nutrition Society*, **63**, 397–403.

Symonds ME, Sebert SP, Hyatt MA *et al.* (2009) Nutritional programming of the metabolic syndrome. *Nature Reviews Endocrinology*, **5**, 604–10.

Symonds ME, Stephenson T, Gardner DS *et al.* (2007) Long-term effects of nutritional programming of the embryo and fetus: mechanisms and critical windows. *Reproduction, Fertility and Development*, **19**, 53–63.

Szepfalusi Z, Loibichler C, Pichler J *et al.* (2000) Direct evidence for transplacental allergen transfer. *Pediatric Research*, **48**, 404–7.

Szepfalusi Z, Pichler J, Elsasser S *et al.* (2000) Transplacental priming of the human immune system with environmental allergens can occur early in gestation. *Journal of Allergy and Clinical Immunology*, **106**, 530–6.

Szyf M, Pakneshan P & Rabbani SA (2004) DNA methylation and breast cancer. *Biochemical Pharmacology*, **68**, 1187–97.

Taitz LS & Byers HD (1972) High calorie-osmolar feeding and hypertonic dehydration. *Archives of Disease in Childhood*, **47**, 257–60.

Tam WH, Ma RC, Yang X *et al.* (2010) Glucose intolerance and cardiometabolic risk in adolescents exposed to maternal gestational diabetes: a 15-year follow-up study. *Diabetes Care*, **33**, 1382–4.

Tan KA, Walker M, Morris K *et al.* (2006) Infant feeding with soy formula milk: effects on puberty progression, reproductive function and testicular cell numbers in marmoset monkeys in adulthood. *Human Reproduction*, **21**, 896–904.

Tanner J (1989a) The organisation of the growth process. In *Foetus into Man: Physical growth from conception to maturity, 2nd edition*. Ware, UK, Castlemead Publications: 165–77.

Tanner JM (1989b) The interaction of heredity and environment in the control of growth. In *Foetus into Man: Physical growth from conception to maturity, 2nd edition*. Ware, UK, Castlemead Publications: 119–64.

Tanner JM & Whitehouse RH (1976) Clinical longitudinal standards for height, weight, height velocity, weight velocity, and stages of puberty. *Archives of Disease in Childhood*, **51**, 170–9.

Tappia PS, Sandhu H, Abbi T *et al.* (2009) Alterations in the expression of myocardial calcium cycling genes in rats fed a low protein diet *in utero*. *Molecular and Cellular Biochemistry*, **324**, 93–9.

Tappin D, Britten J, Broadfoot M *et al.* (2006) The effect of health visitors on breastfeeding in Glasgow. *International Breastfeeding Journal*, **1**, 11.

Tarry-Adkins JL, Martin-Gronert MS, Chen JH *et al.* (2008) Maternal diet influences DNA damage, aortic telomere length, oxidative stress, and antioxidant defense capacity in rats. *FASEB Journal*, **22**, 2037–44.

Taveras EM, Rifas-Shiman SL, Oken E *et al.* (2008) Short sleep duration in infancy and risk of childhood overweight. *Archives of Pediatric and Adolescent Medicine*, **162**, 305–11.

Taylor PD, Khan IY, Lakasing L *et al.* (2003) Uterine artery function in pregnant rats fed a diet supplemented with animal lard. *Experimental Physiology*, **88**, 389–98.

Taylor PD, McConnell J, Khan IY *et al.* (2005) Impaired glucose homeostasis and mitochondrial abnormalities in offspring of rats fed a fat-rich diet in pregnancy. *American Journal of Physiology – Regulatory, Integrative and Comparative Physiology*, **288**, R134–9.

ten Cate B, de Bruyn M, Wei Y *et al.* (2010) Targeted elimination of leukemia stem cells: a new therapeutic approach in hemato-oncology. *Current Drug Targets*, **11**, 95–110.

Tennant PW, Rankin J & Bell R (2011) Maternal body mass index and the risk of fetal and infant death: a cohort study from the North of England. *Human Reproduction*, **26**, 1501–11.

Thomas M & Avery V (1997) *Infant Feeding in Asian families*. London, The Stationery Office.

Thomas B & Bishop J (2007) *Manual of Dietetic Practice*. Oxford, Wiley-Blackwell.

Thompson C, Syddall H, Rodin I *et al.* (2001) Birth weight and the risk of depressive disorder in late life. *British Journal of Psychiatry*, **179**, 450–5.

Thompson JR, Gerald PF, Willoughby ML *et al.* (2001) Maternal folate supplementation in pregnancy and protection against acute lymphoblastic leukaemia in childhood: a case-control study. *Lancet*, **358**, 1935–40.

Thompson RA & Nelson CA (2001) Developmental science and the media: early brain development. *American Psychologist*, **56**, 5–15.

Thompson RL, Miles LM, Lunn J *et al.* (2010) Peanut sensitisation and allergy: influence of early life exposure to peanuts. *British Journal of Nutrition*, **103**, 1278–86.

Thornburg KL & Louey S (2005) Fetal roots of cardiac disease. *Heart*, **91**, 867–8.

Thornburg KL, O'Tierney PF & Louey S (2010) Review: the placenta is a programming agent for cardiovascular disease. *Trophy Research*, **24**, S54–S9.

Thulier D (2009) Breastfeeding in America: a history of influencing factors. *Journal of Human Lactation*, **25**, 85–94.

Thulier D & Mercer J (2009) Variables associated with breastfeeding duration. *Journal of Obstetric, Gynecologic & Neonatal Nursing*, **38**, 259–68.

Tibblin G, Eriksson M, Cnattingius S *et al.* (1995) High birthweight as a predictor of prostate cancer risk. *Epidemiology*, **6**, 423–4.

Tinker SC, Cogswell ME, Devine O *et al.* (2010) Folic acid intake among US women aged 15–44 years: National Health and Nutrition Examination Survey, 2003–2006. *American Journal of Preventive Medicine*, **38**, 534–42.

Tobi EW, Lumey LH, Talens RP *et al.* (2009) DNA methylation differences after exposure to prenatal famine are common and timing- and sex-specific. *Human Molecular Genetics*, **18**, 4046–53.

Todd JM & Parnell WR (1994) Nutrient intakes of women who are breastfeeding. *European Journal of Clinical Nutrition*, **48**, 567–74.

Tomat AL, Inserra F, Veiras L *et al.* (2008) Moderate zinc restriction during fetal and postnatal growth of rats: effects on adult arterial blood pressure and kidney. *American Journal of Physiology – Regulatory, Integrative and Comparative Physiology*, **295**, R543–9.

Touwslager RN, Gielen M, Mulder AL *et al.* (2011) Changes in genetic and environmental effects on growth during infancy. *American Journal of Clinical Nutrition*, **94**, 1568–74.

Townsend E & Pitchford NJ (2012) Baby knows best? The impact of weaning style on food preferences and body mass index in early childhood in a case-controlled sample. *British Medical Journal*, **2**, e000298.

Tunstall-Pedoe H, Connaghan J, Woodward M *et al.* (2006) Pattern of declining blood pressure across replicate population surveys of the WHO MONICA project, mid-1980s to mid-1990s, and the role of medication. *British Medical Journal*, **332**, 629–35.

Turner SW, Campbell D, Smith N *et al.* (2010) Associations between fetal size, maternal {alpha}-tocopherol and childhood asthma. *Thorax*, **65**, 391–7.

Turner SW, Palmer LJ, Rye PJ *et al.* (2004) The relationship between infant airway function, childhood airway responsiveness, and asthma. *American Journal of Respiratory and Critical Care Medicine*, **169**, 921–7.

Tycko B & Morison IM (2002) Physiological functions of imprinted genes. *Journal of Cellular Physiology*, **192**, 245–58.

Tzonou A, Signorello LB, Lagiou P *et al.* (1999) Diet and cancer of the prostate: a case-control study in Greece. *International Journal of Cancer*, **80**, 704–8.

Uauy R & Dangour AD (2009) Fat and fatty acid requirements and recommendations for infants of 0–2 years and children of 2–18 years. *Annals of Nutrition and Metabolism*, **55**, 76–96.

Uauy R, Hoffman DR, Mena P *et al.* (2003) Term infant studies of DHA and ARA supplementation on neurodevelopment: results of randomized controlled trials. *Journal of Pediatrics*, **143**, S17–25.

Uauy R, Mena P & Rojas C (2000) Essential fatty acids in early life: structural and functional role. *Proceedings of the Nutrition Society*, **59**, 3–15.

Udagawa J, Hashimoto R, Suzuki H *et al.* (2006) The role of leptin in the development of the cerebral cortex in mouse embryos. *Endocrinology*, **147**, 647–58.

Ulijaszek SJ, Johnston FE & Preece MA (1998) *The Cambridge Encyclopaedia of Human Growth and Development*. Cambridge, Cambridge University Press.

Umbricht CB, Evron E, Gabrielson E *et al.* (2001) Hypermethylation of 14-3-3 sigma (stratifin) is an early event in breast cancer. *Oncogene*, **20**, 3348–53.

Underwood JCE & Cross SS (2009) Carcinogenesis and neoplasia. In *General and Systematic Pathology, 5th edition*. Edinburgh, Churchill Livingstone: 221–58.

United Nations Children's Fund (UNICEF) (2001) *A League Table of Teenage Births in Rich Nations*. Florence. www.unicef-irc.org/publications/pdf/repcard 3e.pdf (accessed 18 January 2013).

United Nations Children's Fund (UNICEF) (2011) The State of the World's Children 2011. New York, UNICEF.

Vaarasmaki M, Pouta A, Elliot P *et al.* (2009) Adolescent manifestations of metabolic syndrome among children born to women with gestational diabetes in a general-population birth cohort. *American Journal of Epidemiology*, **169**, 1209–15.

Valerio A, Ghisi V, Dossena M, *et al.* (2006) Leptin increases axonal growth cone size in developing mouse cortical neurons by convergent signals inactivating glycogen synthase kinase-3β. *Journal of Biological Chemistry*, **281**, 12950–8.

van Asperen PP, Kemp AS & Mellis CM (1983) Immediate food hypersensitivity reactions on the first known exposure to the food. *Archives of Disease in Childhood*, **58**, 253–6.

Van Assche FA, Holemans K & Aerts L (2001) Long-term consequences for offspring of diabetes during pregnancy. *British Medical Bulletin*, **60**, 173–82.

van Raaij JM, Vermaat-Miedema SH, Schonk CM *et al.* (1987) Energy requirements of pregnancy in The Netherlands. *Lancet*, **2**, 953–5.

van Staa TP, Dennison EM, Leufkens HG *et al.* (2001) Epidemiology of fractures in England and Wales. *Bone*, **29**, 517–22.

van Wijk N, Rijntjes E & van de Heijning BJM (2008) Perinatal and chronic hypothyroidism impair behavioural development in male and female rats. *Experimental Physiology*, **93**, 1199–209.

Vanbillemont G, Lapauw B, Bogaert V *et al.* (2010) Birth weight in relation to sex steroid status and body composition in young healthy male siblings. *Journal of Clinical Endocrinology and Metabolism*, **95**, 1587–94.

Vandenplas Y, De Greef E, Devreker T *et al.* (2011) Soy infant formula: Is it that bad? *Acta Paediatrica*, **100**, 162–6.

Vasilatos SN, Broadwater G, Barry WT *et al.* (2009) CpG island tumor suppressor promoter methylation in non-BRCA-associated early mammary carcinogenesis. *Cancer Epidemiology, Biomarkers and Prevention*, **18**, 901–14.

Vatten LJ & Kvinnsland S (1990) Body height and risk of breast cancer: a prospective study of 23,831 Norwegian women. *British Journal of Cancer*, **61**, 881–5.

Vaupel P, Kelleher DK & Hockel M (2001) Oxygen status of malignant tumors: pathogenesis of hypoxia and significance for tumor therapy. *Seminars in Oncology*, **28**, 29–35.

Vehaskari VM, Aviles DH & Manning J (2001) Prenatal programming of adult hypertension in the rat. *Kidney International*, **59**, 238–45.

Velkoska E, Cole TJ, Dean RG *et al.* (2008) Early undernutrition leads to long-lasting reductions in body weight and adiposity whereas increased intake increases cardiac fibrosis in male rats. *Journal of Nutrition*, **138**, 1622–7.

Venter C, Pereira B, Voigt K *et al.* (2008) Prevalence and cumulative incidence of food hypersensitivity in the first 3 years of life. *Allergy*, **63**, 354–9.

Verhagen H, Andersen R, Antoine JM, *et al.* (2012) Application of the BRAFO tiered approach for benefit–risk assessment to case studies on dietary interventions. *Food and Chemical Toxicology*, **50** Suppl 4, S710–23.

Vickers MH, Breier BH, Cutfield WS *et al.* (2000) Fetal origins of hyperphagia, obesity, and hypertension and postnatal amplification by hypercaloric nutrition. *American Journal of Physiology – Endocrinology and Metabolism*, **279**, E83–7.

Vickers MH, Breier BH, McCarthy D *et al.* (2003) Sedentary behavior during postnatal life is determined by the prenatal environment and exacerbated by postnatal hypercaloric nutrition. *American Journal of Physiology – Regulatory, Integrative and Comparative Physiology*, **285**, R271–3.

Vickers MH, Gluckman PD, Coveny AH *et al.* (2008) The effect of neonatal leptin treatment on postnatal weight gain in male rats is dependent on maternal nutritional status during pregnancy. *Endocrinology*, **149**, 1906–13.

Vickers MH, Ikenasio BA & Breier BH (2001) IGF-I treatment reduces hyperphagia, obesity, and hypertension in metabolic disorders induced by fetal programming. *Endocrinology*, **142**, 3964–73.

Victora CG, Barros FC, Horta BL *et al.* (2001) Short-term benefits of catch-up growth for small-for-gestational-age infants. *International Journal of Epidemiology*, **30**, 1325–30.

Vieth R, Chan PC & MacFarlane GD (2001) Efficacy and safety of vitamin D3 intake exceeding the lowest observed adverse effect level. *American Journal of Clinical Nutrition*, **73**, 288–94.

Vik T, Bakketeig LS, Trygg KU *et al.* (2003) High caffeine consumption in the third trimester of pregnancy: gender-specific effects on fetal growth. *Paediatric and Perinatal Epidemiology*, **17**, 324–31.

Villar J, Abdel-Aleem H, Merialdi M *et al.* (2006) World Health Organization randomized trial of calcium supplementation among low calcium intake pregnant women. *American Journal of Obstetrics and Gynaecology*, **194**, 639–49.

Vizcaino AP, Moreno V, Lambert R *et al.* (2002) Time trends incidence of both major histologic types of esophageal carcinomas in selected countries, 1973–1995. *International Journal of Cancer*, **99**, 860–8.

von Wintzingerode F, Gobel UB & Stackebrandt E (1997) Determination of microbial diversity in environmental samples: pitfalls of PCR-based rRNA analysis. *FEMS Microbiology Review*, **21**, 213–29.

Vortkamp A, Lee K, Lanske B *et al.* (1996) Regulation of rate of cartilage differentiation by Indian hedgehog and PTH-related protein. *Science*, **273**, 613–22.

Vucetic Z, Kimmel J, Totoki K *et al.* (2010) Maternal high-fat diet alters methylation and gene expression of dopamine and opioid-related genes. *Endocrinology*, **151**, 4756–64.

Wachs TD (2009) Models linking nutritional deficiencies to maternal and child mental health. *American Journal of Clinical Nutrition*, **89**, 935S-9S.

Wadsworth M, Butterworth S, Montgomery S *et al.* (2003) Changing Britain, changing lives: three generations at the turn of the century. *Bedford Way papers* Ed. Ferri E, Bynner J & Wadsworth M. London, Institute of Education, University of London.

Wagner CL & Greer FR (2008) Prevention of rickets and vitamin D deficiency in infants, children, and adolescents. *Pediatrics*, **122**, 1142–52.

Wagner CL, Hulsey TC, Fanning D *et al.* (2006) High-dose vitamin D_3 supplementation in a cohort of breastfeeding mothers and their infants: a 6-month follow-up pilot study. *Breastfeeding Medicine*, **1**, 59–70.

Wainfan E, Dizik M, Stender M *et al.* (1989) Rapid appearance of hypomethylated DNA in livers of rats fed cancer-promoting, methyl-deficient diets. *Cancer Research*, **49**, 4094–7.

Wajchenberg BL (2000) Subcutaneous and visceral adipose tissue: their relation to the metabolic syndrome. *Endocrine Reviews*, **21**, 697–738.

Wald DS, Law M & Morris JK (2002) Homocysteine and cardiovascular disease: evidence on causality from a meta-analysis. *British Medical Journal*, **325**, 1202.

Walker BR, Irving RJ, Andrew R *et al.* (2002) Contrasting effects of intrauterine growth retardation and premature delivery on adult cortisol secretion and metabolism in man. *Clinical Endocrinology*, **57**, 351–5.

Walker SP, Wachs TD, Gardner JM *et al.* (2007) Child development: risk factors for adverse outcomes in developing countries. *Lancet*, **369**, 145–57.

Wallace JM, Bourke DA, Aitken RP *et al.* (2002) Blood flows and nutrient uptakes in growth-restricted pregnancies induced by overnourishing adolescent sheep. *American Journal of Physiology – Regulatory, Integrative and Comparative Physiology*, **282**, R1027–36.

Wallace JM, Luther JS, Milne JS *et al.* (2006) Nutritional modulation of adolescent pregnancy outcome: a review. *Trophy Research*, **27**, 61–8.

Wang J, Ma H, Tong C *et al.* (2010) Overnutrition and maternal obesity in sheep pregnancy alter the JNK-IRS-1 signalling cascades and cardiac function in the fetal heart. *FASEB Journal*, **24**, 2066–76.

Wang Y, Hoenig JD, Malin KJ *et al.* (2009) 16S rRNA gene-based analysis of fecal microbiota from preterm infants with and without necrotizing enterocolitis. *ISME Journal*, **3**, 944–54.

Wang YC, McPherson K, Marsh T *et al.* (2011) Health and economic burden of the projected obesity trends in the USA and the UK. *Lancet*, **378**, 815–25.

Ward M, Hutton J, McDonnell R *et al.* (2004) Folic acid supplements to prevent neural tube defects: trends in East of Ireland 1996–2002. *Irish Medical Journal*, **97**, 274–6.

Wardle J, Brodersen NH, Cole TJ *et al.* (2006) Development of adiposity in adolescence: five year longitudinal study of an ethnically and socioeconomically diverse sample of young people in Britain. *British Medical Journal*, **332**, 1130–5.

Wardle J, Haase AM, Steptoe A *et al.* (2004) Gender differences in food choice: the contribution of health beliefs and dieting. *Annals of Behavioural Medicine*, **27**, 107–16.

Warner JA, Miles EA, Jones AC *et al.* (1994) Is deficiency of interferon gamma production by allergen triggered cord blood cells a predictor of atopic eczema? *Clinical & Experimental Allergy*, **24**, 423–30.

Warner MJ & Ozanne SE (2010) Mechanisms involved in the developmental programming of adulthood disease. *Biochemical Journal*, **427**, 333–47.

Waterland RA & Jirtle RL (2003) Transposable elements: targets for early nutritional effects on epigenetic gene regulation. *Molecular and Cellular Biology*, **23**, 5293–300.

Waterland RA, Lin JR, Smith CA *et al.* (2006) Post-weaning diet affects genomic imprinting at the insulin-like growth factor 2 (Igf2) locus. *Human Molecular Genetics*, **15**, 705–16.

Waterland RA & Michels KB (2007) Epigenetic epidemiology of the developmental origins hypothesis. *Annual Review of Nutrition*, **27**, 363–88.

Watkins AJ & Fleming TP (2009) Blastocyst environment and its influence on offspring cardiovascular health: the heart of the matter. *Journal of Anatomy*, **215**, 52–9.

Watkins AJ, Platt D, Papenbrock T *et al.* (2007) Mouse embryo culture induces changes in postnatal phenotype including raised systolic blood pressure. *Proceedings of the National Academy of Sciences of the USA*, **104**, 5449–54.

Watkins BA, Lippman HE, Le Bouteiller L *et al.* (2001) Bioactive fatty acids: role in bone biology and bone cell function. *Progress in Lipid Research*, **40**, 125–48.

Watkins BA, Shen CL, Allen KG *et al.* (1996) Dietary (n-3) and (n-6) polyunsaturates and acetylsalicylic acid alter ex vivo PGE2 biosynthesis, tissue IGF-I levels, and bone morphometry in chicks. *Journal of Bone and Mineral Research*, **11**, 1321–32.

Watson PE & McDonald BW (2007) Seasonal variation of nutrient intake in pregnancy: effects on infant measures and possible influence on diseases related to season of birth. *European Journal of Clinical Nutrition*, **61**, 1271–80.

Waylen A, Ford T, Goodman R *et al.* (2009) Can early intake of dietary omega-3 predict childhood externalizing behaviour? *Acta Paediatrica*, **98**, 1805–8.

Weaver IC, Cervoni N, Champagne FA *et al.* (2004) Epigenetic programming by maternal behavior. *Nature Neuroscience*, **7**, 847–54.

Weaver LT (2008) Infant welfare, philanthropy and entrepreneurship in Glasgow: Sister Laura's Infant Food Company. *Journal of the Royal College of Physicians, Edinburgh*, **38**, 179–86.

Weggemans RM, Zock PL & Katan MB (2001) Dietary cholesterol from eggs increases the ratio of total cholesterol to high-density lipoprotein cholesterol in humans: a meta-analysis. *American Journal of Clinical Nutrition*, **73**, 885–91.

Weichselbaum E & Buttriss J (2011) Nutrition, health and schoolchildren: A British Nutrition Foundation Briefing Paper. *Nutrition Bulletin*, **36**, 295–355.

Weiderpass E, Braaten T, Magnusson C *et al.* (2004) A prospective study of body size in different periods of life and risk of premenopausal breast cancer. *Cancer Epidemiology, Biomarkers & Prevention*, **13**, 1121–7.

Weiler H, Fitzpatrick-Wong S, Schellenberg J *et al.* (2005) Maternal and cord blood long-chain polyunsaturated fatty acids are predictive of bone mass at birth in healthy term-born infants. *Pediatric Research*, **58**, 1254–8.

Weiler HA (2000) Dietary supplementation of arachidonic acid is associated with higher whole body weight and bone mineral density in growing pigs. *Pediatric Research*, **47**, 692–7.

Weinstock M (2001) Alterations induced by gestational stress in brain morphology and behaviour of the offspring. *Progress in Neurobiology*, **65**, 427–51.

Weir EC, Philbrick WM, Amling M *et al.* (1996) Targeted overexpression of parathyroid hormone-related peptide in chondrocytes causes chondrodysplasia and delayed endochondral bone formation. *Proceedings of the National Academy of Sciences of the USA*, **93**, 10240–5.

Wells JC, Chomtho S & Fewtrell MS (2007) Programming of body composition by early growth and nutrition. *Proceedings of the Nutrition Society*, **66**, 423–34.

Wells JC, Hallal PC, Wright A *et al.* (2005) Fetal, infant and childhood growth: relationships with body composition in Brazilian boys aged 9 years. *International Journal of Obesity*, **29**, 1192–8.

Welsh M, Saunders PT, Fisken M *et al.* (2008) Identification in rats of a programming window for reproductive tract masculinization, disruption of which leads to hypospadias and cryptorchidism. *Journal of Clinical Investigation*, **118**, 1479–90.

Wen X, Triche EW, Hogan JW *et al.* (2011) Prenatal factors for childhood blood pressure mediated by intrauterine and/or childhood growth? *Pediatrics*, **127**, e713–21.

Wen Y & Leake DS (2007) Low density lipoprotein undergoes oxidation within lysosomes in cells. *Circulation Research*, **100**, 1337–43.

West CE, D'Vaz N & Prescott SL (2011) Dietary immunomodulatory factors in the development of immune tolerance. *Current Allergy and Asthma Reports*, **11**, 325–33.

Westergaard T, Melbye M, Pedersen JB *et al.* (1997) Birth order, sibship size and risk of Hodgkin's disease in children and young adults: a population-based study of 31 million person-years. *International Journal of Cancer*, **72**, 977–81.

Whalley LJ, Dick FD & McNeill G (2006) A life-course approach to the aetiology of late-onset dementias. *Lancet Neurology*, **5**, 87–96.

Whincup PH, Kaye SJ, Owen CG *et al.* (2008) Birth weight and risk of type 2 diabetes: a systematic review. *JAMA*, **300**, 2886–97.

Whitaker RC (2004) Predicting preschooler obesity at birth: the role of maternal obesity in early pregnancy. *Pediatrics*, **114**, e29–36.

White A, Freeth S & O'Brien M (1992) *Infant Feeding Survey 1990*. London.

White SL, Perkovic V, Cass A *et al.* (2009) Is low birth weight an antecedent of CKD in later life? A systematic review of observational studies. *American Journal of Kidney Disease*, **54**, 248–61.

Whitlock G, Lewington S, Sherliker P *et al.* (2009) Body-mass index and cause-specific mortality in 900 000 adults: collaborative analyses of 57 prospective studies. *Lancet*, **373**, 1083–96.

Wickes JG (1953) A history of infant feeding. IV. Nineteenth century continued. *Archives of Disease in Childhood*, **28**, 416–22.

Widdowson E (1968) Growth and composition of the fetus and newborn. In *The Biology of Gestation*. Ed. Assali N. New York, Academic Press: 1–49.

Widdowson EM (1976) Changes in the body and its organs during lactation: nutritional implications. *Ciba Foundation Symposium*, 103–18.

Widschwendter M, Apostolidou S, Raum E *et al.* (2008) Epigenotyping in peripheral blood cell DNA and breast cancer risk: a proof of principle study. *PLoS One*, **3**, e2656.

Wilcox AJ & Russell IT (1986) Birthweight and perinatal mortality: III. Towards a new method of analysis. *International Journal of Epidemiology*, **15**, 188–96.

Wilkinson LS, Davies W & Isles AR (2007) Genomic imprinting effects on brain development and function. *Nature Reviews Neuroscience*, **8**, 832–43.

Williams EL, Harvey NC, Dennison E *et al.* (2009) Maternal nutrition and bone health in the offspring. *International Journal of Clinical Rheumatology* **4**, 133–45.

Wilson AC, Forsyth JS, Greene SA *et al.* (1998) Relation of infant diet to childhood health: seven year follow-up of cohort of children in Dundee infant feeding study. *British Medical Journal*, **316**, 21–5.

Wilson MR & Hughes SJ (1997) The effect of maternal protein deficiency during pregnancy and lactation on glucose tolerance and pancreatic islet function in adult rat offspring. *Journal of Endocrinology*, **154**, 177–85.

Winsloe C, Earl S, Dennison EM *et al.* (2009) Early life factors in the pathogenesis of osteoporosis. *Current Osteoporosis Reports*, **7**, 140–4.

Wjst M & Dold S (1999) Genes, factor X, and allergens: What causes allergic diseases? *Allergy*, **54**, 757–9.

Wolff GL, Kodell RL, Moore SR *et al.* (1998) Maternal epigenetics and methyl supplements affect agouti gene expression in Avy/a mice. *FASEB Journal*, **12**, 949–57.

Woodall SM, Breier BH, Johnston BM *et al.* (1996) A model of intrauterine growth retardation caused by chronic maternal undernutrition in the rat: effects on the somatotrophic axis and postnatal growth. *Journal of Endocrinology*, **150**, 231–42.

Woods LL, Ingelfinger JR, Nyengaard JR *et al.* (2001) Maternal protein restriction suppresses the newborn renin-angiotensin system and programs adult hypertension in rats. *Pediatric Research*, **49**, 460–7.

Woods LL, Ingelfinger JR & Rasch R (2005) Modest maternal protein restriction fails to program adult hypertension in female rats. *American Journal of Physiology – Regulatory, Integrative and Comparative Physiology*, **289**, R1131–6.

Woods LL, Weeks DA & Rasch R (2004) Programming of adult blood pressure by maternal protein restriction: role of nephrogenesis. *Kidney International*, **65**, 1339–48.

World Cancer Research Fund/American Institute for Cancer Research (2007) *Food, Nutrition, Physical Activity and the Prevention of Cancer: A Global Perspective*. Washington DC, American Institute for Cancer Research.

World Health Organization (WHO) & Food and Agriculture Organization of the United Nations (2003) *Diet, Nutrition and the Prevention of Chronic Diseases: WHO Report of a Joint WHO/FAO Expert Consultation*. Geneva, WHO; Rome, FAO.

World Health Organization (WHO) (1995) World Health Organization's infant feeding recommendation. *Weekly Epidemiological Record*, **70**, 119–20.

World Health Organization (WHO) (2012) Obesity and overweight Factsheet No. 311 (May 2012). www.who.int/mediacentre/factsheets/fs311/en/ (accessed 16 January 2013).

World Health Organization (WHO) (2003) *Global Strategy for Infant and Young Child Feeding*. Geneva, WHO.

World Health Organization (WHO) (2008) *The Global Burden of Disease: 2004 update*. www.who.int/health info/global_burden_disease/2004_report_update/en/index/html.

World Health Organization (WHO) (2005) *Report of a WHO Technical Consultation on Birth Spacing*. Geneva, Switzerland. www.who.int/maternal_child_adolescent/documents/birth_spacing.pdf (accessed 8 January 2013).

World Health Organization (WHO) (2009) *Infant and Young Feeding: Model Chapter for text books for medical students and allied health professionals*. Geneva, WHO.

World Health Organization (WHO) (2011) Diabetes Fact sheet N°312. www.who.int/mediacentre/factsheets/fs312/en/index.html (accessed 18 January 2013).

World Health Organization (WHO) & United Nations Children's Fund (UNICEF) (2009) *Acceptable medical reasons for use of breast-milk substitutes*. Geneva, http://whqlibdoc.who.int/hq/2009/WHO_FCH_CAH_09.01_eng.pdf (accessed 18 January 2013).

World Health Organization (2006) WHO Child Growth Standards based on length/height, weight and age. WHO Multicentre Growth Reference Study Group. *Acta Paediatrica Supplement*, **450**, 76–85.

Wozniak SE, Gee LL, Wachtel MS *et al.* (2009) Adipose tissue: The new endocrine organ? A review article. *Digestive Diseases and Sciences*, **54**, 1847–56.

Wrieden WL & Symon A (2003) The development and pilot evaluation of a nutrition education intervention programme for pregnant teenage women (food for life). *Journal of Human Nutrition and Dietetics*, **16**, 67–71.

Wright A & Schanler R (2001) The resurgence of breast-feeding at the end of the second millennium. *Journal of Nutrition*, **131**, 421S–5S.

Wright C, Lakshman R, Emmett P *et al.* (2008) Implications of adopting the WHO 2006 Child Growth Standard in the UK: two prospective cohort studies. *Archives of Disease in Childhood*, **93**, 566–9.

Wright CM, Cameron K, Tsiaka M *et al.* (2011) Is baby-led weaning feasible? When do babies first reach out for and eat finger foods? *Maternal and Child Nutrition*, **7**, 27–33.

Wright CM, Cox KM & Le Couteur A (2011) How does infant behaviour relate to weight gain and adiposity? *Proceedings of the Nutrition Society*, **70**, 485–93.

Wright CS, Rifas-Shiman SL, Rich-Edwards JW *et al.* (2009) Intrauterine exposure to gestational diabetes, child adiposity, and blood pressure. *American Journal of Hypertension*, **22**, 215–20.

Wu Y, Yakar S, Zhao L *et al.* (2002) Circulating insulin-like growth factor-I levels regulate colon cancer growth and metastasis. *Cancer Research*, **62**, 1030–5.

Wyness LA, Butriss JL & Stanner SA (2011) Reducing the population's sodium intake: the UK Food Standards Agency's salt reduction programme. *Public Health Nutrition*, 1–8.

Xu Y, Williams SJ, O'Brien D *et al.* (2006) Hypoxia or nutrient restriction during pregnancy in rats leads to progressive cardiac remodeling and impairs postischemic recovery in adult male offspring. *FASEB Journal*, **20**, 1251–3.

Xue Q & Zhang L (2009) Prenatal hypoxia causes a sex-dependent increase in heart susceptibility to ischemia and reperfusion injury in adult male offspring: role of protein kinase C epsilon. *Journal of Pharmacology and Experimental Therapeutics*, **330**, 624–32.

Yajnik CS, Deshpande SS, Jackson AA *et al.* (2008) Vitamin B_{12} and folate concentrations during pregnancy and insulin resistance in the offspring: the Pune Maternal Nutrition Study. *Diabetologia*, **51**, 29–38.

Yamashita H, Shao J, Qiao L *et al.* (2003) Effect of spontaneous gestational diabetes on fetal and postnatal hepatic insulin resistance in Lepr(db/+) mice. *Pediatric Research*, **53**, 411–18.

Yi P, Melnyk S, Pogribna M *et al.* (2000) Increase in plasma homocysteine associated with parallel increases in plasma S-adenosylhomocysteine and lymphocyte DNA hypomethylation. *Journal of Biological Chemistry*, **275**, 29318–23.

Yngve A & Sjostrom M (2001) Breastfeeding in countries of the European Union and EFTA: current and proposed recommendations, rationale, prevalence, duration and trends. *Public Health Nutrition*, **4**, 631–45.

Yuasa Y (2002) DNA methylation in cancer and ageing. *Mechanisms of Ageing and Development*, **123**, 1649–54.

Yura S, Itoh H, Sagawa N *et al.* (2005) Role of premature leptin surge in obesity resulting from intrauterine undernutrition. *Cell Metabolism*, **1**, 371–8.

Zamora SA, Rizzoli R, Belli DC *et al.* (1999) Vitamin D supplementation during infancy is associated with higher bone mineral mass in prepubertal girls. *Journal of Clinical Endocrinology and Metabolism*, **84**, 4541–4.

Zaren B, Lindmark G & Bakketeig L (2000) Maternal smoking affects fetal growth more in the male fetus. *Paediatric and Perinatal Epidemiology*, **14**, 118–26.

Zaridze DG & Basieva TH (1990) Incidence of cancer of the lung, stomach, breast, and cervix in the USSR: pattern and trends. *Cancer Causes and Control*, **1**, 39–49.

Zeisel SH (2006) The fetal origins of memory: the role of dietary choline in optimal brain development. *Journal of Pediatrics*, **149**, S131–6.

Zeltner TB, Caduff JH, Gehr P *et al.* (1987) The postnatal development and growth of the human lung. I. Morphometry. *Respiratory Physiology*, **67**, 247–67.

Zimmermann MB (2009) Iodine deficiency in pregnancy and the effects of maternal iodine supplementation on the offspring: a review. *American Journal of Clinical Nutrition*, **89**, 668S–72S.

Zylinska L, Kawecka I, Lachowicz L *et al.* (2002) The isoform- and location-dependence of the functioning of the plasma membrane calcium pump. *Cellular and Molecular Biology Letters*, **7**, 1037–45.

Index

Page numbers in *italics* denote figures, those in **bold** denote tables.